HANDBOOK OF PROGRAM DEVELOPMENT FOR HEALTH BEHAVIOR RESEARCH & PRACTICE

HANDBOOK OF PROGRAM DEVELOPMENT FOR HEALTH BEHAVIOR RESEARCH & PRACTICE

Steve Sussman
Editor

Sage Publications, Inc.
International Educational and Professional Publisher
Thousand Oaks ▪ London ▪ New Delhi

Copyright © 2001 by Sage Publications, Inc.

All rights reserved. No part of this book may be reproduced or utilized in any form or by any means, electronic or mechanical, including photocopying, recording, or by any information storage and retrieval system, without permission in writing from the publisher.

For information:

Sage Publications, Inc.
2455 Teller Road
Thousand Oaks, California 91320
E-mail: order@sagepub.com

Sage Publications Ltd.
6 Bonhill Street
London EC2A 4PU
United Kingdom

Sage Publications India Pvt. Ltd.
M-32 Market
Greater Kailash I
New Delhi 110 048 India

Printed in the United States of America

Library of Congress Cataloging-in-Publication Data

Main entry under title:

Handbook of program development for health behavior research and practice / edited by Steve Sussman.
    p. cm.
Includes bibliographical references and index.
  ISBN 0-7619-1673-3 (cloth)
  1. Health promotion. 2. Health behavior—Research. I. Title: Handbook of program development for health behavior research and practice. II. Sussman, Steven Yale.
  RA427.8 .H365 2000
  613—dc21

                                                              00-011163

01 02 03 04 05 10 9 8 7 6 5 4 3 2 1

Acquiring Editor:	C. Deborah Laughton
Editorial Assistant:	Eileen Carr
Production Editor:	Diana E. Axelsen
Editorial Assistant:	Victoria Cheng
Typesetter/Designer:	Janelle LeMaster
Indexer:	Mary Mortensen
Cover Designer:	Michelle Lee

Contents

Foreword   xiii
   Lawrence W. Green

Preface   xv
   Steve Sussman

Acknowledgments   xviii

Part I
Rationale for a Handbook of Program Development

1. **Rationale for Program Development Methods**   3
   Steve Sussman and Thomas Ashby Wills
   - Why a Science of Health Behavior Program Development Is Important   5
   - History of Behavioral Health and Program Development   8
   - An Overview of Program Development   11
   - Issues for Implementation   23
   - General Discussion   25
     - Commentary   31
       Pekka Puska

2. **Case Study 1**

   Implementing Program Development in a State or Local Health Department: A Smoking Prevention Media Campaign Example   34
   John K. Worden
   Using the Chain Model   36
   Conclusions   46

3. **Identifying and Overcoming Barriers to Empirically Based Health Behavior Program Planning**   48
   Rick Petosa
   Health Promotion: Promise and Undocumented Performance   50
   Barriers to Empirically Based Health Behavior Program Development   54
   Overcoming Barriers to Empirical Program Development   61
   Conclusions   66
       Commentary 1   69
         M. Douglas Anglin and Brian Perrochet
       Commentary 2   73
         Herbert H. Severson

Part II
The Connection Between Theory and Activity Pooling

4. **Praxis in Health Behavior Program Development**   79
   Steve Sussman and Alan N. Sussman
   Definitions   79
   Levels of Theory and Levels of Measurement   83
   How Does Theory Suggest Program Ideas?   84
   Why Do Applied Professionals Provide Only Lip Service to Theory?   86
   Why Is Theory Important for Health Behavior Program Development?   88
   Criteria for Theory Development or Selection   90
   Tying Theory Into Specific Health Areas: Linking Theory With Health Problems   92
   Tying Theory Into Specific Health Areas: Measures and Activities   93
   Discussion   94
       Commentary   98
         Hope Landrine and Elizabeth A. Klonoff

5. **Case Study 2**

   Implicit Cognition Theory in Drug Use and Driving-Under-the-Influence Interventions 107
   Alan W. Stacy and Susan L. Ames

   Principles of Memory Association Applicable to Interventions and Their Evaluation 113

   A Specific Application of Theory in Booster Programming 119

   Summary and Implications 125

6. **Choosing Assessment Studies to Clarify Theory-Based Program Ideas** 131
   Valerie Johnson and Robert J. Pandina

   Conceptual Issues: The Importance of Etiological Research 132

   Questions of Inquiry for Designing an Assessment Study 135

   The Dimensions of an Assessment Study 136

   Pooling Multiple Sources of Information 142

   Decision Criteria When Selecting Assessment Studies for Review 144

   Conclusions 148

   Commentary 155
   Suzanne M. McMurphy and Kim T. Mueser

7. **Pooling Information About Prior Interventions: A New Program Planning Tool** 158
   Carol N. D'Onofrio

   Why Pooling Information About Interventions Is Important 159

   Planning Your Search for Other Interventions 162

   Sources of Information About Other Programs 177

   Conducting Your Search 193

   Reviewing Your Pool of Information About Other Programs 197

   Conclusions: Making Your Intervention Available to Others 200

   Commentary 1 204
   Mary Ann Pentz

   Commentary 2 207
   Stephen L. Hamann

8. **Case Study 3**

   The Program Archive on Sexuality, Health, and Adolescence (PASHA):
   A Study of Activity Warehousing 210
   Starr Niego and James Peterson
   Goals of the PASHA Project 211
   Conclusions 231

Part III
Perceived Efficacy Methods

9. Verbal Methods in Perceived Efficacy Work 237
   Guadalupe X. Ayala and John P. Elder
   Methods of Perceived Efficacy Work 241
   Summary and Conclusion 261
      Commentary 264
        Edward G. Singleton and Jack E. Henningfield

10. **Case Study 4**

    Use of Focus Groups for Adolescent Tobacco Use Cessation 267
    Steve Sussman, Kara Lichtman, and Clyde W. Dent
    Method 272
    Focus Group Results 276
    Discussion 284

11. Nonverbal Methods of Perceived Efficacy 287
    Elahe Nezami, Gerald C. Davison, and Beth R. Hoffman
    Perceived Efficacy Methods 289
    Computerized Assessment 298
    Conclusions 300
       Commentary 303
         Jeffrey L. Kibler and Ronald S. Drabman

12. **Case Study 5**

Use of a Theme Study for Adolescent Tobacco Use Cessation — 307
Clyde W. Dent, Kara Lichtman, and Steve Sussman

Method — 309
Results — 315
Discussion — 316

Part IV
Immediate-Impact Methods and Program Construction

13. Component Studies — 321
Thomas R. Simon, Kris Bosworth, and Jennifer B. Unger

What Are Component Studies? — 321
Types of Relations Among Components — 323
Types of Component Studies — 325
Types of General Questions Asked in Component Studies — 326
How Are Component Studies Conducted? — 328
Conclusions — 341
    Commentary — 345
    Brian R. Flay

14. **Case Study 6**

Project EX Component Study — 348
Kara Lichtman, Clyde W. Dent, Brian Colwell, Dennis W. Smith, and Steve Sussman

Method — 354
Results — 356
Discussion — 358

15. Sequencing Issues in Health Behavior Program Development — 361
William B. Hansen and David G. Altman

Importance of Sequencing — 362
Conceptual Approaches to Sequencing — 363

	Sequencing Level 1: Environment and Life Course Development	367
	Sequencing Level 2: Sequencing Complex Program Elements	374
	Sequencing Level 3: Sequencing Within Single Points of an Intervention	379
	Conclusions	382
	Commentary	387
	Douglas Longshore	
16.	**Pilot Studies**	**391**
	Michael Lynskey and Steve Sussman	
	Methods of Pilot Studies	397
	Design Issues	403
	Evaluation Measures in Pilot Programs	407
	Discussion	416
	Commentary	422
	Shirley M. Glynn	
17.	Case Study 7	
	Development and Pilot Testing of Project SMART	**425**
	Louise Ann Rohrbach, Jill English, William B. Hansen, and C. Anderson Johnson	
	Program Development	426
	First Phase of Pilot Testing	429
	First-Year Implementation of Project SMART	434
	Second Phase of Pilot Testing and Program Implementation	436
	Lessons Learned	438
	Conclusions	444

Part V
Tying Immediate-Outcomes Measures to Longer-Term Outcomes and Conclusions

18.	**Using Meta-Analyses to Improve the Design of Interventions**	**449**
	Stewart I. Donaldson, Gordon P. Street, Steve Sussman, and Nancy S. Tobler	
	Meta-Analysis	450
	Meta-Analysis and Program Development	454

	Some Examples of Meta-Analysis in Health Behavior Research and Practice	463
	Conclusion	465
	Commentary *David Duncan*	467
19.	**Mediator and Moderator Analysis in Program Development** *Stewart I. Donaldson*	**470**
	Developing Conceptual Frameworks	472
	Empirical Confirmation	481
	Some Health Behavior Examples	487
	Conclusion	493
	Commentary *David P. MacKinnon*	497
20.	**Needs for the Future of Program Development** *Steve Sussman, Rick Petosa, and Howard Leventhal*	**501**
	Obstacles to Maintaining an Empirical Program Development Process	502
	A Review of the Chain Model	505
	Future Research Needs	506
	Conclusions	515
	Commentary 1 *Richard I. Evans*	517
	Commentary 2 *Stan Maes*	521
Author Index		525
Subject Index		537
About the Contributors		551

Foreword

In the broad sweep of social and behavioral science applications in medicine, public health, and health promotion, the sciences are maturing rapidly, the applications are progressing more fitfully, but the health results are panning out with frustrating inconsistency. In this volume, Dr. Sussman and his collaborators have tried to put their collective fingers on the link in this chain that seems to have been the weakest—the link between the science and its most appropriate application to ensure the best result. The reason this link is weak has much to do with the variability of the targets—the populations and their circumstances. These circumstances include the particular population's health needs and resources that biomedical scientists and epidemiologists would have us analyze. They also include their cultural traditions that anthropologists would have us understand, their socioeconomic conditions that sociologists and economists would have us appreciate, and the contingencies of their behavior that psychologists would have us consider. In short, the program development link in the theory- and evidence-based planning-to-evaluation chain is an interchangeable link, depending on the delineation of a population and its circumstances.

Science, in this context, refers to the combination of theory, evidence from past applications of the theory, and methods for data collection and analysis appropriate to the particular population, its health issues, and its cultural, socioeconomic, and psychological circumstances. To bring these elements of science to bear on the program development link between planning and evaluation, Sussman et al. offer a more intricate chain made up of six smaller links to repair the weak link of program development. They provide a theoretical and practical rationale for the attention to each of these six steps in program development, theory, and research that underpins the step. Also, for each step, they provide a case study that illustrates the application of the step in a real-world population and health problem. They also invite commentary from recognized theorist-researcher-practitioners in the health field who have dealt with some success with that step or aspect of the program development process.

When all these six steps are added to what they consider a paralyzing array of planning and evaluation processes, many practitioners will react with some diffidence if not resistance. The editors and authors of this book retain a refreshing appreciation of the practicalities of applying theory-based and evidence-based program development methods in real time. They suggest (or recognize the need for) shortcuts, resources, and rule-of-thumb methods to get the essential information required to make professional judgments in the absence of complete information. As these methods and rules of thumb become codified, we may hope for readily retrievable instruments and computer software that will help the practitioner apply them more efficiently.

This book promises to strengthen that weak link between planning and evaluation, offering relevant theory and methods for matching appropriate interventions with the specific needs and circumstances of populations. If practitioners will incorporate these methods into their planning process, they will add credibility and effectiveness to their programs. If researchers will concentrate some of their evaluation efforts to this phase of the planning process, the larger good will be served by the improved guidance available to practitioners, who now must depend heavily on their ability to sort intervention fads and fashions from evidence-based matching of interventions to populations and circumstances.

Lawrence W. Green

Preface

Health behavior program development refers to what goes into the construction of a health behavior program from the point at which it is conceived to the point at which the program is built and ready for a trial. A careful search of alternative texts and journals reveals that there is no one source that is dedicated to presentation of research or practice in this arena. In fact, no forum for consensual systematization of health program development methods exists in health behavior research or practice. Yet, health program development is essential to changing health research and practice needs. As the social climate changes, new approaches to changing health behavior often need development. Program development work also is needed to determine the appropriate constituents of a program for a new population that differs in lifestyle characteristics or risk. Modifications also may be needed in a program as applied to different levels of implementation (e.g., community-wide coalitions vs. clinics).

This volume justifies the importance of engaging in a scientific and systematic practice of health behavior program development. It identifies means to overcome obstacles to development of this arena and offers a consensual model to guide development of programming. This model is referred to as the six-step "program development chain model." This model provides a comprehensive road map (see Table 1.1). It serves as a guide to the creation of new program development methods and evaluation (research) and development of programs based on a compilation of methods and evaluation techniques presented in this text (practice). One goal of this book is to speak to the breadth of health behavior research and practice when describing previous or future needed program development work. Thus, each of the 13 substantive chapters in this text presents examples from two or more health areas. A wide variety of techniques are presented. In addition, case study information is presented in 7 chapters to demonstrate the use of these techniques in action. Many technical terms are introduced in this text. These terms are bolded on their first occurrence to assist in recognition and acquisition of critical material. In all, this handbook provides 20 chapters of detailed and useful information, making it the most complete text of its kind.

The audience for this handbook includes researchers, teachers, public health practitioners/clinicians, students, and policymakers. Persons in the academic community will be very interested in this compendium because it definitely fills a research gap. This work could serve as the basis of some courses in methodology (e.g., design courses, program development courses that as of yet do not exist), as well as provide a needed avenue of investigation.

County health department personnel generally are provided funds to evaluate immediate outcomes. Thus, county health department and other health agency managers and evaluators across different health arenas may hold great interest in this handbook. Those who engage in health program development work at health maintenance organizations, public health departments, or industry will be very interested in using methods presented here. Those policymakers who must decide which data to trust also will be potential readers. Of course, some material, such as meta-analysis, is suited primarily for the research community. However, an attempt was made to place much of this material in a framework that can be understood by educated laypeople. Some practitioners may wish to engage in their own systematic reviews of previous empirical studies, and this text will help them in that endeavor. Because its orientation is methodological, this volume will have international application.

The handbook consists of five parts. The first part provides a justification for the field and consists of three chapters. Chapter 1 provides the history and rationale for engaging in health behavior program development. Chapter 2 presents a case study that shows how to apply the six-step program development model presented in Chapter 1 to the arena of mass media smoking prevention efforts. Chapter 3 presents the hurdles to engaging in program development and how to surmount those hurdles.

The second part of the handbook presents the connection between theory and pooling intervention activities together. The fourth chapter of the text, the first in this part, provides an explanation of the use of theory in program development. Next comes Chapter 5, a second case study, which presents the use of a novel instance of theory—implicit cognition—for drug abuse and driving-under-the-influence (DUI) prevention. Next, Chapter 6 presents the use of assessment studies to fill in gaps in theory regarding what leads to health-related behavior. Assessment studies also can help suggest plausible activities to alter health-related behavior. Chapter 7 discusses many issues and resources relevant to pooling information about prior interventions. Chapter 8, a third case study,

TABLE 1.1   The Six-Step Program Development Chain Model

Step 1: Use a theory that considers antecedents of healthy or unhealthy behavior, considers mediation of the relations between the antecedents and behavior, and identifies program activities that plausibly may act on the antecedents, mediators, or behavior. Engage in assessment studies to fill any gaps in theory. Make sure that community cooperation is achieved (see Chapters 2-6).

Step 2: Go to a resource that systematically pools and warehouses promising activities and pool activities from several sources, or create your own activities, and collect these plausible activities for potential testing (see Chapters 7 and 8).

Step 3: Systematize a set of perceived efficacy studies that can screen among promising activities gathered in the last step for additional program development work. This could be viewed as a program activity "screening" step (see Chapters 9-12).

Step 4: Systematize a set of immediate-impact studies that can provide a means of determining workability of individual program components (e.g., component studies; see Chapters 13 and 14).

Step 5: Systematize program construction and pilot testing of a complete program (see Chapters 15-17).

Step 6: Refine a set of immediate posttest/posttreatment activity measures that are likely to predict target population receptivity and longer-term outcomes (see Chapters 18-20).

provides an example of pooling information for teen pregnancy and sexually transmitted disease (STD) prevention.

The third part of the handbook presents perceived efficacy (i.e., concept evaluation) methods of activity selection. Chapter 9 provides a review of numerous verbal methods of selecting potentially useful activities. Chapter 10, the fourth case study, provides an example of the collection and use of verbal perceived efficacy information (use of focus groups for teen smoking cessation). Next, Chapter 11 provides a review of numerous paper-and-pencil methods of selecting potentially useful activities. Chapter 12, the fifth case study, provides an example of a paper-and-pencil perceived efficacy study (use of theme studies for teen smoking cessation).

The fourth part of the handbook presents immediate-impact studies of activities and program creation. Chapter 13 discusses the main type of immediate-impact study of individual activities or sessions—the use of component studies. Chapter 14, the sixth case study, provides an example of the use of component studies for teen smoking cessation. Chapter 15 discusses issues relevant to sequencing of programming—that is, programs over the life span, sessions in a single program, and activities in a single session. Chapter 16 then discusses use of the pilot study, which tests a full program. Chapter 17, the seventh case study, presents an example of the use of pilot testing for teen drug abuse prevention.

Finally, the fifth part of the handbook discusses finding immediate-outcome measures that will predict longer-term outcome measures and discusses future issues to consider in this arena of health behavior program development. Chapters 18 and 19 present the use of meta-analysis and mediation analysis, respectively, to identify good programming and immediate-outcome measures. Finally, Chapter 20 summarizes the text, suggests mediator and moderator measures that might be most important in health behavior programming, and indicates future issues to attend to by researchers and practitioners.

One interesting aspect of this volume is the inclusion of the seven case studies, which provide practical guidelines on addressing relevant aspects of program development. These case studies provide useful information for discussion, research, and application. A second valuable aspect of this handbook is the inclusion of commentaries at the end of each substantive chapter that is not a case study. Sixteen commentaries are included. These commentaries extend the chapters; that is, they provide additional considerations for researchers and practitioners in the field of health behavior research and practice, as expressed by several leaders in the field. It is our shared vision that this text will become a standard resource for persons in our field in the years to come.

▶ ACKNOWLEDGMENTS

There are a lot of people to thank for helping put together a text of this magnitude. First, I would like to thank several persons at Sage Publications for their efforts. Dan Ruth guided me in the development of the text, and C. Deborah Laughton helped bring the text to a safe landing with the assistance of Eileen Carr, Diana Axelsen, Gillian Dickens, and Janelle LeMaster. Sage maintains a strong and positive interest in bridging important new frontiers in health behavior research and practice. Second, I would like to thank my private grammarian, Susan Perry, now a well-respected book author, for helping to smooth out the chapter bumps. Third, I would like to thank the University of Southern California (particularly Andy Johnson, Malcolm Pike, and Leslie Bernstein), National Institute on Drug Abuse (particularly Larry Seitz and Bill Bukoski), and California Tobacco-Related Disease Research Program (particularly Larry Gruder and Phil Gardiner) for giving me the support and flexibility to complete the editing on this test. Fourth, I would like to thank reviewer Dan Romer, Bill Bukowski, Andrew Baum, and Bruce L. Levin for their suggestions. Fifth, I would like to thank all the book authors and commentary writers for their input. All of these persons are leaders in their fields and have shown great collaborative spirit in development of the text. Some of these persons greatly influenced the shape of my own career, for which I will always be grateful (e.g., Howard Leventhal, Brian Flay, and Richard Evans). Sixth, I would like to thank my wife, Rotchana, and my children, Guang and Evan, for their love and support at home, which helped make the completion of the text a balanced process. Finally, I would like to thank the reader looking through this text, considering its contexts, and engaging in a grand, shared scheme—to improve dramatically the development and outcomes of health behavior programs

Steve Sussman
University of Southern California

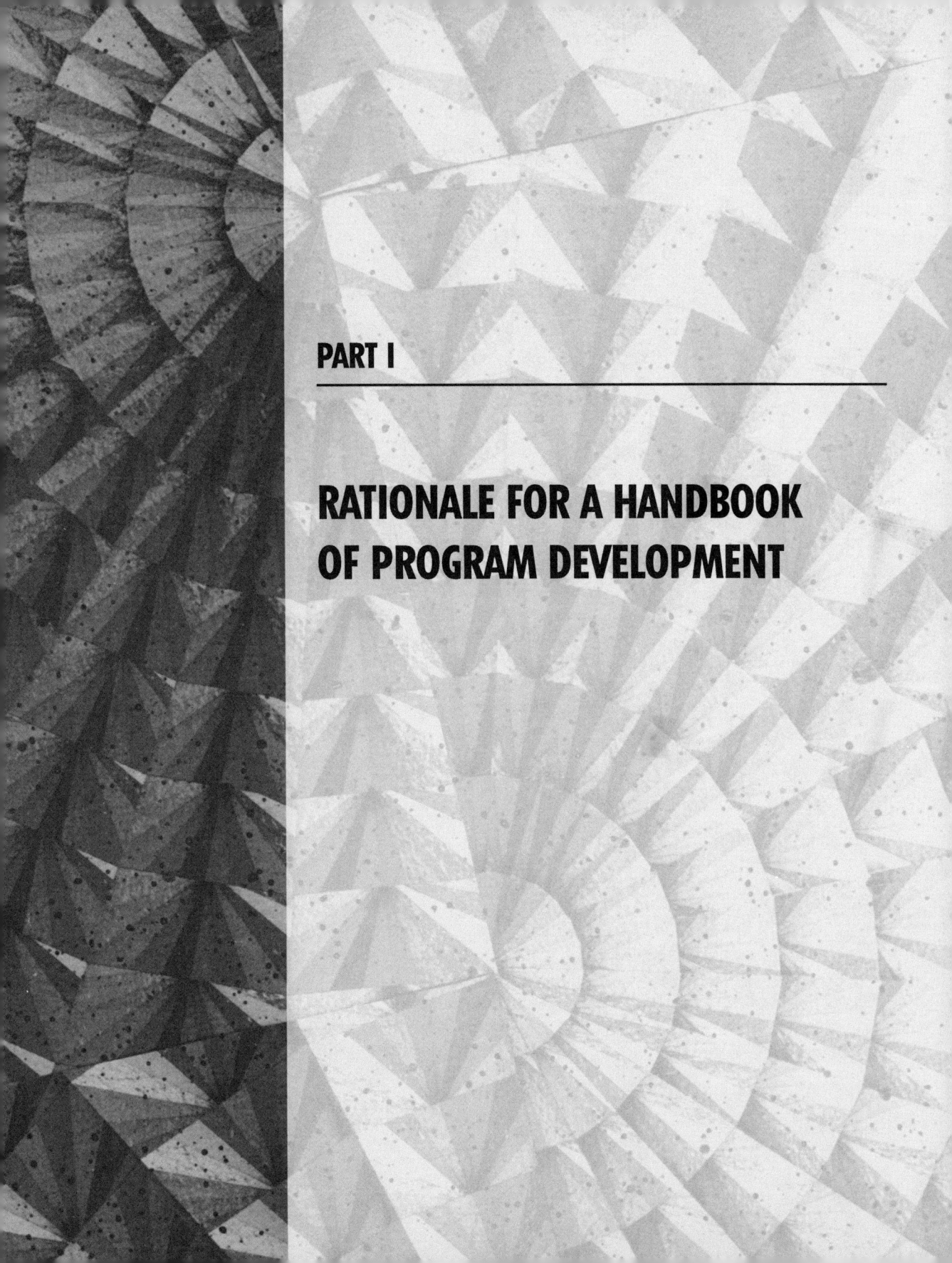

PART I

RATIONALE FOR A HANDBOOK OF PROGRAM DEVELOPMENT

CHAPTER 1

Rationale for Program Development Methods

Steve Sussman
Thomas Ashby Wills

Imagine this scenario: A baby is crawling along the living room floor. You, her parent, watch in anticipation as she braces herself on a chair and stands herself up as if preparing for her first steps. Then, you watch in amazement as your baby begins to walk, then race, through the house. Does this story sound like fiction? Of course, we all know the expression, "You need to learn to walk before you can run." But this truism sometimes seems lost in the purview of those who develop health behavior programs. More often than not, a program is conceived based on a brief needs assessment or theoretical model; then it is expected simply to be constructed and set off on its main trial run. Don't programs need to walk first? In other words, shouldn't a program be evaluated as it is being constructed to make sure the program is maximally solid? We believe it should. The above example may seem too dramatic to some people. But the point is that acquiring a skill, building a structure, or developing a model of effective change involves a series of progressive steps.

This chapter provides an overview of the field of health behavior program development. First, we discuss why it is important to systematize and refine a science of health behavior program development at this time. The history of health behavior program development is described next. Finally, plausible "walking steps" of health behavior program development are described. The rest of the chapters in this handbook explicate these "walking steps" through a chain model of program development. Along with chapters on the phases of program development, case study chapters are presented that provide examples of program development in action. The science and practice of health behavior program development have come of age.

DEFINITIONS

To avoid confusing the readers when we initially refer to a health behavior program or to program development, let us clarify some terms. Here, the term *health behavior program* refers to any program that directly (through education) or indirectly (through environmental modification) intends to modify a behavior that is ultimately relevant for health status, such as cigarette smoking or dietary intake. The term *program,* as defined here, refers to a program of education or action that facilitates healthy behavior. It does not refer to personal or vocational improvement (e.g., university education programs) or computer systems programming. The term *development,* as defined here, is not merely a program description or flowchart, and it does not pertain specifically to outcomes research of newly developed programs. Health program development pertains to "what goes on" when the basic methods of a health behavior program are being conceived (e.g., theory regarding a health behavior; see Chapter 4, this volume) and the outlines for the program approaches that are being developed (e.g., pilot work; see Chapter 16). The goal is to provide the beginnings of a science of program development.

The early phase of program development includes focusing on the theoretical processes that indicate why a program is needed and explaining how a given behavior may be changed in a healthier direction. (The baby stands up.) Middle phases examine program component contents and modalities of implementation to maximize involvement of persons from the intended target group and to clarify hypothesized mediators of change. (The baby walks.) Later phases combine program components, pilot test a complete program, and develop reliable mediator and moderator measures that are likely to predict longer-term outcomes. (The baby begins to trot.)

NEED FOR A COMPREHENSIVE HANDBOOK

In previous health behavior research and practice, program developers have used several types of methods to develop the programming; these include intuitive ideas, theoretical derivations, and trial-and-error approaches. However, in many cases, the development approaches were not documented for others to follow. The rationale for this book is to show how to make explicit, systematize, and evaluate the methods used to develop health behavior programs, affording everyone the opportunity to learn from others' experiences and thereby enhance the building of cumulative knowledge in health behavior research and practice. A single complete source for this information simply did not exist until now (see additional discussion below).

The aim of this handbook is to formalize the area of health behavior program development. Our goals are to provide a forum for discussing the following:

1. the rationale for empirically based program development work;
2. approaches to systemization of effective program development methods;
3. strategies for pooling of program development studies to help identify mediators and moderators of longer-term health program effects;
4. arguments for a systematic, consensual, financially supported program development protocol; and
5. identification of research needs to enhance the scientific status of program development work in health behavior research and practice.

WHY A SCIENCE OF HEALTH BEHAVIOR PROGRAM DEVELOPMENT IS IMPORTANT

We are currently observing, with respect to indicators of morbidity and mortality, the effects of the recent societal emphasis on improvements in health behavior and those of advances in biomedical technology. For example, mortality from heart disease, the number-one killer in the United States, dropped almost 50% between 1975 and 1995 due to social climate changes, introduction of education and treatment programs, medical advances (e.g., bypass surgery), and consequent lifestyle changes such as smoking cessation (Matarazzo, 1984). Thus, there is some evidence for effectiveness of an earlier generation of programs. However, in most cases, the program development methods used to develop these programs were not presented in writing, were presented in obscure technical reports, or were presented only in passing within the context of reporting outcome evaluation studies.

A person with rich experience in an area may intuit an effective program. Is program development, then, an art rather than a science? Certainly, an experienced person can make judgments about what composes an effective program in some area. It is also likely that this person, if effectively prompted, could report the basis for his or her judgments to others. Thus, this is a method, one of expert judgment; the goal is to capture the basis of the expert's judgments so that they can be systematized and evaluated. In other words, program development, even when considered an art, can, through careful quantifying, become a science. The real deficits in current health behavior program development include (a) little systematization of methods, (b) lack of explicit linkages of theories to methods or of one method to other methods within a program, and (c) few ties of immediate-outcome assessments to longer-term outcome assessments. A broadening of attempts to address these issues will advance the scientific basis of health behavior program development (Braverman & Campbell, 1989).

There are at least four reasons why it is important to engage in an empirically based health behavior program development process (see also Sussman, Petosa, & Clarke, 1996). First, a rigorous development process may permit the identification of hypothesized mediators and moderators of program effects (see also Chapter 19, this volume). With regard to mediation, many programs do not act directly on health behaviors; rather, they work by having an impact on mediators such as coping patterns, normative perceptions, and attitudes toward the behavior (e.g., Hansen & Graham, 1991; Hansen et al., 1988; MacKinnon, Johnson, Pentz, Dwyer, & Hansen, 1991; Tobler & Stratton, 1997). Without measurements of these mediators, it is difficult to tell why a program worked or did not work. Moderators (process variables) also should be considered. There is evidence that variables such as homework returns, measures of program enthusiasm, and measures of group interaction precede behavioral changes and are predictive of program outcomes 1 or 2 years later (Sussman et al., 1989; Sussman, Dent, Burton, Stacy, & Flay, 1995; Tobler, 1995; Tobler & Stratton, 1997). The program development process will provide more useful evaluations by focusing attention on mediators and moderators of program effects.

Second, a consensual empirically based process can minimize subjective bias of individual program developers because decisions are made with input from several persons (i.e., multidisciplinary teams). The impact of a particular program activity on mediators of change, including health knowledge, attitudes, and beliefs, may not be tapped adequately through a single person's judgments. Pooling the efforts and judgments of multiple persons may help to develop a better and more generalizable program.

Third, a methodologically rigorous development process can be used to maximize receptivity by target populations (Thoresen, 1984). If a program is not perceived as interesting by participants, it will not be implemented well or attended to. Members of target populations appear to be reasonably good judges of what leads to healthy behavior if they have sufficient information to select among alternative strategies (e.g., Sussman, 1996; Sussman, Dent, Stacy, & Craig, 1998). Thus, focusing on the preferences of consumers tends to translate into behavior change later on.

Finally, health program development is essential for adaptation to historical and cohort factors. As the social climate changes, approaches to modifying health behavior often need continuing development (i.e., programs may become obsolete over time). Program development work also is needed to determine the appropriate components of a program for a new population that differs in lifestyle characteristics or risk. For example, programs focused on social influence processes are relevant to the prevention of adolescent problem behavior among general populations. However, motivation-oriented approaches appear to be more relevant for high-risk youth (e.g., Sussman et al., 1998), and although problem behaviors are correlated (Donovan, Jessor, & Costa, 1988), certain unique antecedents may operate so that different program activities are relevant for different behaviors. As a second example, the concept of the stepped-care approach assumes that different programming has to be developed as a function of how severe a health problem has become (e.g., Brownell & Wadden, 1992). Finally, modifications may be needed for a program applied at different levels of implementation, such as community-wide coalitions versus neighborhood clinics (McLeroy et al., 1993).[1]

The purpose of this book, then, is to provide a forum for consensual systematization of program development methods. In current health behavior research, no such forum exists. Articles of the health program development type are scattered across many journals on substance use, preventive medicine, public health, health education, and evaluation research; however, there is no journal dedicated specifically to program development. Recent program evaluation texts provide information on topics such as conducting needs assessment, obtaining outcome evaluation data, and performing statistical analyses (e.g., Isaac & Michael, 1990; Kettner, Moroney, & Martin, 1990; Miller, 1991; Rossi & Freeman, 1993; Windsor, Baranowski, Clark, & Cutter, 1984), but there is relatively little mention of program development work. For example, Kettner et al. (1990) provide information on engaging in a needs assessment for social services programs, developing hypotheses to set intervention goals, designing social service programs, building an ongoing management information system, establishing costs and values of programs, and evaluating programs. However, this text spends only 3 of 215 pages on formative evaluation. Rather, once an intervention goal is established, the social service program is created without use of formal program development tools.

Miller (1991), in his text on research design and social measurement, describes research issues, methods of data collection, statistical analysis, measurement tools, and funding mechanisms. This text mentions the importance of using theory to guide research, and it discusses some data collection methods that might be used in program development studies (i.e., questionnaires, interviews). However, there is no mention of program development work.

A book by Sussman et al. (1995) includes some material on program development but was focused on a single tobacco use prevention and cessation program, so it is not a comprehensive text of health behavior program development. The present volume aims to be precisely that much-needed comprehensive text.

► HISTORY OF BEHAVIORAL HEALTH AND PROGRAM DEVELOPMENT

Efforts to encourage others to adopt healthy behavior and eliminate unhealthy behavior date back to the dawn of civilization. Knowledge of how to avoid the ravages of poor weather, the importance of rest, what to eat and drink, what not to eat or drink, what areas not to travel in, and other lifestyle regimens were passed down from parents to children within the context of a family, tribe, village, or government. In other words, life experience and cultural practices represent early methods of programmatic health practice. Of course, not all health wisdom reached mass circulation right away; as a popular example, in 1779, James Lind knew that one should eat citrus fruit to prevent scurvy, but his ideas were not adopted on a wide scale for more than 100 years. Conversely, other practices such as bloodletting were widely used but were of dubious value for health promotion (Taylor, Denham, & Ureda, 1982).

The modern public health movement began perhaps as a reaction to the cholera epidemic that spread throughout Europe in 1830. The first International Sanitary Conference was held in Paris in 1851 to try to develop consensus on how to stop this epidemic, but that effort failed. Eventually, use of the method of governmental consensus conferences led to well-organized attempts to put a stop to cholera and other epidemics. In 1872, the American Public Health Association (APHA), the oldest and largest organization of public health professionals in the world, was formed. In 1878, the U.S. Congress enacted a federal law to prevent introduction of infectious diseases into the United States, later extending it to prevent the spread of diseases within national borders. Furthermore, in 1887, the U.S. federal government opened a one-room laboratory on Staten Island for research on disease; this served as the root of the National Institutes of Health (NIH). The forerunner of the Pan American Health Organization (PAHO) was set up in Washington, D.C., in 1902, and prevention and treatment measures against smallpox, typhus, and cholera were attempted in the Americas. In 1912, the Public Health Service was founded, and an emphasis began on investigating and treating diseases stemming from the relationship of people with their environment; neighborhood problems, air pollution, sanitation, and control of infectious diseases were considered.

Over the next several decades, a few programmatic health behavior texts appeared. Health-related texts were often self-published, pertaining primarily to nutrition and spirituality and influenced by works of Christian physiologists from the early part of the 19th century (e.g., Abbott, 1947; MacFadden, 1924). The approach of Alcoholics Anonymous, a 12-step spiritual program text based on a consensus of the experiences of 100 alcoholics, also was published during this period (Alcoholics Anonymous, 1939). In 1939, related federal works in the fields of health, education, social insurance, and human services were joined together under the Federal Security Agency. Some notions of behavioral health were discussed in meetings at this time, particularly how to avoid or cope with infectious diseases. Regarding most behavioral problems, governmental promotions through radio, movie clips, and magazines emphasized the importance of engaging in responsible behavior for the public good (Tuchfeld & Marcus, 1984). Methods of health program development at this time included very limited use of target subject self-report assessments, expert consensus, and interviews. For example, Karl Lashley and John B. Watson, who defined the century-long dominance of physiological and behavioristic psychology, designed a government-thwarted venereal disease education project (Lashley & Watson, 1921).

In 1946, the forerunner of the Centers for Disease Control and Prevention (CDC) was created, initially to monitor the spread and control of infectious disease. In 1948, the World Health Organization (WHO) constitution came into force, and national health organizations, such as the PAHO, became subsumed under WHO. Further organizational progress occurred in 1953, when the Department of Health, Education, and Welfare (DHEW) was created. The Bureau of State Services, Public Health Service, began the unit that supported the development of the health belief model from 1954 onward. The second piece to be developed in that unit was one by Howard Leventhal, on influenza vaccination.

A major step in disease prevention occurred when the Salk polio vaccine was licensed in 1955, and school-based vaccinations nationwide occurred soon thereafter. The Sabin oral polio vaccine was developed in 1960 and provided easier administration and higher participation. The development of weight and mortality tables by the Metropolitan Life Insurance Company in 1960 promised a future of lower insurance rates with better health habits. However, until the mid-1960s, prevention of disease was mainly accomplished through immunization (Matarazzo, 1984). Some of the earliest published work regarding compliance with infection-targeted treatments appeared only in the early 1960s (Epstein & Cluss, 1982).

The release of the first surgeon general's report on smoking and health in 1964 represents a major early statement of the behavioral health movement, even though smoking cessation was discussed on only one page of the report (U.S. Department of Health and Human Services [DHHS], 1964). This text's expansion of statements made 7 years earlier about the relation of smoking to lung cancer highlighted for a mass audience the relation of behavior to a disease process and marked the beginning of a downward trend in smoking among adult Americans. The next year, nutritional programs for the elderly were created under the Older Americans Act. Marking the beginning of a rapid increase of public interest in exercise, Kenneth Cooper (1968) published his first book on aerobics. The work of Lester Breslow and colleagues, based on research from a community sample in Alameda County, California, that began in 1965, was influential in promoting adoption of seven health practices that could increase one's life expectancy: sleeping 7 to 8 hours per day, eating breakfast daily, not eating between meals, not being overweight, not smoking, not drinking too much alcohol, and engaging in regular physical activity (Belloc & Breslow, 1972; Breslow & Breslow, 1993). Beginning in 1965, prolific behavioral modification research was applied to smoking and alcohol cessation and to eating disorders (Blanchard, 1992; O'Leary & Wilson, 1975).

Behavioral health became a more important priority in the later 1970s. In 1974, after years of dissatisfaction with health services, WHO launched an extended program of immunization to protect children from infections such as measles, diphtheria, and tuberculosis. Smallpox was eradicated worldwide in 1978. In 1977, the 13th WHO Assembly encouraged health promotion policies, urging "Health for All by the Year 2000." Since 1979, it became accepted that at least 7 of the 10 leading causes of human death—heart disease, cancer, stroke, nonvehicle accidents, infectious diseases, motor vehicle accidents, diabetes, cirrhosis, arteriosclerosis, and suicide—could be reduced through behavioral means (Matarazzo, 1984; U.S. DHHS, 1990). Organizations that considered different aspects of behavioral health began to proliferate. After branching from the Department of Education, DHEW became the Department of Health and Human Services in 1980. Other new organizational units included the Society for Behavioral Medicine (1978), the Health Psychology Division of the American Psychological Association (1979), the Addictive Behaviors Division of the American Psychological Association (1993), and the Society for Prevention Research (1993). Behavioral health research areas expanded to include exercise, hypertension, headaches, chronic pain, cardiovascular diseases, gastrointestinal disorders, arthritis, medication compliance, and diabetes (Blanchard, 1992).

In 1984, Matarazzo and colleagues published the book *Behavioral Health*. This text summarized the state of the art in behavioral health knowledge and provided a template for future research and practice directions. Numerous theories were discussed, including those pertaining to learning, attitude change, coping and social support, ethnographic factors, human factors knowledge, health education strategies, and communication. Prevention and treatment techniques were discussed, including the use of biofeedback, relaxation training, cognitive-behavior modification, social skills training, time management, placebo or motivation manipulations, compliance-gaining strategies, and use of policy. In addition, theories and techniques were applied to numerous health domains (exercise, diet, smoking, hypertension, dental health, safety, and alcoholism) in various settings (e.g., school, clinic, worksite, home, community-wide).

Very little space in *Behavioral Health* was dedicated to health program development. Several chapters (i.e., Chesney, 1984, chap. 22; Feldman, 1984, chap. 77; Farquhar et al., 1984, chap. 84; Solomon & Maccoby, 1984, chap. 13) discussed topics such as engaging in a needs assessment; conducting audience, media channel, and program analysis; and obtaining audience feedback in planning programs. However, Thoresen (1984, chap. 19) provided the real plea for a science of program development. He noted that self-care or admonitions by authorities did not reliably lead to behavior change, so it was important to find out why these methods did not always appeal to participants. He suggested that a science of program development using ecologically valid and flexible but interpretable designs and involving subjects in the methods of inquiry was essential to the optimization of behavioral health programming.

AN OVERVIEW OF PROGRAM DEVELOPMENT ◀

This section provides an overview of previous program development models and presents an integrated chain model of the program development process. Three models have gained popularity in the research literature over the past decade. One is the social marketing/formative evaluation approach, exemplified by the work of Worden and colleagues (Worden et al., 1988; Worden et al., 1996). This approach generally begins with some theoretical and epidemiological knowledge of the needs of a problem population, based on previous work. The first phase of program development is termed the *diagnostic phase*. Focus group, survey, or interview data are collected from a target population regarding prevalence of the target behavior, attitudes, and lifestyle variables that precede and maintain the behavior (etiology and correlates) and preferred treatment modalities. For the second or *formative phase*, the research team provides program developers with the results of the first phase through summaries compiled into writers' notebooks, along with a list of educational objectives. The program developers then supply a list of potential activities to the research team, who then obtain data on comprehensibility and likability of the activities from ratings by representative target subjects. Finally, in the third or *selection phase*, the results of the previous phase are reviewed by an expert advisory board, and approximately 50% of the activities are retained for implementation (see also Lefebvre & Flora, 1988).

Another perspective is provided by Green's precede-proceed planning model (e.g., Daniel & Green, 1995; Green & Kreuter, 1991, among 400 publications that refer to this model). First, according to this model, the perceived need for remedy of a health problem or encouragement of a healthy behavior is assessed among a target population ("social diagnosis"). Next, available databases are searched, and additional information is collected to ascertain the prevalence of the unhealthy or healthy behavior and its antecedents, such as etiological factors ("epidemiological diagnosis"). Third, behavioral factors amenable to change are identified through available statistical data ("behavioral and environmental diagnosis"). Next, three types of factors are assessed that might modify the target behavior. Predisposing factors are motivation-related variables, enabling factors are variables that help motivation-related variables become realized, and reinforcing factors are variables that maintain behavior change ("educational and organizational diagnosis"). Fifth, practical considerations are addressed that may either support or block implementation of change strategies ("administrative and policy diagnosis"). From this point on, the planning model continues from implementation through outcome evaluation phases, using a perspective that involves a series of iterative program and evaluation phases.

The third model is Sussman's four-step model of empirical curriculum development (e.g., Sussman, 1991; Sussman, Petosa, & Clarke, 1996). Four general steps of program development are proposed. The first step involves adopting and extending a theoretical knowledge base. This step includes adoption of a theoretical perspective to guide the conduct of the research and use of assessment studies to increase knowledge of variables that may facilitate or deter a health behavior. Several different types of assessment studies could assist in identifying systematic relations between antecedent variables and levels of health behaviors and on mediators that might counteract the relations between the antecedents and behaviors, including various cross-sectional, prospective, and experimental studies. The second step is one of pooling program activities from previous work, developing new activities that are hypothesized to target the same set of mediators of change, and adding these new activities to the pool. The third step involves testing individual program activities; that is, this step involves studies of perceived efficacy (i.e., concept evaluation) to screen among a large set of activities, followed by studies of immediate impact (e.g., on knowledge or attitudes). Perceived efficacy studies permit selection of a subset of activities for subsequent immediate-impact testing. The latter step then permits selection of a further subset of activities with favorable ratings. This subset that is retained after use of perceived efficacy and immediate-impact studies is used to compose the program. The final step involves constructing and testing a full program. This step includes issues related to how to combine activities to produce sessions, combine sessions to produce a complete program (e.g., issue of sequence), test the workability of the program, and pilot test the effect of the whole program on a set of immediate-impact variables.

STEPS IN PROGRAM DEVELOPMENT: THE CHAIN MODEL

The three models described above share several overlapping and non-overlapping features but could be combined to provide a more solid linking across different development steps. Therefore, a six-step "program development chain" model integrating these features is proposed (see Table 1.1).

> **TABLE 1.1** The Six-Step Program Development Chain Model
>
> **Step 1:** Use a theory that considers antecedents of healthy or unhealthy behavior, considers mediation of the relations between the antecedents and behavior, and identifies program activities that plausibly may act on the antecedents, mediators, or behavior. Engage in assessment studies to fill any gaps in theory. Make sure that community cooperation is achieved (see Chapters 2-6).
>
> **Step 2:** Go to a resource that systematically pools and warehouses promising activities and pool activities from several sources, or create your own activities, and collect these plausible activities for potential testing (see Chapters 7 and 8).
>
> **Step 3:** Systematize a set of perceived efficacy studies that can screen among promising activities gathered in the last step for additional program development work. This could be viewed as a program activity "screening" step (see Chapters 9-12).
>
> **Step 4:** Systematize a set of immediate-impact studies that can provide a means of determining workability of individual program components (e.g., component studies; see Chapters 13 and 14).
>
> **Step 5:** Systematize program construction and pilot testing of a complete program (see Chapters 15-17).
>
> **Step 6:** Refine a set of immediate posttest/posttreatment activity measures that are likely to predict target population receptivity and longer-term outcomes (see Chapters 18-20).

Program development is only as strong as its weakest link. Health behavior program development involves two central ideas. The first concept is that programs are developed, beginning with certain theoretical notions of participants' crucial needs and relevant mechanisms of change. The second concept is that the movement from theory to the completed program involves a series of steps or stages. What these stages are may vary widely across projects. It is argued here that the Worden, Green, and Sussman models can be integrated with a consideration of methodological demands in program development.

First, concurrent with the assessment of a target population's needs, a theory of program mediation should be developed to address the identified needs. Program activities that plausibly might address these health needs should come to mind. In other words, the program developer should be thinking about antecedents of the health problem behavior, the consequences of the target behavior, and how to counteract the problem behavior, its antecedents, or its consequences. This type of information is contained in the first step of the social marketing model, the first four steps of the precede-proceed model, and the first two steps of the four-step model.

Second, there is a need to systematically pool and warehouse promising activities for new uses. The theory of program mediation developed in the prior step leads one to search for promising activities to test. One should be able to go through a library of activities and pull out useful information. This program development chain step is best reflected in the second steps of the social marketing and four-step models, as well as in the fourth and fifth steps of the precede-proceed model.

Third, there is a need to systematize a set of perceived efficacy studies that can screen among promising activity ideas gathered in the last step for additional program development work. Numerous ideas gathered during the previous step can be contrasted by using methods that are relatively time- and cost-effective. This could be viewed as a program activity screening step. This information is reflected in the first three steps of the social marketing model, the fourth and fifth steps of the precede-proceed model, and the third step of the four-step model.

Fourth, there is a need to systematize a set of immediate-impact studies that can provide a means of determining workability of individual program components. Possibly, the top half of the most favorably rated activities from the previous step would be retained for this one. This information is perhaps best reflected in the second and third steps of the social marketing model, the fourth and fifth steps of the precede-proceed model, and the third step of the four-step model.

Fifth, there is a need to systematize program construction and pilot testing of a complete program. Around 50% of activities from the previous step are retained for this step. Rules of construction, including a consideration of program content and process sequencing, along with a consideration of pragmatics of testing a complete program, should be addressed. Finally, there is a need to refine a set of immediate posttest/posttreatment activity measures that predict longer-term outcomes from short-term measures. Pilot testing outcome measures should be able to predict not only target population receptivity but also longer-term behavior. This step is not just a theoretical necessity but a practical, monetary reality among many local health department program developers. The fifth and sixth steps of the program development chain model are reflected in the third step of the social marketing model, the fourth and fifth steps of the precede-proceed model, and the fourth step of the four-step model.

OVERVIEW OF THEORY OF NEED-PROGRAM LINKAGE: STEP 1 OF THE CHAIN MODEL

Health behavior program development begins with use of theory, an organized set of concepts that suggest the causal mechanism through which an outcome occurs. Theory shows the need for a program and identifies mechanisms of change to promote a healthy behavior or counteract an unhealthy behavior (e.g., van Ryn & Heaney, 1992). The first aspect of the use of theory involves achieving a good understanding of a health or problem behavior. Potential mediators of change are hypothesized as not being sufficiently affected through naturally occurring socioenvironmental events or available programming.[2] Formal needs assessments generally involve a review of the literature and adoption of a theoretical model or models before engaging in empirical procedures. For example, guided by the theory that unstructured and unsupervised time is the mediator of adolescent problem behavior (Richardson et al., 1989), a youth needs assessment survey may address daily activities accessible to youth, youths' enjoyment of different activities, and perceived needs for new means to structure time.

Addressing theoretical work suggests a search for mediators of program effects. The concept of mediation is that the prevention program has an impact on psychosocial constructs that are relevant for producing the problem behavior. A range of theories may be useful for program development work (see Wills & Cleary, in press-b). Family interaction theory may link smoking or alcohol use to conflict in family interactions and lack of perceived support from parents (Wills & Cleary, 1996). Cognitive theories may suggest linkages of problem behavior to consensus perceptions (i.e., perceiving that smoking is very common among agemates when this is not really true) (see Graham, Marks, & Hansen, 1991; Sussman et al., 1988) or relatively favorable images of the typical smoker or alcohol user (Gibbons & Gerrard, 1995; Gibbons, Gerrard, & Boney-McCoy, 1995). Attitudinal theories may suggest how problem behavior is linked to perceived acceptance of the behavior by peers or community members (Brody, Flor, Hollett-Wright, & McCoy, 1998; Petraitis, Flay, & Miller, 1995). Social learning theories suggest how substance use may occur through persons becoming involved with groups of peers who are using (or beginning to use) a substance (e.g., Mosbach & Leventhal, 1988; Wills & Cleary, in press-a). Through acquaintance with relevant theory, the program developer can identify mediator variables that transmit the impact of the program. This knowledge can be crucial for sophisticated designs that measure hypothesized mediators as well as the outcome variable.

The second aspect of the use of theory involves consideration of how to manipulate the problem behavior.[3] Most theory in health behavior research tends to rely on a functional analysis of behavior; the ABCs approach (A = antecedents, B = behavior, C = consequences) (Sussman et al., 1995) dominated early health research with the behavior modification studies conducted in the 1960s. Variables considered as antecedents are perhaps much more broadly based nowadays than in the early behavior modification literature and include a variety of intrapersonal, interpersonal, and environmental variables (e.g., see Newcomb & Earleywine, 1996; Wills, Pierce, & Evans, 1996). Specific theories focus on one or more of the three elements—A, B, or C—and are grouped as either acquisition oriented (targets antecedents; especially true of various prevention models), behavior change oriented (targets behavior; traditional learning theory notions), or consequences oriented (counteracts consequences; health protection models).

Etiologic research is used to extend and refine the application of concepts to a health arena. One popular method of theory operationalization is the use of the semistructured elicitation questionnaire. A series of open-ended questions are asked about theoretical variables. Salient or most frequently mentioned responses are retained for use as measures of the variables, either recorded verbatim or after content analysis (Middlestadt, Bhattacharyya, Rosenbaum, Fishbein, & Shepherd, 1996; Stacy, Galaif, Sussman, & Dent, 1996). Through use of this or other approaches, which can vary in format from unstructured (e.g., ethnographic case studies or observation) (Scrimshaw & Gleason, 1992) to semistructured (e.g., focus groups, task analysis, task forces) to highly structured methods (forced-choice response questionnaires), etiologic researchers begin the empirical process of developing a health behavior program.

Etiologic research also may be valuable for providing evidence about mediator variables. For example, several studies have shown that effects of risk factors (e.g., parental substance use) are mediated through constructs such as self-control ability, academic competence, and attitudinal tolerance for deviance (Wills, Cleary, Shinar, & Filer, in press; Wills, Schreibman, Benson, & Vaccaro, 1994). Acquaintance with this research may assist the program developer in identifying additional dimensions that could be affected by a program and designing components to target those constructs.

Unfortunately, sometimes etiologic work is treated as if it were a separate enterprise from program materials development. Thus, it is not all that surprising in applications of program development that often a theory is adopted, and then program materials are developed, without actually linking the theory to the materials development. Fortunately, functional analysis work, as well as recent stage theory on program planning, does include such a linkage (e.g., Daniel & Green, 1995; Sussman et al., 1995). In particular relevance to program development, assessment studies are used to fill in gaps of knowledge between antecedents, mediators, behaviors, and consequences. Mediation analyses using multiple regression or structural modeling can then be performed to provide specific tests of the hypothesized linkages (see Wills & Cleary, in press-b).

For example, consider the issue of smoking prevention. Let us say that a major antecedent variable includes social influence. Social influence (the A) will increase the likelihood that a youth will be a smoker (the behavior, or B). Furthermore, let us say that a mediator of the relation between social influence and smoking is one's refusal assertion skill (knowing how to say no). Then, one might conjecture that decreasing the effects of social influence through instruction in refusal assertion training could help loosen A-B bonds (acquisition-oriented programming). Consequences (or Cs) include changes among adolescent smokers in lung function and intima-medial coronary artery thickening that indicates increased risk for lung disease and stroke later on in life. An understanding of a chain of consequences may be quite important in secondary prevention efforts and provides the basis for screening-type programs. Alternatively, let us say that the main goal is to focus on breaking the bonds between performing the behavior and suffering the consequences. Such B-C bonds can be severed by removing the C (e.g., low-tar cigarettes, harm reduction) as well as changing the B (quit-smoking programming, behavior-focused programming). These kinds of ideas can be suggested through a combination of relevant theory, prior epidemiologic research, and careful assessment work.

A systematization of etiologic methods would be useful. For example, perhaps some methods are better for identifying certain A-B links than are others. One may conjecture that to obtain information about sensitive topics such as unsafe sexual behavior, anonymous self-report data may be a better means than use of focus groups. Careful etiologic work among those who interact with a target group, gatekeepers of a target group, and key or prototypical members of the group permits the researcher or practitioner better access to the group as an important side effect (Higgins et al., 1996). A detailed presentation of theory in program development can be found in Chapter 4 of this text, and a case study example of theory development is in Chapter 5. A detailed presentation of assessment study work can be found in Chapter 6. Some techniques material of additional interest to those who wish to conduct assessment studies can be found in Chapters 9 and 11, and additional material on mediation analysis can be found in Chapter 19.

ACTIVITY POOLING AND WAREHOUSING: STEP 2 OF THE CHAIN MODEL

This second step of program development involves collecting previously used activities and teaching methods from other projects in related areas that have obtained research support or conceptualizing new plausible activities, which might be useful in the present development context. *Pooling* refers to the collection process: a means of collecting effective program content and process elements. *Warehousing* refers to mechanisms of storing and retrieving program elements. Methods of pooling activities include literature review and recommendations, expert panel ratings, consensus meetings, grant agency reports on grantees, creation of consortiums for service coordination and cross-training, and coordination of target groups or self-help group opinion. Warehousing these activities means that one needs to consider development of reasonable sets of inclusion and exclusion criteria (e.g., topic area applicability), copyright considerations, and territorial interests.

Such tasks currently are being accomplished through small-business grants and other awards from the National Institute on Drug Abuse, Sociometrics Corporation, and Spencer Foundation, as well as other venues (e.g., conferences, technical reports, private company ventures, some journal articles) (e.g., Silvestri & Flay, 1989). For example, one popular prevention strategy is refusal assertion training. Generally, a set of strategies is taught and practiced through role-play scenarios. Refusal assertion training is quite similar in construction across problem behavior programs (e.g., violence, drug abuse, risky sexual behavior). This is one activity that has been documented and warehoused for potential selection as an activity in a new research arena (Drug Strategies, 1996). Program process, as well as substantive content, can be pooled and warehoused. For example, use of the Socratic (interactive) method of teaching is an example of an important process element (Tobler & Stratton, 1997) that can be warehoused for use in new health behavior program applications.

This step also can involve development and pooling of new activities that are hypothesized to counteract certain antecedent variables. New activities would be labeled as plausible but in need of a research base of support (e.g., Sussman, 1996). Activities would be considered relevant to a particular health area based on completed etiologic work and a set of decision rules regarding how these activities plausibly might address this etiologic work. The use of qualitative decision making and analysis is relevant here (e.g., Dey, 1993; Nevo, 1995). Also, new activities can be contrasted against more established activities for subsequent perceived efficacy testing to select program material for a new research arena. A detailed presentation of activity pooling and warehousing can be found in Chapter 7, and a case study example of warehousing is in Chapter 8. A meta-analytic perspective of activity pooling is mentioned in Chapter 18.

PERCEIVED EFFICACY STUDIES: STEP 3 OF THE CHAIN MODEL

Many approaches can be used to screen and select activities. Perceived efficacy studies include focus groups or theme studies (e.g., Basch, DeCicco, & Malfetti, 1989; Dent, Galaif, Sussman, & Stacy, 1996), among other methods, to screen a large number of activities and remove those that definitely would not be received well by the target population. Discussion about the activities, as opposed to actually engaging in the activities, leads to timesaving. This approach alternatively might be referred to as *activity acceptance* or *concept evaluation,* although *perceived efficacy study* arguably is the most precise description for this type of work. We will continue to use this terminology.

The goals of the activity should be stated. One potential criterion for screening among a sufficient number of activities is observed redundancy of activities offered across multiple types of informants (e.g., Higgins et al., 1996). In addition, given a large number of activities, ratings can be made for program interest, comprehensibility, and perceived efficacy to reduce the number that would be retained for further testing (e.g., Worden et al., 1988). One is not assessing exposure, attitude change, or behavior change, per se, but rather perceived quality of the activity. Verbal perceived efficacy methods include use of focus and discussion groups, Delphi techniques, interviews (including variations of structured to unstructured and one-on-one or two-on-one evaluations), use of standardized patients, and expert consensus on perceived efficacious activities. These methods can vary in assessment context (e.g., clinic, home, worksite, computer). An example of one verbal perceived efficacy method is the use of focus groups. Focus groups consist of small groups of subjects who are asked open-ended questions by a trained facilitator to generate ideas. Group discussion may be content coded later on or may be supplemented with a collection of questionnaire data. The strengths of verbal methods are that in-depth information can be acquired, and sensitive topics might be probed (especially in private settings). Also, these methods have potential to serve as a tool to screen among numerous activities, and literacy of the target subject is not at issue. Limitations include the ability to generalize from a perceived efficacy approach to actually doing the activity. Also, expectancy confounds may operate (Sussman, Petosa, & Clarke, 1996); for example, characteristics of the data collector (dress, gender, speech tone) could influence responses and should be controlled.

Paper-and-pencil methods include use of theme studies, role model stories, card-sorting tasks, timed protocols, and self-report questionnaires to identify activities perceived as efficacious. For example, theme studies consist of brief written descriptions of activities that are rated for their perceived interest and efficacy. These activities may be student or researcher generated. Paper-and-pencil methods are best for identifying potentially efficacious activities in some special populations (e.g., the mute) and generally are relatively the easiest data to collect, code, and analyze. These methods also are useful as a screening tool but are limited in terms of ability to generalize these data to actually doing the activity. A detailed presentation of verbal perceived efficacy studies can be found in Chapter 9, and a case study example is in Chapter 10. Also, a detailed presentation of nonverbal perceived efficacy studies can be found in Chapter 11, and a case study example is in Chapter 12.

COMPONENT STUDY (IMMEDIATE-IMPACT) METHODS: STEP 4 OF THE CHAIN MODEL

Immediate-outcome studies test the impact of program activities shortly after administration of a complete program or some of its components. For example, component studies consist of testing the immediate impact of a draft lesson or activity. A component study generally contrasts two or more approaches to affecting a single mediator of behavioral effects. Immediate-impact designs include single-group (e.g., testing multiple activities across groups, perhaps controlling for order or testing effects), quasi-experimental, and experimental tests. Changes in program-related knowledge, attitudes, and beliefs typically are assessed. Also, the same component could be assessed comparing different groups (called a "comparison evaluation study"), a component could be added to an existing program (a "tack-on component study"), or a component could be added and subtracted within a fuzzy set of activities that are assessed iteratively ("action research"). Also, components may be different but provide the same general message ("complementary"), one component may build on another ("building block"), or the same general type of component may be adapted for implementation in different community units ("constellation").

The strength of component study methods is that one can test for effects on potential mediators of change. The weaknesses of this approach are that a lesson or activity is assessed without regard to other activities (lessons could detract from each other when combined), and one is only conducting an immediate-outcome evaluation; hence, effects on longer-term outcomes are less certain. A detailed presentation of component study work can be found in Chapter 13, and a case study example is in Chapter 14.

PROGRAM CONSTRUCTION AND PILOT TESTING: STEP 5 OF THE CHAIN MODEL

There are general guidelines for program construction (Sussman, 1991). These suggest how to combine activities into sessions, including notions of sequence (e.g., provide skills information first, then skills practice, then review), and combine sessions into a program (instill motivation, then provide information and skills, then encourage a commitment to program goals). Also, program development methods could be used to combine material. Such methods include rated preferences of experts and measures of the effects of combining lessons (e.g., additive—effects of a combination of lessons are equal to the sum of their individual effects; synergic—effects of a combination of lessons are greater than the sum of their individual effects; or detractive—effects of a combination of lessons are less than the sum of their individual effects).

Some means of program testing involve qualitative analysis. For example, feasibility studies involve delivering draft lessons or a full curriculum to get subjective judgments of workability. Gross negative subject group effects, such as confusion or lack of receptivity, may be ironed out. The strength of this approach is that a gross evaluation of an entire package under "real-world" conditions is possible. For example, implementation issues can be addressed to prepare for maximum implementation of the program. The weakness of this approach is that mostly "soft data" are collected, which are vulnerable to experimenter bias.

After the complete program is composed from multiple activities, the feasibility and immediate impact of the program are tested (e.g., pilot studies). Pilot studies also include single-group, quasi-experimental, and experimental designs, adding an activity to an existing program, comparison evaluation studies, and action research. The strength of the pilot study is that one can test for effects on potential mediators of change. The weakness of this approach is that one is conducting only an immediate-outcome evaluation; hence, effects on longer-term outcomes are less certain. A detailed presentation of sequencing issues in health behavior program development can be found in Chapter 15. Also, a detailed presentation of pilot studies work can be found in Chapter 16, and a case study example is in Chapter 17.

SELECTING PROGRAM DEVELOPMENT OUTCOME MEASURES TO HELP ASSESS LONGER-TERM OUTCOMES: STEP 6 OF THE CHAIN MODEL

An important additional consideration is the need to select immediate-outcome measures that will predict longer-term outcomes. In principle, program development involves the manipulation of hypothesized mediators of program effects. There is now evidence that certain immediate program outcome variables such as homework returns, enthusiasm, perceived effectiveness, attitude and belief items (e.g., prevalence estimates, attitudes toward the problem behavior), and behavioral intentions precede health behavior changes and are predictive of program outcomes 1 to 2 years later. These variables may mediate program effects.

In particular, an increase in attitudes inconsistent with unhealthy target behaviors statistically mediates relations between type of program and differences in behavior outcomes (Hansen, 1992; Tobler & Stratton, 1997). Methods of selection include empirical reviews (which sometimes suggest how immediate outcomes were related to longer-term outcomes), meta-analysis, and mediation analysis. Little work has been completed in this area of program development, although it is quite important. Several different types of immediate outcomes could be considered for different purposes. For example, marketability or dissemination potential might be measured through variables such as ease of implementation, audience acceptance of program, total cost, or cost-effectiveness. Efficacy of the program might be measured through variables that the program intends to manipulate directly (e.g., norms) or indirectly (e.g., generalized perceived efficacy). A detailed presentation of the use of meta-analysis and the use of mediator and moderator analysis to identify relevant immediate-outcome measures can be found in Chapter 18 and Chapter 19, respectively. A presentation of plausible general mediators and moderators that should be considered for health behavior program development and main trial work is presented in Chapter 20.

LITERATURE SEARCH ON METHODS

Which elements of this program development chain model are addressed most or least often in the research literature? To address this question, MedINFO and PsycINFO searches were completed dating back from 1984 through February 1998. Search terms were *Formative and Research* (or *Formative Research* for MedINFO) and *Health and Program and Development* (or *Health with Program with Development* for PsycINFO). A total of 160 relevant articles were found. Articles from previously searched work ($n = 30$) were added, providing a total pool of 190 articles of the health behavior program development type. Certainly, some additional articles might be found by searching under different terms (*component* or *mediation*, for example), but this search revealed a great deal of the published work in this scientific arena.

Of these articles, 18% were theoretically oriented and suggested that programming might be developed based on a theory. Of the theories presented, 51% took a "stages" or social marketing approach to program development, 11% were cultural type, 9% were functional analysis oriented (behavior oriented), 9% emphasized empowerment-coping-wellness, 6% were ecological (health protection or consequences oriented), and the remainder emphasized goals and obstacles or risk factors. Thus, antecedent-, behavior-, and consequences-oriented theories all were represented.

Of the articles, 23% pertained to assessment for program development. Of these, 51% were needs assessment surveys or interviews; 23% involved collection of ethnographic information (demographics, participant observation, or naturalistic observation); 14% involved use of task forces, inspections, or technical assistance; and the remainder was scattered across different approaches (e.g., case study, task analysis). Of the articles, 41% were relevant to Step 1 of the chain model.

A total of 14% of the articles referred to a pooling of resources or services. Of these, 65% involved coordination of services, 19% involved pooling of resources, and 16% involved consensus meetings. Thus, pooling-type work (Step 2 of the chain model) primarily has involved how one service delivery system has been able to cooperate with another delivery system.

A total of 12% of the articles referred to perceived efficacy studies (Step 3 of the chain model), 82% of which pertained to use of discussion or focus groups. Clearly, relatively little work on perceived efficacy has been completed.

A total of 28% of the articles referred to immediate-impact studies. Of these, 64% were pilot studies, 20% were component studies, and the remainder was scattered across different approaches (e.g., action research, comparison evaluation). In other words, approximately 8% of all studies found reflected Step 4 of the chain model (referred to component study work), whereas 20% of these studies reflected Step 5 of the chain model (referred to program building and pilot work). Clearly, more component study work is needed.

Finally, a total of 4% of the articles looked at predictors of longer-term outcomes; of these few studies (11 articles), 55% were empirical reviews, 25% were mediation studies, and 20% were meta-analyses (Step 6 of the chain model). Very little work examined how program development might translate into longer-term outcomes. In summary, as indicated in published works, prototypical program development work has been antecedent oriented, involving a needs assessment and coordination of services, perhaps involving some focus group work to screen among potential activities and use of pilot testing, and possible use of empirical reviews to get some idea about program mediation. A rather restrictive use of program development strategies is suggested by this literature review.

ISSUES FOR IMPLEMENTATION ◄

There are several challenges for maintaining progress in a science of health behavior program development. One possible barrier is that some researchers and practitioners may assume that the mere mention of a theory or a vaguely described use of one development technique suffices as a means to justify program contents and means of delivery. This is not the case. Use of a health behavior program development process requires investment of time and resources by those who develop the program and those who test it at target subject sites. Ideally, several stages of development are necessary to produce the most effective product.

Resource problems (staff, time, money, facilities) may deter optimal application of a program development process. Yet adequate testing is needed both as components of a program are being developed and as pieces of a program are put together. As an example of the importance of a stage approach, consider instruction in refusal assertion. Refusal assertion training, when taught alone, may actually reduce one's self-efficacy to refuse drug offers because one may fear encountering numerous offers from others. However, when provided with education on prevalence overestimates and lessons on normative restructuring, it may increase efficacy to refuse drug offers (Donaldson, Graham, & Hansen, 1994). Thus, component studies may produce results that vary from what would be expected in a pilot study. Both types of studies may be needed to select and compare "strong" sessions to compose a program.

An empirical approach to program development will be a new and somewhat intrusive approach for those in charge of instruction in a community setting. Considerable attention must be devoted to practical concerns and reservations of that community network (e.g., school administrators and city leaders). Their informed participation is critical to the ultimate success of the empirical approach. Therefore, recruitment, role specification, and training of implementation site staff require careful attention. Even use of technical language needs to be grappled with. How many deliverers of a program would like their clients to be referred to as "target subjects," for example? Ultimately, the quality of the final product depends on the enthusiastic participation of program site staff.

Three considerations that may need to be addressed with uninformed persons include the need for training in program development, perceived costs of program development, and skepticism on how immediate impact might predict longer-term outcomes. It should be noted that few program developers have the training to effectively participate in empirical procedures (e.g., knowledge of sampling, data analysis, and interpretation) (Nevo, 1995). Centralized resources such as this handbook should help remedy this problem.

Second, systematic program development is more expensive initially than merely intuitively coming up with a program. It would not be too difficult to convince persons in the community, though, that a program development process is less expensive in the long run. One may argue that the costs of using a careful development process "up front" would be much less than would be the costs involved in implementing an unsuccessful curriculum (and the need to develop and implement yet a new curriculum). A formal cost-benefit analysis is beyond the scope of this text, although future research might more directly address this issue in program development. (A brief discussion is completed in Chapter 16 of this text.)

Some persons may be skeptical that a program development process has any relevance to long-term impacts because, often, only perceived or immediate impact is assessed. At present, the reliability and predictive validity of such methods are not definitively established. Still, a systematic process is better than relying on the subjective judgments of a few people. Also, as mentioned earlier in this chapter, there is now evidence that certain immediate-outcome variables are predictive of program outcomes (e.g., MacKinnon et al., 1991; Sussman et al., 1995; Tobler, 1995; Tobler & Stratton, 1997; see Chapter 20, this volume). As the field develops, we expect that additional evidence on the reliability of immediate-outcome measures will become available. On the other hand, process or immediate-outcome evaluations should not be viewed as an alternative to long-term outcomes (summative) evaluations—the latter serves as the final basis for accountability of a curriculum (Nevo, 1995).[4] A detailed discussion of barriers to health behavior program development and how to surmount these barriers is presented in Chapter 3 of this text.

GENERAL DISCUSSION ◄

In this chapter, we have outlined the rationale for program development research and some methods for doing it. Program development research steps back from the evaluation of a completed program and aims to provide a systematic process for developing the program. This process uses theoretical information to suggest which variables are necessary for health behavior change, uses several iterative methods of development, and should use the perspectives of several program content specialists to obtain a consensual protocol that minimizes any personal bias of an individual developer.

Also, program development research uses the consumer as an integral part of the process. The views of typical participants are elicited to obtain a fuller understanding of how they perceive their needs and how they regard potential activities that could be included in a program. In addition, the empirical approach of the program development process examines how program activities act when they are combined into a multisession package; rather than assuming necessarily that more is better, the research tries to determine what combination and sequencing of activities will have the most beneficial impact.

An essential part of the program development process is to identify and test possible mediators and moderators in program effects. Through testing variables that are expected theoretically to mediate the impact of a preventive intervention, we can obtain resultant data that provide more useful information about why a program worked or did not work. Using short-term outcomes provides more information through an "early return system" that helps investigators to learn whether a program is having the desired impact on the kinds of factors that help to motivate and consolidate long-term change processes.

The "chain model" summarized in this chapter recognizes that the various program development steps described here have been used to some extent in previous curriculum development and evaluation research. However, the integrated model aims to systematize this process so that the efforts of a program development team will be of maximal value to their colleagues for theoretical understanding and empirical replication. This general model, we believe, is applicable across any number of health settings (school, workplace, community agency, families). The unit of application will vary by setting. For example, we might ask persons about community poverty versus personal income in community-wide versus worksite program development. Still, the same six steps can be applied fruitfully.

The health behavior program development process outlined here may sound like "more work," which is true, and it will benefit from a protocol pursued with support from community groups and funding agencies. We have outlined the reasons why this approach to prevention research provides advantages to the field through more useful feedback to participants and sponsors and through faster gains to the field in cumulative knowledge.

▶ NOTES

1. For example, McLeroy et al. (1993) offer an ecological planning model: (a) develop an understanding of the psychosocial factors affecting the problem, including the interrelationships of factors at different levels of analysis (theories of the specific problem); (b) gather knowledge about previous interventions and their relative effectiveness with various cultural and population groups (theories of intervention); and (c) become aware of the community and cultural context within which the program would be implemented (i.e., consider organizational moderator variables).

2. In other words, unique causal mechanisms need to be addressed such as cultural sensitivity or other ecological concerns (e.g., Daniel & Green, 1995; Green & Kreuter, 1991; Green, Richard, & Potvin, 1996; van Ryn & Heaney, 1992).

3. Philosophy of social science ideas is considered here, including a consideration of how the "abstract" becomes the "concrete" (Sussman, Simon, Glynn, & Stacy, 1996; van Ryn & Heaney, 1992). How does theory become operationalized into entities that can be modified? Rules of operationalization include testability, plausibility, and heuristics. A theory with substance lends itself to a complete test of its components (testability). Each component is assessed ideally by at least two measures. The operationalization should consist of logically valid statements regarding theoretical components (plausibility). Finally, the testing should be such that potential for replication and generalizability and program improvement is maximized (heuristics).

4. Another issue is that the academic profession assigns too little credit to this form of scholarship, compared to research that tests the outcomes of completed interventions (Boyer, 1990; Sussman, Petosa, & Clarke, 1996). Even when investigators support their development of programs with research, their inquiries often rely on strategies such as focus groups and single-group, repeated-measures designs that some in the academic community may consider inferior. Our view is that more credit needs to be given to this endeavor because too little "Phase Two" (National Institutes of Health term for methods development) research has been conducted (Sussman et al., 1995), and we believe that health behavior program development encompasses the essence of the scientific method.

▶ REFERENCES

ABBOTT, G. K. (1947). *The witness of science: To the testimonies of the spirit of prophesy.* Angwin, CA: Pacific Union College.
ALCOHOLICS ANONYMOUS. (1939). *Alcoholics Anonymous.* New York: Alcoholics Anonymous World Services, Inc.

BASCH, C. E., DeCICCO, I. M., & MALFETTI, J. L. (1989). A focus group study on decision processes of young driver: Reasons that may support a decision to drink and drive. *Health Education Quarterly, 16,* 389-396.

BELLOC, N. B., & BRESLOW, L. (1972). Relationship of physical health status and health practices. *Preventive Medicine, 1,* 409-421.

BLANCHARD, E. B. (1992). Introduction to the special issue on behavioral medicine: An update for the 1990's. *Journal of Consulting and Clinical Psychology, 60,* 491-492.

BOYER, E. L. (1990). *Scholarship reconsidered: Priorities of the professoriate.* Princeton, NJ: Carnegie Foundation for the Advancement of Teaching.

BRAVERMAN, M. T., & CAMPBELL, D. T. (1989). Facilitating the development of health promotion programs: Recommendations for researchers and funders. In M. T. Braverman (Ed.), *Evaluating health promotion programs* (pp. 5-18). San Francisco: Jossey-Bass.

BRESLOW, L., & BRESLOW, N. (1993). Health practices and disability: Some evidence from Alameda County. *Preventive Medicine, 22,* 86-95.

BRODY, G. H., FLOR, D. L., HOLLETT-WRIGHT, N., & McCOY, J. K. (1998). Children's development of alcohol use norms: Contributions of parent and sibling norms, children's temperaments, and parent-child discussions. *Journal of Family Psychology, 12,* 209-219.

BROWNELL, K. D., & WADDEN, T. A. (1992). Etiology and treatment of obesity: Understanding a serious, prevalent, and refractory disorder. *Journal of Consulting and Clinical Psychology, 60,* 505-517.

CHESNEY, M. A. (1984). Behavior modification and health enhancement. In J. D. Matarazzo, S. M. Weiss, J. A. Herd, N. E. Miller, & S. M. Weiss (Eds.), *Behavioral health: A handbook of health enhancement and disease prevention* (pp. 338-350). New York: John Wiley.

COOPER, K. H. (1968). *Aerobics.* New York: Bantam.

DANIEL, M., & GREEN, L. W. (1995). Application of the precede-proceed planning model in diabetes prevention and control: A case illustration from a Canadian aboriginal community. *Diabetes Spectrum, 8,* 74-84.

DENT, C. W., GALAIF, E. R., SUSSMAN, S., & STACY, A. W. (1996). Use of the "theme study" as means of curriculum development in continuation high schools. *Journal of Drug Education, 26,* 377-393.

DEY, I. (1993). *Qualitative data analysis.* London: Routledge Kegan Paul.

DONALDSON, S. I., GRAHAM, J. W., & HANSEN, W. B. (1994). Testing the generalizability of intervening mechanism theories: Understanding the effects of adolescent drug use prevention interventions. *Journal of Behavioral Medicine, 17,* 195-216.

DONOVAN, J. E., JESSOR, R., & COSTA, F. M. (1988). Syndrome of problem behavior in adolescence: A replication. *Journal of Consulting and Clinical Psychology, 56,* 762-765.

DRUG STRATEGIES. (1996). *Making the grade: A guide to school drug prevention programs.* Washington, DC: Author.

EPSTEIN, L. H., & CLUSS, P. A. (1982). A behavioral medicine perspective on adherence to long-term medical regimens. *Journal of Consulting and Clinical Psychology, 50,* 950-971.

FARQUHAR, J. W., FORTMANN, S. P., MACCOBY, N., WOOD, P. D., HASKELL, W. L., TAYLOR, C. B., FLORA, J. A., SOLOMON, D. S., ROGERS, T., ADLER, E., BREITROSE, P., & WEINER, L. (1984). The Stanford Five City Project: An overview. In J. D. Matarazzo, S. M. Weiss, J. A. Herd, N. E. Miller, & S. M. Weiss (Eds.), *Behavioral health: A handbook of health enhancement and disease prevention* (pp. 1154-1165). New York: John Wiley.

FELDMAN, R. H. L. (1984). Evaluating health promotion in the workplace. In J. D. Matarazzo, S. M. Weiss, J. A. Herd, N. E. Miller, & S. M. Weiss (Eds.), *Behavioral health: A handbook of health enhancement and disease prevention* (pp. 1087-1093). New York: John Wiley.

GIBBONS, F. X., & GERRARD, M. (1995). Predicting young adults' health risk behavior. *Journal of Personality and Social Psychology, 69,* 505-517.

GIBBONS, F. X., GERRARD, M., & BONEY-McCOY, S. (1995). Prototype perception predicts (lack of) pregnancy prevention. *Personality and Social Psychology Bulletin, 21,* 85-93.

GRAHAM, J. W., MARKS, G., & HANSEN, W. B. (1991). Social influence processes affecting adolescent substance use. *Journal of Applied Psychology, 76,* 291-298.

GREEN, L. W., & KREUTER, M. W. (1991). *Health promotion planning: An educational and environmental approach.* Mountain View, CA: Mayfield.

GREEN, L. W., RICHARD, L., & POTVIN, L. (1996). Ecological foundations of health promotion. *American Journal of Health Promotion, 10,* 270-281.

HANSEN, W. B. (1992). School-based substance abuse prevention: A review of the state of the art in curriculum, 1980-1990. *Health Education Research: Theory and Practice, 7,* 403-430.

HANSEN, W. B., & GRAHAM, J. W. (1991). Preventing alcohol, marijuana, and cigarette use among adolescents: Peer pressure resistance training versus establishing conservative norms. *Preventive Medicine, 20,* 414-430.

HANSEN, W. B., GRAHAM, J. W., WOLKENSTEIN, B. H., LUNDY, B. Z., PEARSON, J., FLAY, B. R., & JOHNSON, C. A. (1988). Differential impact of three alcohol prevention curricula on hypothesized mediating variables. *Journal of Drug Education, 18,* 143-153.

HIGGINS, D. L., O'REILLY, K., TASHIMA, N., CRAIN, C., BEEKER, C., GOLDBAUM, G., ELIFSON, C. S., GALAVOTTI, C., & GUENTHER-GRAY, C. (1996). Using formative research to lay the foundation for community level HIV prevention efforts: An example from the AIDS Community Demonstration Project. *Public Health Reports, 3*(Suppl.), 28-35.

ISAAC, S., & MICHAEL, W. B. (1990). *Handbook in research and evaluation.* San Diego, CA: EdITS.

KETTNER, P. M., MORONEY, R. M., & MARTIN, L. L. (1990). *Designing and managing programs: An effectiveness-based approach.* Newbury Park, CA: Sage.

LASHLEY, K. S., & WATSON, J. B. (1921). A psychological study of motion pictures in relation to venereal disease campaigns. *Social Hygiene, 7,* 181-219.

LEFEBVRE, R. C., & FLORA, J. A. (1988). Social marketing and public health intervention. *Health Education Quarterly, 15,* 299-315.

MACFADDEN, B. (1924). *Eating for health and strength.* New York: MacFadden.

MacKINNON, D. P., JOHNSON, C. A., PENTZ, M. A., DWYER, D. P., & HANSEN, W. B. (1991). Mediating mechanisms in a school-based drug prevention program: First year effects of the Midwestern Prevention Project. *Health Psychology, 10,* 164-172.

MATARAZZO, J. D. (1984). Behavioral health: A 1990 challenge for the health professions. In J. D. Matarazzo, S. M. Weiss, J. A. Herd, N. E. Miller, & S. M. Weiss (Eds.), *Behavioral health: A handbook of health enhancement and disease prevention* (pp. 3-40). New York: John Wiley.

McLEROY, K. R., STECKLER, A. B., SIMONS-MORTON, B., GOODMAN, R. M., GOTTLIEB, N., & BURDINE, J. N. (1993). Social science theory in health education: Time for a new model? *Health Education Research: Theory and Practice, 8,* 305-312.

MIDDLESTADT, S. E., BHATTACHARYYA, K., ROSENBAUM, J., FISHBEIN, M., & SHEPHERD, M. (1996). The use of theory based semistructured elicitation questionnaires: Formative research for CDC's prevention marketing initiative. *Public Health Reports, 3,* 18-27.

MILLER, D. C. (1991). *Handbook of research design and social measurement.* Newbury Park, CA: Sage.

MOSBACH, P., & LEVENTHAL, H. (1988). Peer group identification and smoking. *Journal of Abnormal Psychology, 97,* 238-245.

NEVO, D. (1995). *School-based evaluation: A dialogue for school improvement.* Oxford, UK: Pergamon.

NEWCOMB, M. D., & EARLEYWINE, M. (1996). Intrapersonal contributors to drug use: The willing host. *American Behavioral Scientist, 39,* 823-837.

O'LEARY, K. D., & WILSON, G. T. (1975). *Behavior therapy: Application and outcome.* Englewood Cliffs, NJ: Prentice Hall.

PETRAITIS, J., FLAY, B. R., & MILLER, T. Q. (1995). Reviewing theories of adolescent substance use: Organizing pieces in the puzzle. *Psychological Bulletin, 117,* 67-86.

RICHARDSON, J. L., DWYER, K., McGUIGAN, K., HANSEN, W. B., DENT, C. W., JOHNSON, C. A., SUSSMAN, S., BRANNON, B., & FLAY, B. R. (1989). Substance use among adolescents who take care of themselves after school. *Pediatrics, 84,* 556-566.

ROSSI, P. H., & FREEMAN, H. E. (1993). *Evaluation: A systematic approach.* Newbury Park, CA: Sage.

SCRIMSHAW, N. S., & GLEASON, G. R. (Eds.). (1992). *RAP (rapid assessment procedures): Qualitative methodologies for planning and evaluation of health related programmes.* Boston: International Nutrition Foundation for Developing Countries (INFDC).

SILVESTRI, B., & FLAY, B. R. (1989). Smoking education: Comparison of practice and state-of-the-art. *Preventive Medicine, 18,* 257-266.

SOLOMON, D. S., & MACCOBY, N. (1984). Communication as a model for health enhancement. In J. D. Matarazzo, S. M. Weiss, J. A. Herd, N. E. Miller, & S. M. Weiss (Eds.), *Behavioral health: A handbook of health enhancement and disease prevention* (pp. 209-221). New York: John Wiley.
STACY, A. W., GALAIF, E. R., SUSSMAN, S., & DENT, C. W. (1996). Self-generated drug outcomes in high-risk adolescents. *Psychology of Addictive Behaviors, 10,* 18-27.
SUSSMAN, S. (1991). Curriculum development in school-based prevention research. *Health Education Research: Theory and Practice, 6,* 339-351.
SUSSMAN, S. (1996). Development of a school-based drug abuse prevention curriculum for high-risk youths. *Journal of Psychoactive Drugs, 28,* 169-182.
SUSSMAN, S., DENT, C. W., BRANNON, B. R., GLOWACZ, K. M., GLEASON, L. R., HANSEN, W. B., JOHNSON, C. A., & FLAY, B. R. (1989). The television, school, and family smoking prevention/cessation project: IV. Controlling for program success expectancies across experimental and control conditions. *Addictive Behaviors, 14,* 601-610.
SUSSMAN, S., DENT, C. W., BURTON, D., STACY, A. W., & FLAY, B. R. (1995). *Developing school-based tobacco use prevention and cessation programs.* Thousand Oaks, CA: Sage.
SUSSMAN, S., DENT, C. W., MESTEL-RAUCH, J., JOHNSON, C. A., HANSEN, W. B., & FLAY, B. R. (1988). Adolescent nonsmokers, triers, and regular smokers' estimates of cigarette smoking prevalence: When do overestimations occur and by whom? *Journal of Applied Social Psychology, 18,* 537-551.
SUSSMAN, S., DENT, C. W., STACY, A. W., & CRAIG, S. (1998). One-year outcomes of Project Towards No Drug Abuse. *Preventive Medicine, 27,* 632-642.
SUSSMAN, S., PETOSA, R., & CLARKE, R. (1996). The use of empirical curriculum development to improve prevention research. *American Behavioral Scientist, 39,* 838-852.
SUSSMAN, S., SIMON, T. R., GLYNN, S., & STACY, A. W. (1996). What does "high risk" mean? A psycINFO scan of the literature. *Behavior Therapy, 27,* 53-65.
TAYLOR, R. B., DENHAM, J. W., & UREDA, J. R. (1982). 1. Health promotion: A perspective. In R. B. Taylor, J. R. Ureda, & J. W. Denham (Eds.), *Health promotion: Principles and clinical applications* (pp. 1-18). Norwalk, CT: Appleton-Century-Crofts.
THORESEN, C. E. (1984). Overview. In J. D. Matarazzo, S. M. Weiss, J. A. Herd, N. E. Miller, & S. M. Weiss (Eds.), *Behavioral health: A handbook of health enhancement and disease prevention* (pp. 297-307). New York: John Wiley.
TOBLER, N. S. (1995, June). *Interactive programs are successful: A new meta-analysis.* Oral presentation at the 3rd Annual Meeting of the Society for Prevention Research, Scottsdale, AZ.
TOBLER, N. S., & STRATTON, H. H. (1997). Effectiveness of school-based drug prevention programs: A meta-analysis of the research. *Journal of Primary Prevention, 18,* 77-128.
TUCHFELD, B. S., & MARCUS, S. H. (1984). Social models of prevention in alcoholism. In J. D. Matarazzo, S. M. Weiss, J. A. Herd, N. E. Miller, & S. M. Weiss (Eds.), *Behavioral health: A handbook of health enhancement and disease prevention* (pp. 1039-1040). New York: John Wiley.
U.S. DEPARTMENT OF HEALTH AND HUMAN SERVICES (DHHS). (1964). *Smoking and health: Report to the advisory committee to the surgeon general of the Public Health Service* (Pub. No. 1103). Washington, DC: Public Health Service.
U.S. DEPARTMENT OF HEALTH AND HUMAN SERVICES (DHHS), PUBLIC HEALTH SERVICE. (1990). *Healthy People 2000: National health promotion and disease prevention objectives.* Washington, DC: Author.
VAN RYN, M., & HEANEY, C. A. (1992). What's the use of theory? *Health Education Quarterly, 19,* 315-330.
WILLS, T. A., & CLEARY, S. D. (1996). How are social support effects mediated: A test for parental support and adolescent substance use. *Journal of Personality and Social Psychology, 71,* 937-952.
WILLS, T. A., & CLEARY, S. D. (in press-a). Peer and adolescent substance use among 6th-9th graders: Latent growth analyses of influence versus selection mechanisms. *Health Psychology.*
WILLS, T. A., & CLEARY, S. D. (in press-b). Theoretical models and frameworks for child health research. In D. Drotar (Ed.), *Handbook of research methods in pediatric and clinical child psychology.* New York: Plenum.

WILLS, T. A., CLEARY, S. D., SHINAR, O., & FILER, M. (in press). Temperament dimensions and health behavior. In L. Hayman, J. R. Turner, & M. Mahon (Eds.), *Health and behavior in childhood and adolescence*. Mahwah, NJ: Lawrence Erlbaum.

WILLS, T. A., PIERCE, J. P., & EVANS, R. I. (1996). Large-scale environmental risk factors for substance use. *American Behavioral Scientist, 39*, 808-822.

WILLS, T. A., SCHREIBMAN, D., BENSON, G., & VACCARO, D. (1994). The impact of parental substance use on adolescents: A test of a mediational model. *Journal of Pediatric Psychology, 19*, 537-555.

WINDSOR, R. A., BARANOWSKI, T., CLARK, N., & CUTTER, G. (1984). *Evaluation of health promotion and education programs*. Palo Alto, CA: Mayfield.

WORDEN, J. K., FLYNN, B. S., GELLER, B. M., CHEN, M., SHELTON, L. G., SECKER-WALKER, R. H., SOLOMON, D. S., SOLOMON, C. J., COUCHEY, S., & COSTANZA, M. C. (1988). Development of a smoking prevention mass media program using diagnostic and formative research. *Preventive Medicine, 17*, 531-558.

WORDEN, J. K., FLYNN, B. S., SOLOMON, L. J., SECKER-WALKER, R. H., BADGER, G. J., & CARPENTER, J. H. (1996). Using mass media to prevent cigarette smoking among adolescent girls. *Health Education Quarterly, 23*, 453-468.

CHAPTER 1

Commentary

Pekka Puska

The chapter starts with a story about how a baby learns to walk. A question that greatly concerns the public health expert is what will be the future health of today's baby. Also, what factors influence a baby's health in the future, in the new century? The most serious threat would be nuclear war or a similar major catastrophe. That is why public health professionals should contribute to the efforts to promote peace and prevent violence, as well as promote bodily health. In a more peaceful situation, it is hoped that today's baby probably will enjoy a healthier future than babies of the 20th century. In the developed world, we learned years ago that our major health risks are cardiovascular diseases, cancers, and assorted other noncommunicable diseases. The first public health revolution in the early 1900s brought most of the serious infectious diseases under control. Subsequently, the public health arena became overwhelmingly focused on certain major chronic diseases.

It is less often realized that the same development is now rapidly taking place in the Third World, where most of the world's population lives. In large parts of the developing world, infectious disease epidemics are now increasingly being brought under control. At the same time, lifestyles are changing in unhealthier directions; smoking is increasing, unhealthy diets are emerging, and physical activity is decreasing, for example. Following this development, noncommunicable diseases have now become the major global health problem, not only in the developed but also in the developing world. According to the latest World Health Organization's (1997) statistics, coronary heart disease is the number-one killer in the world. And it will also be responsible for the greatest losses in disability-adjusted life years. Cardiovascular diseases are already responsible for about 30% of the some 50 million annual deaths in the world.

Thus, the message for our baby's future health is clear: The keys to good health are behavioral factors that can prevent the contemporary chronic diseases responsible for most premature deaths and, for much disability, human suffering and economic losses. Unlike the previous infectious disease epidemics, these health problems are not caused by bacterial or viral agents. Previously, they were referred to as diseases of affluence. This term is, however, grossly misleading. It is true that these diseases emerge when traditionally poor societies experience economic growth. But in most populations, most chronic diseases and their risk factors concern particularly the less advantaged parts of the population. Furthermore, along with more recent economic growth, several countries such as the United States and Finland have already achieved major success in reducing these chronic disease epidemics (e.g., Puska, Vartiainen, Tuomilehto, Salomaa, & Nissinen, 1998).

What are the determinants of these contemporary health problems? What is the information needed for our growing baby to enjoy a long and healthy life? There is, no doubt, much more research needed to learn about the full etiology and pathogenesis of these diseases. At the same time, however, extensive international medical research since the early 1950s has revealed solid information about some major risk factors.

These factors are in a strong, consistent, and causal way related to the development of many of our major noncommunicable diseases. Typical of the major disease risk factors is that they closely reflect our lifestyles, such as smoking, certain nutritional habits, physical inactivity, alcohol consumption, and so on. This feature is so strong that these diseases are also commonly called "diseases of lifestyle." In populations in which certain chronic diseases are prevalent, particular harmful lifestyles are usually common. On the other hand, countries that have experienced major positive changes have usually succeeded in reducing these harmful lifestyles. Thus, it is obvious that our baby's future health is very much dependent on what kind of lifestyle he or she will learn in childhood and adolescence, as well as what kind of behavioral changes will take place in adulthood. It is quite obvious that the optimal situation would be to learn in childhood and adolescence the lifestyles conducive to health, as a natural way of living. But medical research has convincingly demonstrated that changing earlier unhealthy lifestyles even relatively late in life can greatly reduce disease risks and promote health.

I hear many readers ask, "Isn't our baby's health in the future greatly influenced by the great achievements in basic medical research, such as in genetics, cell biology, and medical technology?" It is quite obvious that we already see major advances in this field, and major new breakthroughs are likely. Thus, it is really difficult to predict the long-term future. We should, however, realize that even if our advanced clinical medicine can often save the life of a patient, this development does not decrease very much the public health burden of chronic diseases. Expensive clinical medicine is mainly dealing with consequences, not causes, of the chronic diseases. High proportions of our cardiovascular deaths are quite sudden, treatment for many cancers is too late, and so on. Also, major changes in the rates of some chronic diseases in different populations have overwhelmingly been related to major changes in lifestyle, not in clinical treatment.

Our baby may enjoy the beneficial consequences of modern medical services in the future, but at least over the next few decades, his or her health is very much dependent on lifestyles and behaviors. We also should realize that certain behaviors are important in the success of medical services: These include behaviors related to disease detection, compliance with treatment, adherence to follow-up, and rehabilitation. In real life, it is not enough that the doctor makes the right diagnoses and decides on appropriate treatment. The patient has to comply with this.

Another important aspect also emphasizes the importance of lifestyle interventions—namely, cost considerations. Medical and technological developments in new treatment modalities tend to increase our health care costs beyond what our societies can afford. That is why cost-effectiveness considerations have become increasingly important. With ongoing limited resources, we should evaluate the cost-effectiveness of our interventions. The research carried out so far in this field has provided very clear results: A whole range of lifestyle-related public health interventions give cost-effectiveness ratios superior to those of many of the modern highly visible clinical treatment options. Thus, it is likely that in the future, prevention and health promotion programs that aim at lifestyle changes will remain a much less expensive means to increase health than medical care options.

It is obvious that both public health and individual-level health are very much dependent on our capability to influence health-related lifestyles and behaviors. Many people actually have remarked that the major question for our public health work is not "what" we should do but "how" we can apply solid medical knowledge to influence people's behaviors for preventing major chronic diseases and for promoting good health. This is the great challenge for public health, and this endeavor also is frequently referred to as behavioral medicine.

Just after the discovery of the classical risk factors, activities were begun to change them through eliciting behavioral changes. The early programs were based on the simple idea that merely providing information to people would change their lifestyles. Indeed, some people do respond to new knowledge and, accordingly, change their behaviors. But in most cases, we are facing the situation in which knowledge is not dramatically new and information messages have only very limited effects. This is because lifestyles are deeply embedded in the society; they have strong cultural, habitual, addictive, economic, and political roots. It has become quite obvious that changing people's lifestyles and behaviors is not embedded in the field of medical sciences. Instead, behavioral and social sciences, which greatly advanced after World War II, do provide appropriate frameworks. The problem, of course, is that there is no single theory that tells us what to do. And health professionals are often frustrated by the inability of the behavioral sciences simply to tell them what to do. Unfortunately, many, if not most, health campaigns and interventions are carried out with little consideration of the frameworks of behavioral or social sciences. Perhaps program developers did not want to engage in a relatively complicated means to develop programs. However, we also should realize that most of the interventions to change lifestyles have met with only little or modest success. This result can be due to choice of the wrong medical targets, lack of appropriate behavioral frameworks, wrong application of the theories in the given circumstances, or too low an intensity of the intervention, among other reasons.

In response to this situation, the theoretical basis for influencing people's health-related behaviors has begun development. There now are many relevant theories and behavioral frameworks (Matarazzo, Weiss, Herd, Miller, & Weiss, 1984), and public health experts have increasingly become aware of Kurt Lewin's (1951) old wisdom that "there is nothing so practical as a good theory." But major questions remain regarding which theory to choose, how to apply it in given conditions, and how to design appropriate programs. This introductory chapter rightly argues that so far, there has been surprisingly little attention to these aspects that are often so crucial for our health work. The reasons for this neglect are multiple. There are often preexisting and strong ideas, there is urgency about starting the activities, there is a lack of resources for appropriate planning—and there may be a lack of skills for proper program planning. The chapter also rightly argues that there has been an unjustified lack of academic interest in this subject. Most publications demand hard empirical data on study design and evaluation results. Program design, planning, and implementation receive less attention.

The chapter reflects predominantly the U.S. literature on scientific development of programming. This work, indeed, should be congratulated. But what about other countries and cultures? Many of the theories and principles described are universal and should be globally applicable. However, in many cases, local cultures and situations should be considered carefully. I hope that this book would inspire programs and experts in other countries to pay more systematic attention to program planning and implementation and publish their principles and experiences. Information from experiences of different cultures could also tell us more about which principles are universally applicable and how to adapt programming in different local cultures. It is obvious that the next generation of health intervention programs should pay much more attention to systematic principles of program planning and development, including setting quality standards for planning criteria and recording program development activities. That is why this book and future related works will fill a great need and are very much welcomed by the public health community.

REFERENCES

LEWIN, K. (1951). *Field theory in social science.* New York: Harper.

MATARAZZO, J. D., WEISS, S., HERD, J. A., MILLER, N. E., & WEISS, S. M. (Eds.). (1984). *Behavioral health: A handbook of health enhancement and disease prevention.* New York: John Wiley.

PUSKA, P., VARTIAINEN, E., TUOMILEHTO, J., SALOMAA, V., & NISSINEN, A. (1998). Changes in premature deaths in Finland: Successful long-term prevention of cardiovascular diseases. *WHO Bulletin, 76,* 419-425.

WORLD HEALTH ORGANIZATION. (1997). *World health report 1997.* Geneva, Switzerland: Author.

Case Study 1

CHAPTER 2

Implementing Program Development in a State or Local Health Department

A Smoking Prevention Media Campaign Example

John K. Worden

In this hypothetical case study, I will illustrate how the six steps of the program development chain model can be used to structure and document the process of creating a mass media campaign. Because the process of developing, implementing, and monitoring a mass media campaign involves the cooperation of many individuals representing different disciplines and viewpoints, it provides an excellent example of how the structure offered by the program development chain model can be used to conduct an effective program. Without such structure, the process could be chaotic. With this structure, all of the elements should work smoothly together, and by documenting each step in the process, program planners can benefit from lessons learned along the way.

To provide a concrete example of the model in action, I present the process of developing a mass media campaign in the form of a "how-to manual" for program planners at a state or local health department who have been given the opportunity to create a smoking prevention mass media campaign for adolescents. I will begin with an overview of the process and resources required to conduct the campaign, then present the six steps of program development. Although this case study is hypothetical, my colleagues and I have applied many of the techniques discussed in our own work numerous times (e.g., Worden et al., 1988; Worden et al., 1996).

Before we look at the steps to be taken in creating a mass media education campaign, it is important to review various resources at hand in a state or local health department that can be dedicated to campaign development. Very often, public health organizations tend to overlook valuable local resources and call in professional advertising or media professionals to develop and conduct a health education media campaign. Unfortunately, although these professionals understand media, they have not been trained to respond to the needs and interests of persons in at-risk groups for whom the campaign is intended.

To use local resources most effectively for this campaign, we recommend that a partnership be formed between professionals from two areas: those who know about substance use prevention and advertising or media professionals who know how to make creative media materials. Having someone familiar with the problem being addressed will help guarantee that principles learned in previous research about the problem can be employed in the campaign. In the example shown here, several key decisions about campaign design are based on studies using social cognitive theory and social marketing principles to prevent smoking (Bandura, 1977; DeJong & Winston, 1990; Flay, 1981; Flay, DiTecco, & Schlegel, 1980; Flynn et al., 1992; Worden et al., 1988; Worden et al., 1996). To keep the program on course, we recommend that someone in the public health organization stay in charge of the process of developing new messages. This person should work with a panel of health educators and substance use prevention experts to review campaign strategy and help in advising producers who will create the media materials. We also suggest that input from targeted segments of the audience be used at critical points in the creative process—when you are developing message concepts and when you pretest messages at a preliminary stage of production.

Let us consider a picture of the overall campaign development process (see Figure 2.1). First, the public health organization, such as a state or local health department, starts the campaign by analyzing the problem to be addressed by a media campaign and by identifying targeted audience segments (e.g., youth). The public health organization (or contractors hired by them) will then conduct diagnostic surveys and focus groups to determine ideas, lifestyles, and media choices for the target segments.

After reviewing the diagnostic information, the public health organization will brief advertising agency creative staff, writers, or those working for media producers. They will provide clear educational objectives for the campaign and information about lifestyles and media choices of the target audience, and they will contract with one or more ad agencies or producers to create concepts for the campaign messages.

The public health organization will then convene a panel of health education professionals to assist in reviewing concepts received from the agencies or producers. For a smoking prevention project, this panel could consist of a behavioral scientist with expertise in substance use prevention, a school health educator, an adolescent development expert, and a mass communication researcher. The public health organization will use the results of this review to select concepts to be produced in preliminary form.

When preliminary messages are produced, the public health organization will pretest them with persons in the target audience and select the most highly rated message for final production. They also will engage media professionals to help them schedule messages for broadcast, using media preference information gathered during previous surveys of persons in the targeted audience segment. Finally, the public health organization will monitor feedback from the target audience through periodic surveys that ask if the messages are recognized and still have appeal or whether they need to be replaced with other messages addressing the educational objectives.

▶ USING THE CHAIN MODEL

Now, let us look at this process organized according to the six steps of the program development chain model. A brief paragraph is included at each step to provide a clear reference of how the model is applied in this example.

STEP 1: DEFINING THE PROBLEM AND TARGET GROUP NEEDS AND INTERESTS

First, one would develop a theory of target group need and program activity links. Concurrent with the assessment of a target population need, a theory of program mediation would be developed to address this need. Program activities

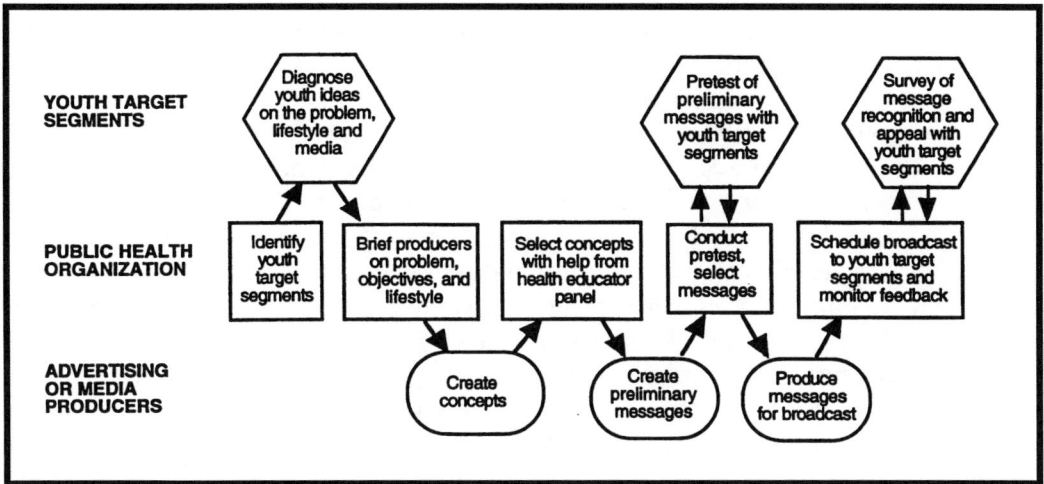

Figure 2.1. Overall Campaign Development Process

that plausibly might address this health need should be generated. In other words, we suggest that needs assessments are never separated from theory.

To begin, clearly *define the problem* in the simplest terms. Here is an example: preventing young people from starting to smoke cigarettes. Once a problem is clearly defined, then *find out what is already known* by doing research to determine (a) what the campaign should say (educational objectives, based on a theory of mediation) and communication strategies, and (b) the types of persons affected by the problem (target groups and their needs and interests).

Educational Objectives and Communication Strategies. Mass media campaigns, like other health education programs, must be built on clearly stated educational objectives. Objectives provide focus for message development based on what is known about factors that influence the target behavior. When selecting educational objectives for the youth in our example, we include four that represent social cognitive theory (Bandura, 1977) because research has found that these factors can influence behavior through the presentation of media spots (Flynn et al., 1992; Worden et al., 1988; Worden et al., 1996). These four objectives are (a) showing positive expectations of nonsubstance use, (b) showing negative expectations of substance use, (c) showing lower occurrence of substance use among the peer group, and (d) showing skills for avoiding tobacco use.

To apply these objectives with youth, we have found that they must be stated more simply, such as the following: (a) It helps to not smoke, (b) smoking causes problems, (c) most kids don't smoke, and (d) how to refuse a cigarette. In planning a campaign, you also will want to consider some strategic communication principles that are recommended from previous research (DeJong & Winston, 1990; Flay, 1981; Worden et al., 1988; Worden et al., 1996), especially in reaching youth with prevention messages.

It is clear that youth respond well to a *variety* of messages. Try to create several ideas that fit into formats they already prefer (e.g., situation comedy and cartoons but also rock videos and straightforward testimonials). Avoid using logos, slogans, or music that would tie the spots together because it has been found that messages appearing to come from different sources are more credible to youth. For variety, it may be best to disperse the production of messages, or spots, among several different production companies. Adults probably prefer variety in messages, too, but they also tend to appreciate a clear reference to the sponsor of the spot, particularly if they want to contact someone to learn more about the topic of the campaign.

For youth, and perhaps for adults, every effort should be made to *avoid exhortations* such as, "Don't smoke!" Instead, following the principles of social cognitive theory, *show successful models* (kids like members of the target group who are a little older and pretty "cool," saying things such as, "I don't smoke and I'm doing fine!").

Avoid Demonstrating the Use of a Harmful Substance. This is an easy trap to fall into, especially if you want to show how to refuse someone offering a cigarette or some other substance. However, if someone is shown using a substance, even those who appear most negative to adults producing the messages could seem positive to some higher-risk youth in the target group. Regardless of what the end of the message may say about the consequences of using a substance, there is great danger in creating an image of anyone using it anywhere in the message because persons viewing the message are likely to be affected by that image, and the take-home message may be that "it's okay to use it."

Identifying Target Audience Segments. Epidemiological research can provide descriptions of the types of persons affected by the problem and identify the *target audiences* who may benefit from a media intervention. For example, to prevent youth smoking, a primary target audience would be youth between the ages of 10 and 15, an age just prior to when most people start smoking. Another target audience for this problem could be parents or persons who sell tobacco, and these groups will require separate campaigns. But for this discussion, we will concentrate on youth.

To make a campaign that will both appeal to and affect this target audience, we must divide them into *audience segments* according to needs and interests that might affect their reception of the campaign. For youth in this age group, audience segments may reflect differences in perceptions and abilities found to be related to gender and stages in human development, so that segments would look like the following: (a) preadolescent boys, ages 10 and 11 (Grades 5 and 6; enjoy physical action, rarely use abstract thinking); (b) preadolescent girls, ages 10 and 11 (Grades 5 and 6; social influences important, rarely use abstract thinking); (c) early adolescent boys, ages 12 and 13 (Grades 7 and 8; enjoy physical action, abstract thinking begins); and (d) early adolescent girls, ages 12 and 13 (Grades 7 and 8; social influences important, abstract thinking begins).

Diagnosing Needs and Interests of Audience Segments. With audience segments identified, it is a good time to learn about their perceptions and interests before designing the campaign. This can be done using brief surveys and focus groups that are planned to get the most information. The first step is to make a brief *survey questionnaire* (see Figure 2.2). From research on the behavioral problem (Step 1), make a list of statements about the problem in terms that can be understood by persons in the targeted segments. In your questionnaire, list the statements and ask persons in each segment how much they agree with them (strongly agree, agree, disagree, strongly disagree). Examples would be the following: (a) Most kids in high school smoke cigarettes, (b) you need to smoke cigarettes to be one of the gang, and (c) if I started to smoke, I could quit anytime I wanted to.

Learn about the interests of the targeted audience segments. In the questionnaire, ask them about their leisure activities, wishes, people they admire, television shows and movies they like, and music they listen to. Also include questions about media used by each segment. Ask them about how often they watch television, which channels they watch most often, and which programs they watch; ask them how often they listen to the radio, which stations, and at what times; and ask them if they often read newspapers, see posters, ride buses with advertising, or use the Internet. Try to find out how often they are exposed to these media.

After you have completed your survey questionnaire, recruit at least three groups of 10 to 20 persons in each of your target audience segments and have them complete the survey questionnaire. Then tabulate the results, and you should have a clear picture of (a) what these persons think of the problem, (b) what interests and inspires them, and (c) what media they use.

On the basis of the survey information, you may now develop your plan for some follow-up *focus groups*. Develop a list of questions that help to explain further *why* persons in this audience segment feel the way they do about the problem, why they enjoy certain interests (along with where they enjoy them and with whom), and why they use the media. Conduct the focus groups with the same groups who completed the survey and audiotape their comments. Transcribe these comments into a written summary.

Compile results of the survey and the summary of comments from the focus groups into a "writer's notebook," which also will include information about

Listed below are activities that you might like to do in your spare time. Check a box next to each activity to tell whether you like to do it a lot, a little, or not at all.

I like to do it	A lot	A little	Not at all
Playing team sports	☐	☐	☐
Going to a party with friends	☐	☐	☐
Swimming	☐	☐	☐

etc.

We all have wishes that we could be a little different than we are. Check the box next to each wish listed below to say whether you wish it a lot, a little, or not at all.

I wish I could be...	I wish it	A lot	A little	Not at all
A better athlete		☐	☐	☐
More popular with boys		☐	☐	☐
Old enough to be on my own		☐	☐	☐

etc.

Now I'd like to ask you about your <u>favorites.</u> What is your favorite...

Movie: _____

Music performer (or group): _____

etc.

Figure 2.2. Sample Survey Questionnaire

message objectives and campaign strategies described earlier. Separate the results for each audience segment, showing the media preferences, leisure activities, wishes, opinions about smoking, and other information in separate sections of the notebook for each group. With this information, writers at the advertising agencies or production companies can develop concepts that clearly address the needs and interests of each segment. This notebook will give you one place to put highly useful information about each of your targeted audience segments, helping you create messages that will reach them, interest them, and should also be effective.

STEP 2: MESSAGE DEVELOPMENT
POOLING AND WAREHOUSING MESSAGES

Second, it is necessary to systematically pool and warehouse promising activities for new uses. The theory of program mediation developed in the prior step leads one to search for promising activities or activity ideas to test. One should be able to go through a library of activities or activity ideas and pull out useful information. However, proprietary interests need to be addressed and potential conflicts overcome.

In this step, we develop a set of activities in the form of media messages, based on the educational objectives, communication strategies, and diagnostic research completed in Step 1. This pool of messages should be highly focused on our objectives while exploring a wide range of needs and interests of our target group. At this step, messages produced by other programs also could be included in the warehousing process for later testing to see if they appear to address similar educational objectives and the needs and interests of the target group. Although the use of existing fully produced messages can be cost saving, one would require permission from the organizations that produced them. The process for developing new messages involves (a) creating message concepts, (b) selecting message concepts, and (c) producing preliminary messages.

Creating Message Concepts. In our example of reaching young people with an effective smoking prevention campaign, we would begin by contracting with ad agencies or production companies to develop several message concepts. These should be written in simple paragraph or script form so that a range of ideas can be created at first and then can be narrowed down to a few "winners" after being thoroughly considered. Creative people at advertising agencies or media production companies who write copy for television or radio commercials often can brainstorm many ideas into brief concepts that can be considered for development into separate 30-second television or 60-second radio messages. By engaging at least two or three advertising agencies or production companies, it is possible to gather in as many as 20 or 30 new concepts.

Selecting Message Concepts. When concepts are received, the health educator panel should be convened by the public health organization. Working with the panel, campaign organizers can review each new message concept for its potential impact on the target group. They should judge how well each message addresses educational objectives, needs, and interests of each audience segment and is consistent with communication strategies. Concepts that pass this test would then be chosen for the next stage of production.

Producing Preliminary Messages. Now it is time to produce the messages in a preliminary form so that they can be presented to representatives of the targeted audience segment. For television, they could be videotaped and rough-edited or presented as a storyboard with sound; radio could be loosely edited, but with some sound effects and music; and print materials could be done as storyboards. All messages would be prepared for testing in the next step.

STEP 3: MESSAGE TESTING—SCREENING AMONG PROMISING ACTIVITIES

Third, there is a need to systematize a set of perceived efficacy studies that can screen among promising activity ideas gathered in the last step for additional program development work. Numerous ideas gathered during the previous step should be able to be contrasted using methods that are relatively time-saving and cost-effective. This could be viewed as a program activity screening step. Activities may be verbal or written in administration or completion.

When the pool of messages (or activities) is prepared in preliminary form, assemble them on separate cassettes or storyboards for presentation to at least three groups of persons in each of the targeted audience segments. Prepare a rating form that includes the message objectives and a measure of how much the person likes each message (see Figure 2.3).

Conducting the Message Test. Before presenting a message, tell the participants to check each of the ideas (reflecting the objectives) that they see portrayed in the message; they may check none or more than one of these ideas. Then ask them to use a 0 to 100 scale to say how much they like the message. Do this for each message, and present the messages in a different random order for each group. Also, request the age and gender of participants for help in fine-tuning message delivery (see Step 5). We have found that two indicators—(a) whether the messages are communicating the ideas you intend and (b) how much the persons in the target segment like the messages—are the best way to predict whether the message will be effective.

Discussing the Messages. After presenting all the messages, it is a good time to review those that were most highly rated to see how they can be improved. Get a show of hands on messages receiving a "75 or above" on the 0 to 100 liking scale. These messages are the most likely to be included in your campaign. Then

Message Number	This message shows that...				HOW MUCH I LIKE THIS MESSAGE (0-100)
	It helps to not smoke	Smoking causes problems	Most kids don't smoke	How to refuse a cigarette	
1					
2					
3					
4 etc.					

Rating scale: 0 10 20 30 40 50 60 70 80 90 100
Don't like it at all   Like it a lot

Age _____

Gender: ___F
___M

Figure 2.3. Sample Rating Form

tape-record comments on what participants liked about the messages, what they did not like, and how they can be improved.

STEP 4: DETERMINING WORKABILITY OF PROGRAM COMPONENTS AND SELECTING MESSAGES FOR FINAL PRODUCTION

Fourth, there is a need to systematize a set of immediate-impact studies that can provide a means of determining workability of individual program components. Possibly, the top half of the most favorably rated activities from the previous step would be retained for this one. Please recall that Step 3 pertains to judgments regarding program ideas or message concepts that are presented in a compact, abridged, preliminary form. Many activity ideas are screened. Subjects rate in part how well they perceive the activity would be received if it were actually carried out. In Step 4, subjects actually experience and evaluate complete media messages.

From the message-testing step, make a summary of the numerical ratings and focus group comments. Try to select a mix of highly rated messages that address a balanced set of objectives, so that all of the objectives can be effectively communicated in your campaign. If you would like a broader perspective to make this selection, you may want to convene your group of professionals who aided in the concept selection (Step 2). Then, review the focus group comments and convey them to producers so that they can use these ideas in fine-tuning the messages during final production.

Some or many messages may be changed considerably. You would now want to test them again after the next or final production with groups of persons from the target audience segment to be sure they have the intended impact. Here, you would present each complete media message component (no longer using storyboards) and measure subjects on immediate impact. You should have your campaign messages completed with the confidence that they are communicating the right ideas to the right people and that the intended audience segment will like them and be likely to attend to them.

STEP 5: PROGRAM CONSTRUCTION—ORGANIZING MESSAGES INTO A CAMPAIGN

Fifth, systematize program construction and pilot testing of a complete program. Perhaps 50% of activities from the previous step are retained for this step. This important step in communicating with your targeted audience segment will be greatly aided by two kinds of information that you will already have gathered in Steps 1 through 4 of the campaign creation process. To use these data, someone in your organization working with a professional who understands message placement in the media can make well-informed decisions on reaching your targeted audience segment most efficiently with enough frequency of message exposure to have an impact.

Using this process, you can launch the first wave of your campaign as a kind of pilot test. Then, based on feedback gathered in Step 6, you can evaluate how well your campaign is being communicated and make changes that will improve its performance. The process for implementing the campaign involves (a) selecting the media, (b) delivering the messages, and (c) determining the campaign intensity and duration.

Selecting the Media. From the diagnostic survey in Step 1, you will have a list of media used by each target audience segment, including the names of television programs in which to place messages, the names of radio stations and times when persons in each segment are listening, and the names of newspapers or other media being used.

Delivering the Messages. From Step 3, you will know which messages appeal most to which audience segment defined by age and gender. Now it is simply a matter of scheduling the messages appealing to each segment in the media during television programs or times when you know these persons are using the media. This can be done either most effectively and, perhaps at greater expense, by using paid advertising, or with less precision by using public service advertising. It always a good idea, however, to use all the information you have on hand about the target audience segment to reach them with messages that you know will interest them and communicate the campaign objectives to them.

Campaign Intensity and Duration. To reach your targeted audience segments, you should plan campaigns for sufficient exposure of messages. Using data from audience research, it is possible to estimate how often persons in the target segments will actually perceive that they have been exposed to each message. A person should see a message at least five times to remember seeing it three times, which most advertising texts suggest is sufficient. If your audience research indicates that about 50% of persons in the targeted segment see a television program, listen to a radio station, or read a newspaper on a given day, we suggest that you double the minimum number of exposures (5) and make sure that the message is run 10 times. If only 30% of the audience uses a medium at a given time, you may need to run 15 exposures. Thinking about the weekly routines of your target segments (which you can explore in focus groups) may take several weeks to space out the exposures for best impact. Many campaigns run for about 2 or 3 months to provide the best visibility so that persons in the target segments will be exposed to enough repetitions of each message to get an impact.

STEP 6: USING AUDIENCE FEEDBACK FOR CAMPAIGN PLANNING—REFINING POSTTREATMENT ACTIVITY SET MEASURES

The final step is to refine a set of immediate posttreatment activity set measures that predict longer-term outcomes. Mediation and meta-analytic work are promising directions to identify important mediators and moderators. To ensure that the messages are of interest to your audience segments and that the campaign is broadcast with sufficient intensity, we suggest that you build into your plans a yearly monitoring survey to see how well your messages are received.

There are two important moderator measures. Find out first if persons in the target audience segment have received your messages by giving them a brief description of each message and asking if they have seen or heard it "a lot," "once or twice," or "never." Second, if the person in the target audience has seen or heard it, ask whether the respondent liked the message "a lot," "a little," or "not at all." Develop some new messages each year, using the process I reviewed earlier, and replace messages that are no longer liked by your target audience segment to keep your campaign fresh and current.

Although it is difficult for a local health department to measure longer-term outcomes such as changes in behavior with the resources at hand, you can measure whether the campaign is having the kind of impact on your target audience that is likely to change behavior. Previous research has indicated that if the campaign messages have been designed to address educational objectives, and if they have good recognition and appeal and have been aired over several years, they are likely to have some positive effect on behavior (e.g., prevent some youth from smoking).

▶ CONCLUSIONS

If your survey indicates that you have good recognition and appeal for the campaign messages but you are unable to show behavior change, even after extended periods of campaign implementation, it is possible that the mediators that you are using—specifically, the educational objectives—may not be appropriate. If these mediators had been based on theory as recommended, it may be more likely that the execution of the campaign could be ineffective. However, it also is possible that conditions had changed with regard to the problem (e.g., youth smoking rates affected by changes in tobacco company advertising), and new mediators should be identified to address the problem. By keeping up to date with recent theoretical developments in your field (e.g., tobacco control strategies), you may identify more effective objectives and strategies to guide your campaign.

▶ REFERENCES

BANDURA, A. (1977). *Social learning theory.* Englewood Cliffs, NJ: Prentice Hall.
DEJONG, W., & WINSTON, J. A. (1990, Summer). The use of mass media in substance abuse prevention. *Health Affairs,* pp. 30-46.

FLAY, B. R. (1981). On improving the chances of mass media health promotion programs causing meaningful changes in behavior. In M. Meyer (Ed.), *Health education by television and radio* (pp. 56-91). Munich, Germany: Saur.

FLAY, B. R., DiTECCO, D., & SCHLEGEL, R. P. (1980). Mass media in health promotion: An analysis using an extended information-processing model. *Health Education Quarterly, 7,* 127-147.

FLYNN, B. S., WORDEN, J. K., SECKER-WALKER, R. H., BADGER, G. J., GELLER, B. M., & COSTANZA, M. C. (1992). Prevention of cigarette smoking through mass media intervention and school programs. *American Journal of Public Health, 82,* 827-834.

WORDEN, J. K., FLYNN, B. S., GELLER, B. M., CHEN, M., SHELTON, L. G., SECKER-WALKER, H. R., SOLOMON, D. S., SOLOMON, L. J., COUCHEY, S., & COSTANZA, M. C. (1988). Development of a smoking prevention mass media program using diagnostic and formative research. *Preventive Medicine, 17,* 531-558.

WORDEN, J. K., FLYNN, B. S., SOLOMON, L. J., SECKER-WALKER, R. H., BADGER, G. J., & CARPENTER, J. F. (1996). Using mass media to prevent cigarette smoking among adolescent girls. *Health Education Quarterly, 23,* 453-468.

CHAPTER 3

Identifying and Overcoming Barriers to Empirically Based Health Behavior Program Planning

Rick Petosa

> *"If you don't keep score, it is only practice."*
> —Vince Lombardi, former coach, Green Bay Packers

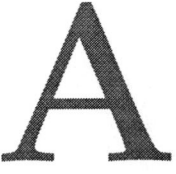pplying Coach Lombardi's principle to the evaluation of health behavior programs would likely be a revealing and unpleasant endeavor. Most health behavior interventions

1. focus on health information dissemination,
2. are designed without assessing the educational needs of the target audience,
3. are designed without benefit of behavioral theories,

4. are designed without being informed by the health behavior research literature,
5. are not field tested before being delivered,
6. are delivered by staff with little to no formal training in health behavior change,
7. are not evaluated for participant learning,
8. are not evaluated for changes in health behaviors, and
9. are not evaluated for changes in health status.

I would venture to infer from Coach Lombardi's quote that the current status of health behavior interventions is "practice" because no one seems to be "keeping score." Furthermore, if we do not make a point of regularly "keeping score," health behavior programs will never be ready for big-league, prime-time action. Which brings us squarely to the purpose of this book—the active promotion of a program-planning model that is grounded in empirical research methods. The empirical approach to health program development "keeps score" or evaluates the effects of health behavior programs at multiple points during the development process. As introduced in Chapter 1 of this book, a sequential, empirically based program development approach permits a solidly linked means of building a program. This approach provides a variety of immediate tangible benefits. First, each element of the intervention is immediately screened and judged by a team of professionals for practicality, theoretical soundness, and a host of concerns to both practitioners and researchers. Also, each element of the proposed intervention is field tested, which allows for an empirical test of the acceptability of program elements to the target audience and implementer-practitioners. Most important, each program element can be tested for its precise, immediate impact on the target audience. This process allows for the continuous refinement of a program. If this empirical approach were used consistently, the maximum feasible effectiveness of health behavior programs could be estimated for different populations, settings, and resource allocations. Thus, this approach could help establish standards of program excellence in a variety of realistic circumstances.

Given the wealth of advantages of empirical program development methods, you would assume rapid and widespread adoption. However, the benefits of this model do not come without costs. With the advantages come substantial changes in the way programs and professionals would operate. The purpose of this chapter is to identify barriers to empirical program development models and suggest approaches to overcoming these obstacles. Ultimately, the chapter attempts to lay a foundation for the widespread adoption of empirical program development methods.

► HEALTH PROMOTION: PROMISE AND UNDOCUMENTED PERFORMANCE

The public health rationale for health behavior change programs remains sound (McGinnis & Foege, 1993; U.S. Department of Health, Education, and Welfare, 1979). If substantial proportions of target populations would alter lifestyle practices, significant reductions in premature death and disease would follow (Belloc & Breslow, 1972; Knowles, 1977; U.S. Department of Health and Human Services [DHHS], 1996). Unfortunately, considerable resource investments in a few "model" health promotion programs typically have produced modest or inconclusive effects on health practices and health status. To make matters worse, most programs are not systematically evaluated; ergo, the question of impact remains unanswered. It is difficult to refer to an established track record of effective practices in health behavior change programming.

Kreuter and Green (1978) have proposed the "poverty cycle of health education" (see Figure 3.1) to illustrate this professional and social transaction. The cycle illustrates how health programs can be caught in a self-perpetuating cycle of low public support coupled with poor-quality, low-impact programs. Inadequate budgets create a context in which staff implement underdeveloped or "canned" programs of questionable quality. Such programs generally produce modest, diffuse, or no identifiable impact on the target population. Inadequate resources also are often cited as a primary reason for having little to no evaluation or program effects. In such cases, professionals or the public have no evidence on which to make informed decisions about program usefulness. In the absence of evidence, policymakers and the public tend to judge such efforts as an investment of dubious value and of low priority. These judgments lead back to inadequate resource support. The cycle is self-perpetuating and would take concerted efforts on many fronts to break.

This book takes the position that practicing professionals share primary responsibility for breaking this frustrating cycle. A practical and effective place to begin is with the adoption of empirically based, systematic program-planning models. Empirical program development models are systematically evaluated at several stages of development and implementation. This process lays the foundation for carefully matching program inputs with target population effects. Over time, this process would link program intensity with variable levels of program impact. These results would directly contribute to breaking the poverty cycle, thereby increasing the ability of health behavior programs to promote the public health.

Although there are potential benefits to empirically based program-planning models, there also are imposing obstacles as well. This chapter will review and

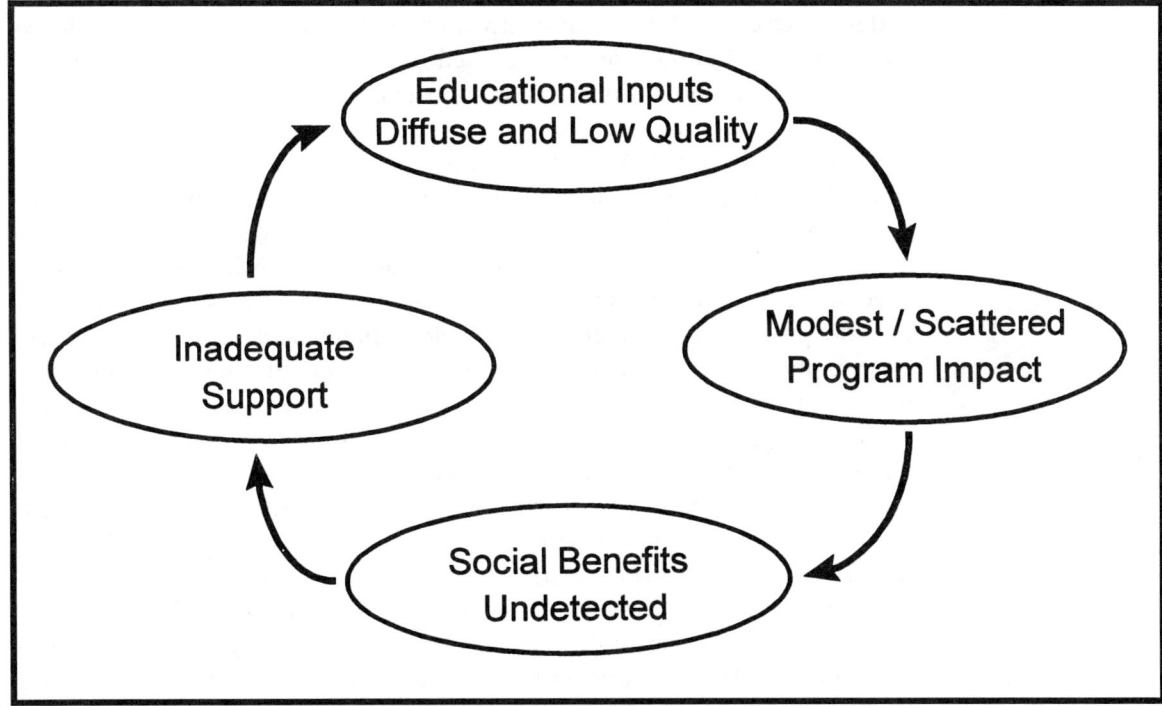

Figure 3.1. Poverty Cycle of Health Education

analyze many of the barriers likely to be faced in using empirically based program-planning models. Once barriers are identified, strategies for overcoming these barriers are discussed. Empirically based health program planning could contribute to breaking the poverty cycle of health promotion as the public becomes convinced that health promotion programs can make a substantial contribution to public health.

HEALTH BEHAVIOR PROGRAM PLANNING: A SYNTHESIS

Health behavior programs can be seen as a collection of planned activities designed to improve health by altering practices of individuals or communities (i.e., systems of interacting individuals). The formality of the program-planning process can range from decisions made by an individual health behavior professional based on personal preferences to a team-based, systematic planning process that carefully assesses the health educational needs of target populations and tailors interventions to ensure high levels of community participation. Time and resource constraints create an environment in which informal methods are more common. But these less formal methods also may be overused whenever practitioners have not been trained in formal needs assessment procedures and community organization strategies.

Green and Kreuter (1991, p. 25) have observed steady progress in moving health behavior program-planning decisions from ones of "expert opinion" to "expert processes." In this analysis, "expert opinion" relies heavily on the observations and experiences of one professional. The individual expert tends to have preferred approaches to programming. Practicing professionals in health behavior program planning come from a wide range of fields (e.g., health science, community organization, education, social work, communications, administration/management, education, or public health). The expert likely has a vested interest in using his or her a priori preferred approaches. Also, the expert may take a rather applied stance toward health programming and focus on how the program is to be implemented rather than why the program should be implemented.

In contrast, expert processes refer to program decision making based on systematic models that can be empirically tested. This approach fosters a climate of collaboration among a variety of disciplines, including public health, health behavior, education, behavioral research, and communications, among others. Expert processes start with carefully targeted outcomes. A systematic analysis seeks to identify modifiable factors that can be demonstrated to produce desired health outcomes. A team-based, expert-processes approach to health behavior program planning is considered an evolutionary improvement in the maturation of the field. It is a rigorous approach that will yield interventions that are carefully tailored to the needs of the target audience and professional staff, and these interventions are grounded in behavioral theory and research. This process should produce interventions that are practical, acceptable, and maintainable. Clearly, these interventions should be more effective in producing changes in health behavior. The empirically based model proposed in this book is an explicit example of using an expert process applied to health behavior program planning.

Figure 3.2 presents a diagram of the six-step program-planning model first described in Chapter 1 of this handbook. This model is a synthesis of the Worden, Green, and Sussman health behavior planning models.

The steps of program planning outlined earlier provide for a systematic approach to the development of effective programs. Used consistently across time, this approach would yield a cumulative body of knowledge about effective approaches to health behavior promotion. Although the potential payoffs are considerable, there are demands created by this planning model. Considerable human and material resources would need to be invested consistently, over time, to support the empirical approach to program development.

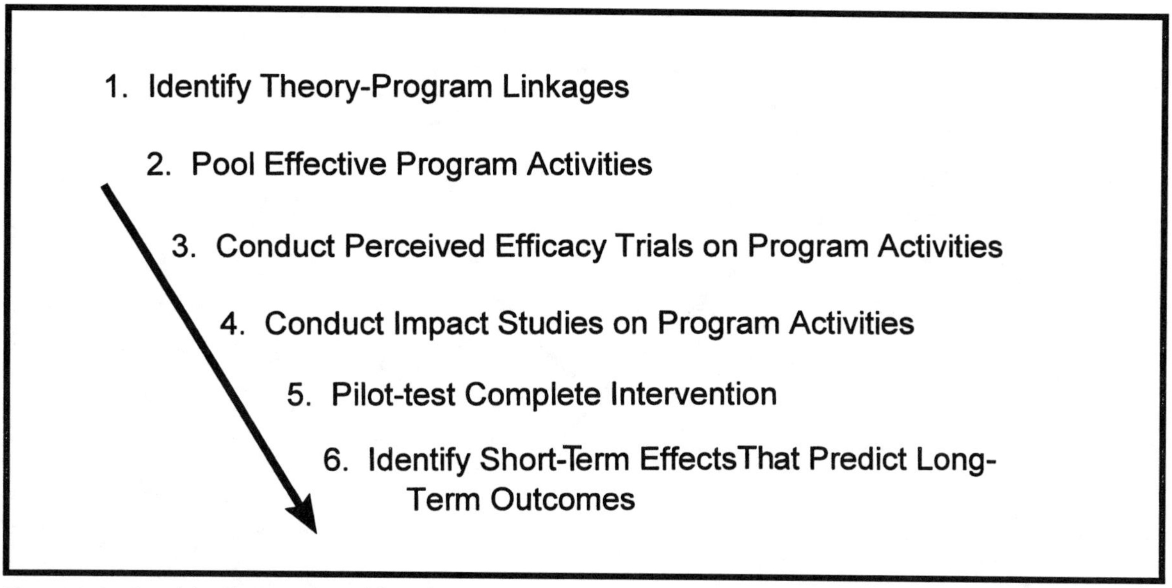

1. Identify Theory-Program Linkages
2. Pool Effective Program Activities
3. Conduct Perceived Efficacy Trials on Program Activities
4. Conduct Impact Studies on Program Activities
5. Pilot-test Complete Intervention
6. Identify Short-Term Effects That Predict Long-Term Outcomes

Figure 3.2. Empirically Based Health Behavior Program Planning

THE INTERPLAY OF PERCEIVED PROGRAM FEASIBILITY AND PERCEIVED PROGRAM EFFECTIVENESS

In general, participants in health behavior program selection and implementation must perceive a program they will use as feasible and efficient. They must believe that the program can be implemented with available resources. At the same time, participants also must perceive the program as effective and worthwhile. They must believe that the program targets valued outcomes and is likely to achieve these outcomes. Unfortunately, sometimes feasibility and effectiveness are treated as interchangeable concepts. Perceptions of measures of program effectiveness have ranged from simple notions of participation to rigorous standards of performance. For some, head counts of the number of people who participate in a program are a necessary and sufficient precondition for program impact (whereas they are just a measure of feasibility). Alternatively, consumer satisfaction models emphasize participants' perceptions of the program as a measure of effectiveness. Still others measure program effectiveness by the degree of change in precursors to health behavior (knowledge, motivation, skills), health behavior change, or measurable changes in health status. Certainly, the missions, training regimens, and compensation of professionals will heavily influence their emphasis on these different perspectives. Empirically based program development models emphasize impact on health behavior by increasing

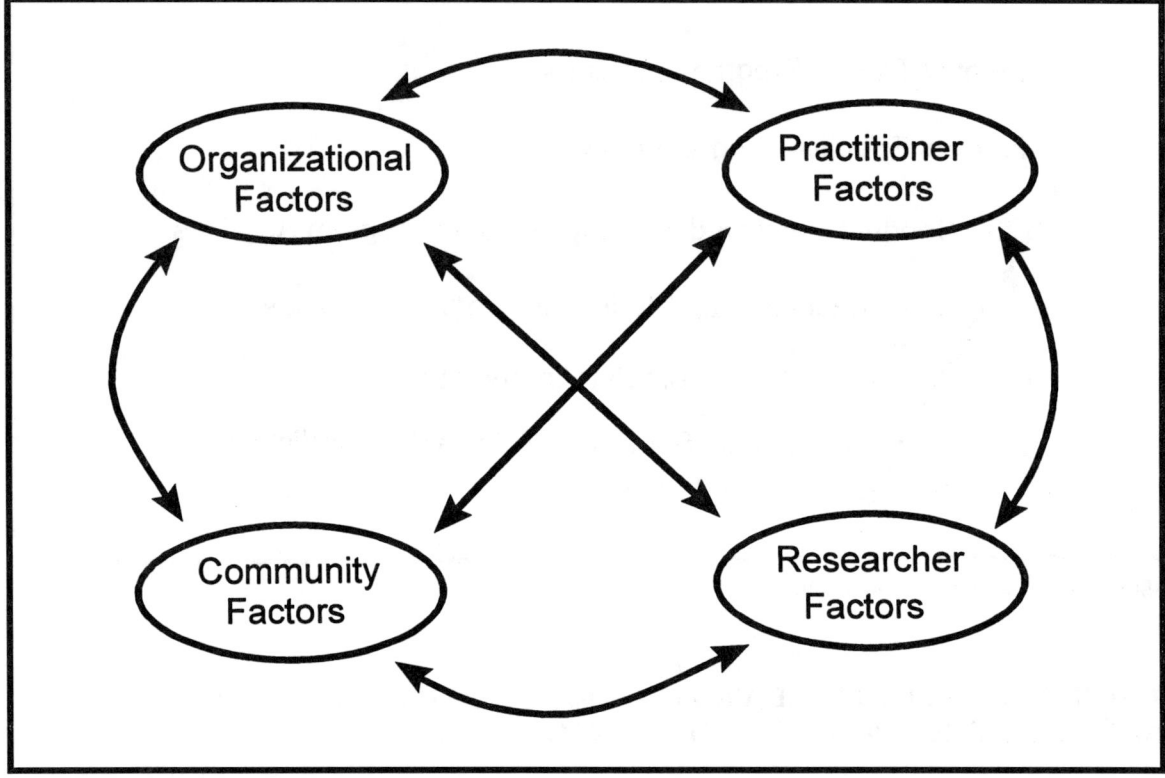

Figure 3.3. Ecology of Health Behavior Programs

program-planning sensitivity to the immediate effects of program activities on precursors of health behavior change.

▶ BARRIERS TO EMPIRICALLY BASED HEALTH BEHAVIOR PROGRAM DEVELOPMENT

An ecological model (see Figure 3.3) is proposed for the analysis of factors that may serve as barriers to empirically based health behavior program development. Each of the four factors represents the interests of groups whose participation is foundational to the success of health behavior programs. Each of these factors can provide resources and impose constraints on each of the other three factors. This continuous process of reciprocal influence among the four factors shapes the nature of the health behavior program that is ultimately designed and delivered. Together, these factors create a context in which health behavior programs evolve and improve or stagnate and die. What follows is a description of each of these factors and identification of potential factor-related barriers to empirically based health behavior program development.

ORGANIZATIONAL FACTORS

Stated broadly, an organization is a functional structure for generating and coordinating the resources necessary to pursue valued goals. Most health behavior programs are designed and delivered in existent organizations in the community (e.g., churches, schools, voluntary agencies, worksites, public health departments, and health care settings). Although each of these organizations exists to serve the public, each setting has a variety of purposes. The primary purpose of health care settings is the diagnosis and treatment of disease. The primary purpose of a worksite is to efficiently provide valued goods or services to consumers. The primary purpose of schools is to educate students in academic disciplines. Please note that each of these health behavior program settings has a primary purpose other than health behavior change. Although the goals of each setting are consistent with health promotion, it remains a **secondary purpose.** In addition, many other support services (e.g., employee assistance programs, health care insurance) also compete for the resources of the organization. Furthermore, organizations have finite resources, and service constituencies possess the potential for infinite demands. It follows that each organization must be mindful of the amount of resources that are devoted to a host of secondary purposes. As a consequence, many organizations find it preferable to adopt existing health behavior canned programs that seem suitable rather than invest the time and money necessary to carefully develop and test a program tailored to their site. How this organizational barrier operates is illustrated by an example derived from experience with school settings. Most schoolteachers' time is consumed by providing direct instruction and management of classroom operations. Program development, evaluation, and research are not a primary mission of schools involved in K-12 grade instruction. It is common to find school staff wary of development and research projects that divert scarce resources away from direct instruction. Many schools feel overwhelmed by requests from outside agencies to conduct research in their classrooms. In response, some schools now employ research review committees to screen projects proposed. A major consideration used by such committees is the amount of classroom instruction time "lost" to the proposed project. The empirically based health behavior program process is a labor-intensive approach that requires considerable investment of staff time. Many teachers would consider reviewing existing curricula materials a more efficient use of time. Researchers often hear teachers remark, "We really aren't interested in research. Tell us what works, and if it makes sense to us, we may adopt it."

To further complicate matters, some innovative health behavior programs seek to go beyond instruction, incorporating environmental or policy-based approaches that further strain the ability of organizations to fully participate. The competition between the primary purposes of these health settings and health behavior programs' secondary status provides a major influence on the organization's support for and ability to deliver health behavior programs.

A key barrier to empirical program development for many organizations would be the **disruption** of established decision-making procedures. Organizations have established formal and informal methods of making decisions regarding health programs and resources to support these programs. Usually, this decision making is a balance between administration, practitioners, and community members. The empirical program development process would likely be perceived as imposing researchers into the decision-making process. Researchers could claim that the data strongly suggest certain changes in health programs. This source of feedback could be seen as disruptive or threatening.

Also included as organizational factors are a host of **funding agencies,** which are involved in established decision making regarding provision of funds. Federal and state governments, foundations, and voluntary agencies serve as examples. Each of these organizations provides resources to support health behavior programs. But each of these organizations has established expectations regarding appropriate use of funds. When funding agencies make decisions regarding health behavior program service, there is a tendency to focus on reaching as many individuals in the target audience as possible. Constraints may be placed on the amount of funds that can be used for developmental work and research evaluation.

There also are **resource problems** (staff, time, money, facilities), which may deter using an empirically based health behavior program development process. In health promotion settings, staff positions generally focus on program delivery. Precious little, if any, staff time is devoted to intervention development. Also, shortages in funds result in fewer staff to take on more tasks than in the past. Other cost considerations in empirical program development pertain to instrument development, data collection, survey coding, data entry, and data analysis. Health promotion organizations may not be equipped for all these tasks. Time, cost, and training issues may limit scope of use. One could reason that the costs of using a careful development process up front would be much less than would be the costs involved in implementing an unsuccessful program. Yet the social costs of ineffective health behavior prevention programs are often hidden by not documenting failure to find immediate or delayed effects or considerable time lags between health behavior changes and changes in health status.

COMMUNITY FACTORS

A community is a collection of people identified by mutually held concerns for the development and well-being of their group (e.g., a neighborhood, a geographic region, or a collection of people who share a common identity [gay community, feminist community, Hispanic community]). Commonly, a city or town is diverse, comprising many different communities. These diverse audiences can shape health behavior programs. Communities have a vested interest in solving health problems, but they also must address a wide range of other social problems, which all compete for a fixed amount of resources. Ultimately, community members must impose constraints on the time, money, and other resources available to any particular program. In this context, it is often difficult to garner adequate resources for empirically based program development models. Political forces may impose resource limits that make evaluation efforts impractical.

Within a community, at least four groups have direct relevance to the consideration of health behavior program development. First, there is the **general citizenry,** who looks at health programming with the eyes of the taxpaying observer. The general citizenry engages in a political discourse about the general purposes and funding levels for health behavior programs. Occasionally, health behavior programs are controversial (e.g., safer-sex programs to prevent HIV in the schools, needle exchange programs, birth control programs). Citizens will engage in a political dialogue about values and the relative worth of engaging in a variety of publicly supported programs. This dialogue ultimately shapes the nature and degree of resource support for a health behavior program (Petosa, 1988).

Special interest groups also may have a direct influence on health behavior programs. Tobacco companies, right-to-life groups, and religious organizations are examples. The general principle of "maximum feasible participation" generally encourages health organizations to openly invite citizens and special-interest groups to participate in public dialogue about the nature and purposes of health behavior programs. It is generally assumed that this input increases public commitment and participation in health programs (Green & Kreuter, 1991). Yet, at the same time, diverse special interests may not agree on a variety of issues that can affect program planning, such as the goals, methods, and target audiences of a program. Generally, special-interest groups in the community will attempt to use political processes to influence program development decisions. The empirical approach could be viewed as undermining the power of political influence and therefore be resisted by such groups.

Another potential source of influence in the community are **private-sector vendors of health behavior program materials.** For example, textbook, multimedia, and health program vendors can exert a powerful influence over programmatic decision making. These vendors preside over a multimillion-dollar industry that produces educational materials with generally high production values and relatively low cost. Rarely are the programs sold by vendors systematically evaluated (although times are changing for some companies with the advent of small-business innovative research programs). Yet these vendors exert considerable influence by providing materials that shape health behavior interventions. This industry provides instructional materials that are easy to use and require small investments of staff time. Clearly, the goal of the textbook or health behavior program industry is to make money by selling materials. To make money, this industry assumes that it must develop products of mass appeal and acceptability. This perspective often leads to the creation and implementation of materials that are inherently conservative. As a consequence, the instructional materials are characterized by traditional methods of instruction, are knowledge based, and avoid controversial topics. It is sobering to remember that behavioral objectives, many health topics, and even decision making may be perceived as controversial in many communities. The concern over controversial topics is heightened when the target audience is composed of minors. The availability of these educational materials can contribute to an environment in which there is little support for empirical program development methods. Many stakeholders could argue that program development steps are unnecessary and expensive when compared to existing programs commercially available.

A fourth party is the **target population** of any health behavior program. The individuals who comprise any target population have preexisting educational and health needs that must be considered. They will possess their own motivations for participation or nonparticipation in health behavior programs. Their willingness to participate in evaluation procedures or program development processes may serve as a limiting factor. A key issue for many consumers is the time commitment involved in participation. Clearly, there are trade-offs between program expediency and program effectiveness (Green, 1986; Green, Wilson, & Lovato, 1986). Professionals involved in health behavior program development need to be cognizant of the amount of discretionary time members of the target population are willing to invest in health behavior programs.

PRACTITIONER FACTORS

The practitioner factor comprises the health behavior program service providers. Professionals from many allied health disciplines deliver health behavior programs (e.g., health educators, nurse educators, exercise physiologists, physicians, health psychologists, social workers, and public health workers). The training of these professionals is diverse. There are few models or theories shared among these professional groups. Many do not receive formal training in health behavior program planning. Only a small percentage of these practitioners receive training in health behavior theory, and an even smaller number receive training in behavioral and educational research methods necessary to empirically validate the effectiveness of health behavior programs. Practitioners may have experiences with characteristics of programs that work and do not work. As a consequence, practitioners develop **implicit heuristics** for making judgments. Often, judgments regarding effectiveness and efficiency of programming are based on impressions of cursory reviews of program materials. Although many of these judgments have sound practical value, they can be inherently conservative and serve as a barrier to program innovation.

It is an educational truism that "educators teach as they were taught." Most health promotion specialists have cultivated areas of content expertise. Based on training and experience, they have preferred methods of instruction. As a consequence, health behavior staff members tend to focus on **didactic methods of instruction** aimed at increasing consumer knowledge of selected health facts and concepts. This **focus on knowledge acquisition** is heightened by time pressures. Most health promotion settings have very limited time to provide direct programming to target populations. For example, a common practice among worksites is to provide health presentations during lunch breaks. Behavior change strategies generally are more time-consuming and labor intensive to instruct when compared to knowledge-based programs. Given these time constraints, it is no surprise that the health specialists place a major emphasis on knowledge acquisition rather than on risk behavior change. In other words, most teachers do not share a behavioral researcher's zeal for health behavior outcomes. The targeting of specific risk behaviors in a theory-driven, empirical program development process may not resonate with health promotion staff.

Practitioners are often more comfortable as **consumers of educational research** rather than as participants in the research process. This preference is in part explained by practitioner experiences in professional preparation programs. Generally, these programs focus on developing expertise in subject content and instructional methods. Only at the graduate level is this expertise refined, and introductory courses in research design and statistics are provided to help teachers develop basic skills to understand educational research conducted by others. The empirical program development model starts with the adoption of a theoretical model of behavior. Practitioners generally are not trained in the application or testing of behavior theories. Few educators have the training to effectively participate in empirical procedures (e.g., knowledge of sampling, data analysis, and interpretation). This lack of training may result in teachers who are uncomfortable with the theory-based or empirical approach. It is common to hear charges of "ivory tower" and "impractical" when research or theory is introduced as a central consideration in program development. Practitioners' lack of experience with scientific methods also may result in feelings of inferiority to any researchers involved in the project. These feelings are not conducive to teamwork or commitment to use an empirical program method. (On the other hand, current demands to use programs that work and availability of resources such as this one may be producing a new generation of research-educated practitioners.)

Practitioners tend to be **"people" people.** They are trained to focus attention on the social, educational, and emotional needs of their program participants. Practitioners develop relationships with participants based on mutual trust and respect. Philosophically, practitioners may express concerns about engaging in a program development process that targets specific health behaviors. Practitioners also are concerned that some participants may feel that prescribed behaviors are being imposed on them. More generally, practitioners are concerned that their program participants' needs may become subservient to the demands of the program-planning and research process. They often remark that this or that approach appears "aggressive" and "coercive." This sets the stage for controversy, politically a no-win situation for practitioners. These philosophical and political concerns are very real for most practitioners.

RESEARCHER-LEVEL BARRIERS

Although researchers are trained in a wide variety of health and research disciplines (e.g., health behavior, education, nursing, medicine, psychology, sociology, and public health), many do not receive formal training in health behavior program planning. There are **few theories commonly accepted** across these professional groups. As a consequence, common assumptions, approaches, and even language are lacking across disciplines. This can increase the communication gap between researchers and practitioners. Many researchers are found in academia, but others are employed in public agencies and private companies.

Most often, researchers' influence over health behavior program planning is indirect. Researchers contribute to the body of literature on health behavior that may inform professionals' program-planning decisions. Researchers also may publish programs that were developed during research projects. In some ideal circumstances, researchers are part of a team in which programs are developed with planned collaboration between administration, program delivery staff, and researchers. But most often, health behavior researchers have only **limited exposure to practitioners and target populations.** This lack of experience can dampen researchers' willingness to commit the time necessary for extended collaboration in the context of a team of health professionals.

Health behavior theory and research methods are wide-ranging and often do not match the immediate, practical needs of practitioners or organizations. For example, a health organization has a vested interest in serving maximum numbers of participants with a focus on consumer satisfaction. Researchers using empirical program development methods would push for resources to be shifted toward extensive program development procedures and evaluation. This shift would result in fewer consumers being served. Researchers are likely to argue that, in the long run, consumer satisfaction may be greater if more effective programs are developed using empirical methods. Administrators and practitioners, conversely, might argue that reaching the most people with programming as soon as possible is the better course of action. At the least, a clear difference in time perspective exists between the needs of researchers and of health organizations.

Researchers' technical expertise in research is often specialized and can contribute to communication gaps with community members, administrators, and practitioners. Researchers often have only limited contact with target populations and the day-to-day operations of health behavior programs. As a consequence, they often may not be fully aware of the practical constraints practitioners and target populations face when interacting with the health behavior program. Taken to extremes, researchers may develop interventions that are so demanding that only a small, select number of consumers would be willing to participate.

Most researchers are accustomed to theory-based research and have **generally focused their energies on summative evaluations.** The methods used in these types of studies tend toward rigorous, time-intensive strategies. Empirical program development methods would need to be less intrusive and focus on rapid-cycle feedback. To accomplish these goals, the evaluation methods would focus on process and may have to sacrifice some degree of rigor to enhance feasibility. Many researchers would be reluctant to make these adjustments for fear of compromising their research or their reputations.

OVERCOMING BARRIERS TO EMPIRICAL ◄ PROGRAM DEVELOPMENT

One of the greatest pains to human nature is the pain of a new idea. It . . . makes you think that, after all, your favorite notions may be wrong, your firmest beliefs ill-founded.

—Bagehot (1873, p. 169)

It is difficult to get a new idea or method adopted, even if it has verified advantages over current approaches. Generally, innovations such as empirical health behavior program development do not sell themselves. This is particularly true when both health organizations and health behavior professionals have established systems for the design and delivery of behavior programs. Diffusion of innovation research has examined factors that facilitate or inhibit the adoption of new ideas. Rogers (1983) has provided both a review of thousands of diffusion studies and a conceptual map for analyzing the processes of the diffusion of innovations. Rogers (1983) defines *diffusion* as "the process by which an innovation is communicated among members of a social system" (p. 5). An innovation is "an idea or practice which is perceived as new by individuals." This section will attempt to apply some of the principles of Rogers's work to a discussion of strategies for overcoming barriers to empirical program development. Although thousands of diffusion studies have been conducted, there is a distinct lack of research examining the diffusion of health behavior program methods. Therefore, the following discussion is a set of inferences based on diffusion of innovation principles. These inferences could best be viewed as a set of testable hypotheses.

According to Rogers (1983), a set of factors associated with the innovation ultimately influences the rate of adoption (i.e., practitioners deciding to implement a particular program). Rates of adoption can range from rapid (a matter of several years) to rejection (the failure of widespread adoption). It can be argued that most innovations in the health behavior arena are not ultimately adopted by most practitioners. Whether this is a comment on a low quality of innovations or a reflection of extraordinary resistance among health behavior professionals remains to be determined by historical analysis. In either case, it is clear that diffusion and adoption of empirical program development methods cannot be assumed. Actions must be taken to actively encourage widespread use. Rogers has identified the following characteristics of innovations that influence adoption rates: (a) relative advantage, (b) compatibility, (c) complexity, (d) trialability, and (e) observability. Each of these five factors will be applied to empirical program development. In addition, the importance of using (f) program champions (Goodman & Steckler, 1989) will be mentioned.

RELATIVE ADVANTAGE

Relative advantage is the degree to which an innovation is perceived as better than current approaches. The empirically based development process integrates program-planning and evaluation processes into an innovative approach to program development. Most practitioners, administrators, community members, and researchers are unlikely to be aware of or understand the need for empirical program development methods because they are novel. It is necessary for professionals who are responsible for health behavior program planning to believe that empirical methods will produce more effective programs. This is a group that generally possesses a considerable investment in professional training and works within organizations that use established procedures and may hold skeptical views regarding program development. It will take considerable effort to create both the evidence and the climate that would enable these professionals to acknowledge and promote the superiority of a more costly innovative method over less costly traditional methods of program planning.

The first step in the dissemination of the approach is the education of researchers and practitioners in the conceptual advantages of and skills necessary to use the approach. Researchers and practitioners will need to assume collaborative leadership roles. First, additional theoretical work needs to be done to develop a variety of specific models of empirically based program planning. These various models will require testing to determine the optimal combination of practicality and rigor necessary for adoption in a variety of community settings. A series of demonstration projects would reveal how to do the various models and the relative effectiveness of each.

Having established a record of tested methods, preservice and in-service training will create a cadre of professionals who are both motivated and skilled in the use of empirically based program planning. Trained practitioners and researchers will need to assume an advocacy role, educating decision makers and community members about the methods and advantages of empirical program development. Eventually, health behavior professionals would need to adopt empirically based approaches as a standard of practice that is incorporated into undergraduate and graduate professional preparation programs, in-service training for existing professionals, and credential-setting mechanisms.

COMPATIBILITY

Compatibility is the degree to which an innovation is perceived as being consistent with existing values, past experiences, and needs of potential adopters. Empirically based program methods integrate evaluation into program planning. In most situations, this involves adding evaluation steps where they did not exist before. There are considerable obstacles in helping practitioners perceive empirical program development as compatible with current practice. Evaluation can produce anxiety among practitioners, if not entire health organizations. Evaluation procedures can imply that individuals and programs are under the microscope. Criticism and the budget ax are seen as an inherent part of the anxiety of program evaluation. Because these beliefs have been supported by many practitioners' experiences, they will need to be directly addressed and successfully resolved. We are essentially asking practitioners to cooperate in increasing the role of evaluation from an occasional, summative experience to an ongoing, regular part of their daily practice. We are asking that evaluation procedures be integrated into program-planning processes, whereas in the past they did not exist. Important, substantive justifications will need to convince practitioners that adding evaluation to program development is worth the effort and resources. Practitioners would need to begin to accept an active role in the design and implementation of evaluation methods. The most important feature of this effort is to replace professionals' view of evaluation as summative and judgmental with evaluation as formative and developmental. Essentially, they would need to accept the idea that health behavior programs would be constantly evolving.

Researchers will need to develop formal, long-term relationships with health promotion organizations to create a climate in which mutual trust can develop. Building long-term relationships with health promotion settings is the best way to understand the specific forces that would support or inhibit the adoption of empirical program development. All involved parties (practitioners, administrators, and researchers) need to come to consensus regarding both the purposes and methods employed. If such collaboration were nurtured, practitioners would be likely to enthusiastically support this new, developmental role of evaluation in health behavior programs. Ideally, practitioners would feel empowered and actively engaged in a continuous, hands-on approach to program refinement. If formative evaluation methods are carefully implemented, practitioners are likely to adopt the role of "experimenting practitioners" (Green, 1986). This expanded role is likely to yield important advances in health behavior methods.

Considerable attention must be devoted to practical concerns and reservations of administrators and practitioners. The empirical approach is likely to take more of their time and resources than traditional methods, which must be planned for. Their informed participation is critical to the ultimate success of the empirical approach. Therefore, recruitment, role specification, and training of staff require careful attention (Petosa & Goodman, 1991). Specific training efforts for staff development would focus on imparting concepts underlying and means of implementing empirical program development methods. All staff should be encouraged to actively participate in a team approach that requires group problem solving regarding how to quickly adjust program and evaluation elements to meet organization goals. Organizations will need to build in reward systems for practitioners who actively engage in empirical program development processes.

COMPLEXITY

Complexity is the degree to which the innovation is perceived as difficult to understand and use. It will be clear to practitioners that empirical planning methods will add complexity to their jobs. Efforts will need to target organizational changes to mitigate practitioners' concerns about the potential intrusive or judgmental nature of empirical program methods. For example, many practitioners have concerns about who will see the formative evaluation results and how they will be used for making decisions. To build trust, administrators, researchers, and practitioners need to arrive at formal policies regarding the patterns of communication of evaluation results. Furthermore, clear limits need to be set on the uses of evaluation results. The purpose of formative evaluation is to refine and improve programs, not determine careers or pass final judgment on a program. Resolving these issues will substantially reduce practitioners' concerns and foster a supportive climate for program development.

Many health behavior practitioners do not have training in evaluation design, measurement, or statistical analysis. As a consequence, they may have concerns about their ability to understand the related evaluation procedures. This lack of training may make procedures appear overly complex and feed fears of the staff. Researchers will need to be particularly sensitive to this issue and make a concerted effort to clearly educate staff on the evaluation methods to be used. An immediate goal is to reduce fears and build trust among team members. Another goal is to build enthusiasm and active participation in the empirical program-planning process.

TRIALABILITY

Trialability is the degree to which an innovation may be implemented on a limited basis. If start-up costs are too high, or if adopters must accept the entire innovation without a trial period, there will be considerable resistance to acceptance. Similarly, if empirical program-planning methods can be broken down into incremental steps, it increases the likelihood that professionals will accept the idea of testing the new approach. Working in teams, researchers and practitioners will benefit from creatively integrating empirical methods. The six-step empirical program-planning chain model (see Figure 3.2) identifies numerous opportunities for evaluation of planning. Most agencies will want to gradually implement aspects of the model to allow for staff to gain experience before making a large commitment of resources.

To enhance trialability, health behavior researchers also may have to expand their conception of program evaluation. They will need to develop expertise in formative evaluation methods. Attention will need to be placed on precisely identifying recipient response to individual program activities and the interaction of these activities in the context of the entire intervention. Attention to segmenting the evaluation protocol also may be necessary. Rather than attempting to complete all levels of evaluation during one trial, evaluation questions would be distributed over a series of trials. A keen sensitivity as to how empirical program development can be conducted without disrupting day-to-day operations of health agencies also is critical. Unobtrusive measures, participant observation, and integration of measures into the educational program are a few ways in which researchers can collect evaluation data without consuming too much intervention time. The research team will need to adjust methods to reflect a more action-oriented, formative evaluation approach.

OBSERVABILITY

Observability is the degree to which the results of the innovation are visible to others. Visibility stimulates discussion and can foster positive feelings about the innovation. Observability provides distinct challenges for administrators, practitioners, and researchers. Empirical program development methods place health programs under the microscope as never before. It provides many opportunities for data collection and subsequent discussion of program impacts. But creating the opportunity for observation is not sufficient. An ongoing program of evaluation reviews and published progress reports will build the perception that "something good is happening." Administration should make an effort to recognize empirical methods and support these efforts as quality product-building processes.

PROGRAM CHAMPIONS

Research by Goodman and Steckler (1989) has established the importance of opinion leaders or program champions in establishing and institutionalizing health behavior programs within an agency. These individuals possess credibility and can influence the decision making of both superiors and subordinates in an organization. Program champions actively seek to motivate other professionals to support a new innovation. It follows that empirical program development would benefit from inclusion of a key member of a target health organization. This individual would be adequately trained to support the proposed innovation knowledgeably and enthusiastically. The goal is to develop a coalition within the organization. This team would work to ensure that adequate resources within the organization are devoted to empirical program development, ensuring successful implementation. This process, led by the program champion, is critical to institutionalizing a new program within an organization.

▶ CONCLUSIONS

Empirically based program development methods have the potential to improve health behavior change interventions. But there are substantial costs and barriers to this new approach. Clearly, empirically based methods are an investment in the long-term improvement of health programs. Systematic efforts would be required in support of this approach. A coordinated approach shared by administrators, researchers, practitioners, and community members is essential for health behavior program efforts but is especially important for empirically based approaches to program development.

The "ecology of health behavior programs model" (see Figure 3.3) illustrates some of the dynamic forces that can support or undermine efforts to develop interventions. These factors continually interact, creating a web of interdependent influence. Actors from each of the factors need to be engaged in a mutually constructive dialogue directed toward the delivery of the most effective health behavior programs for the least cost. Yet, individuals operating within each of these factors often have significantly different agendas and may actively seek to have an impact on the purposes or processes of health behavior programs. Professional responsibility lies with practitioners and researchers to engage organizations and communities in meaningful dialogue during program development. Ultimately, it is the responsibility of health behavior professionals to facilitate a collaborative process that produces effective, socially valued health behavior programs. Breaking the poverty cycle of health education (see Figure 3.1) requires skilled discipline on the part of practitioners and researchers to ensure that programs are of sufficient quality to promote health behavior change to reduce risk of disease. Only consistently effective programs will ultimately influence policy and garner enduring public support. To accomplish this task, one requires systematic planning and regular evaluation to verify that programs are effective. Certainly, once empirical program development becomes adopted by practitioners and researchers, the fruit gained will, itself, create an affinity for this approach. In Vince Lombardi's words, we need to quit practicing and get in the game.

REFERENCES ◄

BAGEHOT, W. 1873/1999. *Physics and politics.* Chicago: Ivan R. Dee.
BELLOC, N. B., & BRESLOW, L. (1972). Relationship of physical health status and health practices. *Preventive Medicine, 1,* 409-421.
GOODMAN, R., & STECKLER, A. (1989). A model for the institutionalization of health promotion programs. *Family and Community Health, 11,* 63-78.
GREEN, L. W. (1986). The theory of participation: A qualitative analysis of its expression in national and international policies. *Advances in Health Education and Promotion, 1,* 407-414.
GREEN, L. W., & KREUTER, M. W. (1991). *Health promotion planning: An educational and environmental approach* (2nd ed.). Mountain View, CA: Mayfield.
GREEN, L. W., WILSON, R., & LOVATO, C. (1986). What changes can health promotion achieve and how long do these change last? The tradeoffs between expediency and durability. *Preventive Medicine, 15,* 508-521.

KNOWLES, J. (1977). *Doing better and feeling worse: Health in the United States.* New York: Norton.

KREUTER, M. W., & GREEN, L. W. (1978). Evaluation of school health education: Identifying purpose, keeping perspective. *Journal of School Health, 48,* 228-235.

McGINNIS, J., & FOEGE, W. (1993). Actual causes of death in the United States. *Journal of the American Medical Association, 270,* 2207-2212.

PETOSA, R. (1988). Educational censorship in school health education. *Journal of School Health, 58,* 414-417.

PETOSA, R., & GOODMAN, B. (1991). Recruitment and retention of schools participating in school health research. *Journal of School Health, 61,* 426-429.

ROGERS, E. M. (1983). *Diffusion of innovations.* New York: Free Press.

U.S. DEPARTMENT OF HEALTH, EDUCATION, AND WELFARE (DHEW). (1979). *Healthy People: The surgeon general's report on health promotion and disease prevention.* Washington, DC: Author.

U.S. DEPARTMENT OF HEALTH AND HUMAN SERVICES (DHHS). (1995). *Healthy People 2000 review: 1994* (DHHS Pub. No. PHS 95-12561). Washington, DC: Government Printing Office.

CHAPTER 3

Commentary 1

M. Douglas Anglin
Brian Perrochet

Being an expert in something does not necessarily mean that you can impart that expertise to other people. Nor does empirically supported knowledge naturally translate into standard practice. Many of the issues responsible for these conundrums, which loom as major obstacles to the transfer of ideas and information from one person or source to some designated recipient, are operative in the larger context of interactions between systems, organizations, or schools of thought. These same issues confound interactions between the world of research and the world of practice. The chapter reviewed in this commentary discusses many communications-related obstacles as they compromise or obstruct rational planning of effective and efficient health promotion programs. In addition to recounting these obstacles, Petosa suggests some broad solutions that might bring the two worlds closer together.

We two reviewers share the notion that the primary issue, both the crux of the problem and the crux of the solution, is *communication,* a not-quite-dead horse that still warrants judicious beating. The communication that is *not* happening is the root cause of the insufficient use of empirical processes in health program development. Also to blame, however, is the communication, as well as the miscommunication, that *is* happening, which is often just as damaging to relationships between researchers and practitioners. Professionals in these separate camps usually have vastly differing perceptions of the needs of clients, communities, and systems and of the ways of creating and implementing effective programs that equitably reflect and efficiently serve those varied needs. When those differing perceptions are poorly represented in the process of defining goals or processes, the consensus-building action that *must* occur is rendered much more difficult because of the flawed communication.

In his chapter on barriers to rational program planning, Petosa describes the divisive dissonance between the two worlds, indicating that it derives from four factors, briefly summarized as the following:

• *Organizational factors.* Specific settings in which programs are devised and implemented have philosophic and logistic orientations that affect the manner of program planning and implementation. Furthermore, organizational resistance to change is intractable and pervasive at all levels.

• *Community factors.* Given the varied interest groups competing for services and resources, planning and action that reflect a "greater good" are compromised, diminishing broad-based support and a lack of faith in the "victor" left standing after the battle of influences has been fought.

• *Practitioner factors.* Often undertrained and underresourced but still required to serve the needs of clients with the inadequate materials and capabilities, practitioners typically resort to nonempirical "implicit heuristics" to guide and assess programs. In addition, time constraints on staff trying to provide optimum services lead to a low priority placed on any research activities that might be incorporated into a program, foiling attempts at generating personnel buy-in that would ensure proper implementation of evaluation measures. Moreover, source funders of services (whether government, foundations, or other) typically do not allocate resources for intensive, on-site, in-service training or permit billable release time for external training.

• *Researcher factors.* This is a very poignant aspect of the author's presentation on factors (and discussed at greater length below). Researchers work *indirectly*, rarely presenting the practitioner with findings, instead publishing articles and reports that the practitioner will probably never see and possibly never benefit from. The evaluation emphasis of research is a lower priority among practitioners, who are still busy doing the real work of providing services to deal with immediate problems. Practitioners' time perspectives are so different from those of researchers that the worlds the two groups inhabit seem to be using different calendars, again leading to incompatible points of view that result in poor communication. As noted for practitioners earlier, source funders of research typically do not allocate resources for the evaluator's time for preparing a presentation of findings in workshop-type settings that allow real learning to occur.

So, the barriers are fairly well understood, not terribly obscure, and yet largely recalcitrant to remediation. As noted in our introductory comments, people will be people; their attitudes, traits, and behaviors certainly influence their decision making on matters of personal concern, and the consequences of these traits at play in the process of deciding larger-scale issues can be ruinous to rational planning or policymaking.

Throughout the reading of this chapter, we were forced to confront the truths (some more implied than explicit) in several of the author's observations about the difficulty surrounding the communications between researcher and practitioner/service provider/program administrator. Petosa noted that several researcher-specific problems severely hindered this communication, which is vitally important in the process of achieving the goal of health planning that is based on rational and logical processes empirically developed and evaluated. Many of the examples of these research-based problems resonated with troubling alarm—he was talking about us, our colleagues, and our profession! As researchers in the conflict-ridden field of drug abuse treatment evaluation, our emphasis always has been on rigorous science that produces relevant findings, usable in the formulation of social policy, criminal justice policy, program planning, and program evaluation. To maintain relevance, we have consistently striven to collaborate with practitioners and service providers, attend conferences and seminars with agency representatives, and interact with community groups that represented the interests of the people who were to be served by the programs and interventions that we were studying or advising. Sadly, the reality of grant deadlines, project management, and administrative burden markedly reduces the time available to practice these convictions.

Even now, after doing our best to understand the perceptions and orientations of most entities involved in studying and serving the needy populations of drug users, we realize that we did not do enough. We believe that no researcher or research group, alone, could overcome the communication problems by unilaterally delving into the many issues pertinent to the nonresearch world. It takes two to tango, and the dance must involve equal partnerships of the researcher and the practitioner. And source funders in both services and research must recognize the need to pay for the music and for the dance lessons.

Petosa suggests as much in his call for greater collaborative roles for both researcher and practitioner. Early education is recommended to incorporate the ethos of research into clinical training, and similar exposure to clinical settings is advised for researchers in training. Specifically regarding evaluation, we need to overcome the natural anxiety that ensues in the practitioner (or anybody) about to be judged. Petosa urges that rather than the evaluation being regarded as an impending criticism, it should be characterized and understood as a regular, ongoing part of daily practice, following the conscientious incorporation of that evaluation into the planning process.

To buttress Petosa's suggestions for overcoming barriers that hinder rational planning, we offer several of our own by way of commentary on the chapter and on the issues raised in it.

- *Egos.* The discomfort that occasionally crops up in interactions between researchers and practitioners often stems from a suspicious defensiveness that must be allayed. The ivory tower is inhabited by many who assert an unwarranted elitism, as we all know, and we must end the presumption of superiority based on academic accomplishment. So, members of each camp must shed their preconceived notions about purported status and place derived from capital letters following a name.

- *Ability.* Awareness and capability must be increased in ongoing self-improvement mechanisms, formal as well as self-directed. Training is a crucial element in the advancement of rational planning—preplanning training to develop the capacities of the involved parties is being suggested and implemented in various fields (e.g., education systems). "Capacity building" of personnel in advance of prospective interagency collaboration is being embraced because it strengthens the ability of institutions to more effectively engage in new works.

- *Time.* Time is the most precious commodity for all of us, and we should recognize that the clocks in the clinics of practitioners run faster than those in the halls of academia or government agencies. Thus, program planning must first account for (and make provision for) the increased time required for implementation of evaluation components so that providers do not experience a threat to their ability to do the work of service delivery.

- *Money.* Because the bottom line is ever more the bottom line, we should pay attention to the issues related to money; dollars can be used as sticks as well as carrots, and to do both is probably appropriate. Research done by the Veterans Affairs (*VERDICT Brief Biannual Newsletter,* 1998) showed that change in medical practice was not produced, as a result of printed-matter information dissemination and medical education due to the absence of a financial incentive to change. In the world of managed care (with all its flawed parts and faulty execution), however, research by Sechrest, Backer, and colleagues has shown that changes in financial strategies result in changes in medical practice—"what's paid for tends to get used" (Sechrest, Backer, Rogers, Campbell, & Grady, 1994). Realistic considerations of the impact of financial incentives—and disincentives—must be entertained by planners.

- *Technology.* Recent technological advances, particularly the Internet, can be valuable parts of planning innovation and practice enhancement. Although Web-based information systems can suffer from lack of accountability of content, the ability to disseminate information quickly and widely has made databases with the best practice guides more available to more people. The many information-sharing opportunities made possible via the Internet represent powerful means of enlightenment and change.

In addressing the public health problems of society, it is the responsibility of all parties to enter into partnerships on equal footings or at least overtly impart a sense of respect and fair dealing with all participants in a planning process. In most cases, guidelines on the creation of partnerships and collaborative arrangements should be clearly codified and shared among personnel at all levels.

CONCLUSION

In summary, Petosa's chapter lays out the role of research-based development, implementation, evaluation, and refinement of health behavior programs, making a good case for the position that rational processes of program planning based on logic and quantifiable measurements will be the best route to efficiency and cost-effectiveness. Those efficiencies may be the primary and sufficient justifications for an empirical approach to planning and developing health programs—standards can be clearly defined, and adherence can be promoted in a formalized structure that responsibly accommodates input from many sources. The issues surrounding the difficulties in making the empirical approach more palatable to the practical world are addressed in a clear, straightforward manner with which any researcher would feel comfortable. This researcher, however, would like the reader to do a bit of the same uncomfortable self-examination that he undertook in response to the chapter's explicit criticism and implicit solutions and then work to make the solutions more explicit and practical. A first step is to remember that we are in the service of people who need help, and our egos must not be permitted to be in the way of devising and implementing the most effective means of providing that help.

▷ REFERENCES

SECHREST, L., BACKER, T. E., ROGERS, E. M., CAMPBELL, T. F., & GRADY, M. L. (Eds.). (1994). *Effective dissemination of clinical and health information.* Rockville, MD: Agency for Health Care Policy and Research.

VERDICT Brief Biannual Newsletter. (1998, Fall). San Antonio, TX: VA Center of Excellence in San Antonio and Charleston.

CHAPTER 3

Commentary 2
Herbert H. Severson

Petosa has very effectively presented a conceptual framework for getting empirically based health programs developed and accepted. The barriers are divided into four factors—organization, community, practitioner, and researcher—that combine to offer an ecological model for illustrating the forces that can deter or enhance the development of health-promoting interventions. This is an important area of consideration because health programs developed within communities or organizations can encourage both ownership of these programs and development of individualized programs for that setting and target population. An allied issue is whether these groups or individuals will adopt versus modify existing programs that have been empirically evaluated under experimental control conditions. My commentary reflects on some of the issues involved in the diffusion and adoption process and how we as behavioral researchers can enhance the adoption of empirically based behavioral health programs.

A key step in promoting health in the United States is the widespread adoption of empirically supported practices. Our knowledge base has grown with respect to intervening for problematic behaviors and has reached a critical mass in a number of areas. This knowledge base could be used to guide our society toward interventions that would substantially reduce the incidence and prevalence of antisocial behavior (Eron, Gentry, & Schlegel, 1994); tobacco, alcohol, and other substance use (Bryant, Windle, & West, 1997); academic failure (Adams & Englemann, 1996); depression (Reinecke, Ryan, & DuBois, 1998); marital discord (Hahlweg & Markman, 1988); teenage pregnancy (Kirby, Barth, Leland, & Fetro, 1991); and diabetes self-care (Glasgow et al., 1999). In short, a better society is within our grasp if we could bring to bear the programs that we know can work and have worked in more limited trials.

Although behavioral and health scientists have developed effective interventions that could significantly improve our population's health, there is a significant gap between empirical evidence and practice. Ultimately, the success of a health promotion effort is dependent on the extent to which these changes in practice occur within the targeted community of providers (Parcel, Perry, & Taylor, 1990). Empirically evaluated programs that have shown acceptable levels of effectiveness need to be broadly adopted to affect the population's health.

The problem is one of diffusion of practice, which has been defined as the "process by which innovation is communicated through channels over time to members of the social system" (Rogers, 1983, p. 5). Research has been completed on the conditions that affect diffusion (Rogers) and evaluation of different methods for disseminating interventions to practitioners (Andrews, Severson, Lichtenstein, Gordon, & Unfried, 1999; Kotke et al., 1990; Richmond & Anderson, 1994). Rogers has evaluated the characteristics of an innovation that influences the speed and extent of the diffusion process: advantage, compatibility, complexity, trialability, and observability, for example. Other research has compared different methods of diffusion such as direct marketing versus personal recruitment (Kotke et al., 1990) and different methods of training, such as workshops versus self-study (Severson,

Andrews, Lichtenstein, Gordon, & Barckley, 1998). Researchers currently debate various ways to promote diffusion of health promotion innovations (Orlandi, Landers, Weston, & Haley, 1990; Parcel et al., 1990), but there is a lack of empirical evaluation of diffusion methods.

Biglan, Mrazek, and Carnine (in press) have described a set of steps that could enhance the likelihood that empirically supported practices get adopted. First, they suggest a registry of prevention trials. There needs to be a repository of clinical trials that is accessible to both the scientific and field communities. There also is a need for standards for identifying useful intervention programs (see Chapter 7, this volume). This lack of consensus has hurt our credibility, and we would all benefit if we could agree on a set of standards. In clinical psychology, Chambless and Hollon (1998) and the American Psychological Association Task Force advocated a set of standards for identifying disseminable treatment procedures. These authors propose that an intervention could be considered efficacious if it has been shown in at least two randomized controlled trials by two different research teams to be superior to other interventions with which it was compared. Although there continues to be a need for more effectiveness trials, in which interventions are tested in real-world conditions, as opposed to efficacy trials that test an intervention under highly controlled conditions, we can still advocate for the adoption of empirically supported practices.

Even if we agree on which programs work, there are few vehicles or organizations to disseminate empirically evaluated practices. As Petosa points out, we need to identify the target of our dissemination. This is not a trivial matter. We need theory-driven research that identifies organizations that might target specific populations. This could also help in monitoring the degree to which an innovation is being adopted by the service providers. Once we target organizations, we need to analyze how to influence them to adopt empirically based practices. Although Rogers (1983) has provided useful analyses of characteristics that impede or foster adoption, we do not know factors that influence organizations to adopt and maintain programs.

One potential influence on an organization would be cost savings from using empirically supported practices. Unfortunately, these cost savings may not accrue to the organization that provided the service because the benefit requires a long-term assessment. Most organizations want to see financial benefits that occur in a short time frame. For example, smoking cessation may help employees live longer, but the benefit of reduced absenteeism from illness and reduced cleaning costs by reducing smoke and tobacco residue are more likely to appeal to an employer as an immediate benefit.

Regardless of the logic and potential benefit, the adoption of health behavior programs rests more on political process than science. Biglan (1998) argues that behavioral scientists need to be involved in advocacy to get behavioral science-based programs adopted. One could argue that advocacy for data-based policies has been most extensive and successful in public health areas such as tobacco control, alcohol use, and AIDS prevention. Behavioral scientists usually are reluctant to be involved in advocacy because it may be perceived that it takes away from their scientific credibility and is a new role for which they are poorly prepared. However, there are ways in which one can advocate for empirically based interventions by joining existing coalitions to influence public policy to adopt proven practices. Researchers can provide information to advocacy groups from the issue and participate in media advocacy to affect policy adoption (Wallach, Dorfman, Jernigan, & Themba, 1993). A compelling example of advocacy by behavioral scientists can be found in tobacco control (Biglan, 1998). Tobacco control advocates have used media advocacy to change public perceptions and encourage the adoption of significant legislation, such as clean indoor air laws, restrictions on youth access to tobacco products, and increases in tobacco taxes. Taking epidemiological data and reframing them into a more compelling message have been a key element in this effort. For example, the number of deaths due to smoking is reframed as equal to "two Boeing 747s crashing every day and killing everyone on board." One could argue that publication of research articles in professional journals has little impact on the public's knowledge of health programs or on the adoption of health programs. What do we have to say that can be used for a newspaper story or press release that may have a broader impact? In essence, we need to be more active in advocating for public policies that apply the research findings of our carefully controlled studies to the benefit of a larger audience.

The ultimate benefit of health interventions is their effect on targeted outcomes. Any intervention needs an ongoing assessment of measurable outcomes that can be used to monitor and evaluate effectiveness. As behavioral scientists, we can offer specific measures that can be used to create a system of accountability as part of an empirical program evaluation.

For those of us who are behavioral scientists interested in promoting the adoption of empirically based health promotion interventions, we should enter into a planful process of getting proven programs diffused into practice. This involves changing our behaviors and being more engaged in the translation of research to practice and being more open in our communication to the public. Behavioral scientists have much to offer now, but we need to be involved in the systematic effort of translating research into public health practice. If we do this, society will benefit from our scientific work, and we can all share the health benefits to our society.

REFERENCES

ADAMS, G. L., & ENGLEMANN, S. (1996). *Research on direct instruction: 25 years beyond DISTAR*. Seattle, WA: Educational Achievement Systems.

ANDREWS, J. A., SEVERSON, H. H., LICHTENSTEIN, E., GORDON, J. S., & UNFRIED, P. (1999, March). *Dissemination of a successful dental office-based smokeless tobacco intervention: Predictors of participation in training*. Paper presented at the annual meeting of the Society of Behavioral Medicine, San Diego, CA.

BIGLAN, A. (1998). *The need for advocacy in translating behavioral science findings into widespread changes in incidence and prevalence of problematic behavior*. Unpublished manuscript.

BIGLAN, A., MRAZEK, P. J., & CARNINE, D. (in press). Strategies for translating research into practice. *American Psychologist*.

BRYANT, K. J., WINDLE, M. T., & WEST, S. G. (1997). *The science of prevention: Methodological advances from alcohol and substance abuse research*. Washington, DC: American Psychological Association.

CHAMBLESS, D. L., & HOLLON, S. D. (1998). Defining empirically supported therapies. *Journal of Consulting and Clinical Psychology, 66*, 7-18.

ERON, L. D., GENTRY, J. H., & SCHLEGEL, P. (1994). *Reason to hope: A psychosocial perspective on violence and youth*. Washington, DC: American Psychological Association.

GLASGOW, R. E., WAGNER, E., KAPLAN, R. M., VINICOR, F., SMITH, L., & NORMAN, J. (1999). If diabetes is a public health problem, why not treat it as one? A population-based approach to chronic illness. *Annals of Behavioral Medicine, 21*, 1-13.

HAHLWEG, K., & MARKMAN, H. J. (1988). Effectiveness of behavioral marital therapy: Empirical status of behavioral techniques in preventing and alleviating marital distress. *Journal of Consulting and Clinical Psychology, 56*, 440-447.

KIRBY, D., BARTH, R. P., LELAND, N., & FETRO, J. V. (1991). Reducing the risk: Impact of a new curriculum on sexual risk-taking. *Family Planning Perspectives, 23*, 253-263.

KOTKE, T. E., SOLBERG, L. I., CONN, S., MAXWELL, P., THOMASBERG, M., BREKKE, M. L., & BREKKE, M. J. (1990). Comparison of two methods to recruit physicians to deliver smoking cessation interventions. *Archives of Internal Medicine, 150*, 1477-1481.

ORLANDI, M. A., LANDERS, C., WESTON, R., & HALEY, N. (1990). Diffusion of health promotion innovations. In K. Glanz, F. M. Lewis, & B. K. Rimer (Eds.), *Health behavior and health education: Theory, research, and practice* (pp. 288-313). San Francisco: Jossey-Bass.

PARCEL, G. S., PERRY, C. L., & TAYLOR, W. C. (1990). Beyond demonstration: Diffusion of health promotion innovations. In N. Bracht (Ed.), *Health promotion at the community level* (pp. 229-251). Newbury Park, CA: Sage.

REINECKE, M. A., RYAN, N. E., & DUBOIS, D. L. (1998). Cognitive-behavioral therapy of depression and depressive symptoms during adolescence: A review and meta-analysis. *Journal of the American Academy of Child and Adolescent Psychiatry, 37*, 26-34.

RICHMOND, R. L., & ANDERSON, P. (1994). Research in general practice for smokers and excessive drinkers in Australia and the U.K.: III. Dissemination of interventions. *Addiction, 89*, 49-62.

ROGERS, E. M. (1983). *Diffusion of innovations* (3rd ed.). New York: Free Press.

SEVERSON, H. H., ANDREWS, J. A., LICHTENSTEIN, E., GORDON, J. S., & BARCKLEY, M. F. (1998). Using the hygiene visit to deliver a tobacco cessation program: Results of a randomized clinical trial. *Journal of the American Dental Association, 129,* 993-999.

WALLACH, L., DORFMAN, L., JERNIGAN, D., & THEMBA, M. (1993). *Media advocacy and public health: Power for prevention.* Newbury Park, CA: Sage.

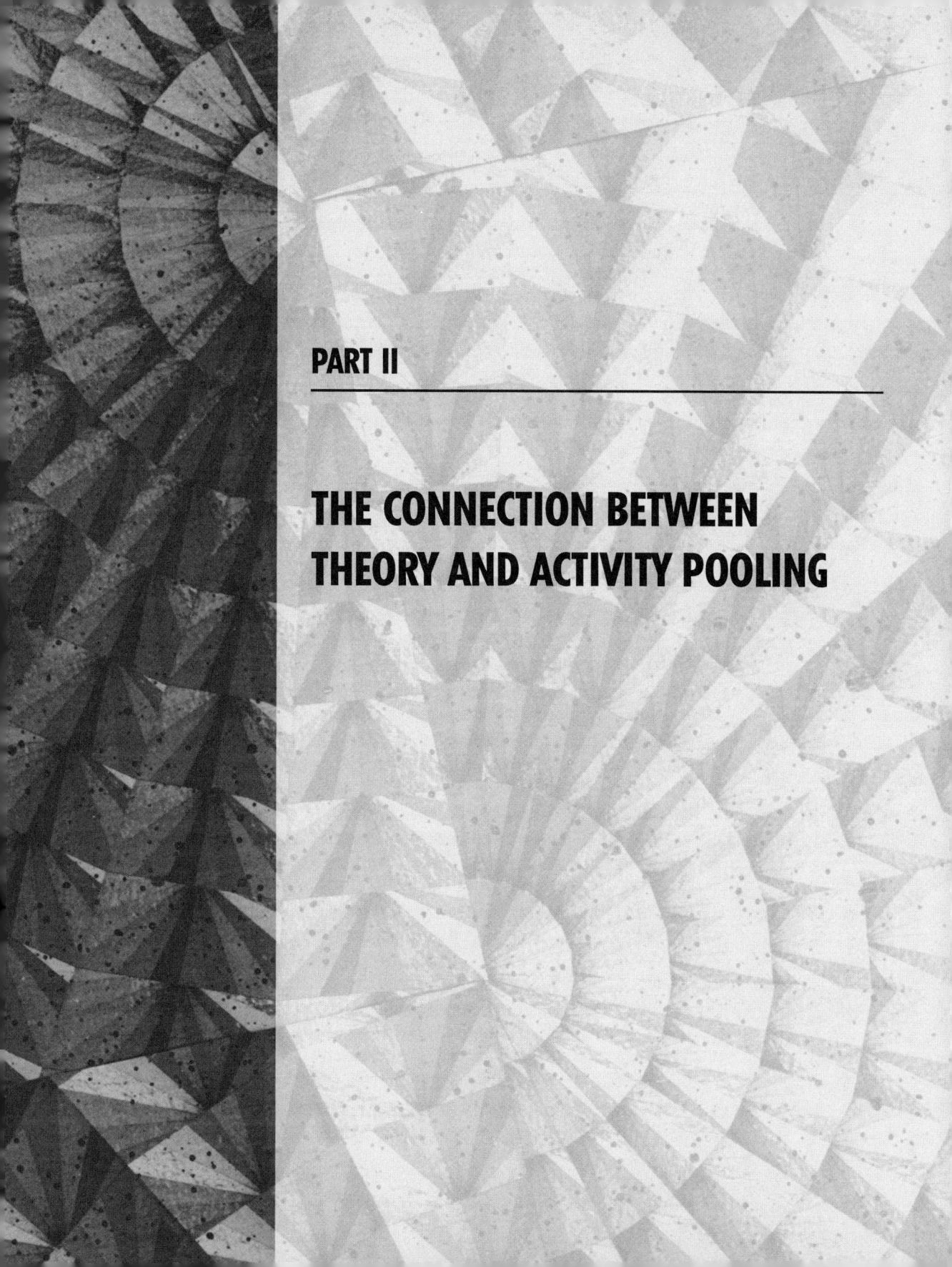

PART II

THE CONNECTION BETWEEN THEORY AND ACTIVITY POOLING

CHAPTER 4

Praxis in Health Behavior Program Development

Steve Sussman
Alan N. Sussman

DEFINITIONS ◄

A health program specialist recognized a problem at his workplace: Others at his workplace were drinking whiskey at work and driving home drunk. In the past week, three coworkers were arrested, and one drove over a pedestrian. Although he realized that there was a problem here, he did not want to upset his coworkers by removing all alcohol from the workplace. So, quickly and without much thought, he removed the whiskey from the cabinets and replaced them with beer. The problem of drinking and driving did not go away. He mused, "Well, back to the drawing board." A real problem here is that he really needed to begin at the drawing board. He needed to carefully study the problem behavior, which was that people were drinking alcohol, then driving. By driving drunk, they could die or kill someone. He thought that filling the cabinet with beer would slow people down. In other words, he had an implicit theory that drinking whiskey led to driving drunk, whereas drinking beer did not. His "theory" was disconfirmed.

He developed a new theory. People at work were stressed out; they drank to relieve the stress. They would drink any alcohol around to relax them; then they had to get home. Now he realized that he needed to either provide a stress reduction program, educate people to not drink before driving, remove all alcohol from the workplace, or provide a shuttle service home. As his theory became more refined, his potential solutions to the problem improved and were more varied.

And all he needed to start out with was a good theory, here a "stress-coping" theory of alcohol abuse.

Health programs should be developed beginning with a **theory,** an organized set of concepts that convey a plausible causal mechanism (history) regarding environmental or behavioral events (Heise, 1975; Rudner, 1966; van Ryn & Heaney, 1992). In other words, a theory is a set of beliefs about causes and effects. For the purposes of this chapter, the words *theory, causal model, paradigm,* and *causal history* are interchangeable. People who identify the need for a program generally think in terms of theory whenever they try to promote a healthy behavior or counteract an unhealthy behavior. The program planner makes assumptions about the nature of the need (i.e., to stop driving-under-the-influence [DUI] arrests and accidents), what caused the need (stress and drinking), which target behavior facilitates or deters the need (drinking, driving), and the ability and means to change the target behavior to meet the need. One may think of a theory as a map. One knows about a terrain (the health behavior). Just looking at all one can look at is not likely to tell anyone anything much. The researcher or practitioner wants to get from Point A to Point B on the terrain. The theory is the map; the theory instructs the person on how to reach Point B. People might as well use theories to their advantage, making them explicit and carefully thought out. One selects things to look at, has beliefs about what causes what, and has beliefs about what can cure the need.

ELEMENTS OF A THEORETICAL MODEL

Hold on; what is theory again? Theory consists of beliefs regarding the relations among a finite set of concepts. Beliefs are hunches about what the truth is. Relations refer to what causes what to happen. Concepts are abstractions that interpret concrete events. These abstractions are subject to change, but the concrete events they represent simply are what they are. Again, theory is a causal history composed of a set of concepts. One may believe that people drink alcohol because they are stressed and alcohol relieves the pressure. The causal history is that subjective stress (a concept that may refer to certain sympathetic nervous system reactions) causes one to consider drinking, the latter leading to relaxation. Alcohol relaxes but also interferes with driving behavior. When one identifies a behavioral event as being healthy or unhealthy, one turns the event (i.e., behavioral movements) into a concept (health promoting or deterring). One may infer that involvement with alcohol-related arrests and accidents is not healthy.

Generally, concepts of events take on different values; they are said to be variables. An individual can be rated as to degree of stress, intoxication, driving impairment, and degree of legal consequence. A person uses his or her beliefs about causal connections to try to solve problems by manipulating causal factors, by changing the values on causal variables to change the values on the outcome variables.

Causes. Causes sometimes are referred to as antecedent variables or predictors when available data as collected do not provide one with adequate evidence that these variables cause the behavior to occur. However, one selects predictors for good reason: for their fit into a planner's map of a health terrain. One could impart a causal explanation regarding the impact of predictors on other events, yet one should be cautious regarding how well supported causal explanations are by the data. Anything that tends to increase the probability of some other thing can be referred to as a cause as long as one assumes that it is always necessary to the causal narrative. Causal variables may potentiate (increase the probability of) or counteract (decrease the probability of) the occurrence of a healthy or unhealthy behavior. Causal variables that potentiate an unhealthy behavior or counteract a healthy behavior are called risk factors. Causal variables that potentiate a healthy behavior or counteract an unhealthy behavior are called protective factors. Stress is a risk factor for DUI behavior in the previous example. When one refers to causes in the health arena, one generally means that a cause (predictor) is part of the causal history of an outcome, not the one and only cause, but that if the cause were manipulated, the outcome would change.

Mediators. Stress does not directly cause DUI behavior, does it? Often, variables also mediate the effects of the causal variables on the outcome variables. These are called mediator or operator variables. A mediator variable may potentiate or suppress/counteract the effects of the causal variable on the outcome variable. In the earlier example, one's expectancies regarding alcohol effects may mediate (potentiate) the effects of subjective stress on drinking alcohol. Stress causes drinking because the person believes that drinking will reduce the stress.

Target Behaviors and Health Outcomes. Finally, there are the target behavior and related health outcomes. Behaviors that directly or indirectly make people healthy or sick are classified as target behaviors. Values may help determine what is healthy or sick. For example, one person may try to keep a person alive at all costs. The person may be in a coma, connected to a life support system. However, others may argue that one should not forestall mortality without a consideration of morbidity (Kaplan, 1984). It is not clear that a person in a coma, nearly brain dead, is having a good-quality life. Together, these four types of variables—causes, mediators, behaviors, and health outcomes—convey a causal mechanism or history.

Causal Mechanisms/Histories. How do these variables convey a causal mechanism? Causes occur before and elicit effects in the presence of a mediator. Without the presence of relevant mediators, the effects will not occur. Mediators intervene or account (at least partially, when statistical tests are applied) for the relations between the cause and the effect. The cause influences the mediator; the mediator influences the effect; and by considering the mediator in a cause-effect model, the relation between the cause and the effect decreases or disappears.

As an example, consider peer dares leading to one's smoking. Obvious ways to avoid addictive smoking and lung cancer include learning how to resist peer dares to smoke so that continued smoking does not occur. However, beliefs that everyone smokes or that one will achieve acceptance of peers by smoking may lead one to smoke even though no obvious peer dares are observed. In fact, the relation between peer dares and smoking may disappear when one considers these cognitive mediators of perceptions that everyone smokes and one will achieve acceptance by smoking (MacKinnon et al., 1991). In other words, peer dares may exert an effect only or partially because the person believes that giving into the dares by smoking will lead to acceptance of peers. (The person may be wrong—who likes a "yes" person? [Sussman, 1989].) If these cognitive misperceptions are changed, maybe one will not smoke. New program strategies other than refusal assertion training may be more fundamental to effective smoking prevention.

Moderators. Finally, persons who engage in health behavior work refer to yet another term, *moderators*. This is another type of variable that will be discussed in more detail in later chapters (e.g., see Chapter 19). Moderators modulate the relation of the cause with the effect. They may or may not themselves have any influence on the effect variables (behavior or health consequence). For example, consider the cause-effect relation of peer dares and one's cigarette smoking. Perhaps, pushes to smoke by others may lead one to smoke. One moderator is susceptibility to peer social influence (Stacy, Sussman, Dent, Burton, & Flay, 1992). Some youth are more or less vulnerable to dares made by other youth. Now, susceptibility to peer social influence may or may not predict later cigarette smoking. However, youth who are not vulnerable to peer dares may not respond to peer dares to smoke.

Summary. A theory provides (a) concepts or interpretations of entities and (b) beliefs about how these concepts are related to each other. In health behavior work, given some assumed values about what is healthy, certain mediator variables potentiate or suppress the effects of risk or protective causal variables on target behavior, which then leads to healthy or unhealthy outcomes. In other words, risk or protective factors manipulate mediators, and the mediators manipulate the target behavior—which leads to a health outcome. Moderators may modulate the strength of effect of the causal variable on the target behavior. Theories provide causal histories or stories about the health outcome. A good theory tells a good story; it does a good job of description, explanation, prediction, or control of an outcome.

LEVELS OF THEORY AND LEVELS OF MEASUREMENT

Interestingly, the lower the level and the narrower the scope of an assertion or set of assertions, the closer it is to direct empirical testing. Such theorizing often consists of little more than inferring empirical generalizations, groupings of predictors. For example, one may find that teenagers report that they engage in smoking, unsafe sex, and drinking to achieve acceptance among peers. One may infer that teenagers engage in risk-taking behavior to achieve acceptance among peers. Now, one could also go to a higher level and broader scope of theorizing. For example, one may infer that teens will try any number of prosocial or anti-social behaviors to achieve acceptance; that is, peer acceptance is a main general motivator among teens. This higher level of theorizing may suggest a wider variety of intervention possibilities than does a lower level of theorizing. (For example, one could suggest that one can achieve acceptance of peers by not smoking and by attending school, that is, by being prosocial.) The goal is to find better maps of the area of interest. The theorist may paste and cut stories about what concepts are and what concepts do (interpretation) to make lower-level theories fit the higher-level theory. A theory covers a set of generalizations, or, at a lower level, a generalization covers a set of data to accomplish something. One theory is better than another, worthy of selection, to the extent that it enables one to achieve his or her goals. These goals include the ability to tell good stories about reality—that is, stories that permit one to broaden and deepen the capacity to describe, explain, predict, and control events. Good beliefs make for effective action.

Level of measurement of a theory refers to the scope of size of observation of variables being studied. At the most molecular level (smallest unit) in health behavior etiology, one considers biological molecules, gene alleles, neurotransmitter functions, or other biological events. At a slightly larger level, one considers intrapersonal processes such as cognition, affect, attitudes, beliefs, perceptions, personality traits and states, and the like. At a larger level, one considers interpersonal processes, which involve a unit of measurement that involves two or more people, such as social pressures and communications. Finally, at the most molar level (largest unit) in health behavior etiology, one considers the broader environment as the unit of measurement, such as organizations, poverty, culture, nationalism, and the like.

Please note that level of a theory is not the same thing as level of measurement. Level of theory refers to the level of abstraction away from the observable. Generally, the more abstract the theory, the wider its scope (the more it explains), the more difficult it may be to test, but the more explanatory power it is likely to have. Level of measurement refers to the number of entities that are represented by the variables that compose the theory. Variables within the human body are considered a smaller level of measurement than are variables that involve multiple persons or organizational units.

The level of a theory may be very concrete (e.g., empirical generalizations about white blood cells and cancer, empirical generalizations about types of crime in neighborhoods) to very abstract (e.g., the molecular biology of cancer, the culture of poverty). Also, the same theory may pertain to a small level or unit of measurement (e.g., human biology) or a very large level of measurement (e.g., neighborhoods). Together, the level of the theory and the level of measurement provide context anchors on a causal history. They describe the level of abstraction of the variables that will be studied and how they will be observed.

▶ HOW DOES THEORY SUGGEST PROGRAM IDEAS?

One could imagine or select an infinite number of theories. All else being equal, the best theory provides the best programs, and, all else being equal, the best programs do the most for the least effort. Effective program planners are good at selecting relevant theories and knowing how to apply them. At present, at least four main general perspectives influence theory construction and suggest program ideas in health behavior research and practice: implicit theory, antecedent oriented, behavior oriented, and consequence oriented. These approaches are not in themselves theory. Rather, they provide a classification; they direct one to different classes of theories or theoretical biases.

IMPLICIT THEORY

A health professional's leap of faith, often based on perceptions of relevance to a target group, determines the direction that a program is planned and constructed. The professional may say that he or she knows how things work because of a "feeling in the gut." Alternatively, he or she may state that "love is what is needed" or may mention that a certain theoretical hunch is "good public relations." Or he or she may say that the notion is just "good common sense." Unfortunately, many such theories (e.g., the "Scared Straight" program, bloodletting, pneumonia vests, mud packs) do not manipulate mediators of change

(Chassin, Presson, & Sherman, 1985; Hayes, 1998). Such implicit theories need to be made explicit and testable to be of any real value to program development. Of course, the criteria of being explicit and testable are important only to the extent that they enhance the applicability of the theory—that is, maximize one's ability to describe, explain, predict, or control behavior.

The other three approaches are explicit appeals to targeting the ABCs of health behavior (Elder & Stern, 1986; Sussman, Dent, Burton, Stacy, & Flay, 1995). The ABCs of health behavior were borrowed from the functional analysis literature of behavior therapy, and they provide different perspectives toward the development of a causal theory with direct applications. These approaches provide a recipe for systematically looking for things one can do before, during, and after the occurrence of the target behavior.

ANTECEDENT ORIENTED

The As refer to antecedents of unhealthy or healthy behavior—that is, what happens before the behavior is performed. For example, an offer of a cigarette, one's perceptions of what it means to refuse an offer of a cigarette, one's desire for popularity, risk-taking tendencies, and upbringing all are potential antecedents of smoking. Theories based on this antecedent-oriented perspective focus on events that may long precede the target behavior. These series of events may pertain to the underlying processes that lead a target population to learn healthy or unhealthy behavior. So-called acquisition-oriented health behavior programming is developed to counteract antecedents (e.g., Chassin et al., 1985; Cowen, 1984). Some researchers consider this type of programming superior to others because it may tap into antecedents that elicit any number of problem behaviors. By counteracting the right antecedent, several behaviors are thereby counteracted (Chassin et al., 1985). For example, smoking and drinking are correlated behaviors. By counteracting misperceptions of peer approval for engaging in risky behavior, several types of drug use might be counteracted. This approach can provide a good story, or map, of behavior.

BEHAVIOR ORIENTED

The Bs refer to the behavior. Behavior-oriented theories are those that have elsewhere been referred to as classical conditioning or instrumental conditioning; they examine the antecedents (stimuli) and consequences (reinforcement) that occur immediately prior to and after the occurrence of a behavior. The behavior is carefully examined regarding its frequency and other characteristics. Behavior change-oriented programming often is aimed at counteracting a specific problem behavior. Three programmatic approaches are subsumed under the behavior-oriented perspective: stimulus control, response control, and reinforcement control. Stimulus control program approaches include use of sensory or informational cues (e.g., lunch bell, instructions) that signal the desired behavior change. Response control program approaches (smoking or not smoking, not inhaling, eating food slowly) pertain to changing the parameters of the behavior directly to exert an effect on health outcomes. Finally, reinforcement control approaches (e.g., rapid smoking as a means to decrease the frequency of smoking behavior) manipulate the consequences of the behavior to elicit a change in the behavior. The behavior-oriented approach differs from the antecedent- and consequences-oriented approaches in that cues and consequences *immediately proximal* to the behavior, or the behavior itself, are addressed.

CONSEQUENCES ORIENTED

The Cs refer to consequences of the behavior—that is, what happens after the behavior is performed. For example, consequences of adolescent smoking include coughing, enjoyment, nausea, or addiction. Consequences-oriented programs are aimed at counteracting consequences of the behavior. Perhaps the most popular of consequences-oriented programs is the health protection model. In this model, consequences are removed from the performance of a behavior. The behavior does not have to change, per se. For example, pill bottle safety caps prevent a young child from being able to successfully open a pill bottle. Although the behavior is not directly targeted, the consequences of the behavior are removed or changed. Over time, the target population may or may not change behavior—in this case, trying to open pill bottles through simply turning a cap.

In summary, there are at least four general types of approaches to address a health behavior problem area. By formalizing (i.e., making explicit and clarifying) the first approach or by framing theories within one or more of the three latter approaches, health professionals can begin to solve health problems. Theory provides the direction for program development.

▶ WHY DO APPLIED PROFESSIONALS PROVIDE ONLY LIP SERVICE TO THEORY?

Thinking in terms of links between variables is not simple. There are at least six reasons that many applied professionals do not use theory carefully in their work. First, there is a break in expertise between theoreticians and applied professionals (Hayes, 1998). Theoreticians tend to think in terms of technical language that pertains to abstract rules and applies to behavior across different situations. Theoreticians may use examples that are removed from important health problems. Applied professionals tend to think in terms of affecting people in specific situations and often are not trained in use of theory. Second, and related to the first point, applied professionals may tend to view theoreticians as living in an "ivory tower" or "in the clouds"; that is, their theoretical thinking is too indirect or untested or unnecessary (van Ryn & Heaney, 1992; see also Chapter 3, this volume). This attitude is unfortunate because theory versus practice is a false dichotomy. A good theory does things.

Third, many applied professionals may view aspects of human health behavior as too complex in causation to be able to apply theory very successfully (Chassin et al., 1985). Indeed, recently developed health behavior theories all explain health behavior change in rather complex ways, potentially beyond any direct applied utility for a specific problem in a specific setting. These theories include the biopsychosocial model (Bernard & Krupat, 1994); community health systems models (e.g., Freimuth & Mettger, 1990; Vicary, Doebler, Bridger, & Gurgevich, 1996); multifaceted definitions of culture (Guarneccia & Rodriguez, 1996); models integrating wellness and social learning (Byrne, Brown, Voorberg, & Schofield, 1994); integration of social, cognitive, and social change theories (Wallerstein & Sanchez, 1994); integration of stressful life events and prevention equation models (Hirayama, Hirayama, & Cetingok, 1993); integration of supply-and-demand reduction approaches (Pentz, Bonnie, & Shopland, 1996); integration of social marketing and reinforcement learning approaches (Lefebvre & Flora, 1988; Sussman et al., 1995; Worden et al., 1988); multilevel approaches (e.g., Marconi & Rudzinski, 1995; McLeroy et al., 1993); and integration of multilevel with cultural, social, and intrapersonal approaches (Petraitis, Flay, & Miller, 1995). Generally, pieces of these theories will be used for a specific health instance. These theories are important in that they begin to suggest broad applicability. However, they are difficult to test right now. The practitioner should be aware of them and know that technology and creativity will permit these theories to have a powerful impact on behavior someday. Until then, it may be okay to use pieces of these theories for different purposes.

Fourth, there sometimes is a tendency among applied researchers to confound causal models with flowcharts. Causation does involve an ordering of events such that a first event (cause) produces an expectation for the occurrence of a second event (effect). In this way, all causal models involve a time element or process. Process models certainly do provide good grounds for deriving causal expectations. However, not all process models are causal. A process model in and of itself simply implies that one thing happens, and then the next thing happens without an indication that the first thing caused the second thing. One may drink a cup of coffee and then drive to work and enter the office. This series of three events may be represented as a flowchart or process model; however, these events are not causally related. Third variables operate, causing each of these variables (e.g., the need to wake up and earn money). Likewise, in health research, a causal model exists only when one variable plausibly elicits another to occur within a context, and alternative potential explanations are considered and controlled.

Fifth, there is a tendency to reference someone else's theory and leave it there. It is not surprising that many applied research studies reference a theory but then do not measure it at all. It also is not surprising that many applied professionals reference a theory and then go on to present a health behavior program that is tangentially related to the theory. In particular, learning theory, social learning theory, self-efficacy theory, and the theory of reasoned action tend to dominate theoretical thought in health behavior research (McCaul & Glasgow, 1985; van Ryn & Heaney, 1992). Although these are great theories, their application to specific instances needs more deliberate purpose than mere lip service to theory. Examining pieces of a theory limits the coverage of the theory to that proportion of the theory that is examined. However, one can use pieces of theories successfully for specific purposes if these pieces work well in explanation, prediction, or control of behavior. Deliberate tying of the theory or pieces of the theory to measurement is needed.

Finally, careful use of theory involves investment of time and effort (Chassin et al., 1985). The researcher or practitioner needs to have some patience to select or create a theory, choose variables to modify and measure, and develop and administer assessment devices. One may have limited time. However, investment of time in theory can lead to good returns. A good theory works; it helps improve one's ability to change a behavior, to maximize a health behavior program.

▶ WHY IS THEORY IMPORTANT FOR HEALTH BEHAVIOR PROGRAM DEVELOPMENT?

Use of theory is important for health behavior program development for at least four reasons. Most important, theory provides a model of causation that enables us to describe, explain, predict, or control behaviors. Careful use of theory makes explicit the hunches that the health professional is making about what is going on with others' behavior (description and explanation), how they are likely to act in the future (prediction), and how they might be best assisted to adopt more healthy behavior (control). Being aware of good causal stories about a health arena enables the program planner to be more in control over the actions undertaken to solve health problems. Those persons who participate in health behavior program development desire ultimately to alter behavior. Remember that the practitioner has no choice about whether to use theory: He or she does. The only question is whether he or she uses it consciously and well. True beliefs about the causal history of a health behavior promote more effective action.

Second, a good theory can be disconfirmed. If a theory does not work well, either desired effects will fail to be achieved or substitution effects may be found (i.e., when the underlying cause is not modified), assuming all the variables in the theory have been measured well. For example, one may propose a theory that youth smoke because of peer pressure or dares. A youth is removed from bad influences and then is engaged in a cessation program. Let us say he or she does not quit smoking. Alternatively, perhaps he or she quits smoking cigarettes by taking up marijuana smoking. This youth is not showing a change in behavior or may be demonstrating substitution of one problem behavior for another. The underlying cause may not be peer pressure per se but perceived peer acceptance, the latter being what really needs to be addressed (see Chassin et al., 1985).

Third, a good theory also permits development of new program ideas or identification of appropriate populations for available program ideas (Chassin et al., 1985). For example, let us say that one believes that perceived peer acceptance mediates the relation between peer pressure and one's drug use. A program is implemented; peer dares are removed by placing the youth away from such influences (e.g., transfer to a new school). The behavior did not improve—the youth was smoking marijuana and probably soon is smoking cigarettes again. One can explain this curious finding—perceived peer acceptance may not have been modified (this possibility can be measured). After testing different plausible possible interventions, one thinks that a normative restructuring lesson might help (Hansen, 1992). Students in this youth's new school are shown two signs: one that says regular smoking is acceptable and one that says regular smoking is not acceptable. Students are told to stand under one of the signs. All the youth in the class stand by the "not acceptable" sign. This youth's perceived peer acceptance for drug use decreases, and he or she stops experimenting with both substances.

Finally, at the very minimum, good use of theory can help one protect against errors in critical thinking. Theory divides up concepts, involves use of different measures to measure various concepts, and orders concepts into functional relationships. Without such carving out of concepts, people may engage in various errors. In particular, they may show confusion in their separation among concepts or misperceive how concepts are related to each other. For example, three types of errors in critical thinking are discussed by Sussman, Simon, Glynn, and Stacy (1996). These errors result from poor theorizing. As a first example, an abstract concept can become reified, that is, treated as a concrete phenomenon. In other words, the concept and a measure of the concept can become treated as if they are one and the same. For example, a youth who exhibits truant behavior may become labeled as high risk. Thereafter, this child may be referred to as high risk, separate from any behavior exhibited. This concept label can then result in poor or incorrect treatment of some individuals. Good theorizing makes it clear that the measure of high risk is only a measure that has error associated with it. Other measures may be needed to provide better content validity of the concept of high risk.

As a second example, a concept may become divided ineffectively into separate concepts (error of division). For example, consider that people treat risk taking, rebelliousness, and sensation seeking as if these are separate concepts. Are they always? Good theorizing may be able to pull together concepts that reflect the same thing.

As a third example, cause and effect can switch orders through circular reasoning. Let us say one observes that a youth is experiencing stress and subsequently can be observed to be a smoker. The youth may be said to smoke because of stress. On the other hand, this smoker who subsequently seems stressed out may be said to be now experiencing stress due to smoking. Which order does the theoretician intend here? Good theory can clarify one's thinking about the ordering of concepts.

Even if one is thinking carefully, however, that does not mean one is working well with a theory. As a caveat, one should consider that very abstract theories become prone to conceptual errors through sheer free falls into the muddle of the concepts involved. Thus, theory is useful for clarifying one's thinking, but clear thinking and theory are not the same thing. It is careful thinking within the context of a good causal history that provides the program planner with the map to continue with further steps of program development.

▶ CRITERIA FOR THEORY DEVELOPMENT OR SELECTION

Everyone has a causal hunch when engaging in health behavior practice. Even if no official theory is specified, health professionals assume that something will produce a change in the health behavior of their clients. What health professionals need to do is to make their hunches explicit. By writing down one's hunches, one is making clear why a program is likely to work and for whom. Thus, the golden rule of theory development and selection is to write down one's ideas.

When writing down one's ideas, at least four criteria might be considered. The main criterion for using any theory is that it should be plausible. In other words, it should fit available observable phenomena well. A theory positing that peer acceptance mediates the relations between peer pressure and one's smoking makes sense. However, it is not particularly plausible that the gravitational pull of the moon serves as the major mediator here.

A second criterion is that a necessary and sufficient number of variables should be included to explain the behavior of interest. In other words, the theoretical model should be developed fully enough to be able to design an intervention that is likely to be effective. One may refer to this criterion as one of completeness or precision. For example, if both perceived peer acceptance and perceived peer use prevalence mediate the relation between peer pressure and youth smoking, program activities will need to be developed that counteract both mediators to maximize program efficacy. Of course, seldom will one know the necessary and sufficient variables for a complete theoretical model; one needs something complete or precise enough to be useful. (*Completeness* and *precision* are used here as a single criterion. Arguably they could refer to two separate criteria.)

A third criterion is that the theory should be testable. If the theory cannot be tested, it reflects only one's belief system, which can vary as much as people vary (Rudner, 1966; van Ryn & Heaney, 1992). The importance of testability cannot be understated, assuming that such testability increases the applicability of the theory. There should be ways to measure each element of the causal history, and one should be able to observe how variation (or direct manipulation) of one variable (the cause) elicits a change in another variable (the effect). For example, let us say that peer dares are the cause of smoking (a direct effects model; no mediator involved). Measures of peer dares could include self-reports that such behavior has occurred, naturalistic observation of such behavior, or implicit cognition-type reports, as examples. These types of measures are discussed in subsequent chapters. (See Chapter 5 for a detailed discussion of implicit cognition. Verbal and nonverbal measures are discussed in Chapters 6, 9, and 11.) Also, smoking behavior can be measured through similar methods of assessment as the cause. Accuracy of self-report of smoking also can be confirmed through use of biochemical validation. When the program is developed, it should induce change in reports of peer dares to smoke, and this change should be associated with changes in smoking.

A final criterion is that a theory should have heuristic value. In other words, a theory should be able to generalize across some settings and situations and should help to generate new ideas or applications. The best theories have better coverage of phenomena; they provide a wider and deeper understanding of the health behavior. For example, peer acceptance as a theoretical component can be used as an explanation of several adolescent risk behaviors across several adolescent groups. However, social learning theory may be applicable across many adolescent and adult behaviors. It may have more heuristic value than a more limited peer acceptance notion. With these four criteria in mind—plausibility, completeness, testability, and heuristic value—one may begin to develop or adapt a theory for use in a health area.

Please remember that if a hypothesis about a causal history is tested and the expected results are not achieved, something has to change. The theory may be wrong or need revision, or the entities used to measure the concepts may be wrong. Of course, even positive results do not mean a theory is true. It means that a theory is useful. A better theory may come along later; it may be even more useful. Also, remember that many theories can be made precise and testable (e.g., one may try to weigh souls); a good theory, however, will work—it will have heuristic value as well. Good theories cover more phenomena better.

▶ TYING THEORY INTO SPECIFIC HEALTH AREAS: LINKING THEORY WITH HEALTH PROBLEMS

There are several means that theory may be linked with health arenas (see Hayes, 1998). We highlight two means. First, a problem may be identified, and then a theory might be found that appears associated with it. Theories that show some evidence for usefulness in that health arena and that might plausibly be linked with the present instance might be selected (van Ryn & Heaney, 1992). This approach can be used successfully. Social influence theory was selected well from basic social psychology research to deal with peer dares to use drugs, for example (Sussman, 1989). However, one may not realize that even identification of a problem area involves implicit assumptions and hunches; even problem identification involves theory. For example, an alcohol drinker may identify his or her blackout the night before as being a normal event, one of being born in the wrong age (e.g., not in the Middle Ages), a moral problem, a behavioral problem, or a disease. How this problem is identified suggests the operation of underlying theoretical notions. Thus, theories should not and cannot simply be superimposed over problem areas. The concepts involved in defining the problem area need to be considered first.

A second means that theories are associated with health areas is to first identify a theory and then search for a problem for its application. In this instance, the problem area would have to fit into the theory, a theoretician would have to be trained well in the problem area to adequately apply the theory, and the assumption is that two fields of study somehow are being married. Certainly, theories have been widely applied to different health problems (e.g., social learning theory). However, what if a phenomenon is not sufficiently explained by a theory? Should the theory be modified, or should part of the phenomenon be ignored? This leads to what Hayes (1998) refers to as the "mutual interest model." Perhaps a relationship may be built between theoreticians and applied professionals based on the contributions made by each to build a theory for a problem area. In

TYING THEORY INTO SPECIFIC HEALTH ◄
AREAS: MEASURES AND ACTIVITIES

this sense, assumptions regarding a problem area are made explicit and fit directly into a structure of causes, effects, and mediators.

Now begins the process of theory building, refinement, and use for solving a health problem. First, each variable in a model should be identified. For example, let us consider youth carrying weapons. Youth may carry weapons for self-protection because of distrust in the efficacy of legitimized protection agents (the police) or to demonstrate a tough, risky social image and earn the respect of their peers. There are two causal variables (self-protection needs and tough, risky image desire), two mediators (distrust of protection agents, need for respect of peers), and one effect (weapon carrying).

Each variable in a theoretical model (causes, effects, mediators) is assessed by one or more measures. For example, desire for self-protection may be measured by feelings of vulnerability to future victimization or self-report measures regarding one's felt need to protect oneself. Distrust of protection agents could be measured by self-reports of one's beliefs that police, school administrators, parents, or community action groups (e.g., Guardian Angels) could protect youth from harm. Weapon carrying could be measured, for example, through self-reports, weapon sales slips, or naturalistic observation. Self-report-type measures could be developed through use of theory-based semistructured elicitation questionnaires (Middlestadt, Bhattacharyya, Rosenbaum, Fishbein, & Shepherd, 1996) or through the many procedures described in later chapters of this volume (e.g., Chapters 6, 8, and 10). The elicitation method involves asking open-ended questions to generate items to measure a theoretical variable. For example, youth might be asked, "How does carrying a weapon protect you?" Responses might include "I feel more power" or "I could injure someone and so they stay away," and items then could be developed to tap aspects of self-protection.

A model is confirmed through etiologic work, particularly in prospective studies, which are able to show the operation of mediators regarding the impact of the causes on the effects (see Chapter 6). Each of the measures used to tap a concept has a certain amount of measurement error associated with it, of course. Also, there may be sources of unexplained variance, third variables that are not known. Still, if a model accounts for more than 10% of the variance (i.e., 10% of the outcome "pie"), the current instance being weapon-carrying behavior, it is likely that a successful intervention can be developed based on this knowledge.

The variables in a causal model suggest potential activities that could be developed. For example, distrust of protection agents is a variable that might be counteracted by using a public relations campaign, different types of community agents (e.g., use of civilian volunteers), or education (e.g., trips to a police station). Researchers who use perceived efficacy studies or immediate-impact studies might be able to discern which activities are relatively likely to be received well by the target population and have an impact on their behavior, as is described in later chapters (see Chapters 9-14). In other words, a good causal model readily facilitates later steps of program development.

▶ DISCUSSION

The transformation of theories within health arenas into specific health behavior activities is the work of later chapters. It is hoped that this chapter provides a framework for understanding why use of theory is important, how to avoid simply giving lip service to theory, and how to make best use of theory. When in doubt, keep it simple. Use one or two causal variables, one or two mediators, and one effect. Build the activity based on how it might counteract the causal variables, perhaps through counteracting the mediators. Importantly, researchers and practitioners should work together to manufacture the best in theory-linked programming.

LIMITATIONS OF SYSTEMATIC THEORY DEVELOPMENT AND CONCLUSIONS

Economists and some health behavior researchers talk of constructing theory in the sense of fitting a bunch of equations to a set of data collected by a firm or government agency. Within this lower-level theoretical view, most such theories apply to groups of persons. They may or may not apply to particular cases; they are empirical generalizations. One works here in terms of probabilities that certain concepts predict other concepts or predict a percentage of the variance of other concepts. Such theories are limited in ability to explain phenomena and in range of application. On the other hand, empirical generalizations can be improved directly by adding another observation to the data set.

Higher-level theory is defined in terms of unobservable and observable phenomena. Higher-level theory is the positing of some unobservable construct and the laws it obeys to explain some set of hypotheses, which refer to observable or measurable phenomena. Using theory in this way is important because it permits one greater explanatory power and range than an empirical generalization approach. However, this higher-level theorizing often immediately brings up certain distinctively philosophical problems. In particular, there is nothing one can do in any direct way to improve theory when considered as such. Simply adding another observation will not necessarily alter the theory. The ability to disconfirm the theory needs to be considered more carefully. Lower-level theories do provide a solid starting point for a higher-level theory because one's use of empirical generalizations as tools of concept development provides a means of developing higher-level theory that is relatively testable.

One best develops a theory for a set of phenomena by coming up with ideas of what might lie behind the phenomena, making them happen. The founders of the atomic theory of matter did not sit down and decide to "make a theory"; rather, it struck them that the observations made in chemistry labs would have been made if matter were made up of smaller elements that came together and broke apart. In other words, progress in theory building often demands not the deployment of available concepts but the creation of new ones by creative imagination. Effective theorizing requires that one walk a fine line between a rejection of the inevitability of common sense and the adoption of the absurd. Experience, intelligence, and energy may lead to wisdom; one can hope so.

In theory development, one first tries to determine what the world is like and why, and only later does one label some of the results of that activity as a "theory." One may think and communicate about what the world is like in the form of a story. The story becomes refined in interaction over time with further empirical work, including some empirical work that never would have happened without the prodding of the theory. Sometimes, this construction is completed without the conscious intention of building a theory; it is done to try to figure out what is going on, as people do the things they do. There is no recipe for good theorizing in the "big picture" except to know one's stuff well and think hard.

Unfortunately, what a field needs for good theorizing is a Newton, an Einstein, a Galileo, a Chomsky, and in health behavior research—perhaps this person has not been born yet. And of course, these persons need certain bases to work from: leisure, freedom from religious and political dogma, and social support. They are like creative artists. Someday, that person will arrive in our field. Also, future technology certainly will provide tools to advance inquiry.

Until that day, the material in this chapter can be of use. Please focus on the perspectives of counteracting antecedents of the health behavior, modifying the behavior of interest, or removing the association of the behavior from its consequences. That is a great start for health behavior program development. And please remember that a good theory will begin with a set of concepts that provides a taxonomy, or principles of classification, for the various entities covered by the theory, which allows for the discovery of lawlike relations between these entities. In so doing, causal histories of events can be defined in terms of past events that conform to the regularities governing the entities so categorized. Theories start with good, useful ideas. These ideas can come from anywhere, so keep your eyes open.

► REFERENCES

BERNARD, L. C., & KRUPAT, E. (1994). *Health psychology: Biopsychosocial factors in health and illness.* Fort Worth, TX: Holt, Rinehart.

BYRNE, C., BROWN, B., VOORBERG, N., & SCHOFIELD, R. (1994). Wellness education for individuals with chronic mental illness living in the community. *Issues in Mental Health Nursing, 15,* 239-252.

CHASSIN, L. A., PRESSON, C. C., & SHERMAN, S. J. (1985). Stepping backward in order to step forward: An acquisition-oriented approach to primary prevention. *Journal of Consulting and Clinical Psychology, 53,* 612-622.

COWEN, E. L. (1984). A general structural model for primary prevention program development in mental health. *Personnel & Guidance Journal, 62,* 485-490.

ELDER, J. P., & STERN, R. A. (1986). The ABCs of adolescent smoking prevention: An environment and skills model. *Health Education Quarterly, 13,* 181-191.

FREIMUTH, V. S., & METTGER, W. (1990). Is there a hard-to-reach audience? *Public Health Reports, 105,* 232-238.

GUARNECCIA, P. J., & RODRIGUEZ, O. (1996). Concepts of culture and their role in the development of culturally competent mental health services. *Hispanic Journal of Behavioral Sciences, 18,* 419-443.

HANSEN, W. B. (1992). School-based substance abuse prevention: A review of the state of the art in curriculum, 1980-1990. *Health Education Research: Theory and Practice, 7,* 403-430.

HAYES, S. C. (1998). Building a useful relationship between "applied" and "basic" science in behavior therapy. *The Behavior Therapist, 21,* 109-112.

HEISE, D. R. (1975). *Causal analysis.* New York: John Wiley.

HIRAYAMA, K. K., HIRAYAMA, H., & CETINGOK, M. (1993). Mental health promotion for South East Asian refugees from the USA. *International Social Work, 36,* 119-129.

KAPLAN, R. M. (1984). The connection between clinical health promotion and health status: A critical overview. *American Psychologist, 39,* 755-765.

LEFEBVRE, R. C., & FLORA, J. A. (1988). Social marketing and public health intervention. *Health Education Quarterly, 15,* 299-315.

MACKINNON, D. P., JOHNSON, C. A., PENTZ, M. A., DWYER, J. H., HANSEN, W. B., FLAY, B. R., & WANG, E. Y. (1991). Mediating mechanisms in a school-based drug prevention program: First-year effects of the Midwestern Prevention Program. *Health Psychology, 10,* 164-172.

MARCONI, K. M., & RUDZINSKI, K. A. (1995). A formative model to evaluate health services research. *Evaluation Review, 10,* 501-510.

McCAUL, K. D., & GLASGOW, R. E. (1985). Preventing adolescent smoking: What have we learned about treatment construct validity? *Health Psychology, 4,* 361-387.

McLEROY, K. R., STECKLER, A. B., SIMONS-MORTON, B., GOODMAN, R. M., GOTTLIEB, N., & BURDINE, J. N. (1993). Social science theory in health education: Time for a new model? *Health Education Research: Theory and Practice, 8,* 305-312.

MIDDLESTADT, S. E., BHATTACHARYYA, K., ROSENBAUM, J., FISHBEIN, M., & SHEPHERD, M. (1996). The use of theory based semistructured elicitation questionnaires: Formative research for CDC's prevention marketing initiative. *Public Health Reports, 111*(Suppl. 1), 18-27.

PENTZ, M. A., BONNIE, R. J., & SHOPLAND, D. R. (1996) Integrating supply and demand reduction strategies for drug abuse prevention. *American Behavioral Scientist, 39,* 897-910.

PETRAITIS, J., FLAY, B. R., & MILLER, T. Q. (1995). Reviewing theories of adolescent substance abuse: Organizing pieces in the puzzle. *Psychological Bulletin, 117,* 67-86.

RUDNER, R. S. (1966). *Philosophy of social science.* Englewood Cliffs, NJ: Prentice Hall.
STACY, A. W., SUSSMAN, S., DENT, C. W., BURTON, D., & FLAY, B. R. (1992). Moderators of peer social influence in adolescent smoking. *Personality and Social Psychology Bulletin, 18,* 163-172.
SUSSMAN, S. (1989). Two social influence perspectives of tobacco use development and prevention. *Health Education Research: Theory and Practice, 4,* 213-223.
SUSSMAN, S., DENT, C. W., BURTON, D., STACY, A. W., & FLAY, B. R. (1995). *Developing school-based tobacco use prevention and cessation programs.* Thousand Oaks, CA: Sage.
SUSSMAN, S., SIMON, T. R., GLYNN, S. M., & STACY, A. W. (1996). What does "high risk" mean? A PsycINFO scan of the literature. *Behavior Therapy, 27,* 53-66.
VAN RYN, M., & HEANEY, C. A. (1992). What's the use of theory? *Health Education Quarterly, 19,* 315-330.
VICARY, J. R., DOEBLER, M. K., BRIDGER, J. C., & GURGEVICH, E. A. (1996). A community systems approach to substance abuse prevention in a rural setting. *Journal of Primary Prevention, 16,* 303-318.
WALLERSTEIN, N., & SANCHEZ, M. V. (1994). Freirian praxis in health education: Research results from an adolescent prevention program. *Health Education Research, 9,* 105-118.
WORDEN, J. K., FLYNN, B. S., GELLER, B. M., CHEN, M., SHELTON, L. G., SECKER-WALKER, R. H., SOLOMON, D. S., SOLOMON, C. J., COUCHEY, S., & COSTANZA, M. C. (1988). Development of a smoking prevention mass media program using diagnostic and formative research. *Preventive Medicine, 17,* 531-558.

CHAPTER 4

Commentary

Hope Landrine
Elizabeth A. Klonoff

Steve and Alan Sussman described the nature of theory, detailed the steps for developing theory, outlined procedures for evaluating the quality of theories, and argued logically and convincingly about the importance of theory for developing effective health intervention programs. Here we simply add two additional points to their cogent presentation. The first is something to be done before creating a theory, and the second is to be done after the theory has been developed.

First, the authors of the prior chapter noted that theories and interventions always address a specific target behavior. We agree that this is necessarily the case but add that defining the target behavior is a difficult process. In the absence of a culturally appropriate definition and conceptualization of the target behavior, theories about that behavior and theory-driven interventions designed to modify it may fail with ethnic minorities but succeed with Whites. Thus, we offer new ways of defining the target behavior so that theories are culturally sensitive and ensuing interventions are effective with a variety of ethnic groups. Carefully defining the target behavior is a step to be taken before developing a theory.

Second, the authors indicated throughout their chapter that we can think of a theory as a map of a terrain, and that a good theory fits the terrain well (i.e., is empirically supported by brute data). Discussing this logical-positivist, correspondence theory of truth is beyond the scope and purpose of this commentary, and hence we simply add this: The map (also) creates both the terrain and the ensuing data in a manner that has consequences for science and society. Thus, we offer additional ways of evaluating a theory in terms of its potential impact. Carefully considering the larger implications of a theory for science, society, and socially constructed reality is the final step to be taken after the theory has been developed.

DEFINING THE TARGET BEHAVIOR

There are two ways that we can think about the target behavior. The first of these has been called *mechanistic* (Biglan, Glasgow, & Singer, 1990; Hayes & Hayes, 1992; Morris, 1988; Pepper, 1942) and is what social and health scientists usually have in mind when they speak of developing theories about and programs to change a target behavior.

Mechanistic Behaviorism. In the mechanistic way of conceptualizing behavior, behavior is understood as superficial, mechanical movements whose name is contingent on the precise features of those movements. For example, "reading a newspaper" is a movement with specific features and so is a type of behavior. "Unprotected anal intercourse" similarly is a specific set of movements and is an additional type of behavior. Behavior is defined and labeled in terms of the precise features of superficial mechanical movements *irrespective of the context in which such movements occur*. Reading a newspaper is a type of behavior and is the same type of behavior irrespective of the social or cultural context in which it appears. Thus, "picking up a newspaper and reading it while riding the subway on one's way to work" and "picking up a newspaper and reading it in the middle of a serious discussion with your significant other" are the same behavior, irrespective of these different contexts. Certainly, different contingencies surround these two episodes of reading the newspaper: The episodes have different causes or antecedents (the A in ABC) and different consequences (the C in ABC), and all would agree with that. Nonetheless, the behavior (the B in ABC) is defined as "reading the newspaper" in both cases. The essence of mechanistic behaviorism, then, is the assumption that movements have a meaning and a label and have one and the same meaning and label, irrespective of the context in which they are exhibited.

This mechanistic view of behavior dominates the social and health sciences, irrespective of whether researchers consider themselves to be "behaviorists." When we theorize about and develop programs to change "risky sexual behavior" or "aggressive behavior" or "smoking," we define behavior in each case as a specific set of superficial, mechanical movements abstracted from their context; we mean constellations of movements that have a label and a meaning irrespective of their context. The name for these various movements is assumed to be inherent in the movements themselves. Behaviors are assumed to have only one label and meaning that they carry with them like designer luggage across time, race, ethnicity, gender, social class, age, and international borders. Hence, when we define and understand *behavior* as superficial-mechanical movements with an inherent meaning irrespective of context, we produce a multitude of "types" or "categories" of behavior out there in the world. We construct (create) C, a social world filled with a multitude of behavioral shoes that everyone everywhere can and does walk in. From this perspective, then, any person of any culture, gender, age, social class, or ethnicity who engages in the specific set of movements is, by definition and necessarily, engaging in the same behavior irrespective of their different sociocultural contexts.

This way of thinking has two serious consequences for our theories about behavior and for the health programs that we develop to change behavior, namely: If behavior is a set of movements that have a label and meaning irrespective of their sociocultural context, such that all people who engage in the movements are engaging in "the same" behavior, then (a) only one theory about "the behavior" is required, and (b) only one intervention is needed to modify it. Given that mechanism dominates health behavior research, this indeed is what health behavior researchers have done and continue to do: We develop a single theory about the target behavior with the assumption that the theory predicts the behavior irrespective of the gender or culture (context) of the individual who exhibits it; then we develop a single intervention to modify that target behavior with the assumption that it will be effective for everyone. More often than not, we find that the theory only predicts the behavior for Whites and for boys and men and does not predict for women, girls, Latinos, and Blacks, let alone Asians or American Indians. Likewise, far too often we find that the intervention was effective for boys but not for girls and for Whites but not for Latinos or Blacks (National Institutes of Health [NIH], 1992). We then wonder where we went wrong, and, whatever theory we develop next to explain the failure of our prior theory and its associated intervention, chances are that we will not see implicit, mechanistic behaviorism as the problem.

Contextualistic Behaviorism. The alternative way of thinking about behavior has been called contextualistic behaviorism or contextualism (Biglan et al., 1990; Hayes & Hayes, 1992; Morris, 1988; Rosnow & Georgoudi, 1986). In the contextualistic way of thinking about behavior, behavior is understood as a meaningful exchange with and in a context. From this perspective, behavior and its context are a single unit. Behavior is not a superficial-mechanical movement irrespective of context but rather is a highly specific act in context. The context is part of the name for the behavior, for the act in context. Consequently, from this perspective, a movement does not have a single label and meaning but rather several different labels and meanings, depending on the context in which it appears because that context is part of what the behavior in context is called.

For example, from a contextualistic perspective, "picking up a newspaper and reading it on the subway on one's way to work" and "picking up a newspaper and reading it in the middle of a serious discussion with your significant other" are not the same behavior; they are not both "reading the newspaper" because their contexts are different. The first behavior is "killing time on the subway" or "avoiding the potentially hostile strangers on the subway by not looking at them," in which the context is part of the name of the behavior. The second behavior is "ignoring your partner" or "letting your partner know that you don't want to have this conversation," in which the context again is part of the name of the behavior. When defined contextually, these are two very different behaviors despite the similarity of the superficial-mechanical movements entailed. These two acts in context are elicited by different stimuli (different As in ABC) and are maintained by different consequences (different Cs in ABC) and so elicit very different responses from others. For example, most people probably would not have a problem with their significant other's picking up a newspaper and reading it on the subway while on the way to work. But most people probably would respond with some irritation at a significant other who picks up a newspaper and reads it in the middle of a serious conversation, during a holiday dinner, while in synagogue or church, or while making love. In the psychology of our everyday lives, we do not label and understand behavior as superficial movements. Instead, we think contextually—we use the context to tell us what the behavior is, what it means, and how to respond. Thus, most people would reject the idea that a partner who picked up a newspaper and started reading it in the middle of a serious discussion was merely "reading the newspaper" and, indeed, would insist that the behavior was everything but that.

Hence, from this perspective, behaviors have no inherent label or meaning, no matter how obvious, thereon-the-surface, self-evident, and inherent in superficial-mechanical movements a label and meaning seem to be. Instead, the label for a behavior is to be discovered empirically through a functional analysis of the behavior; the name for the behavior is to be discovered by examining the contextual antecedents and consequences of it.

Likewise, from this perspective, similar mechanical movements appearing in different contexts are not the same behavior. They are different behaviors, unless an empirical analysis of their discriminative stimuli and contingencies indicates otherwise. As radical as this view may at first seem, it has ample empirical support. For example, studies have shown that even among White couples and families of the 1980s in the United States, whether a movement is labeled *hitting, helping, aggression,* or *affection* is contingent not on the act but on the structure and form of the relationship in which it occurs, on the context. These labels and meanings are socially constructed and negotiated in relationships. The manner in which these labels are applied to specific movements does not generalize across relationships of various types, such that these labels are by and large independent of the movements themselves (see Gergen & Gergen, 1983; Greenblat, 1983; Harre, 1981; Kayser, Swinger, & Cohen, 1984; Lasswell & Lasswell, 1976; Mummendey, Bonewasser, Loschper, & Lenneweber, 1982; Tedeschi, 1984). Such data indicate that ordinary people understand behavior contextually. This suggests that our theories about people's behavior and our interventions designed to modify their behavior should be similarly contextualistic.

The contextualistic way of thinking has two serious consequences for our theories about behavior and for the health programs that we develop to change behavior, namely: If the name for and meaning of behavior are tied to its context such that people of different sociocultural contexts who engage in similar movements are *not* engaging in the same behavior, then (a) multiple theories about the behavior in its sociocultural context are required, and (b) multiple interventions that are tailored to each sociocultural context are needed to modify each specific behavior in context. This, indeed, is what the NIH (1992) concluded about how to improve health behavior theories, research, and interventions for minority groups (although the NIH did not describe the problem as an issue of implicit, mechanistic assumptions). An example of the contextualistic approach to developing theories about and interventions to modify health behavior will clarify these points.

CONTEXTUALISTIC THEORIES AND PROGRAMS

The contextualistic approach entails four steps: (a) We begin with the assumption that when we are observing members of cultures other than our own, we do not know what kind of behavior we are observing; discovering what the behavior is called and means is an empirical question. (b) Hence, we gather information on the antecedents, consequences, and correlates of the behavior *in that context* by talking to people; we then define and label the target behavior as a behavior in a specific sociocultural context. (c) Next, we develop a theory about the behavior in its sociocultural context, following the clear steps that Steve and Alan Sussman so carefully detailed. (d) Finally, we design an intervention that modifies the antecedents, consequences, or both of the specific sociocultural context to create change.

Example: "Unprotected Anal Intercourse." Recent studies have found that the prevalence of AIDS among young Latinas is significantly higher than for other gender-ethnic groups (e.g., Mays & Cochran, 1988). Other studies (e.g., Arguello, 1993) indicate that this ethnic difference is in part a function of differences in the frequency of engaging in unprotected anal intercourse; this specific, risky sexual behavior appears to be frequent only among young, inner-city, unmarried, heterosexual Latinas—especially those who are members of gangs (Arguello, 1993).

The standard, mechanistic-behavioral approach to reducing AIDS among this population would be to define the target behavior as "unprotected anal intercourse." By that we would mean a specific set of movements that anyone anywhere can engage in, with these movements presumed to have the same meaning irrespective of their sociocultural context. The researcher then might develop a reasonable theory of the behavior so defined, based on his or her hunches, namely: that these specific, young, lower-class Latinas lack information about the risks entailed in this behavior and so require AIDS education. A program providing such information then would be designed based on this theory. The program might even be (ostensibly) "culturally tailored"—that is, delivered in Spanish by Latinos. The program would have no effect whatsoever on the behavior, and the researcher would discover that these Latina gang members already knew quite well how AIDS is transmitted (Arguello, 1993). The mechanistic approach yielded a theory and an intervention that did not work. We are left wondering what went wrong.

The alternative approach, the contextual approach, begins with the assumption that the name for this behavior is to be discovered empirically through a careful analysis of its context. The first step is to discover what the behavior in context is and what it means by talking informally to the young Latinas who engage in it. Arguello (1993) and her colleagues at the Center for the Study of Latino Health in Los Angeles did precisely that. What they found was that these young, unmarried, Latina gang members were engaging in anal intercourse to maintain their virginity. As unmarried Roman Catholic women, men demanded that they be virgins when they finally married but also demanded intercourse. Anal intercourse was a solution to these contradictory demands: It was a way for women to have intercourse yet still remain virgins for men who demanded both—in a larger, sociocultural context in which women need the financial support of these men and had negotiated this solution with them. Condoms were not used because condoms were conceptualized as a means of birth control, and birth control is not an issue when intercourse is anal.

When contextually defined as an act in context, the behavior here is not "unprotected anal intercourse" except in the most superficial way of thinking about people. For these Latinas, the behavior is "trying to maintain virginity for but still have intercourse with men who are demanding both," and that surely is not the same behavior that gay men engage in when they exhibit similar superficial, mechanical movements. The contingencies that control the behavior also differ for different groups. For these specific Latinas, the contingency is the aversive consequences of losing your virginity before you are married in a cultural context in which men value women's virginity; the consequence was rendering yourself un-marryable and was viewed by Arguello's (1993) sample as more aversive than the possibility of contracting AIDS.

When defined contextually as "trying to maintain virginity for and simultaneously have intercourse with men who demand both," the context-specific and culturally specific contingencies surrounding this behavior in context are obvious, as are several contextualistic and culturally specific interventions entailing manipulating those contingencies. At the simple level, the intervention could stress the need to use condoms without addressing the act in context. At a more fundamental level, the intervention should be a feminist one that addresses virginity, the sexual double standard, and young Latinos' control of Latinas' sexuality. Arguello (1993) and her colleagues designed such an intervention (i.e., a series of feminist workshops titled "Virginity as Oppression" and "Who Owns Latinas' Bodies?"). These workshops were significantly more effective than any standard AIDS education intervention and led to rejection of the tyranny of virginity and to vaginal intercourse with condoms. Such an intervention (the workshops) would be irrelevant to gay men because their behavior is not the same as the behavior of these Latinas.

The distinction between mechanistic versus contextual approaches to defining the target behavior is similar to the difference between etic and emic approaches to research and theory making, in which these latter terms stem from Pike (1967). The term *etic* refers to the outsider's—the researcher's—perspective and entails defining and interpreting behavior through the researcher's own cultural dictionary and categories. Etic approaches to defining target behaviors have as their hallmark the elevation of observers (researchers) to the status of ultimate "judges of the categories and concepts used in descriptions and analyses . . . [these categories are not] necessarily real, meaningful and appropriate from the native's [the research participant's] point of view" (Harris, 1980, p. 32). Research and theory driven by an implicit etic framework focus on mechanistic movements.

Emic, on the other hand, refers to the insider's—the research participant's—perspective and entails participants' descriptions, definitions, categorizations, and explanations of their behaviors' meaning and function, typically with categories and labels that differ from those of the researcher. Emic approaches to defining target behaviors

> have as their hallmark the elevation of the native informant to the status of ultimate judge of the adequacy of the observer's descriptions and analyses. The test of [the success of emic approaches] is their ability to generate statements that the native accepts as real, meaningful, or appropriate. (Harris, 1980, p. 32)

Research and theory driven by an implicit emic framework focus on contextualized behaviors. Pike (1967) argued that our (notoriously) etic theories must be informed by emic approaches and data. Indeed, Pike argued that only emic data constitute "truth" and saw etic data and definitions as necessary, preliminary evils that provide "access into the system" (p. 38). Specifically, Pike's advice to theorists was that their "etic description gradually be refined, and . . . ultimately . . . replaced by one which is totally emic" (pp. 38-39).

Likewise, then, we suggest that emic or contextual approaches be added to theory making at the very beginning—as the first step—so that the researcher's definition and conceptualization of the target behavior match that of participants. We believe that this is important in all theory making. Thus, for example, at the start of their chapter, the authors provided an example of a bad theory related to drinking in the workplace and driving drunk, as well as its associated failed intervention. We suggest that in that example, the theorist failed to conceptualize and define the target behavior contextually (emically) and that this led to creating the bad theory. Although we believe contextualism to be an essential step in defining the target behavior of all people, we see it as particularly important when developing theories that are meant to apply to multiple ethnic groups.

In summary, we suggest that theories that are meant to apply to the health behavior of a variety of ethnic-cultural groups (a) must define the target behavior in a manner that has meaning for each group and (b) must include predictor, moderator, and mediator variables specific to each group's cultural context. This brings us to the question of what maps do to terrains.

MAPS, TERRAINS, AND THE SOCIAL CONSTRUCTION OF REALITY

A theory may indeed be a map of a terrain, but the theory itself creates—it socially constructs—the terrain. A theory entails imposing interpretations (definitions, categories, and understandings) on behavior. Once we have a theory in mind, we pose questions that take those definitions, categories, and understandings for granted. We do not ask about all variables that might be relevant but only about those we have already defined as relevant; hence, that is all that we discover about the terrain, and the terrain then matches the theory because the theory created it. The great philosopher of science, Charles Taylor (1979), put it this way:

> Let us say that we are trying to understand the goals and values of a certain group . . . we might try to probe this by a questionnaire asking them whether they assent or not to a number of propositions which are meant to express different goals, evaluations, beliefs. But how did we design the questionnaire? How did we pick *these* propositions? Here we relied on our understandings of [our theories about] the goals, values, vision involved. [Because] this understanding can be challenged . . . the significance of our results [is questionable]. (p. 41)

How we ask the questions determines the answers (Schwarz, 1999). A few examples may clarify this point.

Suppose that we have noticed that certain expressive behaviors (consideration for others, passivity) seem to be common among the women we know in our sociocultural context, whereas certain instrumental behaviors (assertiveness, ambitiousness) seem to be common among the men we know in our sociocultural context. We develop the theory that these patterns of behavior are gender related, and so we define them as "feminine" and "masculine," respectively. We then develop a questionnaire to examine the possibility that these behaviors represent femininity and masculinity by testing the extent to which expressive behaviors are endorsed by women and instrumental ones by men. When we find that this indeed is the case, we believe that our theory matches the terrain and that we therefore have discovered something significant about people. There are several problems with this.

The first is that our theory of femininity and masculinity led us to design a survey that asked about expressive and instrumental behaviors alone. Other behaviors that did not fit neatly into the categorization scheme that we imposed on behavior (i.e., academic behavior, values, work-related behavior, diet, exercise, prejudice, and countless other behaviors) were omitted. Because the theory limited our questions, all that we can discover is what we asked. Our data are not brute empirical facts but are theory-laden facts—our data are themselves impositions of categories on behavior, and they are interpretations of behavior (see Morawski, 1985, on this issue). The map fits the terrain because the map created the terrain by sculpting it into a particular form by the questions asked. But this is only the beginning of the problem.

Ten years later, the theory has reached the general public, and thousands—perhaps millions—of people now think of themselves as feminine or masculine. The theory has created the terrain; it has socially constructed reality as a gendered one (Morawski, 1985). Human behaviors that are exhibited by all people are now understood as women's versus men's. The fact that in some cultures (e.g., Japan), the behaviors now categorized as women's are displayed primarily by men is lost. Although we would view it as racist to define those behaviors as "Japaninity," no one sees it as sexist to call them "femininity." Twenty years later, men and women are understood as different "types" of people who display such radically different "types" of behavior that they could be from different planets; "women are from Venus, men are from Mars" becomes a popular phrase. Reality has been changed by the theory and changed in a manner that has negative consequences for a group of people—namely, women (see Morawski, 1985). That both women and men are from Earth and are exhibiting human behavior is simply forgotten.

The theory of stress is a health-related example of how theories construct and change reality. In the 1950s, Hans Selye (1956) theorized that the various upsets that people must adjust to and feel burdened by could all be conceptualized as similar to the strain placed on metal. At the time, the term *stress* referred to physical strain on metal that could be measured objectively and indeed was visible to the naked eye (Pollack, 1988). Selye applied the term *stress* to people. Ten years later, social and health scientists adopted the theory, and thousands of articles appeared on the health impact of stress—an immaterial, ethereal, supernatural force whose existence cannot be empirically demonstrated. In these studies, surveys were designed to ask people about events that are burdensome (now called stressful events), and millions of other events that people experience but that do not fit neatly into the category were omitted. The theory imposed a categorization scheme on experience; it limited the questions that were asked and found answers only to what was asked (i.e., it yielded theory-laden data). Thus, studies discovered that people do indeed find stressful events to be upsetting and to be a burden, and hence the events have consequences for their physical and mental health.

Thirty years later, the theory reached the general public, and millions of people now think of themselves as stressed and interpret events in their lives—and their health—in terms of stress. Employee assistance programs offer stress management, physicians advise patients to reduce their stress, books and tapes about stress abound, stress is a defense in criminal trials, and federal funds for investigating stress exist. The map changed the terrain; the theory altered reality so fundamentally that now everyone knows what stress "is" and attributes a variety of behaviors and outcomes to "it." That all of us experience some events as burdensome and others as uplifting has been forgotten, and we now experience those same events as stressful versus nonstressful. Likewise, that the term *stress* once meant the physical strain on metal has been forgotten as well. Stress is "a modern mythology" created by a theory steeped in Western-industrial cultural values and concerns (Pollack, 1988).

These examples are meant to highlight two points. First, there are no brute, objective facts in any science of human beings; all facts are theory laden and indeed are interpretations of behavior. Specifically, four levels of interpretation enter research. *The first level is the researcher's theory about behavior.* The researcher's interpretations (understandings) of behavior lead to surveys and experiments that are theory saturated (Schwarz, 1999; Taylor, 1979). Researchers' theories also reflect their values, prejudices, social context, gender, and ethnicity (Collins & Pinch, 1982; Knorr, Krohn, & Whitley, 1980; Latour & Woolgar, 1979). Thus, women would never develop a theory that interprets women's behavior as indicative of penis envy, and Blacks would never develop a theory that interprets racial differences in IQ scores as biologically determined. *The second level is that of the research participants* who interpret the survey questions, the researcher's behavior, and their own behavior during the study. These interpretations are powerful variables in how research participants behave (Antaki, 1981; Miller, 1984; Sabini & Silver, 1981). Some subjects try to please the researcher by providing the answer that they believe the researcher desires, others nay-say (endorse the lowest answer), still others yea-say (endorse the highest answer), and others try to outwit the experimenter—with all of these patterns strongly predicted by ethnicity (Landrine, Klonoff, & Brown-Collins, 1992; NIH, 1992).

The third level is that of the researcher who now categorizes (interprets) the research participants' behaviors, answers, and scores when these interpretations may bear little resemblance to what the subjects meant and are biased in favor of the theory (Rabinow & Sullivan, 1979; Taylor, 1979). How researchers interpret participants' behavior is culturally and socially determined and is embedded in their values, context, power, privilege, gender, and need to get published (Collins & Pinch, 1982; Knorr et al., 1980; Latour & Woolgar, 1979). Finally, *the fourth level is the researcher's interpretation of the data from the study.* These data are mute (Feyerabend, 1976) and do not speak for or against any theory. What we take to be the voice of the data is the researcher's interpretation of them. Such interpretations differ significantly, as indicated by ongoing debates over the meaning of data on racial differences in IQ scores.

Thus, studies involving human beings have never yielded or entailed objective observations or brute behavioral data; rather, they have entailed and yielded *in-*

terpretations of interpretations of interpretations of interpretations, each level of which is in part culturally determined and situated. Scientific facts are socially constructed (Latour & Woolgar, 1979). This brings us to our second (and major) point.

Given the many (by and large highly personal) (see Polanyi, 1974) interpretations entailed in theory making and testing, and given that these interpretations socially construct reality—they change the terrain—it is crucial that we are careful about what we theorize. It is critical that theorists consider the larger implications of their theory for the group being theorized about. Theories do not simply lead to interventions that do or do not work; they also lead to public policies, legal decisions, changes in allocation of state and federal funding for various public programs, changes in how people think about themselves, and changes in the relations between various social and cultural groups (Edelman, 1977). Thus, after one has developed a theory (and before testing it), it is important to ask these questions to evaluate the quality of the theory: What does this theory say about my values, biases, and social status? What impact might this theory have on how those I am theorizing about (e.g., women, minorities, teenagers) will be regarded and treated? Is it possible that this theory (my *personal* interpretation and understanding of behavior) may lead to negative outcomes for a group? How will this theory change reality, and are those changes of benefit to society? If one's answer is that one's theory has the potential to harm groups, relations between groups, or society, then the theory is a bad theory.

To Steve and Alan Sussman's list of ways to evaluate a theory, we add the above—namely, that the theory be evaluated in terms of its impact on society. We suggest that a "good" theory is one that advances both science and society, rather than science alone. In addition, Pike (1967) suggested that a "good" theory is one that those who are being theorized about would find to be an acceptable and accurate account of their behavior. To their list of ways to evaluate a theory, we add this emic criterion as well and believe that it can improve the cultural sensitivity of theory and therefore the cultural appropriateness of interventions.

REFERENCES

ANTAKI, C. (1981). *The psychology of ordinary explanations.* London: Academic Press.

ARGUELLO, M. (1993, February). *Developing outreach programs for AIDS prevention with Latino youth.* Paper presented at the Institute for Health Promotion and Disease Prevention Research, University of Southern California Medical School, Los Angeles.

BIGLAN, A., GLASGOW, R. E., & SINGER, G. (1990). The need for a science of larger social units: A contextual approach. *Behavior Therapy, 21,* 195-215.

COLLINS, H. M., & PINCH, T. J. (1982). *Frames of meaning: The social construction of extraordinary science.* London: Routledge Kegan Paul.

EDELMAN, M. (1977). *Political language: Words that succeed and policies that fail.* New York: Academic Press.

FEYERABEND, P. (1976). *Against method: Outline of an anarchist theory of knowledge.* New York: Humanities.

GERGEN, K., & GERGEN, M. (1983). The social construction of helping relationships. In J. D. Fisher, A. Nadler, & B. DePaulo (Eds.), *New directions in helping* (Vol. 1, pp. 7-18). New York: Academic Press.

GREENBLAT, C. S. (1983). A hit is a hit is a hit . . . or is it? In sfamily violence research (pp. 3-12). Beverly Hills, CA: Sage.

HARRE, R. (1981). Expressive aspects of descriptions of others. In C. Antaki (Ed.), *The psychology of ordinary explanations.* London: Academic Press.

HARRIS, M. (1980). *Cultural materialism: The struggle for a science of culture.* New York: Vintage.

HAYES, S. C., & HAYES, L. J. (1992). Some clinical implications of contextualistic behaviorism. *Behavior Therapy, 23,* 225-249.

KAYSER, E., SWINGER, T., & COHEN, R. (1984). Laypersons' conceptions of social relationships. *Journal of Social and Personal Relationships, 1,* 433-458.

KNORR, K. D., KROHN, R., & WHITLEY, R. (1980). *The social process of scientific investigation.* Dordrecht, the Netherlands: Reidel.

LANDRINE, H., KLONOFF, E. A., & BROWN-COLLINS, A. (1992). Cultural diversity and methodology in feminist psychology: Critique, proposal, empirical example. *Psychology of Women Quarterly, 16,* 145-163.

LASSWELL, T., & LASSWELL, M. (1976). I love you but I'm not in love with you. *Journal of Marriage and Family Counseling, 38,* 211-224.

LATOUR, B., & WOOLGAR, S. (1979). *Laboratory life: The social construction of scientific facts.* Beverly Hills, CA: Sage.

MAYS, V. M., & COCHRAN, S. D. (1988). Issues in the perception of AIDS risk and risk reduction activities by Black and Hispanic/Latina women. *American Psychologist, 43,* 949-957.

MILLER, J. G. (1984). Culture and the development of everyday social explanation. *Journal of Personality and Social Psychology, 46,* 961-978.

MORAWSKI, J. G. (1985). The measurement of masculinity and femininity: Engendering categorical realities. *Journal of Personality, 53,* 196-223.

MORRIS, E. K. (1988). Contextualism: The world view of behavior analysis. *Journal of Experimental Child Psychology, 46,* 289-323.

MUMMENDEY, A., BONEWASSER, M., LOSCHPER, G., & LENNEWEBER, V. (1982). It is always somebody else who is aggressive. *Zeitschrift für Sozialpsychologie, 13,* 341-325.

NATIONAL INSTITUTES OF HEALTH (NIH). (1992). *Health behavior research in minority populations: Access, design, and implementation* (NIH Pub. No. 92-2965). Washington, DC: U.S. Department of Health and Human Services, Public Health Service, National Institutes of Health.

PEPPER, S. C. (1942). *World hypotheses: A study in evidence.* Berkeley: University of California Press.

PIKE, K. (1967). *Language in relation to a unified theory of the structure of human behavior* (2nd ed.). The Hague, the Netherlands: Mouton.

POLANYI, M. (1974). *Personal knowledge: Towards a post-critical philosophy.* Chicago: University of Chicago Press.

POLLACK, K. (1988). On the nature of social stress: Production of a modern mythology. *Social Science & Medicine, 26,* 381-392.

RABINOW, P., & SULLIVAN, W. M. (1979). *Interpretive social science.* Berkeley: University of California Press.

ROSNOW, R. L., & GEORGOUDI, M. (1986). *Contextualism and understanding in behavioral science.* New York: Praeger.

SABINI, J., & SILVER, M. (1981). Introspection and causal accounts. *Journal of Personality and Social Psychology, 40,* 171-179.

SCHWARZ, N. (1999). Self-reports: How the questions shape the answers. *American Psychologist, 54,* 93-105.

SELYE, H. (1956). *The stress of life.* New York: McGraw-Hill.

TAYLOR, C. (1979). Interpretation and sciences of man. In P. Rabinow & W. M. Sullivan (Eds.), *Interpretive social science* (pp. 25-71). Berkeley: University of California Press.

TEDESCHI, T. (1984). A social psychological interpretation of human aggression. In A. Mummendey (Ed.), *Social psychology of aggression* (pp. 8-20). Berlin: Springer-Verlag.

Case Study 2

CHAPTER 5

Implicit Cognition Theory in Drug Use and Driving-Under-the-Influence Interventions

Alan W. Stacy
Susan L. Ames

In this chapter, we outline a recently corroborated theory of health behavior and how it can be applied to prevention research. Although it exemplifies important features of theory development described in Chapter 4, it represents a major departure from previous theories of health behavior and from some public health approaches. Indeed, it is sometimes argued that in a public health approach, the exact mechanism responsible for prevention effects may not need to be known. This text and the present authors disagree with this assertion with respect to health-behavior change, noting that public health approaches using inoculations have much basic science backing them. If a complex bioactive agent is uncovered that has certain promising effects as a pos-

AUTHORS' NOTE: This chapter was supported in part by grants DA 10353 and DA 07601 from the National Institute on Drug Abuse.

sible vaccine, intensive research is visually undertaken to isolate the effective component before it is used in clinical trials and eventually as a vaccine. Although the analogy is obviously not complete because of inherent complexities in educational programs in health behavior work, educational programs that are effective can easily drift to ineffectiveness during dissemination if the effective ingredient of the program is not clearly understood. Thus, it is important to fully understand how health behavior programs, such as prevention campaigns, work. To the extent that theoretical mechanisms involved in prevention programming are understood, prevention work can become *prevention science*. To fully understand how prevention programs work, as well as how health-related habits are determined, we need to consider a wide range of plausible alternative processes.

In this chapter, we take the position that most prevention research has addressed only a subset of the etiological processes that may underlie drug use and driving under the influence (DUI) of drugs. For example, most prevention research has focused mostly on several theories from social psychology, social learning, and personality. Theories that have been developed in basic research in memory, neurobiology, learning, and allied fields have been mostly ignored. The present approach focuses on one of these areas derived from basic research: memory and implicit cognition. The theory behind this approach is first outlined in some detail. Then, it is demonstrated how principles from the approach can be applied to interventions and their evaluation. Finally, the approach is applied to a booster intervention in an ongoing drug abuse prevention project among continuation high school students.

EXPLICIT VERSUS IMPLICIT COGNITIVE APPROACHES

Almost all research on cognitive processes and drug use has focused on theories and methods of *explicit cognition*, as defined by Greenwald and Banaji (1995). When explicit cognition is assessed, people are asked directly to introspect about the causes or correlates of their behavior through assessments such as beliefs, expectancies, or attitudes. Because participants are asked directly about these cognitions, these assessments also can be classified as measures of *metacognition*. Theories within this general framework apparently assume that such metacognitions accurately reflect the cognitive processes governing behavior. However, for at least two decades, some have questioned whether such methods could possibly reflect fundamental aspects of human cognition (Nisbett & Wilson, 1977).

Another approach to cognition emphasizes the role of *implicit cognition*. Implicit cognition is revealed when past experience influences responses "in a fashion not introspectively known by the actor" (Greenwald & Banaji, 1995, p. 4). Research on human memory and other areas of cognitive science provides a great number of examples of how implicit cognition is studied. Beginning in the 1970s, researchers in these areas developed paradigms to study the implicit activation of concepts in memory (e.g., Meyer & Schvaneveldt, 1976), and theories were derived to explain how neural activation spreads automatically from one concept represented in memory to highly associated concepts in memory (e.g., Anderson, 1983). A variety of additional measures of implicit cognition have been studied in cognitive science in the 1980s and 1990s. Many of these measures are referred to as assessments of *implicit memory* because they assess memory for previous experiences without asking the subject to deliberately recollect those experiences (for review, see Roediger, 1990). During this same period, numerous theories have been developed to explain implicit memory and other types of implicit cognition phenomena. These theories include, for example, biologically based approaches that model neural networks (e.g., Hopfield & Tank, 1986; Masson, 1995) or that emphasize neurological systems underlying implicit memory (e.g., Squire, 1986; Tulving & Schacter, 1990), as well as approaches that focus on the transfer of memory performance from one situation to another (e.g., Roediger, 1990). Now, a large number of studies document the importance of implicit cognition phenomena, as well as theories that agree on at least some key points in the explanation of these phenomena. The importance of applying these phenomena to applied problems has been underscored since the mid-1980s (Greenwald, 1992; Greenwald & Banaji, 1995; Jacoby & Kelley, 1987; Kihlstrom, 1987). However, applications of this literature only recently have been attempted in health-related research.

One of the primary benefits of implicit cognition theory (ICT) is that measures of implicit cognition can assess cognitive processes that may be unavailable to introspection. Another benefit is that measures can be constructed to be relatively demand free because they do not inquire directly about one's behavior. Also, measures of implicit cognition can be constructed to unambiguously assess memory for the target concepts and their associations, rather than assess self-perceptions of one's own behavior (a confound that plagues research on explicit cognition) (see Feldman & Lynch, 1988). Finally, many implicit cognition measures map very well into formal theories of memory activation, some of which have received continued experimental support. We do not wish to suggest that this approach should necessarily replace research on explicit cognition. Rather, we wish to point out that research on implicit cognition is a largely untapped and promising approach to research on drug use and DUI.

Drug use investigators recently have begun using implicit cognition approaches. For example, Tiffany (1990) used such an approach theoretically by outlining how drug use may be motivated by an automatic memory process. Goldman and his colleagues outlined how alcohol use motivation may be represented by a semantic network of association in memory (e.g., Goldman, Brown, Christiansen, & Smith, 1991; Rather & Goldman, 1994), although implicit cognition assessments were not used. Stacy and his colleagues have shown that manipulations of the accessibility of drug-related cognitions from memory may influence drug use decisions (Stacy, Dent, et al., 1990), and measures of implicit memory for drug effects predict drug use cross-sectionally and prospectively (Ames & Stacy, 1998; Stacy, 1995, 1997; Stacy, Leigh, & Weingardt, 1994). Other research has shown important links between alcohol or other drug use and implicit cognition assessments (e.g., Doherty & Szalay, 1996; Earleywine, 1994; Hill & Paynter, 1992; Stormark & Hugdahl, 1997; Szalay, Inn, & Doherty, 1996). Recently, an implicit cognition theory of HIV risk behavior has been proposed (Stacy, Newcomb, & Ames, 2000). Taken together, these findings are consistent with biological approaches to health behavior motivation (e.g., Jaffe, 1989; Wise, 1988), which see memory processes as fundamental mediators. The implicit cognition framework in health behavior appears to be one of the most promising and neurologically plausible ways to construe and assess these mediators.

Previously published research on cognitive processes in drug abuse prevention (adult or adolescent) has focused entirely on explicit cognition. Much of this explicit cognition research has emphasized "rational human" or classical decision theory approaches (for recent reviews of adolescent drug use research, see Hawkins, Catalano, & Miller, 1992; Petraitis, Flay, & Miller, 1995; for examples of DUI research, see Donovan, 1993; Klepp, Perry, & Jacobs, 1991; Klitzner, Vegega, & Gruenewald, 1988; Turrisi & Jaccard, 1991). "Rational human" approaches assume explicitly that people weigh consequences and that these weightings *readily* influence behavior. Although some errors in weightings are acknowledged (e.g., Jaccard & Turrisi, 1987), explicit cognition approaches do not address memory activation or memory retrieval. Instead, they assume tacitly that all cognitions are equally and immediately accessible from memory to guide behavioral decisions. Theories of memory activation are not consistent with equal or immediate accessibility (for discussion, see Stacy et al., 1994). Explicit cognition frameworks certainly have their place and should be studied. However, the implicit cognition approach also deserves extensive research and may have an explanatory advantage when addressing self-destructive, apparently irrational behaviors.

IMPLICIT COGNITION THEORY IN DRUG USE, DUI, AND OTHER HEALTH BEHAVIORS

In the ICT approach to health behavior (Ames & Stacy, 1998; Stacy, 1997; Stacy et al., 1994), drug use and DUI decisions are influenced strongly by the current pattern of activation of concepts in memory. When one concept, or set of concepts, is strongly activated in memory, it implies that this concept and anything strongly related to this concept in memory are highly accessible. That is, it readily influences one's train of thought, it affects what "pops to mind," and it colors one's current interpretations, judgments, and performance of behaviors related to the concept. Numerous studies outside the drug use research area document that this type of effect occurs; some of these studies were cited earlier in our outline of previous research on implicit cognition.

With respect to drug use, an example will help illustrate how one's pattern of activation in memory can influence behavior. When a teenager wishes to have fun with friends after school or to relax on a Friday night, thoughts about these outcomes (e.g., having fun) are likely to promote a certain pattern of activation in memory, in which concepts previously associated with the outcome become strongly activated in memory. For some individuals, behavioral concepts such as marijuana or alcohol use become strongly activated and most highly accessible; driving activities involved in procuring or using drugs also may become highly activated in memory. In accord with the literature on implicit cognition, people do not have to deliberately recollect what they have done to have fun or relax in the past for this process to operate. Rather, these behaviors pop to mind spontaneously as a result of the prevailing circumstances and strong associations in memory between certain outcomes (or cues) and certain behaviors. We now outline the details of this process and its measurement.

In a number of studies, we have found that implicit measures of memory association provide good measures of the pattern of activation in memory that is elicited by drug-related cues, thoughts, and outcomes (Stacy, 1995, 1997; Stacy, Leigh, & Weingardt, 1993, 1994). In this approach, people differ in the strength of associations in memory between outcomes (e.g., relaxation) and behaviors (e.g., marijuana use), as well as between cues (e.g., seeing a friend) and behaviors (e.g., marijuana use). The strength of these associations determines whether a drug-consistent cognitive state and tendency to use drugs are readily activated by changing circumstances, as outlined below.

Strong outcome-behavior and cue-behavior associations have motivational significance. As introduced earlier, a strong association in memory between a given outcome and a behavior implies that when the outcome is thought about or desired, the behavior becomes strongly activated in memory as a behavioral option. In accord with our previous example, if life events or other cues prompt thoughts or desires related to relaxation, a certain behavioral option (marijuana use) becomes strongly activated in memory in individuals with strong relaxation-marijuana memory associations. Regarding cue-behavior associations, strong associations in memory imply that certain cues (e.g., drug stimuli or events at a party) will readily trigger cognitions related to drugs (for more details, see Stacy, 1995; Stacy et al., 1993). Strong accessibility or activation of a behavioral concept (e.g., marijuana use) is expected to influence subsequent responses, including those involving behavioral decisions (e.g., Fazio & Williams, 1986; Stacy, Dent, et al., 1990) and motor responses (McClelland & Rumelhart, 1985; cf. Tiffany, 1990). Thus, individuals with strong outcome-behavior and cue-behavior associations in memory should frequently be biased in their behavioral decisions regarding this behavior. When a drug-consistent pattern of activation is elicited by cues or thoughts of outcomes, it is unlikely that competing concepts (i.e., healthy alternatives) are simultaneously activated. This view is consistent with the neurological position that many cognitive processes involved in motivation are mutually inhibitory in the brain (Gray, 1987, 1990) and with research on memory documenting inhibitory processes (e.g., Dagenbach, Carr, & Barnhardt, 1990).

This all implies that drug-consistent tendencies become manifested in overt behavior (including drug use and DUI) when a particular pattern of activation is triggered (i.e., by cues, thoughts of outcomes). This pattern influences the ongoing train of thought and drug-related interpretations, thoughts, and desires or urges. Drug use becomes a highly accessible behavioral option and, in Gray's (1990) terms, steers the behavioral activation system toward drug use. This pattern of activation sometimes might be called a type of schema (e.g., Tiffany, 1990) or a type of cognitive set or frame of mind (e.g., Marlatt & Gordon, 1985). However, because of the many different definitions used for each of these constructs and because we focus on implicit cognition, we repeatedly refer simply to the pattern of activation in memory. This is consistent with a variety of theories of memory and is most readily exemplified in neural network models of memory activation (e.g., Hopfield & Tank, 1986; Masson, 1991, 1995).

Many of the theoretical positions in this approach are readily applied to other health behaviors. In addition to ICT approaches to HIV risk behavior (Stacy, Newcomb, & Ames, 2000; Stacy, Stein, & Longshore, 1999), implicit cognition is also suitable for application to dietary, exercise, violence, media, and health compliance areas of research.

IMPORTANCE OF MEMORY AND IMPLICIT COGNITION PROCESSES IN INTERVENTIONS

In ICT, prevention programs that do not take into account the process through which memory activation guides behavior are neglecting an important, perhaps fundamental, process governing the choice of alternative behaviors. For example, in this approach, facts, skills, beliefs, or cognitions about behavioral alternatives acquired in an intervention will not be effective unless they are highly accessible from memory when they are needed most. They must be accessible enough to relatively spontaneously pop to mind when the adolescent is at risk for performing the behavior. If an intervention does not take into account these processes, it may be confounded. For example, an intervention may be designed to change refusal or social skills when it actually changes an association in memory between a peer social situation and something else learned in the program. Details about these possibilities are delineated further below.

PRINCIPLES OF MEMORY ASSOCIATION APPLICABLE TO INTERVENTIONS AND THEIR EVALUATION

CUE DEPENDENCE AND HIGH-RISK SITUATIONS

Memory activation, as a potential instigator of drug use and DUI, does not occur in isolation. The cues that activate memories promoting drug use and DUI must be thoroughly understood. Indeed, contemporary theories of memory (e.g., Anderson, 1983; Hintzman, 1986; Hopfield & Tank, 1986) contend that the pattern of activation in memory is highly dependent on the prevailing set of cues (which take a variety of forms, including features of the physical and social environment, feelings, activation of other concepts or thoughts, etc.). In drug use, a certain set of cues is likely to characterize what has been called a "high-risk situation." A high-risk situation is a particular, identifiable circumstance that reliably precedes drug use and is integrally involved in the motivation to use drugs (Marlatt & Gordon, 1985). Differences in activation or accessibility in different situations can explain, for example, why some cognitions about consequences of drug use may predict drug use (but others do not) or why information presented in a drug abuse intervention may be learned but not applied to drug use situations (Stacy, Dent, et al., 1990; Stacy, Widaman, & Marlatt, 1990).

Information learned in a program is unlikely to influence behavior unless this material becomes part of what gets activated in memory when behavioral decisions are made. An example will help illustrate this point. A teenager may learn the dangers of driving after smoking marijuana during a driver education class, as evidenced by his or her score on a multiple-choice exam. The exam might be constructed in a way that will lead to memory retrieval of available (stored) information, but the exam score does not necessarily reflect how accessible the information will be at a teenage party, where the student may not try to retrieve previously learned information. The learned information has a *chance* of being accessed at the party, but because of incompatibilities in cues or processing operations (e.g., mode of thinking) (see Roediger, 1990) between the party and the learning situation, the information may not be readily accessible. Again, in the implicit cognition framework, the learned information will not influence behavior unless it is accessible during behavioral decisions. On the other hand, memory activation does not guarantee application. Other aspects of an intervention, not addressed in this chapter, must ensure that an individual wants to apply accessed information. Nevertheless, in the present model, memory access in some form is necessary before the information has any chance of being applied.

Previous drug use research has studied and identified a variety of high-risk situations in particular populations—for example, in alcoholics trying to avoid relapse (Marlatt & Gordon, 1985) and in adolescents in treatment for drug abuse (Brown, Stetson, & Beatty, 1989). This line of research has focused on tabulations of verbal descriptions of high-risk situations. These tabulations include descriptions such as, "I drink when I am upset" or "I drink when I am with friends," which are then grouped into larger categories of situations (e.g., negative affect).

In the associative memory framework espoused in ICT, these descriptive characterizations of high-risk situations are useful but, by themselves, are insufficient for the purposes of tapping into the pattern of activation in memory that accompanies a high-risk situation. As outlined earlier, this memory pattern is likely to be activated by a number of cues that converge on drug use meanings and outcomes. These cues potentially include anything that gets processed during a drug use episode (e.g., perceived outcomes, physical objects, people, social events, etc.). Therefore, in this perspective, it is important to characterize the high-risk situation with a variety of cues, not just a verbal description or summary. Furthermore, in an implicit cognition perspective, it is imperative to use procedures that identify cues from the high-risk situation that are strongly associated with drug use in memory. Research on this topic is needed because the protocols used in previous research to characterize high-risk situations (e.g., Annis, 1984) were not designed to tap into cues that are most strongly associated with drug use in memory. Similarly, paradigms used in cue reactivity (Pavlovian conditioning) research are not designed in terms of the implicit cognition framework, although eventually such paradigms might be combined with the present approach. Using the implicit cognition approach, we are now conducting studies that elicit high-risk situations and specific cues from these situations. Our unpublished data collected so far reveal enough individual variation in cues to suggest the use of an individualized approach to elicit cues that characterize high-risk situations.

In the ICT approach to interventions, cues from high-risk situations are used to tie information learned in a program to the cues that precede or instigate drug use and DUI. In this manner, information learned in a program can become more accessible when it is needed most, that is, during high-risk situations. As outlined below, there are at least several ways in which cues can be tied to program information so that they trigger thoughts about program content.

ELABORATION IN PROCESSING

As outlined earlier, the ICT approach to health behavior contends that participants in a program (e.g., for prevention or cessation of drug use) must not only learn program information and skills, but this information also must become highly accessible from memory when health behavior decisions are being made. One primary way to increase accessibility during drug use decisions is to increase memory associations between the "target" (e.g., program) information and cues that characterize high-risk situations. No previous program components in existing prevention programs have been designed specifically to address this issue. Although there is widespread support in the memory literature for the potential importance of this approach, it has not yet been tested in any area of health behavior.

On the basis of our review of the relevant literature, one of the most effective methods of increasing an association in memory is *elaborative processing*. Dozens of studies have provided evidence that when participants conceptually elaborate two pieces of information, these pieces of information become more strongly associated in memory, as reflected in memory performance. For the purposes of this chapter, it is most important to note that elaborative processing reliably affects performance on cued tests of implicit memory for newly acquired associations (e.g., Howard, Fry, & Brune, 1991; Micco & Masson, 1991; Schacter & Graf, 1989), as well as cued tests of explicit memory for new associations (e.g., Micco & Masson, 1991). Effects of elaborative processing on tests of implicit memory for new associations even have been found among some individuals who show severe memory impairment on explicit tests of memory (for review, see Bowers & Schacter, 1993). A variety of different study materials are used to engage participants in elaborative processing (e.g., Micco & Masson, 1991; Schacter & Graf, 1989; Schacter & McGlynn, 1989). Participants' responses to these study materials can be reliably coded to detect individual differences in degree of elaboration (Stein et al., 1982) as a potential mediator of intervention effects. Because elaborative processing affects scores on both implicit and explicit measures of memory, it is best to use implicit (free association) as well as explicit (cued recall, free recall) tests of memory performance in evaluations of memory effects. However, our main interest is in documenting changes in performance on the implicit test because this would provide evidence that implicit cognitive processes are influenced by the procedure. Nevertheless, to the extent that explicit memory also influences behavior, it is important to document effects on explicit memory as well. The reader wishing to apply memory procedures to this area should become very familiar with the different types of memory tests available and their operational definitions, as available in various sources (e.g., Roediger, 1990). Below, we state how these memory measures are operationally defined in our planned intervention.

Elaborative processing has been described metaphorically as the glue that forms new associations in memory (Graf & Schacter, 1989). More technically, the effect of elaboration on implicit memory appears to operate through *unitization,* which involves processing two initially discrete pieces of information as a single, coherent unit (Graf & Schacter, 1989; Micco & Masson, 1991; Schacter & Graf, 1989). Effects of elaboration on explicit memory probably involve additional processes (see Graf & Schacter, 1989). Specific methods of invoking elaboration in processing are described in later sections of this chapter.

REHEARSAL AND FEEDBACK

In addition to elaborative processing, other procedures may help make program content accessible from memory when high-risk situations are encountered. An intervention might include extensive study of newly learned concepts to a criterion followed by repetitive testing of newly learned associates as a means of enhancing memory for the new content and increasing the strength of association. Repetitive testing that includes performance feedback and restudy also has shown large effects on explicit and implicit memory for new associations (Howard, Heisey, & Shaw, 1986) and can be integrated in prevention program interventions. Although evidence of increased association has been found even when participants copy new associative pairs (concepts presented together that have no preexisting association) only once (Micco & Masson, 1991; Reingold & Goshen-Gottstein, 1996), extensive study of such new associates (Dagenbach, Horst, & Carr, 1990) and repetitive exposure to the to-be-remembered associative pairs improve performance on tests of implicit and explicit memory for new associations (Schacter & McGlynn, 1989).

"BACKFIRE" POSSIBILITIES IN INTERVENTIONS: UNINTENDED MEMORY EFFECTS

Many interventions address myths about drug use or review the positive consequences of use, in hopes of countering these misleading or false expectancies or beliefs. If memory processes are not considered during prevention programming, it is possible that such program information could have a reverse effect and lead to increases in memory for positive consequences and myths. An area of basic research in memory has shown that unconscious influences of past presentations of information can increase the probability of mistaking the source of messages and even completely altering the impact of a message. Jacoby, Kelley, Brown, and Jasechko (1989) demonstrated such an effect, which they labeled a "sleeper effect in fame judgments." They used a paradigm in which individuals read lists of famous and nonfamous names and, when asked to judge the fame of those names 24 hours later, participants mistakenly reported nonfamous names as being famous. This "false-fame" effect occurred over time and did not occur on an immediate judgment task (Jacoby, Kelley, et al., 1989). Prior presentation of nonfamous names increased participants' familiarity with the names and the likelihood that these names would be called famous in a later judgment task (Jacoby & Kelley, 1987; Jacoby, Kelley, et al., 1989; Jacoby, Woloshyn, & Kelley, 1989). As time lapsed, participants had difficulty recollecting the source of familiarity of the names they were to judge, yet the names remained familiar.

Investigators recently have applied similar concepts to drug use research, replicating the finding that source misattributions can easily occur over time. Krank and Swift (1994) demonstrated that myths about drug use could be retained as facts after only 24 hours had lapsed. They used an unconscious memory paradigm similar to Jacoby's false-fame paradigm in which participants read a series of myth and fact statements about drug use effects. The statements included whether the information about the alcohol effect was fact or myth. Following exposure to the statements, participants rated the appropriateness of the statements for an adolescent information campaign; this constituted an incidental learning task. Following the incidental learning task, participants' memory for the facts and myths was tested indirectly, either immediately or after a delay of 24 hours. In these indirect memory tests, participants were asked to generate and write down outcomes that first came to mind that could occur from alcohol. In other words, they were asked to generate facts about alcohol effects that popped to mind. The researchers found strong main effects for prior exposure to myth messages and fact messages on the immediate test. Both myth and fact messages were generated more frequently than previously unexposed alcohol effect statements on the immediate test. In addition, myths were generated with less frequency than were facts. This latter finding is in accord with what one might expect because myths involve outcomes that do not occur from alcohol use—they should be listed with less frequency. Importantly, on the delayed test, the difference between reporting of myth and fact statements diminished (i.e., fewer fact statements were generated, and more myth statements were generated). Thus, over time, the likelihood of generating myth statements as true outcomes of alcohol use increased. In essence, participants did not accurately attribute the source of the outcomes (myth or fact) they accessed from memory.

As in the famous-name studies, these results underscore the point that it is easy to forget details about information learned at an earlier time, including details about the source or validity of the information. If these types of memory processes are not taken into account, a similar misattribution of the source of familiar messages could have a negative impact on prevention programming. That is, myths may be retained as facts after the program is completed.

Jacoby, Kelley, et al. (1989) suggested that reinstatement of various aspects of the learning context could help minimize misattribution of the source of a message and may have implications for memory access. Associative elaboration of the source and message during the intervention may foster their joint, implicit reinstatement in memory at later times. In this manner, program information may have the appropriate, intended effect. Another possible way to avoid unintended effects is to minimize interference in memory, caused by presentation of an excessive amount of information or presentation of material without sufficient spacing. If too much unspaced information is presented, the chances of losing essential details (i.e., myth or fact attributions) about that information from memory are increased.

COGNITIVE PROCESSING CONFOUNDS IN PREVIOUS INTERVENTION RESEARCH

Previous prevention research in drug use and most other areas of health behavior has not considered the types of processing that participants engage in during interventions as a possible confound. One intervention condition may encourage elaborative processing, but another condition does not. Yet, the conditions may be summarized in research reports, as well as in the practitioner's mind, as manipulating the content of focus (e.g., coping skills vs. resistance skills or negative consequences information vs. normative restructuring). To the extent that program content is confounded with type of processing (e.g., elaborative vs. not elaborative), memory processes may be responsible for the superiority of one condition over another. The basic research reviewed earlier has shown that elaboration has significant effects on memory performance, on both implicit and explicit memory assessments. Thus, it is a likely confound.

Intervention conditions also vary in the extent to which they address cues that may occur in the high-risk situation, in which drug use is likely. For example, some intervention conditions may address many social features integral to the high-risk situation (e.g., peer use situations), but other conditions may not (typical health effect information). It is very possible that such interventions are manipulating whether social cues are the focus, in addition to the target information. For example, a condition focusing on refusal resistance training manipulates not only skills and knowledge about resistance but also the social cues to which this information is tied. If a second condition focuses on health effect information but does not address social cues, then an intervention manipulating these two conditions is confounded. Target information (resistance vs. health) would be confounded with type of cue (social vs. not social).

Other processing confounds may exist in prevention research. The point is that a memory and implicit cognition perspective opens the door for the consideration of confounds that are not typically considered in these interventions. The zeitgeist in drug prevention research has been based primarily on a small subset of principles from social psychology and social learning theory, rather than on basic research in human memory and cognitive science. This does not imply necessarily that the zeitgeist has been wrong. In fact, the existing prevention paradigms still may be shown to be quite good and possibly even preferable to alternatives. However, the existence of prominent confounds implies that we may not really know why prevention programs are sometimes effective. To progress toward a science of prevention, one must have such knowledge.

A SPECIFIC APPLICATION OF THEORY IN BOOSTER PROGRAMMING

In collaboration with our colleagues (Sussman et al., 1995), we are developing a memory enhancement component as an *adjunct* to comprehensive prevention programs, especially those that target continuation high school or DUI offender groups. The component is not designed as a complete, self-contained intervention program. However, it is designed to be readily appended to existing comprehensive programs, which do not now focus explicitly on any type of memory process. We already have outlined many reasons why these processes should be emphasized.

Because of the widespread evidence for the effectiveness of elaborative processing methods, we hypothesize that these methods will be effective in enhancing associations in memory between high-risk cues and information relevant to the prevention of drug use, drug abuse, and DUI. In the present case study, we outline a specific example of this component, used as a short telephone booster intervention that will be evaluated soon. The booster intervention is designed to help students remember and apply what they learned previously from a classroom-based drug abuse prevention program (Sussman et al., 1995). Because of cost considerations, a short telephone booster intervention was the only type of memory enhancement component we could test in the near future. Nevertheless, this type of intervention illustrates some of the ways in which memory processes can be applied to prevention programs, and a telephone booster component represents a cost-effective, realistic way to begin developing and testing the recommended procedures.

Participants. Participants will be approximately 1,200 continuation high school students enrolled in an ongoing prevention project (Sussman et al., 1995).

Procedures. Students will be randomly assigned to an elaboration study condition or a control condition. When reached by phone, students will be given an explanation of the purpose of the phone call and asked for their voluntary participation in the booster study. They will be asked to find three full-size pieces of blank paper on which to jot a few things down during the session.

Elaboration Condition. In this condition, participants will complete exercises that emphasize elaborative processing. They will receive three sets of exercises, linking three high-risk situations (and specific cues within these situations) to a number of facts learned in the earlier prevention program. The order of situations will be randomized for each subject to fully control for potential order effects (e.g., primacy, recency, or fatigue effects). High-risk cues were taken from two studies on this topic (Ames, Stacy, Sussman, & Dent, 1999; Sussman, Stacy, Ames, & Freedman, 1998). The elaborative processing exercises will use the following strategies and steps.

Step 1

Students first complete a draw-a-picture test (DAPT) (Ames et al., 1999) for one of the target situations. This test allows for the use of individualized cues within a standardized design, in which participants assigned to a given condition receive the same instructions. This test encourages the cognitive re-creation of high-risk cues and contexts, using prompts for images and thoughts that are likely to overlap with those elicited in high-risk DUI and drug use situations. These procedures are in part based on cognitive interview procedures (Geiselman, Fisher, MacKinnon, & Holland, 1985). Students will be asked to complete their sketches on the top half of one of the blank pieces of paper.

As an example of the first situation, students may be asked to

> think of being at home with three or more friends on a Friday night when your parents are not home. Try to form a picture of this in your mind. Quickly sketch out, in simple stick figures, three friends and yourself, in one of the rooms at home. Include any objects or details about the room that come to mind. Label each person with his or her name, but do not tell me any names. Do this very quickly. Don't worry about how good your sketch is. Take 2 minutes to do this.

Step 2

In the second step, students are asked to think about some information involving multiple concepts learned in a group of interrelated lessons in the prevention program, preferably information that can be "chunked" together in some manner. As an example, students might be asked to think about what TRAP stood for in the program (an acronym for stages of drug use involvement taught in the program: trial, recreational use, abuse, and pinned down). The health educator reminds them of the correct response. The students are asked to jot down the words in the acronym and their meanings on the bottom half of their worksheets after being reminded of them.

Step 3

In the third step, the information listed in the second step is integrated with the situation and specific cues from the first step. A variety of issues should be considered when attempting this integration. Basic research on elaboration in memory suggests that students should be given prompts that encourage elaborations that clarify the significance of relationships between cues and the target information and that decrease the arbitrariness of these relationships. Prompts designed in this manner have shown large effects on the enhancement of memory (Stein & Bransford, 1979; Stein et al., 1982; Stein, Littlefield, Bransford, & Persampieri, 1984). A decrease in arbitrariness and an increase in the clarity of the relationship may be accomplished by focusing on *functional* relationships between the cue and target. Theoretically, this approach is akin to classical expectancy approaches that focus on *memories* of functional relationships between cues, outcomes, and behaviors (Bolles, 1972; Tolman, 1932) rather than on beliefs reported on a questionnaire.

Prompts also should encourage the development of integrated, or unitized, thoughts and images about cues and program information. Such procedures combine two initially separate pieces of information (cue and target) into a single cognitive unit, following the gestalt principles outlined in research on implicit and explicit memory for new associations (Micco & Masson, 1991; Schacter & Graf, 1989). When pieces of information become unitized, the presentation of one aspect of that information "redintegrates" (Horowitz & Prytulak, 1969) the rest of the unit—that is, it activates the larger unit as a whole.

One example of an attempt to integrate the concepts in TRAP with the target situation is as follows. Students are asked to imagine that the four people in their sketch are having a conversation about TRAP. In this conversation, each person says what one of the four concepts in TRAP means to him or her. The student is asked to quickly write down what each person said, in one short sentence or phrase. It should be noted that the sentences do not have to be realistic expressions of the people in the sketch to be effective. Rather, it is important that the meanings of each concept are elaborated on in the context of the situation in the sketch.

Step 4

If time allowed, an additional step in this exercise would be the use of repetitive study test trials, which include performance feedback. Repetitive testing that includes performance feedback and restudy has shown large effects on explicit and implicit memory for new associations (Howard et al., 1986). Unfortunately, there is not sufficient time for this step in a 15-minute phone booster intervention involving multiple concepts. The reader should keep in mind that this fourth step could be essential, but its implementation must await future research.

After the completion of Step 3, students in the present booster intervention will complete a second sketch about a second situation chosen from a list of frequent high-risk situations for drug use. The three steps will be followed for this exercise as well. The target information will involve four different concepts, chosen from another set of interrelated lessons taught in the prevention program. Finally, a sketch of a third high-risk situation will be completed, followed by the same three steps, targeting four different concepts from a different set of interrelated lessons. A total of 12 concepts are addressed in the three sets of sketch exercises.

Control Condition. The present case study will use a control condition, in which students are presented with the same 12 target concepts as in the elaboration condition, but one critical component is missing. Students in this condition first complete the DAPT, as in the first step of the elaboration condition. Then, the target concepts are presented in the same manner as in the second step of the elaboration condition. That is, the health educator presents each concept, and the student are asked to write down the concept and its meaning. After one set of four concepts is addressed, a second and third set of concepts are presented, each involving interrelated lessons with four concepts each, as in the elaboration condition. The critical third step of the elaboration condition is not performed in the control condition.

Distracter Task. Immediately after the exercises are completed in both the elaboration and control conditions, a distracter task is completed for 2 minutes. This task should be unrelated to the facts presented earlier and be engaging or difficult enough to capture the students' full attention. It may also serve a second function, such as a short personality or verbal test or an inventory of background characteristics. In the present study, we will use a short, multiple-choice vocabulary test.

Dependent Variable Tests. Immediately after the vocabulary test, participants within each group are randomly assigned to take one of three tests: free recall, free association, or cued recall. All students are asked to get a new blank piece of paper and to put aside any papers they had worked on earlier, where they cannot see them. In all test conditions, students are asked to list information in three blocks. For free recall, participants are instructed as follows for the first block: "Think about four concepts we went over today. Write down the names for these four concepts." After 1 minute, the second block is completed, in which students are asked to think of another four concepts they went over. After a second delay of 1 minute, students are asked to write down four additional concepts from the session. No cues are provided in this condition, consistent with typical instructions for free recall.

For cued recall, participants are instructed as follows: "Think about the first sketch you did today without looking at it, and write down the names of the four people in the sketch, including yourself. Now, next to each name, write down one of the names of the concepts we went over today. The people in your sketch may help you remember a concept." The sketch provides a general cue, and the names of the people provide specific cues to help prompt recall. After a delay of 1 minute, the second block is given, in which students are asked to think of the second sketch, write four names from that sketch, and write down the names of concepts as in the first block. After a second delay of 1 minute, the third block is presented in the same manner as the first two blocks, targeting the third sketch and its concepts.

For the free-association condition, participants are instructed as follows: "Think about the first sketch you did today without looking at it, and write down the names of the four people in the sketch, including yourself. Now, next to each name, write down the *very first* word that person makes you think of." After a delay of 1 minute, the second block is given, in which students are asked to think of the second sketch, write four names from that sketch, and write down the first word each name made them think of as in the first block. After a second delay of 1 minute, the third block is presented in the same manner as the first two blocks, targeting the third sketch and its concepts. Free association is an indirect or implicit test of memory because it does not refer explicitly to a particular study episode and does not ask students to deliberately interrogate their memory. It is well-documented as a useful test of implicit memory; for a brief review, see Stacy et al., 2000.

Wrap-Up. After the completion of the assigned test, students are asked to read the tested words back to the health educator. After the health educator has written down the words, he or she briefly explains more about the purpose of the study. Students are told the following:

> We think the sketches and exercises you completed may help you more spontaneously remember and think about information from the project

when you are in situations with people your age. You may want to review your sketches on your own against the words you wrote down. It may be fun to check yourself and see how many of the words you wrote down match the words on your sketches. Do you have any questions? Thank you very much for your participation in the project.

As this wrap-up reveals, these procedures make explicit the intention of the memory intervention.

Scoring. The words are scored in two ways for program content: exact and gist. In the exact scoring method, words are scored "correct" if they match perfectly the words presented in the booster lesson, except for tense. In the gist method, words are scored as "correct" if the meaning is the same as a concept from the lesson.

PRIMARY HYPOTHESES AND DATA ANALYSIS

On the basis of the literature reviewed earlier, we expect that the results will provide evidence that associations between cues and program concepts have been strengthened in memory when students use elaborative processing to study these associations. Thus, elaborative processing during the experimental manipulation should result in superior performance on cued tests of memory (free association, cued recall), as compared with the control study condition. However, elaborative processing also should have some effects on free recall because this type of processing can result in an increase in "retrieval routes," even when cues are not provided at test (e.g., Anderson, 1983). Nevertheless, because cued tests are more compatible with the way the target facts were elaborated at study, the effects of elaboration should be stronger for cued tests than for free recall. Cued tests may lead to somewhat worse levels of performance than free recall under the control study condition, consistent with transfer-appropriate processing and encoding specificity propositions and research (e.g., Roediger, 1990; Tulving, 1983). These hypotheses imply that both a main effect of study condition and a study-by-test interaction should be found; no main effect of test condition is anticipated. We expect the forms of the interaction and main effect to be roughly consistent with the following two ways of depicting the same effects, shown in Figure 5.1.

Data Analysis. These primary hypotheses will be analyzed using a general-linear model, regression analogue of analysis of variance. Such an analysis will readily allow for the study of individual difference covariates, as well as for the study of the experimental manipulations. Although random assignment of participants

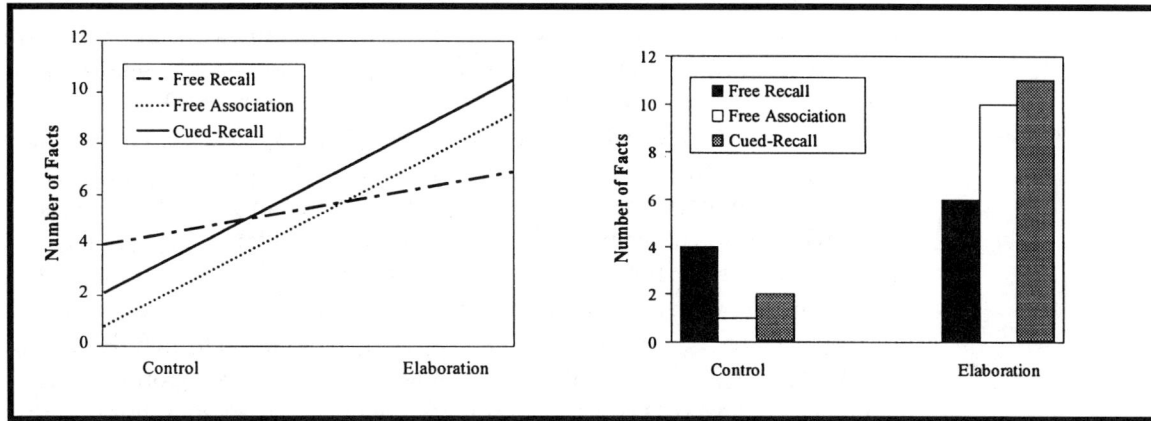

Figure 5.1. Two Different Ways to Depict the Same Hypothesized Effect
NOTE: In both graphs, all memory scores are higher when the study condition is elaboration. However, the strength of this effect varies under different testing conditions (free recall, free association, or cued recall).

to conditions should guarantee that covariates do not confound treatment effects, possible effects of covariates (e.g., previous drug use, ethnicity, acculturation, age, and gender) are still investigated. In the present study, these variables were assessed in an earlier school-based survey that will be linked to the phone booster results. In supplementary analyses, possible moderator influences of the covariates also will be explored, using the regression procedures of Aiken and West (1991) to study interaction effects of individual differences.

SUMMARY AND IMPLICATIONS ◄

The general goal of this case study is to apply implicit cognition theory to a health behavior intervention. The specific goal is to see if elaborative processing exercises increase associations in memory between high-risk cues and program information in a short phone booster program. If such effects are found, evidence would be obtained that program information has become more accessible from memory when high-risk cues are encountered (at least in an experimental procedure). After the completion of this study, additional evaluation of this booster needs to be accomplished to determine if it has effects on drug use behavior over time. Thus, we are planning to conduct additional studies to evaluate the long-term effects on behavior patterns.

Research on ICT and allied memory processes adheres to a very different framework in theory, assessment, and intervention when compared to research from the current zeitgeist in prevention research. This framework argues that we may not yet understand the central determinants of either health behavior decisions or intervention effects. This contention is based on the fact that whole domains of cognitive and learning processes have been excluded from most theory and program evaluation in health behavior. Yet, some key principles from the excluded domains have received consistent experimental support in basic research. Research on these domains may provide important developments in theory and practice, suggesting how memory and implicit cognition concepts may act as complements or alternatives to traditional approaches.

Application of memory and implicit cognition concepts may have pronounced public health benefits, if memory access is indeed as important as these approaches suggest. In addition, nothing in the present theoretical framework is incompatible with public health approaches that focus on providing information to large groups of individuals. Nevertheless, some implementations of this theoretical approach also allow for individualized components, as in the provision of participants' own high-risk cues in the present case study. Within the case study, the instructions across participants are the same within the same experimental condition, allowing for a standardized, well-controlled manipulation while targeting the participants' own salient cues. Other variations of the present case study are feasible, including those that are less individualized but still capture high-risk cues that are common to most participants. Finally, the theoretical framework can be implemented in a variety of ways in addition to those in this case study.

It is important to note that the development of theory and interventions that apply memory and implicit cognition perspectives requires relevant background in the cognitive science of experimental psychology. Working knowledge of allied fields in learning, neurobiology, and experimental social cognition also is helpful. It is our perhaps controversial opinion that most other cognitive or metacognitive approaches to health, which are usually not as well grounded in basic research, have less unconfounded evidence supporting them. It is in the interest of investigator teams developing applied cognitive science approaches to spend considerable time developing the necessary expertise in this area. We believe this requires a good knowledge of current theoretical issues in basic research in memory and implicit cognition, as well as a thorough understanding of measurement and design in these areas. It is one thing to theorize how memory concepts apply to health behavior, as has been done since the mid-1980s (e.g., Baker, Morse, & Sherman, 1987; Stacy, 1986). It is another matter to understand and apply paradigms that unambiguously measure memory associations and access rather than self-perceptions of behavior. These applications pose an exciting challenge to researchers committed to the further development of cognitive theories of drug use, DUI, and health-behavior interventions.

REFERENCES

AIKEN, L. S., & WEST, S. G. (1991). *Multiple regression: Testing and interpreting interactions.* Newbury Park, CA: Sage.

AMES, S. L., & STACY, A. W. (1998). Implicit cognition in the prediction of substance use among drug offenders. *Psychology of Addictive Behaviors, 12*, 272-281.

AMES, S. L., STACY, A. W., SUSSMAN, S., & DENT, C. W. (1999, June). *Multimodal situation assessment in adolescent drug use.* Paper presented at the meeting of the Research Society on Alcoholism, Santa Barbara, CA.

ANDERSON, J. R. (1983). *The architecture of cognition.* Cambridge, MA: Harvard University Press.

ANNIS, H. M. (1984). A basic follow-up package. In F. B. Glaser, H. A. Skinner, S. Pearlman, R. L. Segal, B. Sisson, A. C. Ogborne, E. Bohnen, P. Gazda, & T. Zimmerman (Eds.), *A system of health care delivery* (Vol. 3, pp. 216-234). Toronto, Canada: Addiction Research Foundation.

BAKER, T. B., MORSE, E., & SHERMAN, J. E. (1987). The motivation to use drugs: A psychobiological analysis of urges. In P. C. Rivers (Ed.), *The Nebraska symposium on motivation: Alcohol use and abuse* (pp. 257-323). Lincoln: University of Nebraska Press.

BOLLES, R. C. (1972). Reinforcement, expectancy, and learning. *Psychological Review, 79*, 394-409.

BOWERS, J., & SCHACTER, D. L. (1993). Priming of novel information in amnesic patients: Issues and data. In P. Graf & M. E. J. Masson (Eds.), *Implicit memory: New directions in cognition, development, and neuropsychology* (pp. 303-326). Hillsdale, NJ: Lawrence Erlbaum.

BROWN, S. A., STETSON, B. A., & BEATTY, P. A. (1989). Cognitive and behavioral features of adolescent coping in high-risk drinking situations. *Addictive Behaviors, 14*, 43-52.

DAGENBACH, D., CARR, T. H., & BARNHARDT, T. M. (1990). Inhibitory semantic priming of lexical decisions due to failure to retrieve weekly activated codes. *Journal of Experimental Psychology: Learning, Memory, and Cognition, 16*, 328-340.

DAGENBACH, D., HORST, S., & CARR, T. H. (1990). Adding new information to semantic memory: How much learning is enough to produce automatic priming? *Journal of Experimental Psychology: Learning, Memory, and Cognition, 16*, 581-591.

DOHERTY, K. T., & SZALAY, L. B. (1996). Statistical risk versus psychological vulnerability: Why are men at greater risk for substance abuse than women? *Journal of Alcohol & Drug Education, 42*, 57-77.

DONOVAN, J. E. (1993). Young adult drinking-driving: Behavioral and psychosocial correlates. *Journal of Studies on Alcohol, 54*, 600-613.

EARLEYWINE, M. (1994). Cognitive bias covaries with alcohol consumption. *Addictive Behaviors, 19*, 539-544.

FAZIO, R. H., & WILLIAMS, C. J. (1986). Attitude accessibility as a moderator of the attitude-perception and attitude-behavior relations: An investigation of the 1984 presidential election. *Journal of Personality and Social Psychology, 51*, 505-514.

FELDMAN, J. M., & LYNCH, J. G. (1988). Self-generated validity and other effects of measurement on belief, attitude, intention, and behavior. *Journal of Applied Psychology, 73*, 421-435.

GEISELMAN, R. E., FISHER, R. P., MacKINNON, D. P., & HOLLAND, H. L. (1985). Eyewitness memory enhancement in the police interview: Cognitive retrieval mnemonics versus hypnosis. *Journal of Applied Psychology, 70*, 401-412.

GOLDMAN, M. S., BROWN, S. A., CHRISTIANSEN, B. A., & SMITH, G. T. (1991). Alcoholism and memory: Broadening the scope of alcohol expectancy research. *Psychological Bulletin, 110*, 137-146.

GRAF, P., & SCHACTER, D. L. (1989). Unitization and grouping mediate dissociations in memory for new associations. *Journal of Experimental Psychology: Learning, Memory, and Cognition, 15*, 930-940.

GRAY, J. A. (1987). The neuropsychology of emotion and personality. In S. D. Iversen, S. M. Stahl, & E. C. Goodman (Eds.), *Cognitive neurochemistry.* Oxford, UK: Oxford University Press.

GRAY, J. A. (1990). Brain systems that mediate both emotion and cognition. *Cognition and Emotion, 4*, 269-288.

GREENWALD, A. G. (1992). New Look 3: Unconscious cognition reclaimed. *American Psychologist, 47*, 766-779.

GREENWALD, A. G., & BANAJI, M. R. (1995). Implicit social cognition: Attitudes, self-esteem, and stereotypes. *Psychological Review, 102*, 4-27.

HAWKINS, J. D., CATALANO, R. F., & MILLER, J. Y. (1992). Risk and protective factors for alcohol and other drug problems in adolescence and early adulthood: Implications for substance abuse prevention. *Psychological Bulletin, 112*, 64-105.

HILL, A. B., & PAYNTER, S. (1992). Alcohol dependence and semantic priming of alcohol related words. *Personality and Individual Differences, 13*(6), 745-750.

HINTZMAN, D. L. (1986). "Schema abstraction" in a multiple-trace memory model. *Psychological Review, 93*(4), 411-428.

HOPFIELD, J. J., & TANK, D. W. (1986). Computing with neural circuits: A model. *Science, 233*, 625-633.

HOROWITZ, L. M., & PRYTULAK, L. S. (1969). Redintegrative memory. *Psychological Review, 84*, 519-531.

HOWARD, D. V., FRY, A. F., & BRUNE, C. M. (1991). Aging and memory for new associations: Direct versus indirect measures. *Journal of Experimental Psychology: Learning, Memory, and Cognition, 17*, 779-792.

HOWARD, D. V., HEISEY, J. G., & SHAW, R. J. (1986). Aging and the priming of newly learned associations. *Developmental Psychology, 22*, 78-85.

JACCARD, J., & TURRISI, R. (1987). Cognitive processes and individual differences in judgments relevant to drunk driving. *Journal of Personality & Social Psychology, 53*, 135-145.

JACOBY, L. L., & KELLEY, C. M. (1987). Unconscious influences of memory for a prior event. *Personality and Social Psychology Bulletin, 13*, 314-336.

JACOBY, L. L., KELLEY, C. M., BROWN, J., & JASECHKO, J. (1989). Becoming famous overnight: Limits on the ability to avoid unconscious influences of the past. *Journal of Personality and Social Psychology, 56*, 326-338.

JACOBY, L. L., WOLOSHYN, V., & KELLEY, C. M. (1989). Becoming famous without being recognized: Unconscious influences of memory produced by dividing attention. *Journal of Experimental Psychology: General, 118*, 115-125.

JAFFE, J. H. (1989). Addictions: What does biology have to tell? *International Review of Psychiatry, 1*, 51-61.

KIHLSTROM, J. F. (1987). The cognitive unconscious. *Science, 237*, 1445-1452.

KLEPP, K., PERRY, C. L., & JACOBS, D. R., JR. (1991). Etiology of drinking and driving among adolescents: Implications for primary prevention. *Health Education Quarterly, 18*, 415-427.

KLITZNER, M. D., VEGEGA, M. E., & GRUENEWALD, P. (1988). An empirical examination of the assumptions underlying youth drinking/driving prevention programs. *Evaluation and Program Planning, 11*, 219-235.

KRANK, M. D., & SWIFT, R. (1994). Unconscious influences of specific memories on alcohol outcome expectancies. *Alcoholism: Clinical and Experimental Research, 18*, 423.

MARLATT, G. A., & GORDON, J. R. (1985). *Relapse prevention.* New York: Guilford.

MASSON, M. (1991). A distributed memory model of context effects in word identification. In D. Besner & G. W. Humphreys (Eds.), *Basic processes in reading: Visual word recognition* (pp. 233-263). Hillsdale, NJ: Lawrence Erlbaum.

MASSON, M. E. J. (1995). A distributed memory model of semantic priming. *Journal of Experimental Psychology: Learning, Memory, and Cognition, 21*, 3-23.

McCLELLAND, J. L., & RUMELHART, D. E. (1985). Distributed memory and the representation of general and specific information. *Journal of Experimental Psychology: General, 114*, 159-188.

MEYER, D., & SCHVANEVELDT, R. (1976). Meaning, memory and mental processes. *Science, 192*, 27-33.

MICCO, A., & MASSON, M. E. J. (1991). Implicit memory for new associations: An interactive process approach. *Journal of Experimental Psychology: Learning, Memory, and Cognition, 17*, 1105-1123.

NISBETT, R. E., & WILSON, T. D. (1977). Telling more than we can know: Verbal reports on mental processes. *Psychological Review, 84*, 231-259.

PETRAITIS, J., FLAY, B. R., & MILLER, T. Q. (1995). Reviewing theories of adolescent substance use: Organizing pieces in the puzzle. *Psychological Bulletin, 117*, 67-86.

RATHER, B. C., & GOLDMAN, M. S. (1994). Drinking-related differences in the memory organization of alcohol expectancies. *Experimental and Clinical Psychopharmacology, 2*, 167-183.

REINGOLD, E. M., & GOSHEN-GOTTSTEIN, Y. (1996). Separating consciously controlled and automatic influences in memory for new associations. *Journal of Experimental Psychology: Learning, Memory, and Cognition, 22*, 397-406.

ROEDIGER, H. L. (1990). Implicit memory: Retention without remembering. *American Psychologist, 45*, 1043-1056.

SCHACTER, D. L., & GRAF, P. (1989). Modality specificity of implicit memory for new associations. *Journal of Experimental Psychology: Learning, Memory, and Cognition, 15*, 3-12.

SCHACTER, D. L., & McGLYNN, S. M. (1989). Implicit memory: Effects of elaboration depend on unitization. *American Journal of Psychology, 102*, 151-181.

SQUIRE, L. R. (1986). Mechanisms of memory. *Science, 232*, 1612-1619.

STACY, A. W. (1986). *Attitude and expectancy models of alcohol use: An integration of theoretical perspectives.* Doctoral dissertation, University of California, Riverside.

STACY, A. W. (1995). Memory association and ambiguous cues in models of alcohol and marijuana use. *Experimental and Clinical Psychopharmacology, 3*, 183-194.

STACY, A. W. (1997). Memory activation and expectancy as prospective predictors of alcohol and marijuana use. *Journal of Abnormal Psychology, 106*, 61-73.

STACY, A. W., DENT, C. W., SUSSMAN, S., RAYNOR, A., BURTON, D., & FLAY, B. R. (1990). Expectancy accessibility and the influence of outcome expectancies on adolescent smokeless tobacco use. *Journal of Applied Social Psychology, 20*, 802-817.

STACY, A. W., LEIGH, B. C., & WEINGARDT, K. R. (1993, November). *An individual difference perspective applied to normative associative strength.* Paper presented at the annual meeting of the Psychonomic Society, Washington, DC.

STACY, A. W., LEIGH, B. C., & WEINGARDT, K. R. (1994). Memory accessibility and association of alcohol use and its positive outcomes. *Experimental and Clinical Psychopharmacology, 2*, 269-282.

STACY, A. W., NEWCOMB, M. D., & AMES, S. L. (2000). Implicit cognition and HIV risk behavior. *Journal of Behavioral Medicine, 23*, 475-499.

STACY, A. W., STEIN, J., & LONGSHORE, D. (1999). Habit, intention, and drug use as interactive predictors of condom use among drug abusers. *AIDS and Behavior, 3*, 231-241.

STACY, A. W., WIDAMAN, K. F., & MARLATT, G. A. (1990). Expectancy models of alcohol use. *Journal of Personality and Social Psychology, 58*, 918-928.

STEIN, B. S., & BRANSFORD, J. D. (1979). Constraints on effective elaboration: Effects of precision and subject generation. *Journal of Verbal Learning and Verbal Behavior, 18*, 769-777.

STEIN, B. S., BRANSFORD, J. D., FRANKS, J. S., OWINGS, R. A., VYE, N. J., & McGRAW, W. (1982). Differences in the precision of self-generated elaborations. *Journal of Experimental Psychology: General, 111*, 399-405.

STEIN, B. S., LITTLEFIELD, J., BRANSFORD, J. D., & PERSAMPIERI, M. (1984). Elaboration and knowledge acquisition. *Memory and Cognition, 12*, 522-529.

STORMARK, K. M., & HUGDAHL, K. (1997). Conditioned emotional cueing of spatial attentional shifts in a go/no go RT task. *International Journal of Psychophysiology, 27*, 241-248.

SUSSMAN, S., DENT, C. W., SIMON, T. R., STACY, A. W., GALAIF, E. R., MOSS, M. A., CRAIG, S., & JOHNSON, C. A. (1995). Immediate impact of social influence-oriented substance abuse prevention curricula in traditional and continuation high schools. *Drugs and Society, 8*, 65-81.

SUSSMAN, S., STACY, A. W., AMES, S. L., & FREEDMAN, L. B. (1998). Self-reported high-risk locations of adolescent drug use. *Addictive Behaviors, 23*, 405-411.

SZALAY, L. B., INN, A., & DOHERTY, K. T. (1996). Social influences: Effects of the social environment on the use of alcohol and other drugs. *Substance Use and Misuse, 31*, 343-373.

TIFFANY, S. T. (1990). A cognitive model of drug urges and drug-use behavior: Role of automatic and nonautomatic processes. *Psychological Review, 97,* 147-168.

TOLMAN, E. C. (1932). *Purposive behavior in animals and men.* New York: Appelton-Century-Crofts.

TULVING, E. (1983). *Elements of episodic memory.* New York: Oxford University Press.

TULVING, E., & SCHACTER, D. L. (1990). Priming and human memory systems. *Science, 247,* 301-306.

TURRISI, R., & JACCARD, J. (1991). Judgment processes relevant to drunk driving. *Journal of Applied Social Psychology, 21,* 89-118.

WISE, R. A. (1988). The neurobiology of craving: Implications for the understanding and treatment of addiction. *Journal of Abnormal Psychology, 97,* 118-132.

CHAPTER 6

Choosing Assessment Studies to Clarify Theory-Based Program Ideas

Valerie Johnson
Robert J. Pandina

Program development in health behavior research and practice first entails the use of an etiologic model that involves constituents, including causes or predictors, target population needs, mediators of effects, and expected outcomes. There may be several gaps in knowledge in a proposed model or models involving one or more of these constituents, and these gaps can be filled through what we refer to as "assessment studies." The realm of assessment work in health behavior program development encompasses a multiplicity of domains, including but not limited to (a) the promotion of healthy behaviors (e.g., nutrition, exercise, stress management), (b) the prevention of unhealthy outcomes brought about by unhealthy or high-risk behaviors (e.g., skin cancer due to excess exposure to sun, HIV infection due to risky sexual practices), (c) the treatment or treatments for curtailing or eliminating unhealthy or high-risk behaviors (e.g., cigarette cessation protocols and programs), and (d) the concerns regarding compliance (e.g., continuing to take prescribed medication for high blood pressure) on both the individual and social levels. Although acknowledging the breadth of arenas within this field of health behavior research, in the discussion that ensues, we focus on recent discussion and research in prevention science as the primary context within which to present information on health behavior program development assessment work.

This prevention focus is for good reason. During the past decade, researchers who study and practitioners who implement prevention programming have joined together to argue strongly for the need to create a science of prevention (e.g., Bryant, Windle, & West, 1997; Coie et al., 1993; Loeber & Farrington, 1998; Munoz, Mrazek, & Haggerty, 1996; Pandina, 1998; Reiss & Price, 1996). A cornerstone of this movement is the tenet that prevention interventions should be based on a solid empirical foundation reflecting current knowledge about the etiology of targeted dysfunctional outcomes if they are to be maximally effective (e.g., Coie et al., 1993; Munoz et al., 1996). Proponents of this view are drawn from a wide range of communities of interest, including advocates for the prevention of alcohol and drug abuse, mental and physical diseases, and violence.

▶ CONCEPTUAL ISSUES: THE IMPORTANCE OF ETIOLOGICAL RESEARCH

Undoubtedly, numerous conceptual, political, and practical considerations drive the nascent prevention science movement to look toward etiological research for assistance in the development of intervention approaches. The focus of this chapter is to explore the desirability of, the manner in, and the degree to which etiological research regarding the origins of serious human dysfunctions can and should inform attempts to prevent such dysfunctions. Many of the examples to be used are drawn from the alcohol and drug literature and, to a lesser extent, the arenas of mental health and violence, inasmuch as our primary research interests lie in these areas. However, it is hoped that the general principles outlined here will prove useful to health behavior scientists and practitioners who focus on program development for a wide range of health behaviors and outcomes.

Five salient conceptual issues are important to consider. Although these five issues portray the real need for continuing etiologic assessments, we do acknowledge that any such work to help clarify a theory and help produce a health behavior program is work worth doing even on a small scale with simple means of analysis. First, several decades of etiological research aimed at investigating precursors of a wide range of dysfunctional outcomes (e.g., alcohol and drug abuse, delinquency, mental disease) have identified what appears to be a large set or generative pool of common biological, psychological, and sociological factors that are linked to all such outcomes. Depending on the dysfunctional outcome of interest, these factors may differ in (a) the manner in which they affect outcomes (direct or indirect effects), (b) their strength of impact (low, medium, high), and

(c) their stability (relatively stable or dynamic conditions). Most important, prevention scientists have come to view such variables as **risk and protective factors**, in which risk factors are associated with heightened likelihood of onset and greater severity and longer duration of dysfunction, whereas protective factors are related to enhanced resistance to the risk or dysfunction (Bry, McKeon, & Pandina, 1982; Coie et al., 1993; Hawkins, Catalano, & Miller, 1992; Kannel & Schatzkin, 1983; Mrazek & Haggerty, 1994). These factors appear to form a rough qualitative continuum ranging from simple markers (i.e., surface indicators, including gender and race) to moderators (e.g., augmenting influences such as the presence of a comorbid disease or disorder) to mediators (primary "causal" mechanisms such as exposure to HIV) of dysfunctional outcomes (Pandina, 1998).

An increasing number of prevention programs are developing strategies targeted specifically at altering risk factors (or enhancing protective conditions) empirically demonstrated to be related to both functional and dysfunctional outcomes. Furthermore, these programs are evaluating efficacy, at least in part, in terms of changes in risk and protective profiles as well as in changes in longer-term outcomes. Taken to the conceptual extreme, one desirable outcome of epidemiological research could be the development of a "periodic table" of essential risk and protective elements for different health arenas. Even achieving the modest goal of creating a glossary or taxonomy of factors would be of enormous value to prevention scientists. In a similar vein, etiological research extends to the exploration of the characterization of dysfunctions themselves, including issues related to the developmental course of the dysfunctions. (For example, in drug abuse, see Pandina, 1998; in delinquency, see Moffitt, 1993; in developmental psychopathology, see Cicchetti, 1993.)

Second, no single factor or set of factors, whether drawn from a single domain or combined from across domains, has led to an accepted etiological theory of one form (let alone all forms) of human dysfunction. Instead, risk and protective factor research has led to the development of dozens of creative and often conceptually compelling etiological theories applicable to specific outcomes, as well as a fewer number of more generic theories. (For examples in the drug abuse literature, see Glantz & Pickens, 1992; Hawkins et al., 1992; Lettieri, Sayers, & Pearson, 1980; Petraitis, Flay, & Miller, 1995; for delinquency, see Loeber & Stouthamer-Loeber, 1998; Moffit, 1993; for depression, see Cicchetti & Toth, 1998.) The number of plausible formulations has led to the view that human dysfunctions are likely to emerge from a number of etiological pathways, each with its own character and developmental trajectory. This "several distinct etiologic pathway" perspective suggests that multiple interventions may be needed for what, on the surface, appears to be the same dysfunctional outcome. This hypothesis could account for the apparent limitations in efficacy for some interventions.

Most, though not all, theoretical formulations can marshal some measure of empirical support. The plethora of plausible theories, as well as the wide range and quality of constructs that contribute to these theories, have led to the evolution of a common guiding heuristic paradigm—**biopsychosocial theory** (Ford, 1987; Institute of Medicine, 1996; Pandina & Johnson, 1999). This paradigm views dysfunctional behavior generically as not only a product of specific neurobiological, psychobehavioral, and socioenvironmental factor arrays but also a product of the complex and dynamic interaction of factors. This paradigm's popularity has resulted, in part, from the fact that many dysfunctional outcomes have been demonstrated to be the result of a common set of factors cited separately in a wide range of theories. (For examples of general and specific applications, see Cicchetti & Toth, 1998; Ford, 1987; Heckhausen & Schulz, 1995; Miller, 1978; Shapiro, Schwartz, & Astin, 1996.)

However, to date, this paradigm has afforded only "weak guidance" for etiology in prevention science (see Turkheimer, 1998). We characterize this as weak guidance because no effective algorithm (or method for developing such algorithms) has emerged that allows for identifying unique or generic factor models that include not only the identification of factors (within and across domains) but also the manner in which factors (and domains) may dynamically interact to produce health outcomes. Information about this dynamic processing could and should be used to inform prevention strategies. This is also important because intervention programs could be assessed on the basis of how effective they are in facilitating (or creating the conditions for facilitating) risk reduction and protection enhancement.

Third, as a consequence of the need for more comprehensive models, etiological researchers continue to develop increasingly **sophisticated methods for assessing empirical data** and fitting those data to complex theoretical explanatory models. For example, the measurement and analysis of change play a central role in many areas of clinical and health research. There are many problems associated with the measurement and analyses of longitudinal data, requiring complicated statistical techniques that have been outlined in works concerning structural equation modeling (Bentler, 1988; Jöreskog & Sörbom, 1988), hierarchical linear modeling (Bryk & Raudenbush, 1987), and growth curve modeling (Duncan, Duncan, & Stoolmiller, 1994; Francis, Fletcher, Stuebing, Davidson, & Thompson, 1991), for example. These same evaluative techniques can and are being adapted to the development of interventions and evaluations of prevention trials (e.g., Baron & Kenny, 1986; Bryant et al., 1997; National Institute on Drug Abuse, 1996). Hence, methods evolving in etiological research offer potential advantages to prevention scientists.

Fourth, it is becoming increasingly apparent that the development and assessment of etiologic (i.e., explanatory) and prevention (i.e., intervention) models are complex but interrelated tasks. Given the apparent **interrelationship**

between etiology and prevention, there is a growing belief that prevention trials research can be designed to yield important insight into etiologic theories of causal processes (e.g., West & Aiken, 1997). For example, etiologic theory building typically relies heavily on observations of variability of subjects and their characteristics, often in conjunction with their environments, to achieve a high level of ecological validity. Seldom does such research involve active manipulation, at least at the level of "large model" development. On the other hand, prevention, by definition, involves manipulation through implementation of an intervention. A prevention program that has a well-specified empirically grounded theoretical model that guides it, in terms of risk and protective factors, as well as intervention techniques and the processes that link factors and techniques, could yield important validations of etiological theories. This hybrid paradigm offers much promise for theory testing.

Fifth, as appealing as the new hybrid paradigm is, it is likely that such program tests of grand or large theory will be relatively limited in number compared to more traditional and more modest programs. The reasons for **limited grand theory testing** can be found in the restrictions in budgets (who will pay for large-scale longitudinal studies), the confines of methodological sophistication (in terms of both instrumentation and data analysis), and the ethical issues surrounding human subjects research (including the denial of intervention or treatment to individuals for the purposes of securing a control group). Furthermore, significant information already exists from both venues that could be useful for program planners. Etiology theorists are currently developing methods for combining information from limited trials and model testing. An increasing number of meta-analyses and empirical reviews are being published, covering important health behavior topics (e.g., see Chapters 18 and 19, this volume).

We began with the case for program planners' need to benefit from etiological research and have made the case for the development of a blended model, wherein assessment studies are then used to refine theory and provide information on requisite activities that facilitate maximized health outcomes. The next section of this chapter discusses some of the major dimensions that need to be considered in studies that fall under the general rubric of etiology assessment. These are the "nitty-gritty" of planning for one's assessment needs for a particular health behavior program.

QUESTIONS OF INQUIRY FOR DESIGNING AN ASSESSMENT STUDY

The foci of an assessment study in this phase of program development may be summarized as six questions of inquiry: why, who, where, when, what, and how.

The first obvious focus of any study is the why question pertaining to the particular phenomenon (i.e., *why* this health behavior or phenomenon is occurring and perhaps, just as important, *why* it is *important* to study this behavior). Once the why question has been addressed, it is then necessary to concentrate on the who component of investigation. In terms of *who*, clinical populations have historically provided the sample pool for the study of most physical and mental health disorders. Those who have been diagnosed in some way and have been treated in clinic settings have been studied extensively. In line with the recent prevention science attempt to reach persons prior to—and to prevent persons from—becoming a clinical sample, subjects now are studied prior to becoming obviously symptomatic. To do this, researchers must expand the *where* of the investigation beyond the clinic context. Also, to accomplish this goal of prevention, researchers have found that tracking the developmental progression of human behavior over the life span is informative. In other words, the *when* of investigation has been greatly extended from previous clinical work. The behaviors measured, or the *what* of investigation, now include early predictors of later disorders. Finally, the specific assessment techniques that are used provide answers to the *how* question. For the purposes of conceptualizing these questions of inquiry into a framework, the elements of a study have been partitioned into four dimensions, outlined below.

▶ THE DIMENSIONS OF AN ASSESSMENT STUDY

First to consider is the study's **type of design.** For example, designs may be cross-sectional, longitudinal, or experimental in structure. The second dimension focuses on the **structure of the observations.** The structure ranges from the completely unstructured observation (including data elements such as antidotal information) to the highly structured observation (including standardized inventories). The third dimension is the **level of observation** or unit of analysis. The unit of analysis in any study can include the smallest observable entity found in the biological organism (genetic makeup, tissue capacity, organ functioning, neural networks), the characteristics of an individual (psychological profile, attitudes toward deviance, physical manifestations of a disorder or disease), the interactions of small groups (play among preschoolers, cigarette smoking among teenagers), and the community or culture at large (number of alcohol-related fatal accidents, number of newborns affected by prenatal alcohol abuse, number of gang-related violent offenses). The fourth dimension is that which **characterizes the subject** under study. In the substance abuse and mental health fields, both clinical and nonclinical individuals have been the subject of study, in that researchers recognize the importance of examining both the healthy and "diseased."

DIMENSION 1: TYPES OF DESIGNS

Although a complex discussion of research design is beyond the scope of this chapter, we will summarize some of the general terms used (see Kazdin, 1992, for a detailed review). Studies have been loosely classified in terms of the research question asked. That is, a study can be (a) exploratory, in which the purpose is to develop hypotheses or establish future research priorities; (b) descriptive, that is, when its function is to assess the aspects of a situation (e.g., the prevalence of a population subsample or a health behavior); or (c) inferential, that is, when it is used to test one or more hypotheses.

One important aspect of a study design is how often the subject of interest is evaluated or examined. Data collected at one point in time (i.e., *cross-sectional*) have the advantages of being less expensive to collect, and results can be disseminated more quickly. These types of studies, be they general surveys or tests of specific models, historically have been the pillars of social science research. These data provide a quick snapshot of the topic but are, in a sense, frozen in a particular historical time frame. The limitation of such inquiries is that stability or change in behaviors or disease status cannot be ascertained.

Longitudinal studies are designed to encompass two or more data collection points that track the same group of individuals over time. These studies have the advantage of being able to trace stability and change in a sample. Note that alternative designs (e.g., time series) gather data at multiple points, although not necessarily using the same sample. In the substance abuse and mental health fields, there has been an outcropping of recent longitudinal studies (e.g., Brook, Balka, & Gursen, 1997; Brown, Gleghorn, & Schuckit, 1996; Brunswick & Messeri, 1986; Caetano & Kaskutas, 1995; Dembo, Williams, & Fagan, 1994; Huizinga, Loeber, & Thornberry, 1993; Hussong & Chassin, 1997; Kandel & Davies, 1992; Kaplan & Liu, 1994; Newcomb & Bentler, 1988; Pandina, Labouvie, & White, 1984; Schulenberg, Wadsworth, & O'Malley, 1996; Stacy, Newcomb, & Bentler, 1991). Longitudinal studies with large numbers of subjects, multiple observation points, and minimum attrition rates allow researchers the statistical power needed to conduct sophisticated analyses such as structural equation modeling, growth curve modeling, and the like (see Chapter 16 for a discussion of statistical power). One drawback of large-scale longitudinal studies is that they are expensive to conduct, and the information is perhaps years in the making. Longitudinal studies often generate large and sophisticated databases, but they also require specialized analysis methods to fully use the data they generate.

Perhaps the most structured of the research designs is the *experimental design*. Basic science and medical researchers have used these methods to manipulate conditions or events and to observe changes in the experimental sample compared to the changes (or lack thereof) in a control sample. Experiments have been conducted by substance use researchers on the biological level (e.g., the effects of prenatal alcohol exposure on developing fetuses in mice), the individual level (e.g., the effects of differential blood ethanol levels on task performance), the group level (e.g., the effects of social influences on peer dare behaviors), and the community level (e.g., manipulation of teen buyer appearance and the likelihood of being able to purchase alcoholic beverages at a store). The limitations of the experimental design include the inability to manipulate many naturally occurring phenomena (e.g., peer dares and one's cigarette smoking behavior, number of alcohol outlets per square mile and purchasing behavior) and the fact that every possible factor that may influence outcomes cannot be controlled. This is particularly relevant in studies conducted at the community level. Later in this chapter, a mixed model combining etiology and intervention assessment is discussed. If manipulations are effective and lead to expected alterations in etiological factors or outcome levels, strong evidence is provided for such a factor as being formative. Such hybrid models are relatively rare, and new applications have yet to be fully evaluated.

DIMENSION 2: STRUCTURE OF THE OBSERVATIONS

Incorporated within the design of a study are alternatives regarding the method of data collection. The means in which subjects are observed or data are collected range from the relatively unstructured a priori to the very structured. For the present discussion, we will briefly mention some of these approaches. We refer the reader to Chapters 9, 11, and 16 in this handbook on perceived efficacy and pilot studies for more information on specific assessment approaches. The case study is typically an unstructured, exploratory, or descriptive study in which data are collected on one case (individual) or on a small number of cases. The case study has been a popular format in the social sciences, where it has typically taken the form of the observational study. The unstructured biography of the experiences of subjects can be informative for mapping the etiology of a health problem. One gets a flavor for the gestalt of experiential influences that lead people to engage in different healthy or unhealthy behaviors. Although *case studies* have the advantage of providing in-depth information, they are limited in the number of subjects; that is, generalization to a group of people is limited. Sometimes, no organized data analysis is completed. Therefore, interpretation of the case often is bound by the perceptions of the case study writer. (Examples of case study descriptions in the substance abuse, aggression, or mental health literatures include those reported most recently by Duffy & Miln, 1996; Dunlap & Johnson, 1996; Fairbanks & Candelaria, 1998; Segal & Fairchild, 1996; Wilens, Biederman, & Spencer, 1997.)

Observational studies often have been conducted to corroborate studies that have relied on self-report or structured interview methods. Observations have the ability to examine more fully group interactions and the milieu in which behaviors occur. Observational studies involve the recording of events in their natural settings when they occur, the use of trained observers, and descriptions of behaviors and events (Sussman et al., 1993). One of the limitations of such a design is the sampling frame. For example, by and large, there is no control regarding the number or characteristics of the subjects who appear at the location that is under surveillance. The form that data collection takes must be decided on (standardized forms, handwritten notes, audio or video recordings), and data must be coded in some fashion for future analyses. (Recent examples in the substance abuse and violence fields include the work of Brudenell, 1997; Klinger, 1995; Raja, Azzoni, & Lubich, 1997; Van de Goor, Knibbe, & Drop, 1990.)

Using primarily the techniques of participant observation, case studies, and interviewing, researchers are conducting *ethnographic studies,* which are now entering the mainstream of social research (National Institute on Drug Abuse, 1997). The work of Stahler, Cohen, and Shipley (1993) and Johnson (1993), among others, argues that ethnographic research can be useful for increasing our understanding of unique or hidden populations, as well as our understanding of prevention and treatment processes and outcomes. Purposive (targeted) sampling is generally used rather than random sampling, and sampling may change over time as the research develops. Field observations typically are recorded, and the data are coded and sorted by topics and analyzed for patterns of behavior. These studies can be conducted over a short period of time at relatively little expense. In addition to the use of observations, case studies, and interviews, ethnographic researchers also have used archived documents, memoranda, newsletters, and the like to cull information. Ethnographic research goes beyond analytic description to include an analysis of the knowledge and beliefs that underlie behaviors. Proponents of this methodology contend that hypotheses built on the personal realities of the subject can be spawned and then later tested within an experimental model.

Ethnographic studies in both substance abuse and violent behavior generally have been concerned with describing a particular group's behavior while placing it in the context of values and norms that guide the group. More recent ethnographic studies have been used for research on alcohol and drug use among random samples (Fendrich, Wislar, & Mackesy-Amiti, 1996), workers (Ames, Grube, & Moore, 1997), adolescents (O'Nell & Mitchell, 1996; Parker, 1996), mentally ill (Cohen & Henkin, 1995; Cohen & Koegel, 1996), substance users (Agar & MacDonald, 1995; Joe, 1996; Sifaneck & Kaplan, 1995), and clients in treatment (Stahler et al., 1993).

Focus groups can be viewed as a more structured yet more intimate form of a survey, and they have been a mainstay in private-sector marketing research. More recently, health services researchers are beginning to discover the potential of this type of data-gathering technique (see Clayson, Berkowitz, & Brindis, 1995; Houghton, Carroll, & Odgers, 1998; Klein, Campbell, Soler, & Ghez, 1997; Levine & Zimmerman, 1996). Focus groups typically consist of 4 to 12 people, assembled in a group in which a moderator or facilitator imposes a focused discussion, and qualitative data are provided by members of the group. The focus group interview is conducted as a series of interviews, and similar persons (who usually do not know each other) are chosen to participate based on the purpose of study. The focus group allows for group interaction and insight on why certain views are held or behaviors committed. A variety of published guides (e.g., Krueger, 1994) provide assistance in planning, moderating, and analyzing results of data gleaned from a focus group encounter. These groups tap into the real-life interactions of people and allow a researcher to get in touch with perceptions, attitudes, and opinions in a way that other procedures do not allow. Focus groups have been used in the drug abuse field to identify early warning indicators of the incidence and prevalence of alcohol and drug abuse cases and provide an assessment of the quality of prevention and treatment service provision. An advantage of focus group interviews is that the format allows for probing by a moderator. In addition, the data have face validity, are gathered at a relatively low cost, and are synthesized relatively rapidly. On the downside, interviewers must be highly trained, a group is generally more difficult to assemble and control than an individual interview, data are difficult to code and analyze, and there is a lack of statistical power to conduct sophisticated statistical analyses. (Also, see Chapter 9 on the use of focus groups.)

DIMENSION 3: UNIT OF ANALYSIS (LEVEL OF OBSERVATION)

The research question at hand is itself the fundamental guiding element in the choice of the level of observation. The motivation for and consequences of engaging in different human behaviors, including health practices, have been researched from the tissue level to the cultural level. The levels of observation traditionally have been conceptualized as three tiers (Cicchetti & Toth, 1998; Ford, 1987; Pandina, 1998), somewhat reflective of any biopsychosocial model. At the *tissue level*, researchers in the fields of genetics, biology, biochemistry, and the like have examined the effect of alcohol and other drugs on neural circuits, as well as on brain and organ functioning. Researchers in the basic sciences also have investigated possible organic causes of aggressive behavior.

Psychologists and mental health specialists have examined the *intrapersonal characteristics* of an individual as both cause and outcome of substance use. Measures such as personality states and traits, cognitive functioning, affective symptoms, and developmental competencies such as coping strategies have been rigorously investigated vis-à-vis substance use and violent behavior.

Sociologists, social workers, and anthropologists historically have examined the characteristics of *groups of people.* Such studies have included the antecedents of substance use or violent behavior (i.e., parental hostility/neglect/abuse, deviant peer groups), the effect of substance use on the quality of interactions with others, the co-occurrence or comorbidity of substance use with violent or antisocial behavior, or, at a community level, cultural/racial/ethnic differences in both predictors and outcomes.

DIMENSION 4: CHARACTERISTICS OF THE UNIT

In addition to the assessment design, structure of observations, and level of analysis, the particular characteristics of the subject to be examined are yet another dimension to be considered. One important dimension is the developmental stage of the individual. In the study of the individual, a common proxy for this measure has been the age of the individual. There is also, of course, the *developmental stage* of the disorder or disease. Historically, in the substance use field, there has been a preoccupation with the study of pathological use and dependence, which resulted in restricting much research to adult clinical populations. Obviously, with the realization over the past several decades that the initiation of alcohol, tobacco, and drug use has its roots in the adolescent population, research in this area has taken on a life span approach in which attitudes and behaviors are viewed as changing or being stable over developmental periods ranging from infancy to old age.

Another salient attribute is the *current health status* of the individual. Studies have been conducted on individuals by virtue of the fact that they have been identified as having one or more predisposing risk factors. For example, children of alcoholics have been scrutinized on a variety of risk and protective factors due to the belief that they are at risk for some problematic outcome due to some mechanism of genetic transmission, even though they exhibit no manifestations of a problem. Additional characteristics of an individual that commonly have been used as exogenous, covariate, or *control measures* include aspects of socioeconomic status (education, income, occupation), culture, race, ethnicity, and geographic location.

The next section provides information on how program planners have organized themselves to collect and combine data.

▶ POOLING MULTIPLE SOURCES OF INFORMATION

To more efficiently process the vast knowledge provided by empirical studies, we have attempted to pool multiple separate sources of etiological information. A variety of governmental, private research, academic, and community-based organizations have joined forces in many locations to investigate the etiology of a variety of health concerns. The most common methods among communities of people wishing to pool information are using a task force, a community surveillance study, or a needs assessment. A common statistical method to pool the results from a variety of published studies is termed "meta-analysis." These four approaches are described below.

A *task force* typically comprises individuals who are trained or are in a position of authority to assess needs for a problem at hand, typically within a specific geographic location. Members of the task force may represent agencies or organizations or be common citizens who represent their families and their community. Typically, the task force will engage in a review of the literature, or it will hire an evaluator or organize a group of experts to summarize the literature for it. Then the task force will use the conclusions it makes based on the review that has been completed to recommend additional assessment work or lobby for needed programming. Task forces have helped to define appropriate uses of specific screening tests and diagnostic tools, counseling interventions, and therapies (McGrath, Keita, Strickland, & Russo, 1990; Widiger et al., 1994). Task forces also have identified high-risk groups and conducted statewide surveys of health statuses (Gratz & Claffey, 1996; Stevens, Mott, & Youells, 1996).

Community surveillance studies typically are conducted by a variety of public health-oriented agencies to study the spread, growth, or development of a public health problem. Information from multiple sources is accessed. For instance, for the purposes of mapping alcohol and drug abuse (see National Institute on Drug Abuse, 1998), such sources of data include information from public and private treatment facilities; a medical examiner or coroner; hospital emergency room records; law enforcement records; national, state, and local surveys; and telephone hotline information. Data from a variety of sources are reported in a standardized format to facilitate the review.

Needs assessments are used to determine the need for specific services in a particular geographic area. Most needs assessments are community based. Program planners conducting needs assessments typically rely on a variety of data sources. First, those conducting the assessment must define the problem and determine its magnitude within the geographic area of interest. If the issue concerns the need for the *treatment* of a specific disorder, researchers generally consider incidence and prevalence data. On the other hand, if the focus is on the *prevention* of a problem behavior, disorder, or disease, information concerning those at risk is sought. Planners also identify the demand for services, which will remediate the problem at hand. An inventory of the area services that are currently available to address the problem is documented. This information helps to establish which services are nonexistent and which are lacking. The differences in supply and demand will determine any gaps in the current provision of services. Finally, planners determine which additional knowledge, services, or resources are needed to fill the gaps and then prioritize the needed assessments or services so that resource allocation can be determined (Amodeo & Gal, 1997).

Meta-analysis is a systematic technique that applies statistically sensitive procedures to a literature review in an attempt to make sense of the variety of information coming from studies with varying samples and measurement instruments. Meta-analysis involves the selection, quality assessment, and synthesis of information concerning salient characteristics and outcomes among a group of studies. Many forms of these analyses have been distinguished, but generally they are used to examine (a) the associations among predictors and outcomes, such as gender and alcohol use or age and offender recidivism (e.g., Hanson & Bussiere, 1998; Johnstone, Leino, & Ager, 1996); (b) potential differences in levels of problem behaviors across naturally occurring groups (e.g., Fillmore, Johnstone, Leino, & Ager, 1993); (c) treatment effectiveness, such as the effect of psychotherapy or a prevention intervention (e.g., Agosti, 1995; Tobler, 1992); and (d) the validity of a measurement procedure, such as comparing quantitative with qualitative data or untangling the methodological parameters that moderate effects (e.g., Bushman & Cooper, 1990). (For more in-depth and readable discussions of meta-analysis applications, see Bangert-Downs, Wells-Parker, & Chevillard, 1997; Bickman & Rog, 1998; Cooper & Hedges, 1994; Durlak & Lipsey, 1991; see also Chapter 18, this volume.) Meta-analysis can handle scores of variables from hundreds of studies. The process of conducting a meta-analysis is similar to conducting a literature review, in that the formulation of the research question is key. Proponents of this method argue that the studies used in any meta-analysis must meet or surpass the highest standards of research integrity (Slavin, 1986). Any study included in a meta-analysis must have a high degree of construct or external validity (i.e., the study must be relevant) as well as a high degree of internal validity (i.e., the design of the study must be sound). Etiological and evaluation studies can be rated on a variety of dimensions of quality encompassing sampling strategies (including initial selection, random assignment to conditions, and the amount of attrition suffered), the adequacy and equivalence of measurements (which affects the ability to identify causal relationships between variables), and, when applicable, the integrity of the intervention or treatment. The pitfalls of these types of analyses are the topic of current debate (see Peck, 1995). Practitioners must rely on the meta-analyst's judgment that all included studies have passed methodological standards for inclusion, that the choice of the coding schema is reliable and valid, and that statistical techniques applied to the data are appropriate. In addition, meta-analysis cannot be conducted on all types of studies due to design and sample size limitations (see Chapter 18, this volume, for more information).

▶ DECISION CRITERIA WHEN SELECTING ASSESSMENT STUDIES FOR REVIEW

The previous sections of this chapter have provided an overview of etiological studies—their rationale, foci, dimensions, and methods. The following section reviews some of the central conceptual and methodological criteria to consider when one engages in a *review* of the assessment study literature. The review of completed studies will save much time and effort and should be the main starting point in etiological assessment work. If one chooses to review primary assessment studies, then having an understanding of basic conceptual and methodological issues will help one to organize a search for relevant information and better evaluate the significance of what is reviewed. The reader also is referred to Durlak and Lipsey (1991, p. 297) for an inventory of the relevant steps and issues at each phase of the research process and to Chapter 7 of this volume, which also provides decision criteria for selecting information for review (in the context of pooling prior intervention-type material).

CONCEPTUAL ISSUES

The primary conceptual challenge is developing a firm, well-defined understanding of the questions to be addressed. However, questions, no matter how specific, need to be answered within the theoretical context from which the question arises. Hence, research questions should be grounded in a clear theoretical context. Studies worthy of attention should outline, preferably explicitly, the theory that has guided their data collection. Questions of importance include the following: What was the purpose of the study? What theory were the authors pursuing? What specific hypotheses were being tested? How did the hypotheses (suppositions or propositions that are assumed but not yet proven) test the theory? Who collected the data? Why were the data gathered? In a sense, the theoretical framework is the implicit or explicit acceptable bias of the investigator—the motivation for conducting the research.

Core questions may appear targeted and quite circumscribed; for example, one might be interested in providing documentation about the extent of a dysfunctional outcome (e.g., hazardous drinking) in a given target population (e.g., youth) for the purpose of designing an intervention program. In many cases, even simple questions that appear well defined are embedded in a broader theoretical framework. Consideration of the broader theoretical picture may affect the interpretation of data for one's purposes—in other words, the weight given to the evidence (also see Chapter 4, this volume).

Hence, it is important to select and weigh studies that allow one to understand the theories and hypotheses that are the foundation for the actual empirical investigation. Theories and hypotheses should be articulated and tied to the data being collected. The data gathered should be connected to the hypotheses in a manner that is clearly articulated. Tests of the hypotheses (e.g., statistical analyses) should be tied clearly to the data no matter what the outcome or results. Interpretations of the data and results of any statistical analyses should be carefully articulated and should flow logically from the data back to the hypotheses being tested. Reasonable questions to ask include the following: Does what the author proposes have internal consistency? That is, do the ideas presented hang together systematically and logically, given the assumptions and biases the author has stated? Do the data being used provide a reasonable picture of the theoretical relationships being proposed? Do the assessments make sense; that is, are the proper comparisons among groups or types of individuals being made? Are the comparisons that the author reports fair tests of the hypotheses? Finally, how were the results interpreted by the author?

It is also important to recognize that for most types of human dysfunction that have become targets of intervention, there is, at best, limited consensus as to which theories are "correct." For many outcomes, a number of viable theories are proposed. In approaching any review, it is important to seek out information on a wide range of alternative explanations and to evaluate the empirical support (i.e., evidence) in a comparative analysis. The likelihood is that many studies will be convincing if they satisfactorily address the questions raised above. Individual studies that pass muster should be viewed as viable "opinions." Therefore, it is important that as many such opinions as are available be sought out and evaluated together. Furthermore, it is important to recognize that many researchers conduct programs of research and therefore publish several articles on related topics, often using the same or similar theories, databases, and analytical approaches. It is important to consider the program of research of a given investigator or laboratory as a single "grand" experiment to have an adequate grasp of where that program of research fits into one's own evaluation and how much weight should be given to results. In this regard, it is also valuable to identify studies purporting to test the same theories and related hypotheses but that had been conducted by unrelated investigators or laboratories. Although it is rare to find complete replications of research (especially in the behavioral and social sciences), even partial replications add weight given to theory testing.

Hence, it is important to look at a reasonably broad sample of theories and related empirical tests of theories to have a more complete picture of current thinking related to the problem of interest. Once there is a clear understanding of the manner in which the research question connects within its broader context and a reasonable, though not necessarily exhaustive, set of alternative answers has been identified, it is time to turn the attention to carefully assessing the details of the alternative answers with an eye to constructing the answer of best fit for the questions that have been raised.

METHODOLOGICAL ISSUES

It is no secret that for any investigation, the devil is in the details. Applied to the goal of this chapter, this axiom means that the weight to be given to empirical evidence is closely related to the adequacy of the methods used to form that opinion. For program planners, it is important to pay careful attention to the goodness of fit between the studies reviewed and the specific aims of a review. In other words, in selecting opinions and data for a research question, it is important to choose methodologically sound studies and those that make a good fit for the question at hand. Questions typically run the gambit from estimating the extent and nature of a problem (e.g., rates of drug use in a community, number of cases of HIV-positive individuals) to considering predictors (e.g., sensation seeking) or complete theories (e.g., problem behavior or social learning theory) pertaining to the behavior. The review of a number of conceptual articles or books adds to an understanding of the depth and range of issues that must be appreciated.

The obvious jumping-off point is the assembly of the data. In the case of most questions, this involves culling out empirical articles that seem to match the particular question on a number of parameters. Because many of the problems of program planners are targeted to understanding problems of specific groups (e.g., school-age children, HIV-positive individuals, the homeless), it is best to gather studies with **subjects that are similar to those that are of interest**. Studies employing larger and more representative samples (i.e., sufficient range in age, gender, race/ethnicity, culture, geographic location) are preferred. Often, useful summaries of incidence and prevalence are available from national institutes or from studies sponsored by national institutes. Many such surveys will contain information beyond simple prevalence estimates. These studies typically document the methods used to collect data, instruments, and important estimates of the representativeness of the study. The methodological features of the studies selected must be reviewed carefully. Using one of the many database-searching tools available at university libraries or through the Internet, one will also yield a significant number of leads about relevant studies (e.g., MedLine, PsychINFO).

In addition to grand-scale prevalence surveys, it is also valuable to seek out smaller-scale studies employing purposeful samples that match closely the kinds of targeted individuals. Purposeful samples include individuals who have certain dysfunctions or fit specific risk criteria. These may be drawn from the general population by using special screening techniques (e.g., telephone surveys using selected interview techniques) or may come from a variety of gatekeeping organizations such as hospitals, clinics, or special treatment programs.

Smaller-scale studies employing purposeful samples can be very informative partly because they use subjects of key interest. Also, because the sample sizes are often small, these studies may employ a wide range of measurement probes (i.e., methods such as questionnaire items, standardized inventories, interview notes, etc.) that provide a more in-depth assessment of subjects than what might be assessed through using surveys of large, representative samples. However, it is important to understand how well these informative subjects may represent the general class of target subjects. In particular, attention must be paid to the manner in which these samples are drawn; most such studies will provide estimates of the degree to and manner in which the samples are representative of the identified group. (See Chapters 9-13 of this text for examples of specific methods often used in smaller-scale studies.)

Although most descriptive studies are cross-sectional in nature, a growing number of studies are longitudinal in design. Longitudinal designs permit assessment of temporal patterns and individual change in dependent and independent variables. When possible, it is desirable to include longitudinal studies in any assessment study pool. However, it is necessary to determine how many subjects are retained in the sample. Results of studies with large rates of attrition (i.e., dropouts from the study) can be problematic to evaluate.

In a similar vein, results of experiments conducted in laboratories may be useful for many purposes. For example, studies of characteristics of specific at-risk groups (e.g., children of alcoholics, depressed cigarette smokers, children diagnosed with attention deficit disorder) may provide insight into the nature of risk and protective factors. Often, these studies are limited by sample size and composition. A quick rule of thumb is that a minimum of five subjects per variable is imperative for needed statistical power. Therefore, it might be necessary to gather several such studies and pool results. In this regard, meta-analytic techniques are useful. In fact, practitioners usually can locate a published meta-analysis that focuses on their interests. (The reader is referred to the excellent review by Durlak & Lipsey [1991] or Chapter 18 of this text for practitioners discussing criteria for evaluating meta-analyses.)

Once studies with informative samples have been identified, attention should be focused on the **types of measurement probes** that are applied.

Probes may range from simple questionnaires to standardized inventories and assessment interviews. In some cases, they may include specialized biological testing involving sophisticated techniques; assessment of biological material (e.g., blood, urine, hair) may be included. Irrespective of how simple or complex a given test or battery of tests is, it should be judged by minimum common criteria. First and foremost, probes should be documented in terms of reliability (i.e., the consistency of the measure) and validity (i.e., the extent to which a particular probe assesses the domain of interest). (Although a discussion of these issues is beyond the scope of this chapter, the reader is referred to Kazdin [1992] for a review of reliability, including test-retest, internal and interrater, and validity, including content, criterion, face, convergent, and discriminant.) The constructs that such probes are meant to represent should be clearly and specifically documented. Ideally, constructs should be measured using multiple indicators. Second, investigators should demonstrate that assessments were properly and consistently performed by trained personnel. Third, results of assessments should be provided in sufficient detail and clarity so that what they mean and how they relate to the concepts of interest are understood. If norms are relied on for standardized tests, these should be provided or documentation presented. Differences in measurement metrics (i.e., the quantitative ways in which a variable is coded, as in nominal, ordinal, or interval levels) (see Kazdin, 1992) should be explained to permit evaluation of effect size, not just in terms of whether groups statistically differed.

In summary, key methodological issues can be scaled along two key dimensions: (a) adequacy and diversity of sample characteristics and (b) identification and specificity of theoretical and measurement models. Studies should be selected that have samples of sufficient size and variability to ensure that the full range of the dysfunction of interest and related risk and protective factors can be displayed. Selected studies should represent the full range of theories and models that attempt to explain the nature of the dysfunctional condition and related etiological factors. Studies that attempt to operationalize and measure empirically the dysfunctional condition and related etiological factors should be given high priority for inclusion in any search.

▶ CONCLUSIONS

Our belief is that health behavior program planners who appreciate why and how dysfunctional behaviors occur (i.e., etiological underpinnings) will be in a better position to design programs that can best alter mechanisms and moderators that produce the dysfunctional outcomes. We believe that interventions that are empirically informed regarding the types and strengths of etiological factors have a greater likelihood of affecting behavior and help advance our etiological understanding as well.

Program planners are faced with many problems when asked to provide a review of the current state of knowledge regarding etiological models. Assuming that samples are adequate and appropriate for specific purposes and that measurements are valid, reliable, and are conceptually of interest, the task that remains is wrangling with the results of the search and their interpretation. This is the most challenging and, in some senses, most artful process to be encountered. Every study has limitations of one kind or another. It is important to understand the limits and what they mean when evaluating the results for specific purposes (see Chapters 9 and 11, this volume). Selected studies should make clear statements about which limitations exist in the approach to assessment and the constraints that these place on key interpretations.

Unfortunately, no conceptual formulas or prepackaged computer programs can ensure that the one correct solution to a particular problem or question will be selected. In the final assessment, two simple principles can be used to guide the program planner: the *preponderance of the evidence* and *solution of best fit*. The preponderance principle dictates that the decision (i.e., verdict) should be based on the weight of the most convincing evidence available at the time. The best-fit principle dictates the need to select some etiological representation for a particular situation that most closely parallels the specifics of the particular situation.

In weighing evidence, under the preponderance principle, it is important to gather and examine as many empirical studies as possible that contain information about the subject or problem of interest. The next task is to rate the studies on a number of core criteria. Studies that have sound methodology should be given greatest weight. Once the set of studies to be relied on as evidence is gathered, it is useful to rank order them from those meeting rigorous methodological criteria to those that may be somewhat limited.

The next step is the most difficult and, perhaps, the most subjective. It is necessary to determine if a clear pattern of results is evident, giving greatest weight to those studies that are strongest and most complete. In a sense, the task is similar to putting a puzzle together. The strongest and most comprehensive studies form the outline (i.e., borders) and give structure (i.e., identify the major objects) to the puzzle picture. The outline and structure provided by the strongest studies help to provide a context for placing the supporting (i.e., acceptable but limited) puzzle pieces. Unfortunately, most scientific puzzles have missing pieces, and it is necessary to fill in the blank spaces based on the amount and strength of information available.

The other principle—solution of best fit—attempts to match the patterns uncovered to the particular circumstances for which one wishes to provide a solution. Thus, one must answer the following question: How closely does the generic picture constructed fit with the circumstances of the problem of interest?

For example, if one wishes to design an intervention program, a series of questions need to be addressed: How closely do the targets of intervention (e.g., seventh graders in an urban environment, high school athletes, female delinquents) in the study set match those in my circumstance? Are the conditions in which interventions took place similar? Can the interventions be delivered in the same manner? What is the expected outcome? In other words, one must define the outline and image of the specific situation and determine the degree to which the general puzzle pieces can be used to form the picture you want.

This chapter has emphasized the need to focus assessment through the lenses of critical questions and has provided guidance as regards methods to formulate such questions. We have offered guidance in assembling and evaluating evidence currently available and in determining how to select the best evidence available to address the problem at hand. In the end, it is believed that choices will be better if the tools provided here are used to build answers. There are probably no perfect solutions, but there are those that best fit a particular circumstance.

▶ REFERENCES

AGAR, M., & MACDONALD, J. (1995). Focus groups and ethnography. *Human Organization, 54,* 78-86.

AGOSTI, V. (1995). The efficacy of treatments in reducing alcohol consumption: A meta-analysis. *International Journal of the Addictions, 30,* 1067-1077.

AMES, G. M., GRUBE, J. W., & MOORE, R. S. (1997). The relationship of drinking and hangovers to workplace problems: An empirical study. *Journal of Studies on Alcohol, 58,* 37-47.

AMODEO, M., & GAL, C. (1997). Strategies for ensuring use of needs assessment findings: Experiences of a community substance abuse prevention program. *Journal of Primary Prevention, 18,* 227-242.

BANGERT-DOWNS, R. L., WELLS-PARKER, E., & CHEVILLARD, I. (1997). Assessing the methodological quality of research in narrative reviews and meta-analyses. In K. J. Bryant, M. Windel, & S. G. West (Eds.), *The science of prevention: Methodological advances from alcohol and substance abuse research* (pp. 405-429). Washington, DC: American Psychological Association.

BARON, R. M., & KENNY, D. A. (1986). The moderator-mediator variable distinction in social psychological research: Conceptual, strategic and statistical considerations. *Journal of Personality and Social Psychology, 51,* 1173-1182.

BENTLER, P. M. (1988). Causal modeling via structural equation system. In J. Nesselroade & R. B. Cattell (Eds.), *Handbook of multivariate experimental psychology* (pp. 317-335). New York: Plenum.

BICKMAN, L., & ROG, D. J. (Eds.). (1998). *Handbook of applied social research methods.* Thousand Oaks, CA: Sage.

BROOK, J. S., BALKA, E. B., & GURSEN, M. D. (1997). Young adults' drug use: A 17-year longitudinal inquiry of antecedents. *Psychological Reports, 80,* 1235-1251.

BROWN, S. A., GLEGHORN, A., & SCHUCKIT, M. A. (1996). Conduct disorder among adolescent alcohol and drug abusers. *Journal of Studies on Alcohol, 57,* 314-324.

BRUDENELL, I. (1997). A grounded theory of protecting recovery during transition to motherhood. *American Journal of Drug & Alcohol Abuse, 23,* 453-466.

BRUNSWICK, A. F., & MESSERI, P. (1986). Drugs, lifestyle, and health: A longitudinal study of urban black youth. *American Journal of Public Health, 76,* 52-57.

BRY, B. H., McKEON, P., & PANDINA, R. J. (1982). Extent of drug use as a function of number of risk factors. *Journal of Abnormal Psychology, 91,* 273-279.

BRYANT, K. J., WINDEL, M. J., & WEST, S. G. (Eds.). (1997). *The science of prevention: Methodological advances from alcohol and substance abuse research.* Washington, DC: American Psychological Association.

BRYK, A. S., & RAUDENBUSH, S. W. (1987). Application of hierarchical linear models to assessing change. *Psychological Bulletin, 191,* 147-158.

BUSHMAN, B. J., & COOPER, H. M. (1990). Effects of alcohol on human aggression: An integrative research review. *Psychological Bulletin, 107,* 341-354.

CAETANO, R., & KASKUTAS, L. A. (1995). Changes in drinking patterns among Whites, Blacks, and Hispanics, 1984-1992. *Journal of Studies on Alcohol, 56,* 558-565.

CICCHETTI, D. (1993). Review: Developmental psychopathology: Reactions, reflections, projections. *Developmental Review, 13,* 471-502.

CICCHETTI, D., & TOTH, S. L. (1998). The development of depression on children and adolescents. *American Psychologist, 53,* 221-241.

CLAYSON, Z., BERKOWITZ, G., & BRINDIS, C. (1995). Themes and variations among seven comprehensive perinatal drug and alcohol abuse treatment models. *Health & Social Work, 20,* 234-238.

COHEN, A., & KOEGEL, P. (1996). The influence of alcohol and drug use on the subsistence adaptation of homeless mentally ill persons. *Journal of Drug Issues, 26,* 219-243.

COHEN, E., & HENKIN, I. (1995). Substance abuse and lifestyle among an urban schizophrenic population: Some observations. *Psychiatry, 58,* 113-120.

COIE, J. D., WATT, N. F., WEST, S. G., HAWKINS, J. D., ASARNOW, J. R., MARKMAN, H. J., RAMEY, S. L., SHURE, M. B., & LONG, B. (1993). The science of prevention: A conceptual framework and some directions for a national research program. *American Psychologist, 48,* 1013-1022.

COOPER, H., & HEDGES, L. V. (1994). *The handbook of research synthesis.* New York: Russell Sage.

DEMBO, R., WILLIAMS, L., & FAGAN, J. (1994). Development and assessment of a classification of high-risk youths. *Journal of Drug Issues, 24,* 25-53.

DUFFY, A., & MILN, R. (1996). Case study: Withdrawal syndrome in adolescent chronic cannabis users. *Journal of the American Academy of Child and Adolescent Psychiatry, 35,* 1618-1621.

DUNCAN, T. E., DUNCAN, S. C., & STOOLMILLER, M. (1994). Modeling developmental processes using latent growth structural equation methodology. *Applied Psychological Measurement, 18,* 343-354.

DUNLAP, E., & JOHNSON, B. D. (1996). Family and human resources in the development of a female crack-seller career: Case study of a hidden population. *Journal of Drug Issues, 26,* 175-198.

DURLAK, J. A., & LIPSEY, M. W. (1991). A practitioner's guide to meta-analysis. *American Journal of Community Psychology, 19,* 291-332.

FAIRBANKS, J., & CANDELARIA, J. (1998). *Case studies in community health.* Thousand Oaks, CA: Sage.

FENDRICH, M., WISLAR, J. S., & MACKESY-AMITI, M. E. (1996). Mechanisms of noncompletion in ethnographic research of drugs: Results from a secondary analysis. *Journal of Drug Issues, 26,* 23-44.

FILLMORE, K. M., JOHNSTONE, B. M., LEINO, E. V., & AGER, C. R. (1993). A cross-study contextual analysis of effects from individual-level drinking and group-level drinking factors: A meta-analysis of multiple longitudinal studies from the Collaborative Alcohol-Related Longitudinal Project. *Journal of Studies on Alcohol, 54,* 37-47.

FORD, D. H. (1987). *Humans as self-constructing living systems: A developmental perspective on behavior and personality.* Hillsdale, NJ: Lawrence Erlbaum.

FRANCIS, D. J., FLETCHER, J. M., STUEBING, K. K., DAVIDSON, K. C., & THOMPSON, N. M. (1991). Analysis of change: Modeling individual growth. *Journal of Consulting and Clinical Psychology, 59,* 27-37.

GLANTZ, M., & PICKENS, R. W. (Eds.). (1992). *Vulnerability to drug use.* Washington, DC: American Psychological Association.

GRATZ, R. R., & CLAFFEY, A. (1996). Adult health in child care: Health status, behaviors, and concerns of teachers, directors, and family care providers. *Early Childhood Research Quarterly, 11,* 243-267.

HANSON, R. K., & BUSSIERE, M. T. (1998). Predicting relapse: A meta-analysis of sexual offender recidivism studies. *Journal of Consulting and Clinical Psychology, 66,* 348-362.

HAWKINS, J. D., CATALANO, R. F., & MILLER, J. Y. (1992). Risk and protective factors for alcohol and other drug problems in adolescence and early adulthood: Implications for substance abuse prevention. *Psychological Bulletin, 112,* 64-105.

HECKHAUSEN, J., & SCHULZ, R. (1995). A life-span theory of control. *Psychological Review, 102,* 284-304.

HOUGHTON, S., CARROLL, A., & ODGERS, P. (1998). Young children, adolescents and alcohol—Part I: Exploring knowledge and awareness of alcohol and related issues. *Journal of Child & Adolescent Substance Abuse, 7,* 1-29.

HUIZINGA, D., LOEBER, R., & THORNBERRY, T. P. (1993). Longitudinal study of delinquency, drug use, sexual activity, and pregnancy among children and youth in three cities. *Public Health Reports, 108,* 90-96.

HUSSONG, A. M., & CHASSIN, L. A. (1997). Substance use initiation among adolescent children of alcoholics: Testing protective factors. *Journal of Studies on Alcohol, 58,* 272-279.

INSTITUTE OF MEDICINE. (1996). *Pathways of addiction: Opportunities on drug abuse research.* Washington, DC: National Academy Press.

JOE, K. A. (1996). The lives and times of Asian-Pacific American women drug users: An ethnographic study of their methamphetamine use. *Journal of Drug Issues, 26,* 199-218.

JOHNSON, P. B. (1993). The value of ethnographic alcohol studies: A psychologist's perspective. *Social Science & Medicine, 37,* 27-30.

JOHNSTONE, B. M., LEINO, E. V., & AGER, C. R. (1996). Determinants of life-course variation in the frequency of alcohol consumption: Meta-analysis of studies from the collaborative alcohol-related longitudinal project. *Journal of Studies on Alcohol, 57,* 494-506.

JÖRESKOG, K. G., & SÖRBOM, D. (1988). *LISREL VII: A guide to program and applications.* Chicago: SPSS, Inc.

KANDEL, D. B., & DAVIES, M. (1992). Progression of regular marijuana involvement: Phenomology and risk factors for near-daily use. In M. Glantz & R. Pickens (Eds.), *Vulnerability to drug use* (pp. 211-254). Washington, DC: American Psychological Association.

KANNEL, W., & SCHATZKIN, A. (1983). Risk factor analysis. *Progress in Cardiovascular Disease, 26,* 309-332.

KAPLAN, H. B., & LIU, X. (1994). A longitudinal analysis of mediating variables in the drug use-dropping out relationship. *Criminology, 32,* 415-439.

KAZDIN, A. E. (1992). *Research design in clinical psychology.* Boston: Allyn & Bacon.

KLEIN, E., CAMPBELL, J., SOLER, E., & GHEZ, M. (1997). *Ending domestic violence: Changing public perceptions/halting the epidemic.* Thousand Oaks, CA: Sage.

KLINGER, D. A. (1995). The micro-structure of nonlethal force: Baseline data from an observational study. *Criminal Justice Review, 20,* 169-186.

KRUEGER, R. A. (1994). *Focus groups: A practical guide for applied research.* Thousand Oaks, CA: Sage.

LETTIERI, D. J., SAYERS, M., & PEARSON, H. W. (Eds.). (1980). *Theories on drug abuse: Selected contemporary perspectives.* Rockville, MD: National Institute on Drug Abuse.

LEVINE, I. S., & ZIMMERMAN, J. D. (1996). Using qualitative data to inform public policy: Evaluating "Choose to De-Fuse." *American Journal of Orthopsychiatry, 66,* 363-377.

LOEBER, R., & FARRINGTON, D. P. (Eds.). (1998). *Serious & violent juvenile offenders: Risk factors and successful interventions.* Thousand Oaks, CA: Sage.

LOEBER, R., & STOUTHAMER-LOEBER, M. (1998). Development of juvenile aggression and violence: Some common misconceptions and controversies. *American Psychologist, 53,* 242-259.

McGRATH, E., KEITA, G. P., STRICKLAND, B. R., & RUSSO, N. F. (Eds.). (1990). *Women and depression: Risk factors and treatment issues: Final report of the American Psychological Association's National Task Force.* Washington, DC: American Psychological Association.

MILLER, J. G. (1978). *Living systems.* New York: McGraw-Hill.

MOFFITT, T. E. (1993). Adolescence-limited and life-course persistent antisocial behavior: A developmental taxonomy. *Psychological Review, 100,* 674-701.
MRAZEK, P. J., & HAGGERTY, R. J. (Eds.). (1994). *Reducing risks for mental disorders: Frontiers for preventive intervention research.* Washington, DC: Institute of Medicine, National Academy Press.
MUNOZ, R. F., MRAZEK, P. J., & HAGGERTY, R. J. (1996). Institute of Medicine report on prevention of mental disorders: Summary and commentary. *American Psychologist, 51,* 1116-1122.
NATIONAL INSTITUTE ON DRUG ABUSE. (1996). *National conference of drug abuse prevention research: Presentation, papers, and recommendations* (NIH Pub. No. 98-4293). Rockville, MD: National Institutes of Health.
NATIONAL INSTITUTE ON DRUG ABUSE. (1997). *International epidemiology work group on drug abuse* (NIH Pub. No. 98-4208B). Rockville, MD: National Institutes of Health.
NATIONAL INSTITUTE ON DRUG ABUSE. (1998). *Assessing drug abuse within and across communities: Community epidemiology surveillance networks on drug abuse* (NIH Pub. No. 98-3614). Rockville, MD: National Institutes of Health.
NEWCOMB, M. D., & BENTLER, P. M. (1988). *Consequences of adolescent drug use.* Newbury Park, CA: Sage.
O'NELL, T. D., & MITCHELL, C. M. (1996). Alcohol use among American Indian adolescents: The role of culture in pathological drinking. *Social Science & Medicine, 42,* 565-578.
PANDINA, R. J. (1998). Risk and protective factor models on adolescent drug use: Putting them to work for prevention. In National Institutes of Health (Ed.), *National conference on drug abuse prevention research: Presentation, papers, and recommendations* (pp. 17-26). Washington, DC: National Institutes of Health.
PANDINA, R. J., & JOHNSON, V. (1999). Why do people use, abuse and become dependent on drugs? Progress toward a heuristic model. In M. Glantz & C. R. Hartel (Eds.), *Drug abuse: Origins and preventions* (pp. 119-148). Washington, DC: American Psychological Association.
PANDINA, R. J., LABOUVIE, E. W., & WHITE, H. R. (1984). Potential contributions of the life span developmental approach to the study of adolescent alcohol and drug use: The Rutgers Health and Human Development Project, a working model. *Journal of Drug Issues, 14,* 253-268.
PARKER, H. (1996). Young adult offenders, alcohol and criminological cul-de-sacs. *British Journal of Criminology, 36,* 282-298.
PECK, R. C. (1995). Inherent problems of meta-analysis. *Addiction, 90,* 1589-1591.
PETRAITIS, J., FLAY, B. R., & MILLER, T. Q. (1995). Reviewing theories of adolescent substance use: Organizing pieces in the puzzle. *Psychological Bulletin, 117,* 67-86.
RAJA, M., AZZONI, A., & LUBICH, L. (1997). Aggressive and violent behavior in a population of psychiatric inpatients. *Social Psychiatry & Psychiatric Epidemiology, 32,* 428-434.
REISS, D., & PRICE, R. H. (1996). National Research Agenda for Prevention Research: The National Institute of Mental Health Report. *American Psychologist, 51,* 1109-1115.
SCHULENBERG, J. E., WADSWORTH, K. N., & O'MALLEY, P. M. (1996). Adolescent risk factors for binge drinking during the transition to young adulthood: Variable- and pattern-centered approaches to change. *Developmental Psychology, 32,* 659-674.
SEGAL, S. D., & FAIRCHILD, H. H. (1996). Polysubstance abuse: A case study. *Adolescence, 31,* 797-805.
SHAPIRO, D. H., SCHWARTZ, C. E., & ASTIN, J. A. (1996). Controlling ourselves, controlling our world: Psychology's role in understanding positive and negative consequences of seeking and gaining control. *American Psychologist, 51,* 1213-1230.
SIFANECK, S. J., & KAPLAN, C. D. (1995). Keeping off, stepping on and stepping off: The steppingstone theory reevaluated in the context of the Dutch cannabis experience. *Contemporary Drug Problems, 22,* 483-512.
SLAVIN, R. E. (1986). Best-evidence synthesis: An alternative to meta-analytic and traditional reviews. *Educational Research, 15,* 5-11.
STACY, A. W., NEWCOMB, M. D., & BENTLER, P. M. (1991). Cognitive motivation and drug use: A 9-year longitudinal study. *Journal of Abnormal Psychology, 100,* 502-515.
STAHLER, G. J., COHEN, E., & SHIPLEY, T. E. (1993). Why clients drop out of treatment: Ethnographic perspectives on treatment attrition among homeless male "crack" cocaine users. *Contemporary Drug Problems, 20,* 651-680.

STEVENS, M. M., MOTT, L. A., & YOUELLS, F. (1996). Rural adolescent drinking behavior: Three-year follow-up in the New Hampshire Substance Abuse Prevention Study. *Adolescence, 31,* 159-166.

SUSSMAN, S., HAHN, G., DENT, C. W., STACY, A. W., BURTON, D., & FLAY, B. R. (1993). Naturalistic observation of adolescent tobacco use. *International Journal of the Addictions, 28*(9), 803-811.

TOBLER, N. S. (1992). Drug prevention programs can work: Research findings. *Journal of Addictive Diseases, 11,* 1-28.

TURKHEIMER, E. (1998). Heritability and biological explanation. *Psychological Review, 105,* 782-791.

VAN DE GOOR, L. A., KNIBBE, R. A., & DROP, M. J. (1990). Adolescent drinking behavior: An observational study of the influence of situational factors on adolescent drinking rates. *Journal of Studies on Alcohol, 51,* 548-555.

WEST, S. G., & AIKEN, L. S. (1997). Toward understanding individual effects in multicomponent prevention programs: Design and analysis strategies. In K. J. Bryant, M. Windel, & S. G. West (Eds.), *The science of prevention: Methodological advances from alcohol and substance abuse research* (pp. 167-209). Washington, DC: American Psychological Association.

WIDIGER, T. A., FRANCES, A. J., PINCUS, H. A., FIRST, M. B., ROSS, R., & DAVIS, W. (Eds.). (1994). *DSM-IV sourcebook* (Vol. 1). Washington, DC: American Psychiatric Association.

WILENS, T. E., BIEDERMAN, J., & SPENCER, T. J. (1997). Case study: Adverse effects of smoking marijuana while receiving tricyclic antidepressants. *Journal of the American Academy of Child and Adolescent Psychiatry, 36,* 45-48.

CHAPTER 6

Commentary

Suzanne M. McMurphy
Kim T. Mueser

Enhancing the rigor of prevention programs and fine-tuning treatment efforts toward the maximization of behavioral outcomes are a critical development in the future of health behavior research and practice and, more specifically, prevention science. The results from several longitudinal studies examining the interactive effects of risk and protective factors on unhealthy behavioral outcomes have provided an abundance of data with which to inform the development of prevention programs. However, making sense of the available data and determining which studies provide reliable and valid information are not easy tasks. The argument for basing prevention programs on empirical knowledge obtained from available etiological studies, making judgments about the quality of these studies, and reviewing the criteria for the development of prevention-based research are critical contributions made by Johnson and Pandina in their chapter. In our commentary, we discuss the points made by the authors and raise several issues that emerge from their discussion.

Johnson and Pandina provide an excellent discussion of the importance of using etiological research to inform the development of prevention programs. They point out that prevention programs often are created without a strong conceptual or theoretical foundation, as little information in the literature has been useful in guiding specific program composition. These authors note that the dominant paradigm—the biopsychosocial theory—has, to date, provided only weak guidance for the development of prevention programs. This is in part due to the multitude of factors identified in the theory and the complexity with which these factors interact. Even with the evolution of increasingly specified statistical models, the multitude of possible ways with which the factors in the biopsychosocial model may interact still does not provide the level of specificity necessary to suggest directions to be taken for prevention program creation.

Recent longitudinal studies have provided a substantial amount of information on the predictors and pathways for a number of dysfunctional behavioral outcomes. Johnson and Pandina argue that the creation of a "periodic table" of these identified risk and protective factors would be a useful taxonomy for prevention programs. Moreover, the authors suggest that the specificity of an algorithm identifying the relevant predictive factors and the dynamic interaction among these factors would provide the most useful information in the development of prevention programs.

The idea of constructing a taxonomy of risk factors that could serve as a basis for prevention programs is unique and creative. One question this suggestion raises is whether the drive toward greater specificity in theory is in fact the most effective strategy for enhancing the applicability of etiologic research for prevention program development. Most predictive studies develop theories based on an examination of developmental processes examined retrospectively. The factors thought to form the basis of predictive pathways to various behavioral outcomes are examined post hoc at the aggregate level. The causal patterns that are identified by predictive theories may be too deterministic to be used for prevention programs that must respond to a wide range of individual and environmental factors.

Furthermore, individuals who participate in prevention programs may not yet exhibit identified behaviors or a specific composite of risk and protective factors suggested by etiological studies. Although etiological-based research can identify a set of factors that, over the course of a pathway, affect the dysfunctional outcomes, the models cannot yet identify the stability of these factors, including the timing, intensity, or content critical for intervention to modify those factors. Therefore, the more restrictive the intervention, the less effective it may be at the individual level. Prevention programs may need to be more general and multifaceted to most effectively respond to the broad range of individuals and targeted behaviors.

Striving to achieve greater specificity with etiological research to enhance prevention programs may be further complicated by the statistical methods used to construct the models. Statistical modeling favors parsimony over breadth and thus may exclude factors that are not statistically significant within a specified aggregate model but are influential at the individual level. For prevention program development, narrowly focused interventions that target a small number of risk and protective factors, supported by rigorous but largely post hoc tests of etiological theories, may be vulnerable to neglecting important (but less statistically significant) pathways. These alternative pathways may be dropped as nonsignificant in conventional model fitting, but their lack of statistical strength may be the result of lower measurement reliability or their overlap with other, more statistically significant pathways, rather than their failure to influence the behavioral outcomes in some individuals.

Perhaps greater unanimity among the variety of causal pathways has not and cannot be achieved because a deterministic model in fact cannot be developed with individual accuracy. Thus, enhanced statistical specificity in etiological models may actually reduce applicability for prevention programs. This would argue, instead, for the creation of prevention programs based on more general models, including a wide variety of identified risk and protective factors, to be most effective.

This does not, however, negate the point made by Johnson and Pandina that prevention programs should become more rigorous in using the knowledge obtained from etiological studies. For example, etiological studies can provide guidance to prevention programs in sharpening their outcome measures and targeting their interventions to more closely address those outcome measures. The development of more defined outcome measures for prevention programs, together with specific interventions for reducing risk and enhancing protective factors based on those identified in the etiology literature, would enhance the rigor of prevention programs. In addition, information from studies such as meta-analyses could assist prevention programs in examining the characteristics of their participants and discerning whether the interventions applied in their programs coincide with evidence of effective treatment models. The use of etiologic research as a tool for the refinement of prevention programs outcomes in a heuristic rather than prescriptive manner would facilitate the application of interventions responding to behavior and needs at the individual level.

To further develop the applicability of etiological models for prevention science, researchers can use prevention programs that provide a significant contribution to the field by testing etiological theories, as argued by the authors. These hybrid programs, which use etiological research to inform the development of program intervention components and develop the mechanisms for testing these theories through rigorous program intervention, would be extremely beneficial for the prevention field. The authors provide a number of helpful decision points for making the selection of appropriate methodological designs.

Finally, the authors provide an excellent discussion of the limitations of designing and implementing a sophisticated longitudinal study. These limitations need not hinder the goal of assessing the applicability of etiological theories for the design of prevention programs and the use of prevention data in informing theory development, as in the hybrid paradigm suggested by the authors. Indeed, it is clear that the success of theory development, the design of prevention programs based on general risk and protective factors, and the evaluation of those programs are ongoing and interactive and need to be examined in the context of the same study to result in the greatest gain in knowledge. The chapter authors have provided an important review of this process and of how etiological research can inform the development of prevention programs.

CHAPTER 7

Pooling Information About Prior Interventions

A New Program Planning Tool

Carol N. D'Onofrio

Interventions previously developed by others offer a gold mine of useful information and ideas for planning a new health behavior program. However, reflecting a general lack of attention to methods of intervention development (Bartholomew, Parcel, & Kok, 1998), researchers in the fields of health promotion and health education have been slow to recognize this resource. Although a number of program planning models have been set forth (Bartholomew et al., 1998; Centers for Disease Control and Prevention [CDC], 1995; Dignan & Carr, 1987; Green & Kreuter, 1991; Sussman, 1991), only the model recently advanced by Sussman, Dent, Burton, Stacy, and Flay (1995) identifies examining other programs as a specific step in intervention development. To date, no systematic procedures have been suggested for accomplishing this task as part of the program-planning process.

This chapter represents an initial attempt to fill this methodological gap. The opening section identifies six ways that reviewing other programs can contribute to the development of a new intervention. The following section will help you focus your search for other programs by discussing specific types of information you may want to seek and by illustrating how this information can be applied in planning your own intervention. The third section identifies numerous sources of information about behavioral health interventions, as well as strengths and limitations associated with each source. Fourth, methods for locating, retrieving, and organizing programmatic information are described. The fifth section discusses methods for reviewing the assembled pool of information. Finally, the concluding section provides some tips to ensure that your program will be available as a resource to others who develop interventions in the future.

These guidelines are grounded in well-established principles of program planning and thoughtful consideration of ways in which the program development process could be enhanced by a systematic review of other interventions. The specific techniques identified are drawn directly from personal knowledge and experience, as well as from insights gained through interactions with many program developers and evaluators over the years. Notwithstanding, these methods have not yet been formally tested, and resources for intervention pooling are rapidly changing.

Readers who use these suggestions, therefore, are encouraged to consider how they could be improved and to share this thinking. As with other scientific advances, the development of effective and efficient methods for reviewing other programs will require successive cycles of formulating recommendations, attempting to apply them in practice, critically assessing the results, drawing conclusions, and identifying potential improvements. Accordingly, this chapter should be regarded as a starting point both (a) for individuals and teams who recognize that reviewing information about other programs can help them to design their own interventions and (b) for a collaborative multidisciplinary effort to develop new and improved methods through which such a review can be accomplished.

WHY POOLING INFORMATION ABOUT INTERVENTIONS IS IMPORTANT

Collecting and analyzing information about other interventions related to the program you are developing enables you to benefit from the critical thinking and creativity that others have invested in planned efforts to improve health status. Moreover, the experience of others in implementing and evaluating these programs provides invaluable information about what does and does not work in practice. Recommendations made by expert committees and others who have conducted their own review of programs can help to ensure that the intervention you develop is at the cutting edge of practice. Further consideration suggests that knowledge obtained from reviewing such information can contribute to intervention development in at least six specific ways.

STRENGTHENING THE RATIONALE FOR YOUR PROGRAM

Examining how others present the need and rationale for programs similar to the one you want to develop can help you to build a persuasive case for your own intervention. Reviewing other programs also may uncover issues that you need to address or further fact-finding that would be desirable to substantiate the validity of your key premises and assumptions.

In addition, you may come across some strategies for preventing or controlling a health problem that are entirely different from those you have considered. Evidence about the extent to which each strategy has been successful with particular target populations will help you to select and justify the approach most likely to be effective with the community or group you hope to serve. Such a review also may help you to determine which group most needs your program or is most likely to benefit from it. If you are committed to working with a particular community or segment of the population, reviewing other programs also can help you to examine the relative importance of the problem you plan to address compared to other issues needing intervention. On reflection, you may decide that the program you are proposing has less merit than another idea. If not, reasons for pursuing your initial concept should be clearer.

Similarly, as you and your planning team consider why other programs included particular elements, you will elucidate a detailed picture of the theories and assumptions underlying each intervention and how these premises were translated into practice. Engaging in such critical analysis for an entire pool of interventions will reveal the strengths and weaknesses of each component, thus clarifying your reasons for including some of these elements, modifying others, and determining that certain ones do not merit further consideration. Questions and issues not adequately addressed by prior program developers also will become apparent. These gaps represent opportunities for you to make improvements, as well as to contribute new knowledge to the emerging field of health intervention science.

DEVELOPING A DETAILED INTERVENTION PLAN

Once you have decided on your general approach, closer review of prior interventions will help you to plan the specifics of your intervention. These include determining what content will be conveyed to your target group, how this content will be translated into key messages, and how these messages will be framed for optimum impact. Because simply providing information seldom changes health-related behaviors, you also need to consider what methods you will employ to ensure that messages command attention, are understood, and are internalized in a way that leads to action. In addition to developing your logic for these decisions, reviewing other programs may identify activities and materials that can be incorporated directly into your intervention. Sometimes, you also will find descriptions of effective methods for activity and materials development.

IDENTIFYING PROGRAMMATIC ISSUES THAT NEED TO BE ADDRESSED

Information about factors that affected the implementation, acceptance, and effectiveness of similar programs in other locales can help you to identify issues that your program plan must address to be successful. For example, accounts of difficulties in recruiting volunteers for a cancer screening program in the inner city might prompt you to consider using different methods of recruitment, enhanced incentives, or the employment of paid workers. Reports that others have encountered complications in transporting older youth to work with younger children should alert you to the importance of arranging transportation logistics in cross-age peer education programs.

ESTIMATING TIME AND RESOURCE REQUIREMENTS FOR PROGRAM DEVELOPMENT

As the previous examples imply, reviewing other interventions also will help you to estimate the scope of work involved in delivering your program and related time and resource requirements. In addition, such a review will help you to assess the time and resources needed for planning. When the pool of other relevant interventions is large, you may be able to identify many "building blocks" that you can apply in constructing your own program (also see the discussion of "building-block" components in Chapter 13, this volume). On the other hand, when the pool is quite small, you will need to create most of your program from scratch. Knowledge about the programmatic resources available to you may affect the scale of the program you initiate, the time you allot for program development, or your decision to continue.

The director of an out-of-school youth organization learned this the hard way when she successfully bid on a county contract to help young children establish smoke-free zones in their homes and family cars. After a year of very hard work designing and implementing an entirely new intervention at multiple sites, she commented, "If only I had known that there was so little material on how to do this, I never would have undertaken this project." Searching for relevant models before the contract was negotiated would have helped both the youth director and county personnel to realize that substantial program development work was needed and that starting with a small pilot project made more sense than launching a multisite initiative. Beginning with a smaller program would have enabled the youth director to experiment with solutions to the difficulties encountered, preserved her creative energies for long-term involvement in tobacco control, and provided a realistic basis for budgeting the time and resources needed to implement the program throughout the county.

BUILDING SUPPORT FOR YOUR PROGRAM

Because reviewing other interventions clarifies the purpose, nature, and significance of your program, this will help to focus and energize the team responsible for its development and delivery. Enhanced precision in planning also will help you to win support for your intervention from agency administrators, community groups, funding agencies, and professional leaders. Including intervention elements that others have found effective will bolster the credibility of your program and confidence in its chances for success. At the same time, the ability to identify unique features of your intervention can arouse interest in its innovative qualities and potential for achieving greater impact.

PLANNING A MEANINGFUL EVALUATION

Reviewing other programs also can assist you in planning an evaluation that is meaningful to your intervention team and to the people served, as well as to the larger field. Because the propositions on which your program is based will be clearly articulated, their validity can be tested. Outcomes of interest to various audiences can be anticipated, and related evaluation measures often can be identified. Examining other programs also can alert you to factors that may mediate these outcomes, including issues in program implementation, the reactions of participants to particular program components, and changes in the larger social environment. Such information can help you to plan a process evaluation focused on the issues most likely to be important, as well as to avoid avenues of inquiry that are unlikely to be productive.

▶ PLANNING YOUR SEARCH FOR OTHER INTERVENTIONS

Information about health behavior programs is available from a number of sources; however, rarely will you find everything you need or want to know consolidated in one place. For this reason, you should identify the types of information you are seeking before initiating your quest for intervention models and ideas. Developing such an outline will help you to focus your search, define key words for exploring databases, sort through the citations that surface, guide further fact-finding, decide which information to add to your pool of program ideas, and organize the resources you are assembling for ease of later application.

The progress you already have made in planning your program is likely to influence the number and range of programs you decide to review. If your thinking is still exploratory, you may wish to structure a review that will help you consider which health problems your program should address, what population group it should target, the theoretical framework that will guide your intervention, and the change strategies that it will employ. If decisions have been made about one or more of these basic program parameters, you may want to restrict your review to interventions sharing similar boundaries.

Narrowing your search will make it more efficient but less likely to challenge your basic planning assumptions. A broader search will be more time-consuming but will strengthen the rationale for your intervention by enabling you to identify more programmatic options and to consider why your approach is preferable to other alternatives. Consequently, even if you have made some preliminary planning decisions, you may want to test your thinking by beginning your review with a broad reconnaissance of other programs. When you are satisfied that the need and rationale for your program are solidly justified, you can filter out those programs or intervention elements that you wish to examine in greater detail. However, you also may find that examining other interventions causes you to reconsider planning decisions that you thought had been settled. If this occurs, try not to be frustrated and keep an open mind, for planning is an iterative rather than a linear process.

To begin creating a plan for your search that is tailored to your needs, draw a matrix with three columns on scratch paper. Use the rows in column 1 to jot down questions, issues, and tasks involved in planning your intervention. In column 2, write key words or phrases that may help you to locate programs relevant to each of these topics. Column 3 should be used to identify possible sources of information about these programs. At this stage, do not worry about organizing the content of the matrix or eliminating duplicate entries, for in planning as in weaving, strands of information are brought forth as they contribute to developing an original and unified whole. Also, be sure to record all of your questions, even if these concern decisions already made.

Table 7.1 illustrates such a matrix constructed during an early meeting of a group responsible for developing a telephone counseling intervention to promote adherence to breast screening recommendations by women whose sisters were diagnosed with breast cancer in the San Francisco Bay Area (Bloom, Stewart, & Lee, 1998). Because the need for this program was already well justified, this group focused on detailed planning of the intervention. The issues and questions raised led members to search for other programs showing how counseling can be adjusted to perceived risk and readiness for screening. They also sought programs demonstrating how to increase motivation for taking action, develop skills for talking with one's doctor, reinforce positive behaviors, and make telephone referrals. Although in planning this project, the principal investigators determined that counseling should be provided to sisters regardless of where they reside, the intervention planning team was concerned about identifying appropriate referral resources in distant communities. Members therefore decided to search especially for programs in which long-distance referrals had been made. They further noted that if adequate procedures could not be identified, the target group for the program might need to be narrowed.

The rest of this section provides a more detailed discussion of ways that reviewing other programs can assist with two main aspects of intervention development: (a) developing and justifying your intervention concept and (b) designing a detailed program plan. As you review this material, flesh out column 1 of your matrix by noting additional questions and issues you need to consider in developing your intervention. If you think of key words that might help you to identify relevant programs, jot them down in column 2. Later sections of this chapter will assist you in completing column 3.

DEVELOPING AND JUSTIFYING YOUR INTERVENTION CONCEPT

A health behavior program is justified by evidence that modifying particular behaviors in a defined population will promote health, prevent a problem, or reduce the magnitude and severity of its consequences. Your decision to develop a program undoubtedly was inspired by such a vision. Perhaps you checked out this concept by discussing it with health experts and community informants, by examining data on the prevalence of the problem and the behaviors of interest, or by reviewing reports in the scientific literature (e.g., note the discussions in Chapters 4-6, this volume). If so, you undoubtedly honed your thinking about the population to be targeted, the behaviors to be changed, and the health benefits to be achieved.

Nevertheless, when an idea excites you, it is natural to seek information that supports it. If potential problems are identified, you devote your energies to finding ways they can be overcome. As a result, you may make some unfounded assumptions, overlook flaws in your program concept, or fail to consider more effective approaches. These blind spots may not be revealed until you encounter difficulties in implementing your program or in finding resources to support it. Reviewing other programs can help you to avoid these pitfalls and make a per-

TABLE 7.1 Example of Planning Matrix to Develop a Telephone Counseling Intervention

Issues and Questions	Key Words	Sources of Information
How should counseling be adapted when women have not thought about or denied their risk of breast cancer?	Risk perception Counseling	Genetic counselors Literature search
How many issues can be addressed in telephone counseling?	Telephone counseling	Cancer Center Programs Cancer Information Service Literature search
Women's rate of clinical breast exam (CBE) may depend more on their doctor's behavior than on their own.	Physicians and CBE	Physician education programs
Counseling should help women to talk with their doctor.	Doctor-patient communication	Patient education programs
Counseling needs to motivate women to take action.	Motivational interviewing	Programs at Stanford and Dana Farber Cancer Center
Women are likely to be at different stages of change for screening.	Interventions tailored to stages of change	Cancer screening and other programs based on Prochaska and DiClemente's (1984) model
What are the risks of counseling women who are already anxious?	Risk perception Counseling Anxiety	Counseling based on Janis and Mann's (1977) theory of decision making under stress Counseling based on coping theory of Lazarus and Folkman (1991)
How can resources be identified for referral, especially if women live out of state? Should women who live out of state be excluded?	Telephone referrals Referral resources	American Cancer Society has new program. Literature search
Some women contacted may already adhere to screening recommendations.	Reinforcement of positive behavior	

suasive case about the need for your intervention. Addressing questions that occur as you review the rationale for other interventions will solidify the logical foundation for your program and enable you to justify it more effectively to others.

Strengthening the Rationale for Your Program. By reviewing the justification for programs similar to the one you want to develop, you can strengthen the rationale for your own intervention. As you conduct this review, identify the arguments you find most compelling and study how these were crafted. Observe what evidence was cited to support each assertion. Be concerned about the extent to which conclusions drawn from the evidence are supported by the scientific community and persons knowledgeable about the population group to be targeted. In addition, keep track of questions left unanswered and propositions based on flawed logic or incomplete information. This will help you to assess limitations in potential models for your intervention, as well as to identify holes in your own reasoning that need to be addressed.

After you examine the rationale for other interventions, critically review your own program idea and the premises on which it is based. Strengths and weaknesses in your reasoning should quickly become apparent. Perhaps you can make a more convincing case simply by reorganizing your argument or by adding references to back up unsupported statements. However, some questions probably will arise that require further thought and investigation. As you gather further information about the problem and ways in which it affects a specific community, your original concept for the program may begin to shift. Regardless of whether this happens, addressing questions that occur as you review the rationale for other interventions will solidify the logical foundation for your program and enable you to justify it more effectively to others.

Examining Alternatives for Framing the Problem. Although research in biology, medicine, epidemiology, and other disciplines identifies behavior changes that would prevent or reduce a health problem, further analysis is often needed to determine how the gap between "what is" and "what ought to be" can best be narrowed. One type of useful analysis involves examining alternative ways to frame the problem.

Rittel and Webber (1973) call many health and social problems "wicked" because they can be formulated in different ways, every problem can be considered symptomatic of another, boundaries are difficult to define, and there is no precisely right or wrong solution. Rather than struggle with these ambiguities, planners tend to pick the explanation that is most plausible to them and that best fits the program concept that they want to develop. Because the way the problem is framed determines the path to its resolution, different and potentially more effective approaches to intervention usually are not considered. Examining programs organized in response to alternative conceptualizations of the problem can help you to avoid this analytic trap. Nevertheless, because such programs may be identified or described in rather different terms, locating them may require that you first identify different ways of approaching the health problems that they address.

A simple case involves a behavior that causes multiple health problems. For example, unprotected sexual intercourse increases risk for unwanted pregnancy, HIV infection, and other sexually transmitted diseases (STDs). Because the biomedical aspects of these problems have been studied independently, most health behavior programs developed to prevent them also are problem specific. This is appropriate in that each health issue has unique characteristics and preventive alternatives; however, sexual abstinence or condom use reduces risk for them all. An option for program development, therefore, is to promote behavior that prevents all three problems instead of a specific disease or condition (Coyle et al., 1996). To examine the pros and cons of these alternatives, you should search for interventions aimed at preventing each of the *problems* caused by a behavior (unwanted pregnancy, HIV, other STDs), as well as programs aimed at preventing or delaying the *behavior* (sexual intercourse), those promoting *behavior modifications* to prevent negative health outcomes (abstinence, condom use), and those emphasizing the *desired outcome* (safe sex).

Identifying alternatives for naming programs with similar behavioral objectives obviously helps to expand your search for relevant intervention ideas. However, keep in mind that differences in labels may reflect deeper variations in the rationale underlying the programs retrieved and therefore in their content and structure. For example, disease-oriented interventions may emphasize the health consequences of a behavior and the importance of risk avoidance. Programs named for the behavior to be prevented or modified may devote relatively more attention to patterns and conditions of current behavioral performance. Other interventions may concentrate on the benefits of the behavior being promoted. Each of these perspectives contributes to analyzing the challenges of change, and therefore considering all of them will assist you in making well-reasoned decisions about the content to be emphasized in your intervention.

Testing and Supporting Your Assumptions. As you examine the initial rationale for your program, you are likely to identify some inadequately supported assumptions. More evidence is needed to test these assumptions and to assure yourself—and others—that they are not weak links in your plan. Data from statistical reports, epidemiological studies, and surveys of health behavior are commonly used to meet this need; however, other interventions also can be sources of pertinent information. Program experiences elsewhere that corroborate your expectations can be cited to justify your premise, but those that do not will alert you to the possible need to rethink it.

For example, suppose you observe that most workers in a large office complex have sedentary jobs and appear overweight. Knowing that lack of physical activity is a risk factor for coronary heart disease and premature death (U.S. Department of Health and Human Services [DHHS], 1996), you are interested in proposing an employee exercise program to the complex manager. You have found data indicating that about one in four U.S. adults does not engage in any physical activity (U.S. DHHS, 1996), but activity levels of workers in the complex have not been studied. Before approaching the manager, you need more evidence to support your assumptions that workers such as those in the complex get insufficient exercise and would respond favorably to a program encouraging physical activity.

Locating exercise programs directed to similar populations of employees in other areas may help you on both counts. Data from preintervention surveys and, if available, from control groups used in other interventions could be used as a convincing proxy for information about the exercise habits of local workers. Similarly, data on participation rates in other programs could be used to estimate the local response. In addition, information about the extent to which exercise patterns changed as a result of the program would help to predict the effectiveness of your intervention.

Selecting and Justifying the Target Group for Your Intervention. As the preceding example indicates, when you already have a target group in mind for your intervention, reviewing other programs can help you to assess the need for your effort, as well as probable receptivity to it. Examining programs directed at a variety of problems in similar populations also may indicate what priority the people affected accord to the issue your intervention will address. In addition, you may pick up clues about ways to gain access to your target group, possible sources of resistance, and adaptations in approach needed for persons varying in age, gender, ethnicity, socioeconomic status, geographic region, or other characteristics.

Such analysis also can be useful when you need to select one of several groups to whom your program might be directed. Although epidemiologic studies and surveys are indispensable in identifying communities and population segments at greatest risk for a health problem and most severely affected by it, not all of these groups have the same potential for change (Ockene, Sorensen, Kabat-Zinn, Ockene, & Donnelly, 1988). Comparing the extent to which similar programs have modified the behavior of persons in each candidate group can help you to determine where your intervention is likely to have the greatest impact.

For example, if your goal is to improve nutrition and physical fitness, you might want to examine the relative effectiveness of programs aimed at instilling positive dietary and exercise habits early in childhood and of those that attempt to affect food choices and activity patterns during major life transitions, such as during adolescence or pregnancy. You also could consider targeting adults whose weight, dietary intake, and sedentary lifestyle increase their risk of disease or, among those already ill, its exacerbation. Even if you decide to develop your program for a group that has been relatively unresponsive to prior interventions, reviewing this pool of programs may help you to identify the weaknesses responsible so that they can be corrected.

Reviewing programs targeting the same behavior in different groups also may help you to justify your population focus. Thus, familiarity with the effects of poor eating and exercise habits on the development of chronic disease points to the importance of developing healthy behavioral habits in children and adolescents. Conversely, increased insight into how patterns of eating and exercise are established early in life underscores the need for special programs to address the difficult task of modifying these behaviors in adulthood.

Choosing Your Change Strategy. Very often, the decision to develop a health behavior program is inspired by a creative intervention idea. Although this concept may be the genesis of an original and effective intervention, commitment to a particular change approach also can be a source of bias in planning. Reviewing other programs can help you to avoid this problem by ensuring that you examine a spectrum of strategies for effecting change. Moreover, comparing other strategies with the one you have in mind will assist you in selecting the approach most likely to be effective, acceptable, and feasible in your situation. For example, if your aim is to increase fruit and vegetable consumption among the elderly, your initial plan might have been to hold cooking demonstrations and recipe exchanges in a senior activity center. However, learning about another program may suggest that a community gardening project would be more effective in increasing not only fruit and vegetable consumption by older people but also their physical and social activity.

DESIGNING A DETAILED PLAN FOR INTERVENTION

After you have determined what health problem your program will address, what population group it will target, what behaviors it will aim to change, what theoretical framework will guide your intervention, and what general strategy of change it will employ, you are ready to begin the detailed design of your intervention.

This involves many challenging tasks; however, reviewing other programs again can be of assistance. As in developing and justifying your basic intervention concept, the purpose of reviewing other programs as part of detailed intervention planning is to identify and evaluate possible alternatives for each decision you must make. Accordingly, you may want to gather information from other programs about the following topics.

Program Participants. Information about the age, gender, ethnicity, socioeconomic status, and other characteristics of groups targeted by other programs is important in helping you to determine ways in which your intended target group is similar or different. This analysis will assist you in assessing whether content and methods used in another intervention are appropriate for your target group, as well as whether similar intervention results can be expected. For example, due to regional differences in the type of firearms available and how they are used, an effective gun control program developed for rural youth in the Mississippi Delta probably could not be directly exported to youth living in the Los Angeles inner city. Nevertheless, principles and concepts applied in the first program may provide a solid basis for developing the latter one.

Also note exclusion or eligibility criteria for program participation and the actual number of persons involved in each program because these factors have implications for the logistical and resource requirements of intervention delivery, as well as for program evaluation. Examining the recruitment procedures used in relation to the proportion of eligible persons who participated in an intervention may assist you in assessing the effectiveness of various techniques for making members of a target group aware of a program and enrolling them in it. Studying variations in participation rates by age, gender, ethnicity, current patterns of behavior, and other characteristics is important for identifying subgroups that other programs have had difficulty reaching. Formulating possible explanations for low levels of program enrollment, erratic attendance, and high dropout rate may enable you to identify the problems responsible so that these can be addressed in your intervention.

If you intend to collect data for program evaluation, inspecting the methods and materials used to provide informed consent in other programs also may contribute to the development of your procedures for protecting human subjects and for obtaining informed consent as part of the recruitment process. If your program is designed for minors, you especially may want to compare participation rates in programs using an active versus what some researchers have referred to as a passive parental consent procedure (i.e., including only those youth whose parents sign forms consenting to their participation vs. including all youth except those whose parents sign forms refusing their participation). The finding that requiring active consent reduces the number of at-risk children involved in a smoking prevention program (Severson & Biglan, 1989; Sussman et al., 1995) necessitates careful consideration of the consent procedure to be used. One that threatens to reduce and bias participation will affect not only the nature of the intervention that you plan but also the external validity of its evaluation and prospects for its dissemination in the future.

Intervention Setting. Information about the settings for other interventions may provide some fresh ideas about the organizations and facilities through which your program could be delivered. If you already have identified a preferred setting, examining other programs may identify important considerations in selecting specific sites, effective methods of site recruitment, and ways of ensuring site cooperation and accessibility. Reviewing programs delivered in similar settings also may expand your understanding of how a site can be involved in intervention, as, for example, when a school-based program is implemented not only in classrooms but also in schoolwide assemblies, in the cafeteria, and through student activities organized at school but conducted at home and in the community.

In addition, obtaining information about barriers to program implementation in particular settings can assist you in choosing feasible intervention methods and in planning the logistics of intervention delivery. For example, if you discover that one session of a school-based program had to be cut because of an unannounced fire drill, you should make advance arrangements with the principal to complete delivery of your program in case of such a contingency. Likewise, if you plan to have groups view a videotape at community centers, reviewing other programs that have done this will prompt you to check the availability of working audiovisual equipment and electrical outlets at the facilities you plan to use. If problems are discovered, you might change the location where groups meet, present content in a way that does not require equipment, or make arrangements to have project equipment and extension cords transported to the centers.

Program Length and Duration. Charting the number and frequency of sessions, activities, or participant contacts in other programs, as well as the total time required for program delivery, will assist you in planning the length, scheduling, and duration of your intervention. Ideally, both the length and pacing of a program should be based on a knowledgeable analysis of the processes involved in changing the targeted behavior. Although research in this area is still in its infancy, if other factors affecting change are adequately controlled, comparing the outcomes of programs differing in length and schedule of intervention may help you to estimate the results that can be expected with a given level of program exposure. When this is not possible, examining a pool of prior interventions will at least enable you to tap the thinking of other program developers about the minimum time required for an intervention to have an effect, as well as about optimum intervals between intervention sessions. For example, a number of programs for youth now include a core curriculum, as well as reinforcing booster sessions delivered several months later.

Of course, the time devoted to an intervention also is affected by many practical matters, including the availability of participants, the commitments that those who control the intervention setting are able to make, and limitations on resources for the development and implementation of your program. Clarity about the minimum time requirements for your intervention and knowledge about the length of similar programs in other locales will assist you in planning and negotiating arrangements.

Specific Behavioral Objectives. Reviewing the behavioral objectives set for other programs and the amount of change they actually achieved will enable you to establish a range of possible change targets for your program. Some reports may identify reasons for setting certain behavioral objectives at a given level either in describing the program or in presenting power calculations for program evaluation. If not, then identifying factors that affected the outcomes achieved by these interventions and determining how similar factors are likely to affect your program may help you to establish appropriate behavioral targets. For example, you might consider whether the amount of change observed was influenced by the initial prevalence of risky behavior in the target population, the change strategy used, and the duration and intensity of intervention.

Be sure to pay close attention to the times when behavior change was measured. Typically, differences between the behavior of a group receiving a program and a control group observed immediately after delivery of an intervention will expand or narrow as more time passes. Behavioral assessments conducted 1, 2, or more years after the program has been implemented therefore are critical in determining when intervention impact peaks, as well as how long effects endure.

Program Theory. If you have not yet chosen a theoretical framework to guide development of your program, reviewing other interventions will assist you in identifying promising theories to consider. You also may discover how two or more theories can be combined to guide program development. Comparing the outcomes achieved by interventions based on different theories may help you to choose between them; however, when results are disappointing, be careful not to blame the theory for flaws in its application. To avoid this pitfall, match the content and methods of each program to tenets of the theory that guided its development. Then identify components of the theory that were not applied, for some programs draw only on popular concepts, omitting others that the theory regards as critical to change. Also, assess how well tenets of the theory have been translated into practice, noting particularly skillful applications, as well as those that appear awkward or incomplete. Finally, check how well the theory worked in practice by determining whether changes were effected in key mediating variables (e.g., the development of refusal skills) and whether these changes, in turn, were related to achievement of the desired behavioral outcomes. Such analysis can assist you not only in selecting a theory to guide development of your intervention but also in determining how your application of that theory can be strengthened.

You also should list the conditions or factors that each theory considers to be a critical determinant of behavior because behavior change is effected by altering these determinants. Depending on the theory used, such mediator changes may include the acquisition and internalization of new knowledge, the modification of attitudes and beliefs, or the development of new skills. Practice in performing the desired behavior in situations in which risky or unhealthy behaviors are common also is often considered important. In addition, an intervention may aim to change the behavior of others who influence the target group or to make environmental and institutional changes that encourage the desired behavior or make the performance of unhealthy behaviors more difficult (e.g., Golaszewski, Barr, & Cochran, 1998).

Some intervention planners establish a series of subobjectives to specify which behavioral determinants will be changed. These subobjectives are then displayed in a hierarchy showing how they relate to each other and to the desired behavior change. If this has not been done for interventions that you review, you may want to translate their program theory into this format. Then, as previously described, by comparing the program's subobjectives to tenets of its theory, you can determine how completely and skillfully the theory has been applied.

This is pioneering work. Although some planning frameworks incorporate the application of theory, and various theories themselves have been used as guides to intervention development (e.g., Glanz, Lewis, & Rimer, 1996), only recently have efforts been made to identify issues in applying theory to practice and to describe methods through which this can be accomplished (D'Onofrio, 1992; Hochbaum, Sorenson, & Lorig, 1992; also see Chapter 4, this volume, on theory development). The experience of program developers in applying theory has not been studied—or even generally acknowledged—as a valuable source of methodological insight. Argyris, Putnam, McLain, and Smith (1985) have made important contributions by distinguishing espoused theory from theory-in-use and by developing methods for making both types of theories explicit. However, this body of work does not examine how practitioners draw on formal theories of behavior, and the Argyris principles of action science have not been used in research on health program development.

Program Modalities. The modalities of an intervention, or the ways in which it is delivered, constitute the structure through which theory is translated into practice. Although this structure may be quite simple, interventions have multiple modalities, each of which may contain one or more elements. These modalities may be delivered in sequence, as when a community-wide lead poisoning prevention program is introduced with a media campaign and then followed by the formation of neighborhood action groups and the screening of individual children. Modalities also may be delivered concurrently, as when a classroom curriculum is accompanied by schoolwide activities, homework assignments, and a newsletter for parents (see Chapters 13, 15, and 16 in this volume for examples of program modalities).

Program Content. Closely reviewing the content included in other interventions will reveal what factual information, instructions, advice, warnings, encouragement, or other messages are considered important in effecting change. Identifying the main messages of a program is important in determining how they are related both to the theory that guides an intervention and to other information provided.

Although tracing these linkages can be tedious, doing so is necessary to understand the reasons for including particular content in an intervention and for delivering this content in a particular sequence. Because, to date, little systematic attention has been devoted to specifying exactly which knowledge is important in changing a given behavior in a designated population group, you may find that the rationale for the content contained in some programs is weak or underdeveloped. On the other hand, Sussman and colleagues (1993; Dent et al., 1995) tested the effects of including or excluding specific types of social influence messages in a school-based smoking prevention curriculum. More such research is needed to inform the development of effective interventions. In the meantime, rigorously reviewing the content of other programs will provide you with a valuable template and important background information for deciding which messages your program should deliver.

In addition to examining the messages used in other programs, you should study how these messages were framed for the audience to which they are directed, as well as any problems encountered. Basic considerations are whether a message awakened interest and how it was understood. Thus, you may find that admonitions not to behave in a certain way ("Don't be a couch potato") were less effective than messages that identified the desired behavior and its positive effects ("Running makes me feel good and look better").

You also should search for information about terms that might be offensive to or misinterpreted by persons differing in age, education, ethnicity, or region. For example, childhood safety programs frequently teach young children not to talk with strangers. However, interactions with preschool youngsters involved in one such program indicated that this message was not well understood. Some children thought that only big and ugly people could be strangers. Others identified a stranger as someone whom they had never seen before. As a result, none of these youngsters felt the need for caution around a pleasant-appearing person who stopped two or three times to watch them play. In contrast, children who defined a stranger as anyone whom they did not already know became fearful of meeting new people, regardless of the circumstances.

Program Methods. Reviewing other programs can help you to identify a variety of methods that might be used to communicate the content of your intervention and to achieve its subobjectives. In some cases, these methods will be prescribed by the theoretical framework used to guide development of an intervention; however, some health behavior programs rely on theories that do not explain the processes through which determinants of behavior are developed or modified. In such instances, planners typically apply other frequently unspecified theories and principles in selecting and developing methods. These might include, for example, providing incentives for participation, personalizing information, delivering messages through multiple channels of communication, repeating these messages at critical intervals, actively engaging participants in problem solving, asking participants to make a personal commitment to change, setting personal goals, mobilizing social support, teaching new skills, providing opportunities for practice with constructive feedback, reducing barriers to behavioral performance, and monitoring and rewarding progress.

Examining how these and other methods have been used in prior programs will help you to understand the purposes each can serve. Because methods can be applied in many ways, you also should note how, when, and where a method was used to achieve a particular effect. Moreover, you should study how methods were combined within various program components because more than one approach usually is needed to help program participants internalize the content of an intervention, integrate new skills into their daily lives, and make other changes necessary for adoption of the desired behavior.

Program Activities. Reviewing other programs will provide you with many ideas for activities and ways that they can be structured. In fact, depending on the health problem and population group your intervention will address, you may be dazzled by the array of discussion techniques, puzzles, role-plays, games, quizzes, computer-based simulations, community projects, and other imaginative activities that you discover. Although you may be tempted to create your intervention by cobbling together the activities you like best, designing an effective intervention requires greater rigor.

Developing activities is perhaps the most challenging task in intervention development because it is in this process that theory and methods are applied to practice. Each activity must convey content that you have identified as essential to your intervention and contribute in other ways to achieving one or more of its subobjectives. The entire package of activities must contain all of the elements needed to achieve the behavioral objectives established for your program. In addition, each activity must attract and hold the interest of your target group, be meaningful in its own right, and result in a sense of accomplishment as it is completed. Each activity and the set as a whole also must be culturally and developmentally appropriate for your target group, compatible with the intervention setting, and feasible to implement with the time and resources available to you. This is a tall order!

Before reviewing other programs, you may find it helpful to list all the criteria that activities in your intervention will need to meet. You can then rate how well specific activities developed by others satisfy each requirement. Also, look beneath the surface features of activities to study how they are constructed and how, when, and where specific methods were applied. Analyzing how activities are sequenced within a program modality and how modalities relate to each other may provide additional insights that will aid you in structuring your own intervention (see Chapter 15, this volume, on sequencing).

To obtain further assistance, search for information about the processes through which activities were developed in other programs. For example, some teams begin activity development by reviewing the objectives and subobjectives of their intervention, its key messages, and a spectrum of possible methods. They then generate ideas for possible activities by brainstorming. After this, activity outlines are developed for the most promising concepts. These are discussed and evaluated against standard criteria, leading to suggestions about how activities might be strengthened. Regardless of the preliminary process followed, advanced drafts of activities usually are tried out in focus groups or in the actual intervention setting and then revised and retested (see Chapters 9 and 11, this volume, on verbal and nonverbal methods in perceived efficacy).

Program Materials. Many interventions include supportive print or audiovisual materials such as a guide for program leaders, a workbook for participants, pamphlets to take home, and videotapes, charts, or other media used in conjunction with specific activities. Reviewing other programs will identify the many purposes for which materials might be used and the variety of formats that they might take. Directly examining materials developed for other interventions will enable you to determine precisely what content was included and how this was presented. Usually, you also will obtain some creative design ideas.

Some program developers have written articles sharing their experience in materials development (e.g., Biglan, James, LaChance, Zoref, & Joffe, 1988; Sabogal, Otero-Sabogal, Pasick, Jenkins, & Pérez-Stable, 1996); however, such resources are still relatively rare. Nevertheless, if you can talk directly with individuals who have been involved in creating materials for an intervention, you are likely to pick up additional tips about the processes through which these were developed, pretested, produced, and distributed, as well as about the time, talents, and costs involved (see Chapters 9-17, this volume).

Program Delivery. Reviewing other programs also may help you to develop detailed plans for implementing your intervention. For example, if you are developing a school-based program for youth, you must decide who should lead it. Examining a pool of prior interventions will show that such programs have been facilitated by many types of personnel, including regular classroom teachers, highly trained health educators, research assistants, college students, law enforcement officers, school nurses, and volunteers. Further review will reveal that hiring and training your own staff will result in greater fidelity of program implementation than depending on people not under your direct supervision. However, relying on personnel who are not an enduring part of the school system reduces the potential for follow-up teaching and may increase program costs, thus raising questions about the feasibility of institutionalizing and disseminating your intervention. Awareness of the trade-offs involved will help you to make an informed decision from the alternatives available to you.

In addition, you may obtain information that will assist you in estimating the personnel, time, facilities, and other resources required to deliver your program, and you may learn how to translate these requirements into a budget and time schedule. You also may identify techniques for recruiting, training, supervising, and mentoring the personnel who will deliver your program and for establishing the organizational infrastructure needed to monitor and coordinate each aspect of program implementation. Then, too, you might identify specific approaches that are effective in gaining the cooperation of key gatekeepers in the intervention setting, as well as some potential barriers that should be considered in implementation planning.

Program Evaluation. Determining how your program will be evaluated is another important aspect of detailed intervention planning. Although reviewing the evaluation designs and methods used in other programs can assist you with this task, discussing specific observations that would be useful and how they might be applied is beyond the scope of this chapter. A general suggestion is to examine how issues encountered in planning your evaluation have been handled in evaluating similar programs. (Much assistance in this regard can be found in Chapter 16, this volume.)

SOURCES OF INFORMATION ◄ ABOUT OTHER PROGRAMS

When you have identified the planning questions and issues that you want to examine, you are ready to search for information about other programs relevant to these topics. This section identifies potential sources of such information, including the published literature, technical reports, expert guidelines, conferences, funding agencies, clearinghouses, newsletters, commercial publications, community experience, the Internet, and direct contact with program developers. As you continue reading, fill in the third column of your matrix by noting the sources most likely to provide the programmatic information you seek (see Table 7.1). Keep in mind that each source has both strengths and limitations.

REPORTS OF SPECIFIC INTERVENTIONS

Most journal articles about specific programs report positive results from outcome evaluations. Although these articles usually provide fairly detailed information about program participants, the evaluation methods used, and the outcomes observed, the intervention itself may be described quite briefly. Nevertheless, such an overview, coupled with evaluation findings, can help you to identify interventions that you want to review in greater depth. Footnotes about author affiliations and reprint requests may assist you in contacting program developers directly.

The references cited also may lead you to additional papers of interest. These might describe the theoretical basis for the intervention or perhaps report the results of its process evaluation. Published case studies of programs, although rare, can provide valuable insights into processes of intervention development, issues that may arise, and factors likely to affect program evolution (e.g., Zapka et al., 1992).

Although peer-reviewed journal articles are the most credible source of information about the effectiveness of health programs, they have several limitations. Because considerable time is required to evaluate an intervention and then to prepare and publish a quality paper reporting results, most journal articles concern programs developed and implemented several years earlier. Journals also are unlikely to accept papers about programs that were not rigorously evaluated or that produced few, if any, measurable effects. In addition, from time to time, a particular model of intervention so dominates the field that programs based on other approaches may not be favorably received by editors and reviewers.

OVERVIEWS OF HEALTH PROGRAMS

Journal articles providing an overview of health programs addressing a particular problem or population group also may contain information useful in intervention development. For example, in examining changes in U.S. government funding for program development, Jansen, Glynn, and Howard (1996) identified effective and promising approaches to the prevention of alcohol, tobacco, and other drug use. Another approach is illustrated by articles reporting the results of national surveys on the frequency of worksite health promotion activities, related trends, and factors affecting program availability (Fielding & Piserchia, 1989; Grosch, Alterman, Petersen, & Murphy, 1998; McGinnis, 1993).

META-ANALYSES

As the number of evaluated programs has grown, techniques of meta-analysis originally applied in clinical research (L'Abbe, Delsky, & O'Rourke, 1987) increasingly have been used to assess the effects of health behavior programs across population groups and intervention sites. If you are fortunate enough to find a meta-analysis relevant to the program you are developing, it will jump-start your review of other interventions.

In preparing for meta-analysis, the investigative team typically seeks published and unpublished evaluations of programs addressing a particular health issue, determines which of these meet prespecified criteria, and then provides an overview of these interventions. Although the selection criteria used may exclude some programs with good ideas, those included probably will be highly relevant to your review. The meta-analysis report usually identifies these programs and summarizes their major features. For example, Dolan-Mullen, Ramírez, and Groff (1994) published a table listing study citations, settings, intervention strategies, smoking cessation rates, and risk ratios for 11 evaluated prenatal smoking cessation programs. Although the relative effectiveness of intervention components could not be assessed with this number of studies, the authors reported a number of observations of clear value to the program developer. For example, they noted that all studies included in the analysis used a pregnancy-specific smoking cessation manual rather than a general one. Chapter 18 of this text provides a more detailed discussion of the use of meta-analysis in program development.

ARTICLES ON INTERVENTION METHODS

Some journal articles critically assess particular intervention methods or approaches. For example, Robison (1998) recently reviewed four major problems associated with the use of incentives to provide positive reinforcement for desired behavior. Johnson, MacKinnon, and Pentz (1996) have examined the pros and cons of aiming to change multiple behaviors or a single one through school-based drug abuse prevention programs. Ways to integrate supply-and-demand reduction strategies for drug abuse prevention also have been discussed (Pentz, Bonnie, & Shopland, 1996).

ARTICLES ABOUT THE HEALTH PROBLEM YOUR PROGRAM WILL ADDRESS

Although journal articles reporting surveillance data and research on health problems usually do not discuss implications for intervention, the occasional exception may identify sources of information about programs relevant to your review. To illustrate, a recent report on the prevalence of diagnosed diabetes among American Indians and Alaskan Natives referred to a clinical trial being conducted by the National Institute of Diabetes and Digestive and Kidney Disease to evaluate three diabetes prevention interventions. This same article also described the establishment of a National Diabetes Prevention Center in Gallup, New Mexico, that will (a) provide guidance and technical support in diabetes prevention and control strategies to American Indian and Alaskan Native communities throughout the United States and (b) develop, evaluate, and disseminate culturally appropriate community-based interventions. Also mentioned were grants to tribal governments to help develop and implement innovative interventions to prevent diabetes and its complications (CDC, 1998).

Some journals include a section devoted to brief reports from practitioners. These can help you to identify individuals currently working on interventions of interest to you. You also may learn something about the approach they are taking and issues that particularly concern them.

BOOKS FROM THE FIELD

Books also may contain valuable information for intervention development. For example, a volume by Sussman et al. (1995) comprehensively reviewed the research, thinking, and methods used in developing the prevention and cessation components of Project Towards No Tobacco Use (Project TNT). Other books have critically examined multiple programs addressing particular health issues and then extracted lessons learned from these efforts.

In one such contribution, Dryfoos (1990) reviewed research on adolescent behaviors that increase risk for health and social problems; analyzed interventions to prevent adolescent delinquency, substance abuse, pregnancy, and school failure; and then identified implications for prevention programs at the community, state, and federal levels. She also compared her findings with Schorr's (1988) assessment of programs that successfully helped disadvantaged children and families, a casebook of 14 model programs identified by a task force of the American Psychological Association (Price, Cowen, Lorion, & Ramos-McKay, 1988), descriptions of local programs prepared by the National League of Cities (Kyle,

1987), and the Amherst Wilder Foundation's analysis of prevention programming in human services (Mueller & Higgins, 1988). Although the insights in such books may make them a valuable resource for many years, they also may become outdated as research, policy, and intervention approaches advance postpublication.

TECHNICAL REPORTS

Technical reports published by government agencies and other organizations may be another source of useful information for program developers. Such reports address a variety of issues and usually contain more detailed data and analyses than journal articles or books. Reports that review the scientific evidence about the health effects of particular behaviors can be instrumental in establishing the need for intervention, as exemplified by the 1964 report to the surgeon general on the health consequences of smoking (U.S. Department of Health, Education, and Welfare [DHEW], 1964). This document launched a series of surgeon general's reports on the health effects of smoking, but the role of adult and youth education in addressing these problems was not considered until 1979 (U.S. DHEW, 1979b). Then, the 1989 report devoted an entire chapter to smoking prevention, cessation, and advocacy activities, in addition to which another chapter considered how smoking control policies and programs may interact (U.S. DHHS, 1989). The 1994 report on smoking prevention among youth was the first to be organized around a programmatic focus (U.S. DHHS, 1994).

As the preceding example indicates, surveillance data and research on health problems are often reported without identifying implications for intervention. Since the late 1970s, the U.S. Public Health Service has bridged the resulting gap by mobilizing resources across government agencies and in the academic community to review the scientific evidence on an array of health problems and to identify related directions for health promotion and disease prevention (U.S. DHEW, 1979a). The first wave of this work provided the basis for a technical report establishing an agenda of health objectives for the nation to be accomplished by 1990 (U.S. DHHS, 1980). An expanded review process involving 22 expert working groups, almost 300 national organizations, all state health departments, and public review and comment by more than 10,000 people led to the issuance of a new report in 1991 that set national health objectives for the year 2000 (U.S. DHHS, 1991). As of this writing, preparation of objectives for the next decade is actively under way (U.S. DHHS, 1998; http://web.health.gov/healthypeople/2010). In the interim, periodic reports and a Web site (http://odphp.osophs.dhhs.gov/pubs/hp2000) provide updates on progress toward achieving the year 2000 objectives.

Some technical reports are dedicated solely to programs addressing health problems or opportunities for prevention. These may discuss issues in intervention development and delivery, describe and evaluate specific programs, and even outline the contents of selected interventions. The National Technical Information Service (http://www.ntis.gov) maintains a bibliographic database that provides citations for many such reports, including, for example, ones on state, regional, and national occupational health and safety programs. Technical reports also can be identified by contacting agencies that issue them, by searching the Internet and library databases, and inquiring whether different research groups have such reports among their unpublished documentation.

CONFERENCES AND PROFESSIONAL MEETINGS

Papers presented at conferences and workshops, as well as proceedings from these meetings, are often timely sources of information about new programs, as well as about recently completed and ongoing research with programmatic implications. The annual International Conference on AIDS exemplifies efforts to make the latest advances in research and interventions widely available with minimum delay.

Conferences or workshops are more likely to provide information about a newly defined health problem than books or peer-reviewed journal articles. During the 1980s, for example, mounting concern about the prevalence of assault and homicide; child, elder, and spousal abuse; and rape and sexual assault prompted the U.S. Department of Health and Human Services and the U.S. Department of Justice to organize a conference on violence as a public health problem. After sharing information about various forms of violence, participants formulated recommendations both for prevention and services to victims (U.S. DHHS, 1986). Conference proceedings contained citations of relevant studies published at that time, but these were relatively few. Subsequently, of course, the literature on violence has burgeoned.

In considering whether to base your program on information reported at conferences and workshops, you should remember that these findings have not yet been subjected to rigorous peer review, and therefore they later may be questioned or disputed in the scientific community. Basing your program on research conclusions that are not yet widely accepted carries the risk that the changes you aim to achieve will not, in fact, affect the health problem and that you will be criticized for undertaking a program based on flimsy science. On the other hand, if new scientific findings turn out to represent a breakthrough, using them as the foundation for your program could hasten their benefit to the public and identify you as a visionary intervention leader.

GUIDELINES AND RECOMMENDATIONS

Government agencies and other organizations sometimes convene expert committees, hold consensus conferences, or initiate other collaborative efforts to produce guidelines or recommendations for clinical practice or health programs. If you are developing a behavioral intervention, you should be familiar with programmatic guidelines pertaining to it. Applicable clinical guidelines also are important if you are planning a program that involves health services. For example, guidelines specifying the age and other characteristics of individuals who should be inoculated against preventable diseases identify groups that should be targeted by programs to increase immunization levels. Other clinical guidelines provide standards for planning service delivery and monitoring its quality.

The CDC maintains a database of more than 400 documents providing guidelines and recommendations for the prevention and control of many public health threats (http://wonder.cdc.gov/wonder/prevguid/prevguid.html). Although most of these guidelines concern clinical and environmental measures, this database contains some programmatic guidelines, including ones for school-based programs to prevent tobacco use and to promote exercise and healthy eating (http://www.cdc.gov/nccdphp/comprehe.htm). Development of evidence-based clinical treatment guidelines has now progressed to the point that the Agency for Healthcare Research and Quality, in partnership with the American Medical Association and the American Association of Health Plans, also has established a National Guidelines Clearinghouse as a public resource (http://www.guidelines.gov). Other clinical and programmatic guidelines may be found in professional publications or obtained through the agencies that sponsored their development.

When you are working with guidelines, it is important to consider the quality of the scientific evidence on which they are based, when they were developed, the experience and qualifications of those who participated, the process used, the mission of the sponsoring agency, and any other factors that may have influenced the recommendations produced. The strongest guidelines are based on expert consensus about scientific findings indicating that a particular practice or procedure produces a desired outcome with no serious side effects. The feasibility of implementing these practices on a widespread scale at reasonable cost also may be considered. When relevant scientific evidence is conflicting or insufficient, another alternative is to base guidelines on expert consensus about best practice.

As demonstrated by heated controversy about the age at which women should begin regular mammography screening, problems can develop when differing interpretations of research result in conflicting guidelines issued by different agencies (Ernster, 1997). For this reason, you should be familiar with all sets of guidelines pertaining to the intervention you are planning, as well as with any minority opinions issued by those who participated in guideline development.

You also should attempt to ascertain what evidence was considered in developing guidelines for health programs because although the scientific basis for clinical guidelines is usually made explicit, less research has been done on behavioral interventions, results seldom are definitive, and the studies considered in developing recommendations frequently are not identified. Consequently, guidelines for health programs more often reflect a consensus of opinions about what works than agreement that the effectiveness of recommended practices has been solidly demonstrated.

RESOURCE BOOKS AND MANUALS

Some agencies and commercial firms have produced resource materials to assist workers in the field to develop a health program. These materials may be presented as user-friendly guidelines, often presented in manuals or workbooks outlining specific steps to be taken in designing, implementing, and evaluating a program within a school, community, or other setting. For example, in 1998, the California Department of Education published an action guide for creating safe and drug-free schools and communities. To highlight the need for school-based programs and to establish a framework for planning, the initial chapter of this guide displays a related national education goal in the initial chapter and then discusses legally mandated school responsibilities, the purpose and organization of the guide, key findings from research on drug prevention programs, and department guidelines for program design. The next chapter discusses specific legal requirements for school districts.

The third chapter describes the action steps for planning, integrating these practical guidelines with related legal requirements, principles of effectiveness, and information about additional resources. The following two chapters identify and discuss exemplary, promising, and ineffective prevention practices, and the concluding section provides abstracts of related research and evaluation studies. Appendixes offer further information about prevention resources, legislation, performance indicators, and sources of financial support (California Department of Education, 1998).

Another type of resource book or manual provides an array of activities that can be included in a health program or used to supplement it. *Kids Act!*, a collection of activities that involve middle school students in advocacy against tobacco use, is one such resource recently produced by the Health Information Network of the National Education Association with support from the Robert Wood Johnson Foundation. Four different advocacy activities are included for each middle school grade, with adaptations for different ability levels, opportunities for integration into subjects taught in the regular school curriculum, and rubrics for assessing student performance. Appendixes identify additional resources for teachers and students and contain an outline showing how activities are related to National Learning Standards in English language arts, health, social studies, science, and mathematics. Also included are a video, stickers for teachers to use at their discretion, and a parent advocacy guide to be sent home with students (National Education Association, 1998).

Such materials can assist program developers in many respects. Because these resources typically are produced with the assistance of an advisory committee, step-by-step guidance for program planning often reflects intimate knowledge about the intervention setting and effective ways to function in this environment. Consolidated information about legal requirements affecting the targeted organizations, other guidelines they are expected to follow, and related goals and principles set forth by bodies that influence them are a great convenience for planners and probably enlightening to those with limited experience in the intervention setting. In addition, activities frequently contain good ideas that are feasible for intended users to implement and formatted according to their preferences. The resources listed may help you to identify other programs and materials that will be useful in planning.

However, not all resource books and manuals are as carefully developed as those described earlier, and even the best ones have some serious weaknesses. Most important, guidelines about the elements essential to program effectiveness are not rigorously anchored in behavioral theory. Similarly, activities in resource binders are compiled without regard to how they should be combined and timed to achieve a behavioral effect. Although those who produce resource materials usually claim that their goal is to promote positive health behaviors, the effectiveness of programs based on these resources is rarely, if ever, evaluated. Instead, when evaluations are conducted, they focus on the acceptability and use of materials. The danger of this approach is that the individuals who use resource books and manuals are led to believe that they are effectively reducing health risks. Because the number of tested health programs is limited, a corollary peril is that those who develop and use resource books and manuals may not recognize the need for continuing efforts to develop more effective interventions.

CLEARINGHOUSES AND RESOURCE CENTERS

A number of government agencies and some other organizations have established clearinghouses that gather, store, and disseminate information about health problems and programs. All the sources of information discussed earlier may be included. Most of these agencies also stock hard copies of training manuals, videotapes, and other materials that may be reviewed on site, downloaded from the Internet, purchased, or possibly borrowed for brief periods. In addition, some clearinghouses will answer questions, conduct customized searches for programs and bibliographic citations, provide technical assistance, and facilitate contact among persons with shared interests. Organizations that perform a variety of these functions may be known not as clearinghouses but as resource centers.

Information about clearinghouses operated by agencies within the U.S. Department of Health and Human Services is available through the Government Information Locator Service (http://www.hhs.gov/progorg/airm/newhhsgils.htm), a Web page describing these resources (http://waisgate.hhs.gov), and also the Web sites of specific agencies and institutes. In addition, the Department's Office of Minority Health serves as a national resource and referral service on minority health issues (http://www.omhrc.gov), and its Office on Women's Health operates the National Women's Health Information Center, which provides access to more than 80 federal health clearinghouses and hundreds of private-sector organizations (http://www.4woman.org). The Educational Resources Information Center (ERIC) within the U.S. Department of Education operates 16 subject-specific clearinghouses and maintains document collections in about 3,000 locations, as well as an answering service on the Internet (http://www.ed.gov/EdRes/EdFed/ERIC.html). Although ERIC does not have a clearinghouse for health programs, these can be readily identified by searching the center's databases. Other resource centers and clearinghouses may be identified through searches on the Internet and by information obtained through sponsoring agencies and professional networks.

Such resources often enable you to access a great deal of programmatic information quickly. However, the nature of the information you receive may be affected by the mission and policies of the agency sponsor. For example, the National Clearinghouse for Alcohol and Drug Information contains a vast array of prevention and treatment programs, but because the federal government has a "no-tolerance" policy toward drug use, it contains no interventions for individuals who use alcohol or other drugs experimentally or in moderation. When a clearinghouse or resource center does not voluntarily communicate the criteria and conditions governing its acquisitions, you should inquire about them.

The amount and quality of programmatic information you receive from a clearinghouse or resource center also will vary with the methods each organization uses to identify, review, select, acquire, catalogue, and distribute materials. Clearinghouses that aim to be inclusive may retrieve so many references that sorting through them to identify materials related to your interests can be very time-consuming. When you finally finish, you may discover that descriptions of some interventions are still incomplete or that materials from some program components are missing. Although smaller centers can be searched more quickly, their collections may be unbalanced or outdated, particularly if they acquire most materials through donations.

Most clearinghouses and resource centers operated by the federal government offer free services and are accessible to the general public, but sponsor policies may limit access to other centers. For example, only persons working on tobacco prevention and control projects funded by the California Department of Health Services may use the excellent Tobacco Education Clearinghouse it supports. Also, although anyone may obtain a catalogue of materials and sales are unrestricted, those not working on state-funded projects are charged a higher price. Reliance on part-time staff and limited hours of operation may reduce access to smaller clearinghouses and resource centers, but these agencies also may be forced to charge a fee for service.

PROGRAM ARCHIVES

Because you are interested in intervention development, you may have been assembling your own collection of health behavior programs and materials over the years. If you work for a health department, a voluntary agency, an educational institution, a research institute, a business, or some other organization involved in health promotion and disease prevention, your employer probably also has stockpiled materials developed or distributed under its auspices, as well as perhaps others that it requested or that arrived unsolicited. Hands-on access to these materials is likely to be convenient, and so it may make sense to begin your search for other interventions here. However, some programs relevant to your interests may not be included, and unless considerable time and thought have been invested in developing these collections, the resulting hodgepodge may be of limited value to you.

A readily accessible warehouse of complete and carefully selected intervention packages obviously would be of great assistance to program developers, but to date, few such resources are available. One pioneering exception is the Program Archive on Sexuality, Health, and Adolescence (PASHA), established by the Sociometrics Corporation, a research and development firm specializing in social science research applications (http://www.socio.com). The purpose of PASHA is to "facilitate cost-effective replication of evaluated prevention programs that work, eliminate wasted effort spent 'reinventing the wheel' and encourage ongoing scientific evaluation of programs to ascertain the robustness of each program's effectiveness (or lack thereof) across different study populations." A Scientist Expert Panel selects the programs included in PASHA for their demonstrated effectiveness in changing teenage sexual behaviors that affect their fertility and risk of contracting HIV and other sexually transmitted diseases.

As of this writing, 23 PASHA program packages are available for purchase. Each package contains a complete set of program materials, a user's guide prepared by archive staff, and resources for reevaluating the program. For the first year, program staff also offer free telephone technical support on program implementation and evaluation. Information about PASHA programs, their developers, and initial evaluation reports is available online. However, because purchase appears to be the only option for reviewing a package in detail, costs may be formidable for program developers who wish to examine a number of interventions. Another disadvantage of such archives is that they contain only programs of developers who have agreed to distribution through this channel. PASHA, as an example of a program pooling approach (Step 2 of the chain model), is discussed in detail in Chapter 8.

FUNDING AGENCIES

Grant-making agencies often provide information about health behavior programs currently being developed, implemented, or evaluated with their support. Descriptions of projects funded by the federal government can be requested under the Freedom of Information Act (http://www.hhs.gov/about/infoguid.htm#2). Other organizations may list grants awarded in their annual report, in newsletters, or in a special report about a particular funding initiative. These reports also often may be obtained by requesting them from the granting agency. Some agencies, such as the Robert Wood Johnson Foundation (http://www/rwjf.org), provide information about funded projects on their Web sites.

Program information from funding agencies frequently is subject to two limitations. First, summaries may be too abbreviated to offer much guidance for program development. Second, the information provided usually concerns a *proposed* intervention rather than one that has been fully developed. Because initial ideas usually are modified as detailed programs are planned and then actually implemented, you may need to contact the program developer for updated information. Alternatively, you can wait until a final project report is submitted. Again, agencies of the federal government must provide you with a copy of such reports when you request them under the Freedom of Information Act. Other granting agencies and some program developers may be willing to share final reports and possibly periodic progress reports as well.

In addition, as mentioned earlier, granting agencies occasionally prepare comprehensive analyses of all projects completed under a specific initiative or during a given time period (e.g., Jansen et al., 1996; Mueller & Higgins, 1988; Tjerandsen, 1980). These resources often provide a valuable perspective on the strengths and weaknesses of prior program efforts and promising directions for the future.

NEWSLETTERS

Newsletters from professional organizations and other agencies frequently contain information about health programs. For example, the Cherokee Nation's substance abuse program was described in a recent issue of *Closing the Gap*, a newsletter of the Office of Minority Health (Oxendine, 1998). Midwife training programs and other strategies to reduce maternal mortality in the developing world were reported in a special issue of *Outlook*, a newsletter published by the Program for Appropriate Technology in Health (Nguyen, 1998).

Although newsletters can be helpful in identifying interventions under development and currently in the field, follow-up usually is necessary to obtain a detailed description of the program and its evaluation. Summary indications of effectiveness may be included in newsletter stories, but more information about methodology is needed to assess the validity and reliability of the findings reported.

FLYERS AND BROCHURES

Flyers promoting conferences and training programs are another potential source of information about health programs. For example, the mail carrier recently delivered a brochure about a 2-day training seminar with continuing education credit to prepare teachers to implement "Wise Guys," a program developed in North Carolina to promote sexual responsibility in young males (Family Life Council, 1998). Another flyer invited attendance at a professional meeting where presentations will be made about several health programs recently initiated in different parts of the country.

Although such materials may identify interventions potentially related to the one you are developing, more information about them is clearly needed. Names and addresses listed on flyers provide tangible leads for further fact-finding. You also might decide to attend a conference that appears especially relevant. If you are unable to do this, inquire whether abstracts will be published as part of the meeting program and, if so, request a copy. Also ask whether printed conference proceedings or audiotapes of presentations will be available and how these can be ordered.

COMMUNITY PROGRAMS

Most of the resources previously discussed contain considerable information about community-based health programs in the United States and other countries. In addition, some Web sites facilitate real-time exchange of information among residents of communities planning or implementing interventions to address particular issues. For example, Join Together was established as a national resource for communities working to reduce substance abuse and gun violence (http://jointogether.org).

Sources of information about programs currently being implemented or previously conducted in a particular community are more difficult to identify, and indeed these may be quite idiosyncratic. Moreover, although process-oriented models of program planning emphasize the importance of community participation (CDC, 1995; Dignan & Carr, 1987), scant attention has been devoted to methods for identifying and reviewing local programs within a participatory community planning context. Remedying this situation is important because development of a new community intervention should build on lessons learned from prior community experience. Familiarity with programs currently being implemented in the community also may help planners to avoid the resistance that can be generated when a new initiative is viewed as duplicating or competing with existing efforts. A case study of the Worcester AIDS Consortium by Zapka et al. (1992) suggests that studying community partnerships and coalitions may be especially fruitful.

Methods are especially needed to deal with the dilemmas that arise when people in the community want to take action on a problem that has not yet been the subject of systematic scientific inquiry or that scientific studies indicate is caused by factors other than those identified. To concerned constituencies, the problem is real and requires intervention. They may be convinced that they know both the source of the problem and the action needed, as, for example, when citizen groups become convinced that industrial waste is contaminating their water supply and causing the deaths of children. Even when they are ultimately proven right, without scientific evidence demonstrating cause and effect, efforts to control the problem may result not in a program but in a legal battle like that chronicled in the award-winning book, *A Civil Action* (Harr, 1995).

COMMERCIAL SOURCES OF INFORMATION

A growing number of health programs and related health promotion materials are available from for-profit and not-for-profit businesses. A few program developers have established their own small companies to disseminate their interventions. Programs distributed by larger publishers may have been developed in-house, through contracts with writers, or by academics and others who want to make their programs widely available. Regardless of their origin, these products are usually marketed using sophisticated techniques, including the widespread distribution of full-color catalogues and brochures, displays at professional meetings, clever Web pages, personalized sales visits, offers of free trial use, complementary copies for libraries, and gifts or entertainment for those who make major purchasing decisions.

Although information about commercially distributed programs is attractive and readily available, the quality of these interventions may be difficult to determine. When you identify a program of interest, you should inquire about how it was developed, the theory on which it is based, and how its effectiveness has been evaluated. In some cases, the publishers may be able to refer you to peer-reviewed journal articles or other documents reporting this information. Even so, claims of effectiveness for programs developed, evaluated, and marketed by the same individual or company often are regarded with skepticism.

Regardless of these issues, reviewing commercially distributed programs may trigger many ideas for the development of your own intervention. Publishers employ an impressive array of creative talent to ensure that their programs will appeal to targeted user groups or market segments, and, for this reason alone, they merit close examination. In addition, content is often thoughtfully selected and well presented, questions for discussion or homework may be excellent, graphics and packaging are likely to be imaginative, and an inviting portfolio of ancillary exercises and materials usually is included.

An increasing number of businesses also produce pamphlets, posters, workbooks, refrigerator magnets, pins, and other items promoting an array of positive health behaviors. In some cases, these materials can be customized by imprinting your own slogan or logo. Because you probably could not produce similar materials for the same or lower cost, you may wish to consider purchasing some of them for use in your program. A potential disadvantage, however, is that using copyrighted materials in your intervention may increase the difficulty of obtaining a separate copyright for it.

Other commercial resources of potential use to program developers include the warehousing of effective interventions, as already described, and the provision of electronic search services. Cambridge Scientific Abstracts, for example, will search its own extensive databases and those of its reputable publishing partners and then make results available in several electronic formats (http://www.csa.com).

THE WORLD WIDE WEB

With development of the Internet, you can now electronically search for much information about health programs that previously could be accessed only through time-consuming library searches, written and telephoned requests, mailings, and visits to clearinghouses or program sites. Relevant journal articles, books, and other print resources can be identified by searching various databases, including the National Library of Medicine's MEDLINE, the American Psychological Association's PsycINFO, and those established by public and university libraries, clearinghouses, resource centers, and other agencies. Full text for an increasing number of journal articles, books, newsletters, and reports is also available online.

As indicated throughout the preceding discussion, many agencies—including departments of government, voluntary agencies, foundations, clearinghouses, and resource centers—also make information about health programs available on their Web sites. In addition, Web sites dedicated to specific health problems and population groups have been established. Other sites have been created to facilitate exchange among members of professional groups. And there are sites for practitioners, regardless of background, who share common programmatic interests. Most of these sites contain links to other Internet locations providing related information. For example, the Web site for the National Women's Health Information Center (http://www.4women.gov) links to more than 1,000 sites, including all federal agencies and publications on women's health, as well as hundreds of government-screened private organizations. The Web page for the American Public Health Association (http://www.apha.org/resources/index.html) provides a gateway to Internet resources on AIDS, children's health, community health promotion, reproductive health, cancer, and a variety of other health topics.

If you have not searched the Internet before, library staff, self-help manuals, and the browser on your computer can help you get started. Most search engines and databases also provide specific instructions for users, as well as tips for solving problems encountered. Lists of Internet locations of potential interest to readers are often published in professional journals and newsletters, and many individuals also circulate lists of their favorite Web sites. When you find a Web page that you may want to visit again, create a bookmark for quick access. However, because the Internet is very dynamic, you should be aware that new Web pages appear all the time, but other sites are not regularly updated or just vanish.

Although the Internet is an amazing resource, hours can slip by as you explore its wonders. Therefore, when you initiate a search, be sure that you have your purpose clearly in mind. Also, learn to evaluate Web sites because their value and reliability vary. Some sites have been established to help you think critically about Web resources (http://www.library.ucla.edu/libraries/college/instruct/web/critical.htm), determine the credibility of a particular site (http://www.sph.emory.edu/WELLNESS/abstract.html), and assess the quality of the health information provided (http://mel.lib.mi.us/health/health-evaluating.html).

DIRECT CONTACT WITH PROGRAM DEVELOPERS

Despite all the other resources available, the individuals who developed an intervention are likely to be the best source of information about it. You therefore may attempt to contact program developers directly with your questions, but unless you know them personally, this experience may be frustrating. Most people who plan and test health behavior programs have many other responsibilities and keep very busy schedules. Although they are likely to be pleased by your interest in an intervention, after its evaluation was completed, they probably went on to other projects now requiring their attention. Requests to send information or copies of materials have to be sandwiched in with other demands.

You can increase your chances for a timely reply by asking brief, specific questions that can be answered quickly. Remember that many program developers work for universities and other organizations that seldom provide resources and an effective infrastructure for program dissemination. Responding to your request may receive low priority if this requires digging through files, duplicating papers, and preparing packets for mailing. Even arranging time and space for you to review materials on-site may be viewed as too time-consuming. You can reduce these barriers by offering several options for reply and by providing your postal and e-mail addresses, as well as your telephone and facsimile numbers. Enclosing a preaddressed stamped envelope also may be helpful. In addition, you might inquire about talking with a program developer at a conference or some other place where usual work pressures are less likely to intrude. Another strategy is to request contact information for people who worked under the program developer's direction on the intervention components of greatest interest to you.

CONDUCTING YOUR SEARCH ◄

Awareness of the numerous resources that provide information about health programs underscores the importance of developing a purposeful search strategy. Before starting the hunt, you should examine column 1 of your matrix and prioritize the types of information you need. Then, from column 3, select the sources most likely to produce this information. If you begin by searching computer databases, use key words from column 2 as appropriate to identify relevant reports and other resources.

If your first pass through a database surfaces only a few references, enter other key words and repeat your search. If results are still disappointing, move on to explore another source of information.

On the other hand, if the number of references identified is overwhelming, restrict your search by adding key words and try again. For example, the phrase "nutrition program" surfaced 21,905 results in a search of ERIC, but adding "evaluat" reduced the number of citations to 77. Note that entering the stem common to "evaluate," "evaluated," and "evaluation" identified references containing any one of these words.

When you have created a promising list of citations, pause to review them. If abstracts or program descriptions are included, these can help you to select specific reports and materials for review. Otherwise, you may need to scan a variety of source materials to identify those that contain information pertinent to your program. To keep this task manageable, begin with the most promising titles. Periodically take stock of what you have discovered and use this assessment to refine plans for continuing your search. At any given point, you might decide that closely examining the programs you already have identified would provide you with valuable guidance for locating additional information. Alternatively, you may prefer to continue your search for relevant citations so that you can retrieve or request those from a particular journal or other resource at the same time.

FINDING INFORMATION ABOUT A PARTICULAR PROGRAM

As you acquire a document or set of materials related to an intervention that you want to review, label it with the name of the program and its primary author, as well as any other identifier that you will use to file and retrieve such resources. If you are working from a copied document, also make sure that the complete bibliographic citation is written on it. Then scan it for information that will help you to learn more about the program, obtain a complete set of program materials, and, if you so decide, request permission to incorporate certain ideas or activities in your own intervention. This information should be entered on a tracking sheet for each program, such as the one illustrated in Table 7.2.

Although you may choose different headings and another format, tracking a program clearly requires noting its title, any abbreviated names by which it may be known, the names of program developers, and contact information for them. Recording the time period during which the intervention was developed and field-tested will help you to estimate when reports about it may have been published so that you can search databases efficiently. In addition, if a program has undergone successive rounds of development, evaluation, and revision, noting the dates of major modifications will help you to trace the changes made, as well as reasons for them.

Information about the purpose of the program, its target group, and major features should be briefly summarized in a way that will help you to locate reports

TABLE 7.2   Sample Tracking Sheet for Locating Information About an Intervention

Program name(s) and years of development/revision:

Developer(s) and author(s):
    Name
    Affiliation
    Address
    Telephone
    Fax
    e-mail

Purpose, target group, and brief description:

Field test(s)/evaluation:
    Year
    Population
    Location
    Intervention setting
    Results

Other reports and sources of information:

Names and locations of organizations that use or have used the program

Publisher/distributor:
    Name
    Address
    Telephone
    Fax
    e-mail

Materials available, cost, and copyright:

Questions/missing information:

and materials. Including the details to be considered in your review is not necessary. Noting references to other reports about the program will facilitate finding them, and recording the names and locations of organizations that have implemented the program may help you to obtain copies of materials that you can review. However, if you can identify an agency that actively distributes the program, this will be the best resource for obtaining the latest and most complete version. Both its cost and the resources available to you will determine whether you can afford to acquire it. You also should determine whether the program and its supporting materials are copyrighted because this may prohibit you from duplicating copies even for limited use in the review process. Finally, listing unanswered questions about the program and specific types of information you are missing will guide your search for additional resources.

MONITORING AND MANAGING THE SEARCH PROCESS

Although tracking sheets will assist you in locating further information about specific programs, you also need a mechanism for managing your search and monitoring its progress. Creating another matrix will enable you to do this efficiently, and later this also will facilitate the systematic review of the reports and materials you are assembling.

To construct this second matrix, make a separate row for each type of information you are seeking and then enter phrases describing these topics in the far-left column. This column should look very much like column 1 of the matrix used to plan your search (see Table 7.1), although topics may be consolidated or expanded. Now make another column for each program that you intend to review and write the name of the program in the column heading. You can draw this matrix on a large sheet of scratch paper, but working with a table or spreadsheet on your computer will make it easier to adjust the size of rows and columns, as well as to add or delete them as the need arises.

Information about each document or set of materials that you intend to review should then be entered in the matrix. To do this for a report, you need to locate the column for the program discussed, scan the contents of the document, and, as you find topics listed in a matrix row, enter the document's identifier in the appropriate cell. An article that contains several types of information should be referenced in each relevant cell so that its identifier appears repeatedly. The identifier for a review article, meta-analysis, or other report that contains information about several interventions also should appear in multiple columns corresponding to all the programs discussed. Intervention materials should be indexed in a similar manner, although almost always they will be specific to a single program and therefore be identified in only one column.

Table 7.3 illustrates the basic format for such a matrix. In the interests of brevity, only a few review topics and programs are displayed, and the information is hypothetical. To indiciate that this matrix design can be modified as you see fit, several rows refer to particular program components so that interventions containing them can be identified at a glance. Also note that cells in some rows contain not only identifiers but also summary phrases describing designated program features. Including such phrases on your matrix provides a quick overview of the interventions you are finding.

Inspecting this matrix as it develops will help you to identify additional information you need, thereby focusing the next stages of your search. Thus, using Table 7.3 as an example, you can quickly see that only one article is cited for each of the programs listed in the last two columns. You therefore might search databases for additional references, using as key words first the name of each program and then the names of those who authored the articles already in your possession. You also might call or write the authors, inquiring whether the program they wrote about earlier has been evaluated and, if so, how a report of findings might be obtained.

How broadly you search and how long you continue will be determined not only by the types of information you are seeking but also by the number of relevant interventions you find. Few prior programs may be available if the health problem your intervention will address is newly defined or if minimal resources have been invested in behavioral approaches to prevent and control the problem. Conversely, you may find literally hundreds of programs developed to reduce risk factors for health problems that greatly concern the public. In either case, your challenge is to obtain information about programs that will contribute to the development of your own intervention. When you reach the point of diminishing returns, do not hesitate to terminate your search. In deciding when to do this, remember that additional time will be needed to review the materials you have acquired and that completion of this task must be coordinated with your overall schedule for program development.

REVIEWING YOUR POOL OF INFORMATION ◄
ABOUT OTHER PROGRAMS

Developing a new intervention requires making a series of planning decisions. The reason for reviewing other programs as part of this process is to identify and evaluate options for each of these choices. This may be done in stages as your planning progresses, or you may prefer to examine the entire pool of information

TABLE 7.3   Example of Matrix Indexing Sources of Information About Health Programs

Topic	Programs "Never Too Old"	"Healthy Aging"	"Fun & Games for Seniors"
Need for program	Phi et al. (1998)	Beta and Zeta (1996)	Alpha (1995) Delta and Rho (1997)
Target group	Female African Americans, age ≥ 65 Omega (1999)	Male and female Whites, age ≥ 55 Beta and Zeta (1996)	Males and females, multiethnic, age ≥ 65 Delta and Rho (1997)
Intervention setting	Inner-city senior center Omega (1999)	Suburban senior center Beta and Zeta (1996)	Residents of retirement community Delta and Rho (1997)
Theoretical framework	Multiple theories Phi et al. (1998)	Health belief model Beta and Zeta (1996)	Social learning theory Delta and Rho (1997)
Change strategies	Experiential learning, social support Phi et al. (1998)	Presentations and group discussion Beta and Zeta (1996)	Role models, self-efficacy, individual goal setting, incentives Delta and Rho (1997)
Program length and duration		Six biweekly sessions 3 months Beta and Zeta (1996)	Ongoing events Delta and Rho (1997)
Behavioral objectives	Lower cholesterol Low-fat, high-fiber diet Phi et al. (1998) Omega (1999)	Low-fat, high-fiber diet Beta and Zeta (1996)	Increase physical activity Delta and Rho (1997)
Exercise component			Many sports, competitions Delta and Rho (1997) Promotional flyer, 1996
Nutrition component	Group meal preparation and dining Gamma (1997)	Guest speakers, films, meal planning Beta and Zeta (1996)	
Health screening component	Health fair Gamma (1997)		
Other components	Family involvement Gamma (1997)		
Mass media	Radio Gamma (1997)		
Other methods	Gamma (1997)		
Evaluation	Process evaluation Omega (1999)		

you have collected about other programs all at once. In the latter case, the options you identify would be considered as related planning decisions are considered.

Although the timing of these two approaches differs, the recommended procedure does not. Proceeding systematically, you should pick a topic identified in column 1 of the matrix summarizing your pool of information. Then, pull all documents identified in the corresponding row, keeping all resources about the same program together. Next, *review* the documents you have pulled to determine how the issue of interest was handled in each program for which you have information. *Combine your findings* to identify all alternatives that have been tried before. Then evaluate the *strengths and weaknesses of each alternative*, considering criteria important in the development of your intervention. As you proceed, you are likely to think of *modifications* that would improve a prior approach or of other ways that the issue could be addressed. Jot down these ideas and subject them to the same critical evaluation. Both the depth of your analysis and the volume of ideas generated will be increased if you involve others in this review. Two or three of you might examine the same set of materials independently and then compare your findings. Or each member of your intervention planning team might be assigned to review and report on different programs as the basis for a group discussion.

Resources listed in each row of your matrix should be reviewed in the same way. Essentially, then, you will dip into your pool of information about other interventions many times, on each occasion withdrawing and reviewing only those resources related to a particular planning issue. Eventually, however, decisions made about specific elements of your program must be integrated into a cohesive whole. At this point, you may want to examine other interventions more comprehensively to study how they were structured. A program-by-program review can be readily accomplished by examining the references listed in each column of your matrix.

Questions may come up that you did not anticipate when you were planning your search for other interventions. If so, familiarity with the programs described in your pool of information still may enable you to find some possible answers. Simply make another row on your matrix for each additional issue that you want to explore and look through all the resources you have assembled for relevant references (see Table 7.3). In addition, because your questions will now be very specific, you might return to the sources of information you found most helpful and search for programs addressing these new issues.

If another program that you review contains ideas, specific content, activities, or materials that you want to use in your own intervention, be sure that you obtain the developer's written permission to borrow these elements, respect any conditions attached, and provide appropriate credits. This is essential if the program or some of its elements have been copyrighted, and it is a professional courtesy, even if they have not.

▶ CONCLUSIONS: MAKING YOUR INTERVENTION AVAILABLE TO OTHERS

At last your intervention has been developed, implemented, and evaluated! However, your work is not completed until you make your program available to others. A first step is to obtain a copyright for it because this provides protection against careless use or adaptation, as well as against outright plagiarism. Another task is to determine how your intervention will be published and distributed. If evaluation has demonstrated positive behavioral effects, you might arrange to submit your program for review by an organization such as the Centers for Disease Control and Prevention, which has formal criteria and procedures for designating model programs that are then actively disseminated by an experienced contractor. You also might inquire about the interest and capabilities that other organizations, including your employer, have in publishing and distributing your program. Reviewing the program tracking sheets you made early in your search for other interventions will help you to identify agencies and firms that distribute related programs.

From each interested agency you identify, obtain detailed information about the criteria used to select materials for dissemination. Also determine how your program might be altered in the publication process, how it would be formatted and packaged, the audiences to whom it would be marketed, the marketing strategies that would be used, when marketing would begin, and what voice you would have in these decisions. And you should discuss projected costs with the purchaser, the royalties you would receive, and the estimated number of programs that would be purchased in each of the next several years. Before making a final decision about which program will distribute your intervention, you might want to review research about factors affecting program dissemination (e.g., Rohrbach, D'Onofrio, Backer, & Montgomery, 1996) and talk with developers of other programs whose materials are distributed by the organizations you are considering.

Although arranging for the distribution of your intervention will make it available to potential users and, through them, to expanding numbers of people who will benefit from program participation, dissemination plans are unlikely to target those who are developing new interventions. To ensure that your program and the lessons that you learned in creating it contribute to the advancement of intervention science, you should reflect on your experience in identifying and reviewing other interventions relevant to your program development effort. Consider the sources of information you found most useful and contribute to them by publishing articles and reports about your program, making conference presentations, and submitting stories to newsletters.

Talk and write not only about the design of your intervention and the results it achieved but also about the processes through which it was developed and tested, the issues you encountered, and the lessons you learned. Sharing your insights will help to refine a new approach for systematically drawing on the knowledge, creativity, and hard work of yourself and others as an important foundation for the development of new health behavior programs.

REFERENCES

ARGYRIS, C., PUTNAM, R., McLAIN, A., & SMITH, D. (1985). *Action science: Concepts, methods, and skills for research and intervention.* San Francisco: Jossey-Bass.

BARTHOLOMEW, L. K., PARCEL, G. S., & KOK, G. (1998). Intervention mapping: A process for developing theory- and evidence-based health education programs. *Health Education & Behavior, 25,* 545-563.

BIGLAN, A., JAMES, L. E., LaCHANCE, P., ZOREF, L., & JOFFE, J. (1988). Videotaped materials in a school-based smoking prevention program. *Preventive Medicine, 17,* 559-584.

BLOOM, J. R., STEWART, S. L., & LEE, M. (1998, February). *Risk notification for women at high risk for breast cancer.* Grant application to the University of California Breast Cancer Research Program.

CALIFORNIA DEPARTMENT OF EDUCATION. (1998). *Getting results: Developing safe and healthy kids: Part I. California action guide to creating safe and drug-free schools and communities.* Sacramento: California Department of Education, Healthy Kids Program Office.

CENTERS FOR DISEASE CONTROL AND PREVENTION (CDC). (1995). *Planned approach to community health: Guide for the local coordinator.* Atlanta, GA: U.S. Department of Health and Human Services, Public Health Service, Centers for Disease Control and Prevention, National Center for Chronic Disease Prevention and Health Promotion.

CENTERS FOR DISEASE CONTROL AND PREVENTION (CDC). (1998). Prevalence of diagnosed diabetes among American Indians/Alaskan Natives—United States, 1996. *Morbidity and Mortality Weekly Report, 47,* 901-903.

COYLE, K., KIRBY, D., PARCEL, G., BASEN-ENGQUIST, K., BANSPACH, S., RUGG, D., & WEIL, M. (1996). Safer Choices: A multicomponent school-based HIV/STD and pregnancy prevention program for adolescents. *Journal of School Health, 66,* 89-94.

DENT, C. W., SUSSMAN, S., STACY, A. W., CRAIG, S., BURTON, D., & FLAY, B. R. (1995). Two-year behavior outcomes of Project Towards No Tobacco Use. *Journal of Consulting and Clinical Psychology, 63,* 676-677.

DIGNAN, M. B., & CARR, P. A. (1987). *Program planning for health education and health promotion.* Philadelphia, PA: Lea & Febiger.

DOLAN-MULLEN, P., RAMÍREZ, G., & GROFF, J. Y. (1994). A meta-analysis of randomized trials of prenatal smoking cessation interventions. *American Journal of Obstetrics and Gynecology, 171,* 1328-1334.

D'ONOFRIO, C. N. (1992). Theory and the empowerment of health education practitioners. *Health Education Quarterly, 19,* 385-403.

DRYFOOS, J. G. (1990). *Adolescents at risk: Prevalence and prevention.* New York: Oxford University Press.

ERNSTER, V. L. (1997). Mammography screening for women ages 40 through 49: A guidelines saga and clarion call for informed decision-making. *American Journal of Public Health, 87,* 1103-1106.

FAMILY LIFE COUNCIL OF GREATER GREENSBORO, INC. (1998). *Wise guys: Male responsibility program training* (Brochure). Greensboro, NC: Author.

FIELDING, J., & PISERCHIA, P. (1989). Frequency of worksite health promotion activities. *American Journal of Public Health, 79,* 16-20.

GLANZ, K., LEWIS, F. M., & RIMER, B. K. (1996). *Health behavior and health education: Theory, research, and practice* (2nd ed.). San Francisco: Jossey-Bass.

GOLASZEWSKI, T., BARR, D., & COCHRAN, S. D. (1998). An organization-based intervention to improve support for employee heart health. *American Journal of Health Promotion, 13,* 26-35.

GREEN, L. W., & KREUTER, M. W. (1991). *Health promotion planning: An education and environmental approach.* Palo Alto, CA: Mayfield.

GROSCH, J. W., ALTERMAN, T., PETERSEN, M. R., & MURPHY, L. R. (1998). Worksite health promotion programs in the U.S.: Factors associated with availability and participation. *American Journal of Health Promotion, 13,* 36-45.

HARR, J. (1995). *A civil action.* New York: Random House.

HOCHBAUM, G. M., SORENSON, J. R., & LORIG, K. (1992). Theory in health education practice. *Health Education Quarterly, 19,* 295-313.

JANIS, I. L., & MANN, L. (1977). *Decision-making: A psychological analysis of conflict, choice, and commitment.* New York: Free Press.

JANSEN, M. A., GLYNN, T., & HOWARD, J. (1996). Prevention of alcohol, tobacco, and other drug use: Federal efforts to stimulate prevention research. *American Behavioral Scientist, 39,* 790-807.

JOHNSON, C. A., MacKINNON, D. P., & PENTZ, M. A. (1996). Breadth of program and outcome effectiveness in drug abuse prevention. *American Behavioral Scientist, 39,* 884-896.

KYLE, J. (Ed.). (1987). *Children, families and cities: Programs that work at the local level.* Washington, DC: National League of Cities.

L'ABBE, K. A., DELSKY, A. S., & O'ROURKE, K. (1987). Meta-analysis in clinical research. *Annals of Internal Medicine, 107,* 224-233.

LAZARUS, R. S., & FOLKMAN, S. (1991). The concept of coping. In Monat, A., R. S. Lazarus, et al. (Eds.), *Stress and coping: An anthology* (pp. 189-206). New York: Columba University Press.

McGINNIS, J. (1993). 1992 national survey of worksite health promotion activities summary. *American Journal of Health Promotion, 7,* 452-464.

MUELLER, D., & HIGGINS, P. (1988). *Funders' guide manual: A guide to prevention programs in human services.* St. Paul, MN: Amherst Wilder Foundation.

NATIONAL EDUCATION ASSOCIATION. (1998). *Kids act! A guide for middle school teachers.* Washington, DC: National Education Association, Health Information Network.

NGUYEN, T. (Ed.). (1998). Safe motherhood [Special issue]. *Outlook, 16.*

OCKENE, J. K., SORENSEN, G., KABAT-ZINN, J., OCKENE, I. S., & DONNELLY, G. (1988). Benefits and costs of lifestyle change to reduce risk of chronic disease. *Preventive Medicine, 17,* 224-234.

OXENDINE, J. (1998). Cherokees build a healthy nation. In U.S. Department of Health and Human Services (Ed.), *Closing the gap* (p. 9). Washington, DC: U.S. Department of Health and Human Services, Office of Minority Health.

PENTZ, M. A., BONNIE, R. J., & SHOPLAND, D. R. (1996). Integrating supply and demand reduction strategies for drug abuse prevention. *American Behavioral Scientist, 39,* 897-910.

PRICE, R. H., COWEN, E. L., LORION, R., & RAMOS-McKAY, J. (1988). *14 ounces of prevention.* Washington, DC: American Psychological Association.

PROCHASKA, J. O., & DiCLEMENTE, C. C. *The transtheoretical approach: Crossing traditional boundaries of change.* Homewood, IL: Dow Jones/Irwin.

RITTEL, H. W., & WEBBER, M. M. (1973). Dilemmas in a general theory of planning. *Policy Sciences, 4,* 155-169.

ROBISON, J. I. (1998). To reward? . . . or not to reward? Questioning the wisdom of using external reinforcement in health promotion programs. *American Journal of Health Promotion, 13,* 1-3.

ROHRBACH, L. A., D'ONOFRIO, C. N., BACKER, T. E., & MONTGOMERY, S. B. (1996). Diffusion of school-based substance abuse prevention programs. *American Behavioral Scientist, 39,* 919-934.

SABOGAL, F., OTERO-SABOGAL, R., PASICK, R. J., JENKINS, C. N. H., & PÉREZ-STABLE, E. J. (1996). Printed health education materials for diverse communities: Suggestions learned from the field. *Health Education Quarterly, 23*(Suppl.), S123-S141.

SCHORR, L. (1988). *Within our reach.* New York: Doubleday.

SEVERSON, H. H., & BIGLAN, A. (1989). Rationale for the use of passive consent in smoking prevention research: Politics, policy, and pragmatics. *Preventive Medicine, 18,* 267-279.

SUSSMAN, S. (1991). Curriculum development in school-based prevention research. *Health Education Research: Theory and Practice, 6,* 339-351.

SUSSMAN, S., DENT, C. W., BURTON, D., STACY, A. W., & FLAY, B. R. (1995). *Developing school-based tobacco use prevention and cessation programs.* Thousand Oaks, CA: Sage.

SUSSMAN, S., DENT, C. W., STACY, A. W., SUN, P., CRAIG, S., SIMON, T. R., BURTON, D., & FLAY, B. R. (1993). Project Towards No Tobacco Use: 1-year behavioral outcomes. *American Journal of Public Health, 83,* 1245-1250.

TJERANDSEN, C. (1980). *Education for citizenship: A foundation's experience.* Santa Cruz, CA: Emil Schwarzhaupt Foundation.

U.S. DEPARTMENT OF HEALTH AND HUMAN SERVICES (DHHS). (1980). *Promoting health/Preventing disease: Objectives for the nation.* Washington, DC: U.S. Department of Health and Human Services, Public Health Service.

U.S. DEPARTMENT OF HEALTH AND HUMAN SERVICES (DHHS). (1986). *Surgeon General's workshop on violence and public health: Report* (DHHS Pub. No. HRS-D-MC 86-1). Rockville, MD: U.S. Department of Health and Human Services, Public Health Service, Health Resources and Services Administration, Bureau of Maternal and Child Health and Resources Development.

U.S. DEPARTMENT OF HEALTH AND HUMAN SERVICES (DHHS). (1989). *Reducing the health consequences of smoking: 25 years of progress: A report of the surgeon general.* Rockville, MD: U.S. Department of Health and Human Services, Public Health Service, Centers for Disease Control, Center for Chronic Disease Prevention and Health Promotion, Office on Smoking and Health.

U.S. DEPARTMENT OF HEALTH AND HUMAN SERVICES (DHHS). (1991). *Healthy People 2000: National health promotion and disease prevention objectives* (DHHS Pub. No. PHS 91-50212). Washington, DC: U.S. Department of Health and Human Services, Public Health Service.

U.S. DEPARTMENT OF HEALTH AND HUMAN SERVICES (DHHS). (1994). *Preventing tobacco use among young people: A report of the Surgeon General.* Atlanta, GA: U.S. Department of Health and Human Services, Public Health Service, Centers for Disease Control and Prevention, National Center for Chronic Disease Prevention and Health Promotion, Office on Smoking and Health.

U.S. DEPARTMENT OF HEALTH AND HUMAN SERVICES (DHHS). (1996). *Physical activity and health: A report of the surgeon general.* Atlanta, GA: U.S. Department of Health and Human Services, Centers for Disease Control and Prevention, National Center for Chronic Disease Prevention and Health Promotion.

U.S. DEPARTMENT OF HEALTH AND HUMAN SERVICES (DHHS). (1998). *Healthy People 2010 objectives: Draft for public comment.* Washington, DC: U.S. Department of Health and Human Services, Office of Public Health and Science.

U.S. DEPARTMENT OF HEALTH, EDUCATION, AND WELFARE (DHEW). (1964). *Smoking and health: Report of the advisory committee to the surgeon general of the Public Health Service* (PHS Pub. No. 1103). Washington, DC: U.S. Department of Health, Education, and Welfare; Public Health Service; Center for Disease Control.

U.S. DEPARTMENT OF HEALTH, EDUCATION, AND WELFARE (DHEW). (1979a). *Healthy people: The surgeon general's report on health promotion and disease prevention* (DHEW PHS Pub. No. 79-55071). Washington, DC: U.S. Department of Health, Education, and Welfare; Office of the Assistant Secretary for Health and Surgeon General.

U.S. DEPARTMENT OF HEALTH, EDUCATION, AND WELFARE (DHEW). (1979b). *Smoking and health: A report of the surgeon general* (DHEW Pub. No. PHS 79-50066). Washington, DC: U.S. Department of Health, Education, and Welfare; Public Health Service; Office of the Assistant Secretary for Health; Office on Smoking and Health.

ZAPKA, J. G., MARRACCO, G. R., LEWIS, B., McCUSKER, J., SULLIVAN, J., McCARTHY, J., & BIRCH, F. X. (1992). Inter-organizational responses to AIDS: A case study of the Worcester AIDS Consortium. *Health Education Research, 7,* 31-46.

CHAPTER 7

Commentary 1

Mary Ann Pentz

The D'Onofrio chapter on using available knowledge to build health behavior programs has much to recommend it. It is first and foremost a practical how-to guide that takes the program planner from a process of clarifying program objectives and health behaviors, searching available databases for existing programs that might be relevant to these objectives and behaviors, and, finally, assessing the relative fit, full or partial utility, and generalizability of existing programs to a new program in terms of targeted audience, resources, and setting (implementation) conditions. Along the way, the chapter also attempts to address advantages and limitations of this process, particularly regarding available databases for existing programs.

This commentary is organized into three parts: chapter emphasis on program theory, evaluation, and accessibility; alternative typologies for evaluating program relevance; and consideration of program adoption, implementation, and diffusion. The commentary concludes with suggestions for information that authors of research might include in future studies and publications to aid program planners.

EMPHASIS ON THEORY, EVALUATION, AND ACCESSIBILITY

The author recommends that the program planner should try to identify which theory or theories underlie each reviewed program and then refer to the theory to identify variables that can serve as mediators of behavior change or interim outcomes for potential evaluation. This point is critical and perhaps should be stated as a requirement rather than a suggestion for the program planner's review. A program planner armed with a theoretical rationale for how a program is expected to work, as well as how behavior change is expected to occur, is in a better position to argue for both adoption and evaluation of that program. A major question, though, is whether most program planners are sufficiently familiar with psychosocial theories of health behavior change to identify the theoretical underpinnings of a particular program. It might behoove the authors of currently available, evidence-based programs to include information about theory when responding to a program planner's request for those programs.

Evaluation also should be key to a program planner's decision to use a particular program. A recent trend on the upswing is considering promising programs in which evidence-based programs either are not available or have not been tried with a particular audience that is of interest to the program planner. The potential danger in considering promising programs is that *promising* is open to interpretation. For example, a governor may decide to adopt and promote Drug Abuse Resistance Education (DARE) as a promising program based on its wide acceptance in communities, or a school health education specialist may adopt group counseling rather than a smoking cessation program for adolescent smokers because it is more familiar. These criteria do not address the intent of federal guidelines for promising programs, which is the potential of programs for directly changing health behavior and attention to the need for careful evaluation.

Finally, accessibility should be emphasized more. Authors of programs should release specific information about when programs and training will be available and at what cost. Information about some types of programs will be more straightforward to provide than others. For example, a school or parent program with a finite set of materials and training package should have a specific cost and schedule. However, programs that require an extensive organizational process, such as a community organization program or a student assistance program, may have costs and timelines that depend on an individual community's or school's leadership capabilities.

ALTERNATIVE TYPOLOGIES

D'Onofrio's chapter recommends that one or more program planners categorize programs on the basis of several practical considerations that are intended to help match a program with the program planner's needs, including similarity of target audience, target health behavior, and setting conditions, among other factors. Additional typologies also could be considered, based on components currently suggested by research as contributing to effectiveness. For example, regarding youth program contents, most effective health behavior programs address and counteract negative social influences on youth behavior, including peer pressure, and, when relevant, media influences. A program planner could check each program for inclusion of such contents. Similarly, regarding process of delivery, most effective programs depend on interactive methods of instructions based on social learning theory, including modeling, role-playing, group discussion, and extended practice. Each program could be rated according to whether such active methods of instruction are used and what proportion of the program relies on such methods. Finally, in addition to evidence of generalizability of application, as D'Onofrio has mentioned, a typology should include timeliness of the program in terms of whether it has been revised or edited and when. Our own experience suggests that even the best youth prevention programs could use revision and updating at least every 3 years. If a program looks worthwhile for adoption by the program planner but has not been revised recently, the planner might offer the author revision on-site, perhaps in return for a reduced program fee or evaluation, if such an arrangement does not violate copyright.

CONSIDERATION OF ADOPTION, IMPLEMENTATION, AND DIFFUSION

It is flattering to an author to consider that his or her program is wanted and may be disseminated widely outside of a research context and after a research phase of program testing has ended. However, the author has or should have at least three major concerns about widespread dissemination that relate to quality of implementation and, subsequently, effectiveness of the program.

First, one should ponder whether the program planner's constituency community, school, agency, or other delivery unit is really ready to adopt and implement the programs. Today, a flurry of requests for evidence-based programs derives more from release of federal and state funds that are contingent on a community adopting such program than from the community's in-depth knowledge and desire for such programs. A lack of readiness likely will show up later as failure or delay in program implementation.

Second, one should consider whether a program, if adopted, will be implemented the way it was designed to be implemented. For example, outcome results that move an untested program to the status of an evidence-based program are based on that program being implemented with a particular number of sessions, by particular implementors, using particular methods of instruction and training and full content. Unfortunately, a longstanding tendency of communities and schools is to want to pick and choose pieces of a program as if from a menu, ostensibly for the purpose of tailoring the program to fit their perceived unique needs. The original program author and the program planner can make no claims as to likely program effectiveness if a menu approach is used. Responsibility for maintaining the integrity of the program probably lies with the program planner, at least in written instructions to potential program users, especially if the planner is considered the champion or major promoter of the program in his or her community.

Third, one may be concerned about diffusion, which also relates to quality of implementation. An analogy of the "post office" game is helpful here. One person in a circle whispers a story to the adjacent person, who passes the story on until it comes full circle. The story related back to the original storyteller is likely to be very different from the original story in word, context, or other parameters simply because of the human, personalizing influence we all have. The same process is true for diffusion of programs, in which communities or schools originally trained by a program's author train others, often in sequences, and end up distributing materials with incorrect, little, or no training passed on. If a program planner expects diffusion to occur, he or she might arrange for a program budget to include annual refresher training for trained implementors, new training for new program implementors, and more intensive certification training of a master set of implementors if a training-of-trainers model will be used to disseminate the program. In any case, the point is to refer to original training protocols as much as possible.

SUGGESTIONS ON HOW RESEARCHERS MIGHT HELP PROGRAM PLANNERS

It is already common practice to address methodological limitations in the conduct of a research study when submitting a proposal or publishing results. Noting these limitations is helpful to other researchers who attempt similar studies, but it is not particularly helpful to a program planner. In gauging the feasibility of introducing a particular program into his or her setting, a program planner could benefit from a research paper that specifies the process and limitations of adoption and implementation that were encountered during testing of the program. Authors could provide this information by including adoption and implementation limitations in the discussion section of publications, as well as more details about the process of recruitment of subjects, organizations, and settings in the methods section. Finally, a substantial number of authors of evidence-based programs are researchers who learn from their first test of a program and then go on to refine, expand, or otherwise change the program for testing in new research trials. A program planner may not be aware of these new refinements, which may take several years to reach publication. If the researcher has kept a log of program planner requesters and users and has adequate mailing or e-mail resources, he or she might provide brief periodic updates about refinements to the planner.

CHAPTER 7

Commentary 2

Stephen L. Hamann

This commentary on pooling information about prior interventions as a new program planning tool will present three elements. A general discussion of behavioral intervention processes will be presented. Next, two examples will be presented of the types of problems that occur when interventions are not properly grounded in accumulated knowledge and practice. Then, the implications of pooling information from prior interventions in circumstances in which there are major constraints on resources will be discussed. One of the reasons the above elements were selected for discussion is that the process of pooling information for interventions is still very new, and therefore it is better to present the potential uses of this process than my own initial and incomplete application. In addition, my own experience has been primarily in service environments such as school-based and community-based projects, and I feel information from this setting will be useful.

BEHAVIORAL INTERVENTION PROCESSES

To understand the importance of pooling information about behavioral interventions, one must understand that intervention research has had a long, historical development. There are both large comprehensive interventions and small, restricted interventions. In both, researchers have moved from black-box, input-output models to complex, multivariate, multipath models. In fact, one common indication of research sophistication is that complex modeling is used in planning and testing behavioral research. This emulation of physical science research has produced some benefits in characterizing behavioral research results. Unfortunately, quantitative approaches also have many limitations in providing clarity regarding chains of behavior that result in benefit or harm. In this regard, methodologists continue to try to develop clever ways to perform critical appraisal, so that researchers and practitioners can feel confident about the validity of research findings (Downs & Black, 1998).

Often, this quantitative approach is not sufficiently grounded in applied settings, and practitioners hope research in practice settings will confirm experimental or quasi-experimental research results. More and more often, however, qualitative research often is used separately or together with quantitative research in applied settings to uncover underlying mechanisms responsible for observed outcomes. Health service, school, and even community programs have begun to use evaluation research approaches that provide important behavioral data for analysis and the resolution of other equivocal research findings. Also, networks of governmental and nongovernmental agencies collect data beyond reporting requirements for social policy formulation.

In addition, there has been some progress in broadening the behavioral research perspective so that disciplines such as economics, geography, and political science have come to play more of a role in the consideration of large interventions and whole-systems approaches (Popay & Williams, 1998). This whole-system approach has opened the possibility of various types of action research, including theory-laden approaches in complex behavioral settings (Gottfredson, 1984). In short, the information age will provide greater opportunities for behavioral change because there can be greater clarity about how things work from collaborations across disciplines (knowledge based) and across settings (data based) and because both quantitative and qualitative measures now provide better historical, contextual, and processual data.

PROBLEMS FROM MY OWN EXPERIENCE

Although it is clear that opportunities such as pooling information for behavioral interventions can strengthen behavioral change, present evidence shows several kinds of problems. Two problems in planning and evaluating research are *fixed aggregation* and *standards of assessment*. Fixed aggregation is the unfortunate tendency to accept aggregated knowledge as if it applied to all persons at all times in all settings. Although this is hardly new, it is extremely common but appearing in newer forms. I am often impressed by academic works that are "expert" or involve meta-analysis, which contain a careful consideration of numerous studies, including hundreds of references, detailed tables, and statistical analysis. They often provide important results but lead to unwarranted generalizations. For example, a recent study reviewed the psychosocial factors related to adolescent smoking (Tyas & Pederson, 1998). It found that adolescent smoking was associated with 20 psychosocial variables. These are interesting findings, but because they are based on a lot of isolated studies, the authors point out the inconsistency of variable definitions, lack of multivariate modeling to test hypotheses, and lack of consideration of theory-driven approaches examining a broad range of important variables. The only variable unequivocally not related to adolescent smoking was gender. This further strengthens my point about overgeneralization because adolescent smoking is related to gender in Thailand, where I live (Goldberg, 1999). Men smoke, but women do not (approximately 45% vs. 2%). A better job of considering the mapping of the epidemiology (persons, place, and time) of aggregated information on effective interventions is necessary. Pooling information that involves careful consideration of a wide range of behavioral variables could prevent this type of error.

Another problem that has surfaced in considering complex interventions is the matter of assessing evidence of effectiveness ("standards of assessment"). Several researchers have pointed out that behavioral research is often poorly planned, funded, and executed because not enough time and effort are expended on defining the target behavior, developing the intervention, and evaluating and extending the results to the population of concern (Fishbein, 1996; Mant, 1996; Nutbeam, Smith, & Catford, 1990). This is not simply a problem of methodology. It is a problem of giving too little and asking too much. Here, again, the epidemiology of behavioral research is often inadequately considered, resulting in disappointing results. This is a great tragedy because important behavioral changes are not adequately measured. In many countries, special institutes for behavioral research have not been but must be established to place an importance on the dynamics of effectiveness requirements, so results for public policy are properly framed and appreciated (Kelleher, 1995). The pooling of information for conceptualizing, justifying, designing, and carrying out behavioral interventions can address many of the effectiveness problems in which there has not been an understanding of the unique features of behavioral interventions. The use of pooling is a collaborative approach that can help provide a more focused, policy-relevant emphasis to concerns about effective behavioral research.

WHERE RESOURCES ARE LIMITED

It is logical to assume that where resources are limited, people would need to pool resources from other sources to survive. Unfortunately, the truth is that many program planners would rather die than work collaboratively with others. I exaggerate, but only slightly.

It is beyond the scope of this commentary to explain all the reasons why this is so. Disciplinary differences would lead the list, followed by a long list of circumstances that reward program planners for acting alone.

It is better to invite people to work together by design than to try to force them to work together. I believe that pooling information on interventions is a way to have people work together so they can contribute their own expertise and learn something new. Because I believe that education, research, and service are seamless, integrated information-related tasks, individuals, groups, and communities can be included in this ongoing process of pooling information for human interventions. Problems provide the gist of powerful instruments of cooperation. Asking the right question regarding a future-oriented behavioral goal is often the most crucial part of appraisal. Those who have many answers must learn a process of generating behaviorally important questions about interventions. Everyone has this same problem, and now they have a new process to address it.

REFERENCES

DOWNS, S. H., & BLACK, N. (1998). The feasibility of creating a checklist for the assessment of the methodological quality both of randomized and non-randomized studies of health care interventions. *Journal of Epidemiology and Community Health, 52,* 377-384.

FISHBEIN, M. (1996). Editorial: Great expectations, or do we ask too much from community-level interventions? *Journal of the American Public Health Association, 86,* 1075-1076.

GOLDBERG, M. (1999). *Adolescent smoking in Thailand.* Unpublished manuscript, Pennsylvania State University.

GOTTFREDSON, G. F. (1984). A theory-ridden approach to program evaluation: A method for stimulating researcher-implementer collaboration. *American Psychologist, 39,* 1101-1112.

KELLEHER, C. (1995). Editorial: Health promotion: Shades of Lewis Carroll. *Journal of Epidemiology and Community Health, 49,* 1-4.

MANT, D. (1996). Health promotion and disease prevention: The evaluation of health service interventions. In M. Peckham & R. Smich (Eds.), *Scientific basis of health services* (pp. 171-177). Philadelphia, PA: American College of Physicians.

NUTBEAM, D., SMITH, C., & CATFORD, J. (1990). Evaluation in health education: A review of progress, possibilities, and problems. *Journal of Epidemiology and Community Health, 44,* 83-89.

POPAY, J., & WILLIAMS, G. (1998). Editorial: Partnerships in health: Beyond the rhetoric. *Journal of Epidemiology and Community Health, 52,* 410-411.

TYAS, S. L., & PEDERSON, L. L. (1998). Psychosocial factors related to adolescent smoking: A critical review of the literature. *Tobacco Control, 7,* 409-420.

Case Study 3

CHAPTER 8

The Program Archive on Sexuality, Health, and Adolescence (PASHA)

A Study of Activity Warehousing

Starr Niego
James Peterson

After two decades of research on the development, implementation, and evaluation of teen pregnancy prevention programs, several recent in-depth reviews have identified promising strategies for reducing adolescent pregnancy (Frost & Forrest, 1995; Institute of Medicine, 1995; Kirby, 1995, 1997; Kirby et al., 1994; Miller, Card, Paikoff, & Peterson, 1992; Moore, Sugland, Blumenthal, Glei, & Snyder, 1995; Philliber & Namerow, 1995). Similarly, researchers in the field of adolescent STD/HIV/AIDS prevention have reviewed multiple studies to identify effective interventions (Aral, 1994; Fisher & Fisher, 1992; Holtgrave et al., 1995; Kelly, 1994). These studies demonstrate that carefully planned and targeted interventions can reduce adolescents' sexual risk behaviors. The programs that offer the greatest promise of effecting behavioral change (a) begin intervention delivery by early to mid-adolescence, when youth are 10 to 15 years old, undergoing sexual maturation, and first confronting peer pressure to engage in sexual behavior; (b) match the duration, intensity, and content of the intervention to specific objectives, as well as to participants' age and risk level; (c) incorporate role-playing, modeling, and skill-building exercises; (d) involve parent and peer support; and (e) combine encouragement of abstinence with support for use of contraception or sexually transmitted disease (STD) protection by sexually active teens.

In our view, programs found to be effective in scientifically rigorous evaluation studies offer excellent starting points for practitioners working with their own groups of teens. To make these interventions available, we have developed the Program Archive on Sexuality, Health, and Adolescence (PASHA), a collection of 30 pregnancy and STD/HIV/AIDS prevention programs.[1] For each intervention participating in the collection, PASHA staff members have prepared a comprehensive, user-friendly package containing all of the materials needed to implement the program, along with questionnaire, data collection, and consultant list resources to assist practitioners in evaluating the effectiveness of the program they have selected. In this chapter, we describe PASHA's goals and methods and share lessons learned in the process of assembling, field-testing, and disseminating these materials. Then we describe follow-up projects to strengthen health promotion intervention and evaluation activities. Finally, in the concluding section of the chapter, we step back from the project to discuss, more broadly, the ways in which researcher-practitioner collaborations can advance our understanding and application of risk prevention and health promotion.

GOALS OF THE PASHA PROJECT ◀

Development of the PASHA collection has been guided by four goals:

1. to identify promising teen pregnancy and STD/HIV/AIDS prevention programs;
2. to package each promising program in a set of comprehensive, attractive, and user-friendly materials for practitioners;
3. to field-test each program in a new setting, with a different group of teens (i.e., try to provide a replication and reevaluation of these programs); and

212 ▶ THEORY AND ACTIVITY POOLING

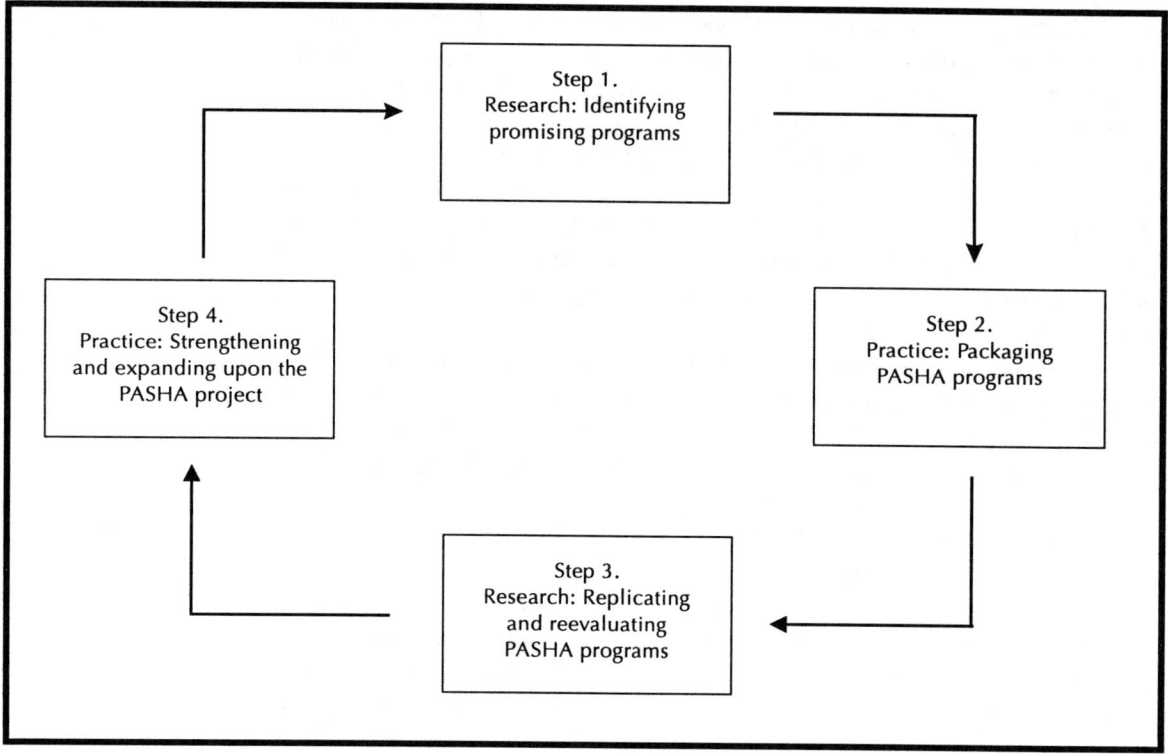

Figure 8.1. The Research-to-Practice Cycle

4. to strengthen and promote the PASHA collection resources for dissemination.

Together, these goals comprise the research-to-practice cycle, shown in Figure 8.1. The cycle illustrates the iterative process guiding the selection, packaging, replication, and dissemination of effective programs. As explained below, each stage builds on the preceding one, as new information from researchers and practitioners is cumulatively integrated into the collection.

In addition, the cycle represents the collaborative exchange that can occur between researchers and practitioners, who may work in different settings and use different methods and tools but, at the core, have closely related goals for health promotion. Researchers and practitioners push one another forward in an iterative cycle of ever-improving program development (see Figure 8.1). Our efforts in the PASHA project challenged us to forge closer ties between these groups. In the process, the benefits of such collaboration became clear.

STEP 1: IDENTIFYING PROMISING PROGRAMS

In assembling the PASHA collection, identifying promising programs was our first step and the one on which the scientific credibility of the project rested. To assist us in our work, we established a five-member Scientist Expert Panel of nationally known pregnancy prevention and/or STD/HIV/AIDS researchers.[2] Through oral and written communication, we reached consensus with the panel on the following set of criteria by which to assess the effectiveness of candidate programs.

Target Population Age. To be considered as a candidate, a program had to be aimed at an appropriate age group. We required that the intervention serve adolescents or young adults between ages 10 and 21 for pregnancy prevention programs and STD/HIV/AIDS programs. Within these years, many individuals engage in sexual experimentation and intercourse with multiple partners and thus put themselves at particularly high risk for STD/HIV/AIDS infection.

Appropriate Evaluation Methods. We further required evidence of a scientific evaluation of the program. This included a follow-up assessment at least 6 months following the end of the intervention period (for pregnancy prevention programs) or at least 3 months postprogram (for STD/HIV/AIDS prevention programs). We required a briefer follow-up period for the infection-related programs to be able to include a manageable number of such studies in the pool under consideration.

Use of a comparison group—preferably but not necessarily a randomly selected control group—also was desired for the evaluation. Yet, in identifying candidate programs, we erred on the side of inclusion. We recognized that programs serving particular high-risk groups (e.g., runaway, homeless, or gay youth) might face unusual hurdles in designing and carrying out evaluation research, such as having a target population too small to divide into independent treatment and comparison groups. Rather than establishing absolute criteria, we chose to have the scientist panel weigh the limitations of a quasi-experimental design against the value of specialized prevention programs (which may not have comparison groups included in their evaluations).

Positive Behavioral Impact. As evident in the review studies cited earlier, researchers have agreed that positive changes in teens' sexuality-related behavior, rather than just in their knowledge or attitudes, are necessary for a program to be judged effective. Accordingly, we required that candidate programs demonstrate a statistically significant positive impact on at least one of the behavioral outcomes listed in Table 8.1.

TABLE 8.1   Indicators of Program Effectiveness

Evaluation data demonstrating the program's positive impact for one or more subgroups of adolescents on at least one of the fertility or STD-related behaviors are listed as follows:
- Postponing sexual intercourse
- Decreasing the frequency of sexual intercourse
- Decreasing the number of sexual partners
- Increasing contraceptive use (at first intercourse, most recent intercourse, or every intercourse)
- Increasing use of effective STD/HIV/AIDS prophylactic method (at first intercourse, most recent intercourse, or every intercourse)
- Substitution of lower-risk for high-risk sexual behaviors
- Increasing STD/HIV/AIDS prevention-related behaviors (i.e., increasing condom purchasing, increasing voluntary condom carrying)
- Preventing pregnancy or STD/HIV/AIDS

For programs aimed primarily at children age 15 or younger, demonstrated positive impact on at least one of the following was accepted as preliminary evidence of effectiveness:
- Fertility- or HIV/STD-related refusal/negotiation skills
- Intentions to engage in one or more of the behaviors cited above
- Values and attitudes favoring the worthwhile nature of one or more of the above behaviors

Nevertheless, we recognized that in many U.S. communities, it might not be appropriate or acceptable to gatekeepers to measure the sexual behaviors of younger teens. For this reason, our effectiveness criteria were relaxed somewhat for interventions aimed at youth age 15 or younger. Here we accepted evidence of a positive impact on sexuality-related refusal or negotiation skills, intentions, values, or attitudes as preliminary indicators of effectiveness. In contrast to changes in knowledge, these outcomes have shown an association, over time, with a reduction in adolescent sexual risk behavior (D'Angelo & DiClemente, 1996; Fisher & Fisher, 1992; Rotheram-Borus, Mahler, & Rosario, 1995).

Program Searches and Expert Ratings. Our next task in the selection process was to conduct a comprehensive search of the literature to identify programs that might meet the above criteria. A variety of the methods were used, including online database searches (with MEDLINE, PsycINFO, and Sociofile), personal contacts, telephone calls to funding agencies, and published announcements in practitioner-oriented newsletters. During this process, we applied one screening measure: existence of a paper documenting the evaluation in a scientifically acceptable manner. This paper need not be published in a peer-reviewed journal, but it did need to provide a description of the intervention, as well as the evaluation research methods, measures, and outcomes (as described earlier) in a scientifically acceptable manner. The unpublished manuscripts that met these criteria included doctoral dissertations, papers submitted to journals, and final reports prepared for granting agencies and foundations. Across all sources, 55 interventions were identified and entered into our candidate pool.

For each candidate program, PASHA staff prepared a set of "briefing documents." These materials included a three- to five-page summary of the theoretical rationale for the program, its curriculum or activities, and the methods and findings of the evaluation study. Also included with the briefing documents were the original reports or journal articles from which the summary was produced. A full set of documents was sent to each panel member, whose charge was to review and rate the candidates, applying our effectiveness criteria. Again, it is important to note that our criteria were not absolute; rather, we relied on the panel's judgment in weighing the merits of often imperfect but "real-world" research. In looking across candidates, for example, panel members needed to determine how a small but significant change with a large sample size compared to an observed change of greater magnitude but for a small group of participants (i.e., consideration of statistical power issues; e.g., see Chapter 15 discussion of statistical power). Or, as noted earlier, they needed to consider how the absence of a comparison group limited the interpretability of a study's findings.

Similarly, we employed a simplified rating system that relied on one overall priority score, rather than multiple subscales. For each candidate, members of the scientist panel were first asked to consider and comment on the following elements of the study: (a) research and evaluation design, (b) data collection methods, and (c) analytical procedures. Then they were asked to assign a priority score between 1 (low) and 10 (high), with scores of 7 or above indicating that the candidate merited inclusion in the collection. Panel members were further asked to abstain from voting on any intervention(s) with which they had been directly involved. We averaged scores across the five panel members and selected into the collection those with a median score of 7 or higher and a mean of at least 6.6. Of the 55 candidates, 30 met this standard. The names and developers of these programs are listed in Tables 8.2 and 8.3. (For more information about the selected interventions, see Card, Niego, Mallari, & Farrell, 1996.)

The Diversity of the PASHA Collection. Before proceeding to Step 2, it may be helpful to take a brief look at the collection. Tables 8.2 and 8.3 show the original setting, approach, components, and duration of each program and together illustrate the diversity of the interventions. First, the collection is evenly divided between pregnancy and STD/HIV/AIDS prevention. Among the pregnancy prevention programs, 11 focus on primary prevention, and 4 aim to prevent or delay a second birth among adolescent mothers. In addition, 7 are primarily school based, 5 are clinic based, and 3 are community based. All of the STD/HIV/AIDS prevention programs aim to prevent STD infection. Among these initiatives, 5 are primarily school based, 2 are clinic based, and 8 are community based. Readers will note that

(text continues on page 220)

TABLE 8.2 PASHA Teen Pregnancy Prevention Programs

Program	Original Site	Approaches	Components	Length/Number of Sessions	Available From PASHA
Barth: Reducing the Risk	School	Abst, Skills, Cont Ed, Sex Ed	Adult, Group, Lect, Role	12 hours/16 sessions	Yes
Bolig: Project Taking Charge	School	Abst, Skills, Life Opt, Sex Ed, Self-Eff	Adult, Group, Lect, Role, Video	Approximately 50 hours/30 sessions	Yes
Danielson et al.: Reproductive Health Counseling for Young Men	Clinic	Abst, Skills, Sex Ed	Role, Video	1 hour/1 session	Yes
Eisen et al.: Teen Talk	School	Skills, Cont Ed, Sex Ed	Group, Lect, Role, Video	12 to 15 hours/6 sessions	Yes
Herre: Teen Outreach Program	Community organization	Skills, Life Opt, Sex Ed	Group	1 school year/1 session per week	No; call (215) 572-9463
Howard et al.: Postponing Sexual Involvement	School	Abst, Skills, Cont Ed, Sex Ed	Group, Lect, Peer, Role, Video	10 hours/10 sessions	No; call (404) 616-3515
Jay et al.: Adolescent Compliance in the Use of Oral Contraceptives	Clinic	Cont Ed, Cont Acc	Peer	4 hours/4 sessions	No
Olds et al.: Elmira Nurse Home Visiting Program	Clinic, community organization	Skills, Cont Ed, Life Opt, Sex Ed	Adult, Case, Group	Pregnancy until 4 years postpartum/approximately 22	No
O'Sullivan et al.: A Health Care Program for First-Time Adolescent Mothers and Their Infants	Clinic	Skills, Cont Ed, Sex Ed	Case, Video	Pregnancy until 1.5 years postpartum/not applicable	Yes

Program	Setting	Approach	Components	Duration	Evaluated
Polly McCabe School: A School-Based Intervention Program for Adolescent Mothers	School	Skills, Cont Ed, Life Opt, Sex Ed	Group, Lect	Pregnancy to delivery/ not applicable	No
Rabin and Seltzer: Queens Medical Center's Teenage Program	Clinic	Skills, Cont Ed, Life Opt, Sex Ed	Case, Group	Pregnancy to age 20/ not applicable	Yes
Search Institute: Human Sexuality—Values & Choices	School	Abst, Skills, Cont Ed, Sex Ed	Adult, Group, Lect, Role, Video	11 to 13 hours/15 sessions	Yes
Vincent: School/Community Program for Sexual Risk Reduction Among Teens	School, Clinic, Community organization	Abst, Skills, Comm, Cont Ed, Cont Acc, Life Opt, Sex Ed, Self-Eff	Adult, Group, Lect, Role, PSAs	1 year minimum/ not applicable	Yes
Winter: New Adolescent Approach Protocols: Tailoring Family Planning Services to Meet the Special Needs of Adolescents	Clinic	Skills, Cont Ed, Cont Acc, Sex Ed	Adult	5 hours minimum/3 sessions	Yes
Zabin: School-Linked Reproductive Health Services (The Self Center)	School, Clinic	Skills, Cont Ed, Cont Acc, Sex Ed	Adult, Group, Lect, Role, PSA	1 year minimum/not applicable	Yes

NOTE: **Approach:** Abst = abstinence; Skills = behavioral skills development; Comm = community involvement; Cont Ed = contraceptive education; Cont Acc = contraceptive access; Life Opt = life options; Sex Ed = sexuality and STD education; Self-Eff = self-efficacy/self-esteem. **Components:** Adult = adult involvement; Case = case management; Group = group discussion; Lect = lectures; Peer = peer counseling or education; PSAs = public service announcements; Role = role-play; Video = videotape.

TABLE 8.3 PASHA Teen STD/HIV/AIDS Prevention Programs

Program	Original Site	Approaches	Components	Length/Number of Sessions	Available From PASHA
Basen-Engquist: Safer Sex Efficacy Workshop	School	Skills, Cont Ed, Sex Ed, Self-Eff	Group, Peer, Role	3 hours/1 session	Yes
Fisher et al.: AIDS Risk Reduction for College Students	School	Skills, Cont Ed, Sex Ed	Group, Lect, Peer, Role, Video	6 hours/3 sessions	Yes
Hobfoll et al.: AIDS Prevention and Health Promotion Among Women	Clinic	Skills, Cont Ed, Cont Acc, Sex Ed, Self-Eff	Group, Role, Video	6 to 8 hours/4 sessions	Yes
Jemmott et al.: Be Proud! Be Responsible!	Community organization	Skills, Cont Ed, Sex Ed, Self-Eff	Group, Lect, Role, Video	12 to 16 hours/1 to 6 sessions	No; call (212) 732-4437
Kipke et al.: AIDS Risk Reduction Education and Skills Training Program	Community organization	Skills, Cont Ed, Sex Ed	Group, Lect, Role	5 hours/3 sessions	Yes
Levy et al.: Youth AIDS Prevention Project	School	Abst, Skills, Cont Ed, Sex Ed	Adult, Group, Lect, Role, Video	14 hours over 2 years/15 sessions over 2 years	Yes
Main et al.: Get Real About AIDS	School	Abst, Skills, Cont Ed, Sex Ed, Self-Eff	Group, Lect, PSAs, Role, Video	10 to 15 hours/14 sessions	Yes
Magura et al.: Rikers Health Advocacy Program	Community organization	Skills, Cont Ed, Sex Ed, Self-Eff	Group, Lect, Role	4 hours/4 sessions	Yes

Program	Setting	Components	Approach	Duration	Available
Remafedi: Youth and AIDS Project's HIV Prevention Program	Community organization, clinic	Skills, Cont Ed, Sex Ed	Case, Group, Lect, Peer, Role, Video	5 hours+/3 sessions + optional meetings	Yes
Rickert et al.: A Clinic-Based AIDS Education Program for Female Adolescents	Clinic	Skills, Cont Ed, Cont Acc, Sex Ed	Lect, Video	1 hour/1 session	Yes
Rotheram-Borus: Adolescents Living Safely: AIDS Awareness, Attitudes and Actions for Gay, Lesbian, & Bisexual Teens	Community organization	Skills, Cont Ed, Cont Acc, Sex Ed	Case, Group, Lect, Role, Video	30 to 40 hours/ 20 sessions	Yes
Rotheram-Borus: Adolescents Living Safely: AIDS Awareness, Attitudes and Actions for Reducing HIV Risk Behavior Among Runaway Adolescents	Community organization	Skills, Cont Ed, Cont Acc, Sex Ed	Case, Group, Lect, Role, Video	30 to 40 hours/ 25 sessions	Yes
New England Research Institute: Poder Latino: A Community AIDS Prevention Program for Inner-City Latino Youth	Community organization	Skills, Comm, Cont Ed, Cont Acc, Sex Ed	Group, Lect, Peer, PSAs	1 year minimum/not applicable	Yes
St. Lawrence et al.: Becoming a Responsible Teen	Community organization	Skills, Cont Ed, Comm, Sex Ed, Self-Eff	Group, Lect, Role, Video	12 to 16 hours/8 sessions	No; call (800) 321-4407
Walter et al.: AIDS Prevention for Adolescents in School	School	Abst, Skills, Cont Ed, Cont Acc, Sex Ed, Self-Eff	Group, Lect, Role, Video	6 hours/6 sessions	Yes

NOTE: **Approach:** Abst = abstinence; Skills = behavioral skills development; Comm = community involvement; Cont Ed = contraceptive education; Cont Acc = contraceptive access; Life Opt = life options; Sex Ed = sexuality and STD education; Self-Eff = self-efficacy/self-esteem. **Components:** Adult = adult involvement; Case = case management; Group = group discussion; Lect = lectures; Peer = peer counseling or education; PSAs = public service announcements; Role = role-play; Video = videotape.

these settings categories are not mutually exclusive; a few of the interventions were launched as partnerships across two different settings, and one was coordinated across all three types of settings.

Behavior Change Approach. Within the PASHA programs, we identified eight different theoretically based approaches to behavioral change. On average, four separate approaches are woven together in each intervention. Three approaches were found in most of the collection: behavioral skill development, sexuality education, and contraceptive education; they appeared in 29, 29, and 27 of the participating programs, respectively. Nine programs promote abstinence for teens, though only 2 (both aimed at middle-school teens) use an "abstinence-only" approach, but the others combine support for abstinence with information about or access to contraception.

Components. PASHA programs incorporate up to eight specific components, or educational activities, in their curricula. The typical program integrates four or more components, most often group discussions, lectures, role-play exercises, and video presentations. It is noteworthy that the most popular approaches and components in PASHA programs are those recommended by researchers.

STEP 2: PACKAGING PROGRAMS

Following program selection, our next set of tasks involved the acquisition and packaging of curriculum materials. We began by inviting the developer(s) of each selected intervention to participate in the project by making their program and evaluation materials available for dissemination through PASHA. Because the concept of *program archiving* (warehousing) was new to many of these researchers, several raised questions about the project. Two were particularly common: (a) How would authorship and copyright be handled? (b) If the original program materials were out of date, could new ones be substituted? In response to the first question, we explained that the original developers and evaluators would be credited as the authors of the program package. They could also hold on to the copyright, if they desired. Many chose to, but others, who had moved on to new research endeavors, preferred that we take responsibility for producing and distributing all materials ourselves.

To address the second question, we did agree to include revised or updated program materials in the package. After reviewing some of the original items, we recognized that they had become dated and, in some cases, inaccurate. Yet, we also recognized that it was a particular intervention that had been found effective, and it was this intervention that we wanted to promote. Thus, we took care to explain in the program guide what had been changed and why. For two programs (one primary pregnancy prevention and one STD/HIV/AIDS prevention), the original materials were also included, along with recommendations for possible substitutions.

As is evident above, we worked individually with the creators of each program to construct a suitable arrangement for their participation. At times, this process was slow, requiring several phone calls and discussions among PASHA staff members and program developers that stretched out over a period of weeks. Yet, in the end, most of the programs selected for the archive did choose to participate. Developers or distributors of 23 of the 30 programs have agreed to make their materials publicly available through PASHA. Moreover, of those that chose not to participate, 4 are publicly available from the original developers or a commercial distributor; consequently, practitioners now have access to 27 of the 30 programs identified by PASHA. (The 3 programs not available at this point include (a) a primary pregnancy prevention program that tested the use of oral contraceptives in a "natural experiment" rather than a planned behavioral intervention, (b) a secondary pregnancy prevention program that lacks the financial and human resources to document work that was completed several years ago, and (c) a secondary pregnancy prevention program in which the original developer is currently seeking funding for large-scale replication.)

For the 23 participating programs, our next task was to develop the program packages. To ensure consistency across the collection, we had each program package follow a standardized template. The package contains a complete set of all of the materials needed to implement the program (e.g., curriculum manual, student workbook, videos, and activity sheets), together with a program guide prepared by our staff. The program guide introduces the theoretical rationale for the intervention, describes the original field study, and provides suggestions for implementing and evaluating the program, including timing, training, and any additional materials that will be needed (e.g., VCR, TV). In addition, three resources are provided to help practitioners reevaluate the effectiveness of the interventions, should they choose to do so. The first is the instrument or set of instruments used in the original field study. Though highly skilled practitioners may choose to use them, in many cases, these measures are more time-consuming and theoretically complex than is necessary or appropriate. For this reason, we include in each package a copy of the Prevention Minimum Evaluation Data Set (PMEDS), a generic questionnaire that is suitable for evaluating most teen pregnancy and STD/HIV/AIDS prevention programs. For simplicity, the core of this modular instrument focuses on measures of the PASHA effectiveness criteria listed in Table 8.1. In addition, the survey is designed for use at pre-, post-, and follow-up assessments. Demographic measures and a tracking form also are included. Supplementary modules in PMEDS contain measures appropriate for specific kinds of interventions, such as STD education programs, programs emphasizing communication skill building, or programs emphasizing abstinence.

Our third and final evaluation resource was developed to assist the many practitioners who want more hands-on assistance. To meet this need, we have assembled a directory that provides a state-by-state listing of evaluation consultants.

Several steps were taken to ensure that each program package would be comprehensive, user-friendly, and visually appealing. First, we upgraded or enhanced many of the items provided to us by the original developers of the interventions. This typically involved use of desktop publishing or graphic design software to reformat existing text. In three cases, in which original materials had been lost, the program developers consulted with us to reconstruct individual lesson plans and activities. A three-step review process provided a further check on our work. A Practitioner Advisory Panel[3] was asked to review the content and design of sample packages and suggest ways we might improve their usability. Panel members reviewed each package, completed a usability evaluation questionnaire, and met as a group to discuss their evaluation results with PASHA staff. In addition, for each program package, we sent draft materials to the original developers and asked that they certify the accuracy of our work. Our third and most comprehensive form of review is the PASHA field test, described below.

STEP 3: REPLICATING AND REEVALUATING PROGRAMS

Following completion of the program packages, we returned to the research part of our framework with the launch of the PASHA replication and reevaluation study. Field-test sites were recruited across the country, at public schools, health departments, juvenile rehabilitation facilities, and Planned Parenthood clinics. Program leaders were asked to implement the intervention, ideally with 75 or more youth. We offered telephone technical support to assist them with any questions or concerns they might have in setting up, implementing, or evaluating the program.

Our first aim of the field test was to gain feedback on the usability of the materials; indeed, before assessing effectiveness, we needed to know whether the interventions had been faithfully implemented, what kinds of changes had been made, and why. One underlying question was whether programs could be "packaged" and made usable for practitioners. In addition, we wanted to investigate whether the programs that had been found effective in one setting would remain so when they were used in new settings and with new groups of teens. And we hoped to document our work within the research-to-practice cycle, especially through our collaboration with practitioners to implement and evaluate the prevention programs. Thus, the PASHA field test comprised both an implementation and outcome evaluation. Below, we highlight key elements of the study; for a more thorough discussion of the methods, analyses, and findings, see Niego,

Park, Kelley, Peterson, and Card (1998), the report from which the following discussion is drawn.

To collect implementation data, we developed a simple log that asked leaders to indicate for each session or activity whether it had been implemented "as is," "with changes," or "not at all." We further asked that they explain the reasons for any changes or omissions they had made. A separate questionnaire asked for instructors' comments and feedback on each element of the program package, as well as their assessment of how well prepared they felt to implement and evaluate the intervention. To collect pre-, -post-, and 6-month follow-up data for youth, we used a shortened and simplified version of PMEDS, focusing on the PASHA effectiveness criteria. Finally, at the conclusion of the study, we conducted debriefing interviews to gain a deeper understanding of each leader's experience with and perceptions of the field-test process.

Fulfilling these responsibilities required an ambitious investment of time and energy by the program leaders. Perhaps not surprisingly, we found the volunteers to be a highly skilled, resourceful, and motivated group of individuals. They were confident in their abilities and eager to take on new challenges. In exchange and gratitude, we offered each site a $500 implementation and a $300 evaluation stipend, along with the program package, which they could keep and use again following the field test. For many leaders, the materials themselves were of great value; several told us that their annual curriculum budget would be exhausted, or nearly so, by the $195 purchase price for a typical PASHA package.

Not all of the 23 programs were included in the field test. Specifically, we decided not to test the 2 secondary prevention programs, focusing our interest instead on primary prevention. Also, for practical reasons, 5 of the STD/HIV/AIDS prevention programs were not included. These reasons were the following: (a) the anticipated difficulty of obtaining cooperative participants in college-age populations (2 programs), (2) an intervention that lasted a year too long for the available field-test time (1 program), and (c) the difficulty of recruiting sufficient numbers of youth for programs aimed at narrowly defined, high-risk groups (2 programs). In all, therefore, we aimed to field-test 16 programs.

From the outset, our desire to conduct rigorous, scientifically valid evaluations came up against real-world issues, including shortages of time and money and difficulties tracking and retaining youth across multiple sites. For example, it proved infeasible to recruit and collect comparison data at each participating site; instead, our first compromise was to use a synthetic comparison group constructed from data in the Add Health Survey (described below). We also found that most sites, particularly those serving high-risk teens, could not gain access to as many as 75 youth, the number calculated to provide reasonable statistical power for tests of program effectiveness. Still others were forced to shorten or cancel their interventions due to unanticipated changes in personnel, funding, approval, or scheduling. In the end, 13 groups took part in the study, testing 12 different interventions at a wide variety of sites. Twelve of these groups eventually provided sufficient data for analyses of implementation, and 6 provided at least minimal data for an outcomes analysis, as summarized below.

Question 1a. Can Programs Be Packaged? Assessment of the Program Packages. At all sites, practitioners generally found the program materials in the packages to be clear and usable. In a few cases, instructors found that individual activities were confusing or materials, usually a video, were out-of-date. Five program leaders found it necessary to adapt items to better meet the needs of their teens. For example, the instructor of an STD/HIV/AIDS prevention program significantly expanded the amount of group discussion to keep her teens interested; for the same reason, she added to the curriculum a visit with an HIV-positive person. Another instructor, also leading an STD/HIV/AIDS prevention program, invented a new title and theme for the intervention and combined the three sessions into a single, full-day workshop. These and the other program leaders reported that the clarity of the PASHA products made it easier for them to modify materials for their group.

Practitioners rated the comprehensiveness of PASHA program packages highly. A few suggested adding some how-to materials to enhance particular kits. This was particularly true for the two practitioners who implemented programs based on a conceptual model—as opposed to a step-by-step curriculum. In addition, in their debriefing interviews, many practitioners told us that they would benefit from more information about the how-tos of implementation and evaluation, such as gaining approval to use a program, retaining students, engaging students in discussions and skill-building activities, and overcoming opposition to program or survey content.

It is interesting to note that few test sites took full advantage of the telephone technical support that we offered. We did speak with nine participating sites to resolve concerns about scheduling, approval, and evaluation materials—before their actual implementations began. Yet, only two leaders requested assistance during the course of their program; one ran into trouble with confidentiality procedures for the evaluation surveys, and the second found participants to be highly critical of particular survey questions. Similarly, although we offer free technical assistance to purchasers of PASHA materials, we have logged only one call asking for such assistance. Most PASHA calls are prepurchase calls. In about 20% of these cases, callers want guidance selecting an appropriate intervention to meet their needs.

Volunteers in the PASHA field test gave high marks in rating the clarity and usefulness of the materials, and, in the absence of external obstacles, they were able to implement them faithfully. Across the 12 sites for which data are available, the implementations were generally smooth and proceeded according to instructions. We found that interventions that follow step-by-step lesson plans appear to work best, especially for educators with limited time for preparation and outside research. Some of the PASHA packages, particularly those designed as comprehensive, community-wide interventions, provide a template or suggested set of protocols, rather than a ready-to-use intervention. Though these may be fine for experienced and confident practitioners, others may feel overwhelmed by the need to customize and expand on what is provided in the package. We further learned that packages can be strengthened by inclusion of more real-world experiences so that users may anticipate and overcome potential barriers to full program implementation. To address the need for more experience-based material, then, we are incorporating into the program guides some of the experiences of our test sites.

Question 1b. Can Programs Be Packaged? Fidelity to Original Implementation. A second part of the "usability" question, and equally critical to our outcome evaluation, was to determine how faithfully practitioners implemented the programs. We found that the degree of fidelity to the original programs varied across the sites. Some program leaders modified lesson content to better meet the perceived needs of their teens; others scaled back or eliminated activities because of time and resource constraints or community objections. Overall, across the 11 test sites for which the necessary data were obtained, we found that 4 implemented programs with *high fidelity*, meaning that they made few or no changes to the program. "Few" changes include modifying activity content slightly or enhancing program activities with other materials. The 4 sites that showed *medium fidelity* made more substantial changes, eliminating larger portions of the program or revamping entire lessons. Among the 3 *low-fidelity* sites, practitioners did not implement major portions of the program. It is interesting to note that of the 3 field-test sites classified under low fidelity, 2 are model-based programs, and 1 involves a lengthy, 27-lesson curriculum.

Question 2. How Effective Are the Programs? We have analyzed outcome (posttest and/or follow-up) data for 7 of the 13 participating test sites. One intervention program was tested at 2 sites, so these 7 sites tested six different interventions. Among those sites excluded from the analysis, several had not completed collecting posttest data from youth by the time our project concluded. Others, due to either low initial sample sizes or high attrition, did not have enough participants tested both before and after the intervention to qualify for analysis. Another site with pre- and posttest data was disqualified from the analysis because it was a short 3-hour intervention, so behavioral change could not be expected. Thus, we acknowledge that our findings are necessarily partial and preliminary, clearly requiring additional investigation and analysis. These findings are presented below, but first let us take a brief look at two methodological considerations: the Add Health comparison group and the use of exact tests.

Comparison Data. Because of the logistical challenges of finding a comparison site for each field-test program, we decided to create synthetic comparison groups using a national sample of adolescents: the 1994-1996 National Longitudinal Survey of Adolescent Health (Add Health). The Add Health study, which examines the general health and well-being of U.S. teens, includes dependent variables such as teen pregnancy, STD and HIV/AIDS infection, diet and nutrition, eating disorders, depression, violent behavior, intentional injury, unintentional injury, suicide, exercise, health service use, and health insurance coverage. To match the demographic characteristics of each field-test site, we standardized the Add Health sample using four weighting variables simultaneously: gender, age, Hispanic ethnicity, and primary racial identification.[4]

Exact Tests. When a data set is small or its variables are not distributed according to a normal (bell-shaped) distribution, its cross-tabulation tables contain many empty cells, or its cases tend to have the same value or order on pairs of variables (e.g., both high, both medium, or both low), it is preferable to calculate a significance level using a test statistic based on the exact distribution of the data. Such tests allow for the calculation of an accurate p value without relying on assumptions about the underlying distribution of the data that may not actually be met. For the PASHA field-test analyses, we used several different exact tests, depending on the level of measurement of the variables (see Niego et al., 1998, for more information). In addition, we chose to perform one-tailed tests, hypothesizing that field-test participants would show more favorable scores than their Add Health counterparts.

For those basic PASHA field-test sites that participated in the analysis, descriptions of each site and study participants can be found in Table 8.4. Under the column labeled "Field-Test Sites," readers will note that for one intervention, two field-test sites are listed. This occurred because the AIDS Prevention for Adolescents in School program was implemented at two separate school sites. The number of participants varies widely across sites. The Reducing the Risk program obtained the largest sample size, with 113 teens completing the pretest and 6-month follow-up test. At other sites, the numbers were much lower, with three programs reporting less than 10 true panel participants. Though the youths' ages ranged from 14 to 20 years, most were between 15 and 18 years old. All but one site had primarily White participants. Two sites were all female, and one was all male. The others, though mixed, had higher numbers of female participants.

Evaluation Findings. Of the seven sites, four provided pretest and posttest data only, whereas three sites also provided follow-up data 3 to 6 months after the end

TABLE 8.4 Characteristics of Participants in PASHA Field-Test Analysis

Program	Field-Test Sites	Number	Age	Sex	Race/Ethnicity
Primary pregnancy prevention programs[a]					
Tailoring family planning services to meet the special needs of adolescents: New adolescent approach protocols	Teen health clinic, Northeast	7	15-18	100.0% female	71.4% White 28.6% Black
Reducing the Risk	Planned Parenthood affiliate, southern high schools	113	15-17	52.2% female 47.8% male	95.6% White 3.5% Black 9% Native American
Teen Talk	County hospital, midwestern high school	13	14-16	76.9% female 23.1% male	15.4% White 84.6% Black
STD/HIV/AIDS prevention programs[b]					
AIDS prevention for adolescents in school (Site 1)	High school, West	44	15-17	61.4% female 38.6% male	59.1% White 27.3% Asian 13.6% other
AIDS prevention for adolescents in school (Site 2)	High school, Northeast	8	15-19	100.0% female	50.0% White 12.5% Black 37.5% other
Rikers Health Advocacy Program (RHAP)	AIDS service organization, Midwestern juvenile rehabilitation facility	26	13-18	100.0% male	80.8% White 15.4% Black 3.8% Native American
Adolescents Living Safely: AIDS Awareness, Attitudes, & Actions for Gay, Lesbian and Bisexual Adolescents	County health department, Pacific Northwest	9	14-20	55.6% female 44.4% male	75.0% White 25.0% Asian

a. Outcome variables measured for pregnancy prevention programs included initiation of sexual activity,, number of partners,, use of contraception at first sex and at last sex,, consistency of use of contraception,, and pregnancy.
b. Outcome variables measured for STD and HIV/AIDS prevention programs included use of STD prevention methods at first and last sex,, consistency of use of STD prevention methods,, STD incidence,, and HIV/AIDS incidence.

of the intervention. Analyses examined the results for each site separately. To broadly characterize the results at the three sites where follow-up data were collected, we found that program participants generally showed positive outcomes on several measures of pregnancy prevention-related behaviors, relative to their Add Health peers. These included postponing sexual intercourse (e.g., 76% vs. 54% remained sexually inactive), decreasing reported number of sexual partners (e.g., an average at follow-up of 2.8 partners vs. 5.7), increasing use of contraception at first and most recent intercourse (e.g., 88% vs. 69% at follow-up), and preventing pregnancy (e.g., no pregnancies reported vs. 13% reporting a pregnancy). Regarding the measures of STD and HIV/AIDS prevention-related behaviors, at two of the three follow-up sites, teens did show a positive increase in consistent use of STD protection; the increase was statistically significant at one of these sites.

Next we consider the findings for the four sites where only pre- and posttest data were collected. Here the analysis was limited to five of the effectiveness criteria—namely, number of partners, contraceptive and STD prevention at last sex, and consistency of contraception and STD prevention. The other criteria, such as "postponing sexual intercourse," could not be properly tested without a comparison group because the desirable direction is "no change," a null hypothesis when comparing the same subjects at two points in time. Although some results were measured in the positive direction, none was significant. The lack of significance could be explained by a number of factors. First, there was very little time for behavioral change between the administration of the pre- and posttests. Some outcomes, such as contracting STDs and HIV/AIDS, will not show up over the short term. The lack of significance is also in part due to the smaller sample sizes; although exact tests are more accurate than asymptotic tests, the level of significance still is affected by the sample size. It is also possible, of course, that these particular programs as implemented in the PASHA field test simply were ineffective. However, the statistical power to detect a true effect was too low to speculate seriously on the effectiveness of the programs.

STEP 4: STRENGTHENING AND EXPANDING ON THE PASHA PROJECT

From the outcome data analyzed to date, it is evident that we have only partially addressed our original research questions. Although it was possible to achieve some knowledge of the ease of implementing these programs, assessment of outcomes simply could not be successfully completed at most sites. Nevertheless, we have learned much about the possibilities for greater researcher-practitioner collaboration in developing, implementing, and evaluating prevention and health promotion programs. Indeed, as we reach the final stage in our framework, our involvement in PASHA has spawned or added impetus to several new projects being carried out at Sociometrics Corporation, the developer of PASHA.

First, however, we want to comment briefly on the importance to the archive of the Practitioner Advisory Panel. We recruited this group of public health professionals, program directors, and agency officials to provide feedback on the PASHA program package and field-test materials. Through these tasks, the panel served as a conduit in two directions. The first was to reflect back to us the educators' and clinicians' perspectives on their experience with using our materials. In particular, the panel functioned as a source of information about the practical challenges of managing program implementation and evaluation. One of the lessons learned is that this is a common failure point in the replication of otherwise successful programs. At the same time, the panel served as a conduit by informally promoting archive resources to their colleagues. Having helped us to develop and improve the materials, the panel shaped them in ways that would enhance their value to practitioners. They were therefore inclined to promote the use of these materials among their own constituencies. In addition, panel members have served to open opportunities—through invitations to meetings, conventions, and workshops—for demonstration and dissemination of information about the program archive resources. We envision and look forward to continued collaboration with such panels in our new endeavors, as described below.

Activity Sourcebook. In addition to preparing individual program packages, we have developed a sourcebook containing activities selected from interventions in the collection. The selection criteria were the following: focus on an appropriate age group, risk level, or environment; clarity of activity goals; replicability; theoretical rationale; effectiveness; and student engagement.

Each activity is described in terms of purpose, appropriate target group, and method of implementation. Although each activity has not necessarily been individually evaluated as to its specific effectiveness, all have been selected from evaluated and effective programs. The sourcebook, therefore, offers ready access to the "why" and "how-to" of several dozen activities included in effective programs. Program administrators could use these to supplement existing programs or to fashion new ones.

Field-Test Book. We also have prepared a monograph sharing lessons learned in the PASHA field-test process. The heart of this book focuses on the experiences of program leaders in schools, communities, and clinics nationwide. Drawing on their experiences, we offer practical strategies for setting up, implementing, and evaluating promising teen pregnancy and STD/HIV/AIDS prevention programs.

Also included is a concise summary of the field-test research, with analysis and findings from the project's outcome evaluation. Among the issues discussed are the challenges and opportunities for conducting evaluations at different levels (process to outcome)[5] under varying field and resource conditions.

Archive of Effective Drug Abuse Prevention Programs for Youth. In discussions with practitioners, many have asked for program packages in other areas of health promotion. Building on the lessons learned in the PASHA project, we have launched an archive of alcohol, tobacco, and drug abuse prevention programs. A significant addition to the package template will be a CD-ROM tutorial to provide users with instruction and guidance in setting up, implementing, and evaluating each intervention. We hope that this tool will further assist practitioners in delivering high-quality prevention programs.

The Institute for Program Development and Evaluation. Indeed, the need for training in program development, implementation, and evaluation has become apparent through our experience in the PASHA project. We are therefore designing a training institute that will provide continuing education credits through both in-person courses and distance learning. The institute will provide interactive instruction in both practice and evaluation research. Courses are being designed specifically to focus on conducting evaluation research in applied settings and to enable practitioners to draw on the results of their own and others' research in developing new programs or improving existing ones. The target audience for the institute is practitioners rather than researchers, but the focus is explicitly on the intersection of research and practice. The staff will be drawn from Sociometrics staff and other researchers who are actively engaged in serving practitioners, and they will draw on the advice and insights of practitioners, including our Practitioner Advisory Panel, in developing course material.

A latent function of the institute will be to strengthen the network of practitioners who are trained in and sensitive to the research-to-practice interaction cycle. In addition, following the conclusion of the institute, we will be offering technical assistance to practitioners as they attempt to bring the lessons of their courses to bear on their day-to-day practice at the local level.

Electronic Comparison Data Source Book. We are also expanding our work with synthetic comparison groups, testing the feasibility of developing a software program to easily construct such groups. As explained earlier, such groups are developed by weighting the national sample to match the local intervention group on key demographic characteristics. Once the national sample is reweighted, it can be used as a point of comparison for the intervention group in a posttest comparison or follow-up comparison design. Although clearly inferior to an experimental design with random assignment (a rarity in small program evaluations), it often can be as good as or superior to a local comparison group that is developed through demographic matching.

Our aim is to enable practitioners to access national data sets online, enter a statistical description of the demographic characteristics of their intervention group, select outcome variables from the national data that match data they are collecting on their sample, and then obtain a set of weighted tables of the outcomes from the national data that are synthetically matched to their own sample. If such a resource can be developed, it would enhance the ability of local program administrators and evaluators to locate and use appropriate comparison data for their local evaluations.

CONCLUSIONS

LESSONS LEARNED

The case study presented earlier is only the beginning of potential ways to improve health promotion interventions through the research-to-practice cycle. In closing, let us consider the lessons we have learned from the PASHA project, particularly and more broadly the program archiving process.

1. Programs can be packaged for use by practitioners. We found that field-test volunteers were able to implement the interventions included in PASHA program packages, and they generally felt well prepared to do so. They also rated the clarity and usefulness of these materials highly. In addition, we learned that interventions that follow step-by-step lesson plans appear to work best, especially for educators with limited time for preparation and outside research. In contrast, the packages that contained only a template or suggested set of protocols, rather than a comprehensive curriculum, appear to be best suited for experienced, confident practitioners.

2. Program developers do support the program-archiving process. As noted earlier, 23 of the 30 programs selected for PASHA have participated in the project. Of those that elected not to participate, 4 are available through commercial distributors, and for these interventions, the need for and value of a PASHA package are less clear.

3. Packages can be strengthened by including more "real-world" experiences. In their debriefing interviews, practitioners told us that they would benefit from more information about the "how-tos" of implementation and evaluation, such as gaining approval to use a program, retaining students, engaging stu-

dents in discussions and skill-building activities, and overcoming opposition to program or survey content. It is interesting to note that few test sites took advantage of our telephone technical support. Similarly, we receive few calls from purchasers of PASHA materials, though assistance is provided free of charge. To address the need for more experience-based material, then, we are incorporating into the program guides some of the experiences of our test sites. We also are launching the Institute for Program Development and Evaluation (as noted earlier) to provide direct, comprehensive training to practitioners.

4. The archiving process is labor intensive and time-consuming. The quality of the materials that we received from developers varied considerably, and most required significant work to make them clear and attractive. At the same time, we recognized that we had to keep the price of the packages low if they were to be within reach of practitioners. In part, this problem may be remedied through technology. Materials that were provided to us in electronic formats were far simpler to upgrade. We would expect this to become more common as future interventions take advantage of new technologies.

5. Evaluation continues to be a tremendous challenge in real-world settings when resources are limited. Though we have developed simplified measurement tools for the PASHA programs, this is just one of many elements in an evaluation study. In the PASHA field test, recruitment, retention, and approval all proved to be tremendous stumbling blocks and ultimately limited, to a significant degree, the quality of our study. Just as researchers have devoted much effort to developing effective interventions, we must also investigate ways of strengthening and facilitating evaluation activities.

THE RESEARCH-TO-PRACTICE CYCLE

Too often, research enterprise and health promotion interventions are carried on in separate worlds. Little information passes across the barriers raised by differing perspectives, languages, and priorities. But at a deeper level, these two enterprises are linked and have much to gain from closer cooperation. The research-to-practice cycle illustrated in this case study is one model for how closer ties can be fashioned that benefit both basic understanding of underlying social processes and practical understanding of what makes for effective intervention.

What Research Has to Gain From Practice. The case study has illustrated many ways in which the research enterprise gains from involvement with practice. By forging a link with health promotion programs, researchers gain a rich laboratory for testing. New sites with different characteristics, new populations, and new sets of external constraints provide rich opportunities to test the robustness of prior results comparing multiple studies. Theories developed under highly controlled study conditions may be tested in the real-world situations encountered in evaluation research.

More important, practice can contribute much to the ultimate goal of research: the development of productive theories and models for understanding reality. For example, applied research may show that project management is as important as intervention design when it comes to effectiveness, suggesting the need to incorporate organizational variables in a more complete model for understanding effects. This has been one of the lessons of our field tests and evaluations. Similarly, the importance of other variables, which are often left out of narrowly focused efficacy work, may become evident in a practice setting. Examples include the state of the economy, the shape and structure of the health care delivery system, the local cultural context of the intervention, and the human and capital resources available to program administrators. Thus, practice may be a rich source of new ideas for the development of better theories, particularly because practice by its nature deals with the full range of social, economic, organizational, contextual, and personal factors that shape individual and group behavior.

In addition, practitioners can provide the qualitative database of experience and organic knowledge that researchers need to be apprised of when interpreting quantitative results. This may be especially so when the results are at variance with what the underlying theory or model predicts. For example, consider an intervention originally found to be effective with sexually active teens, due in large measure to its explicit discussion of particular contraceptive methods (e.g., Depo Provera, Norplant). If this intervention were implemented at a time and place that coincided with media coverage of controversial aspects of these new contraceptive methods (e.g., side effects such as irregular bleeding or chronic fatigue), youth might fail to heed the program's lessons in this context. Feedback to researchers from practitioners is needed to help explain potential variance in program outcomes.

What Practice Has to Gain From Research. At the same time, the practical enterprise has much to gain from cooperation with research. Indeed, our experience has shown that practitioners are aware of and actively seek research results that will help them mount more effective programs. First, the selection of interventions may be guided by what research has shown to be the best programs. This reduces the tendency to either reinvent interventions or make up new ones without guidance. The use of the national Scientist Expert Panel of researchers in this case study is a prime example of how this can take place. Having selected a program shown to be effective elsewhere, evaluation research may be used as a very effective tool for program development and adjustment. Such research provides evidence for effectiveness and, when done carefully, may even be able to point to those aspects of a program that are particularly effective (or not) and which population subgroups are most likely to benefit. This information is invaluable for fine-tuning programs and for checking results against original outcome goals.

Perhaps the primary benefit of research is to provide an objective picture of program results. Too often, participant and staff enthusiasm for an intervention is taken as prima facie evidence for effectiveness, whereas enthusiasm may primarily reflect personal investment in the program or intangible benefits (e.g., community relations) that have little to do with stated program goals. In the end, the business of health promotion interventions is to promote health; if they fail in this, as shown by objective research results, no one—participants, administrators, or funders—will maintain their motivation to continue the effort. Indeed, the funders of intervention programs increasingly are requiring research-based evidence of effectiveness as a condition of continued support. Thus, a program increases its funding potential greatly if research has demonstrated its effectiveness (also see Chapter 3, this volume).

Through interaction with researchers, practitioners may gain a better understanding of the effects of moderating variables that researchers have learned to look for and take into account in assessing a program's impact. For example, practitioners could learn that the demographic composition of program participants compared to that of the pool of potential participants may have a major influence on the direction and size of program effects.

In the model illustrated by this case study, we served as a broker between the worlds of the practitioner and the researcher. Though originally trained as researchers, we have worked to gain practical experience through program archiving, evaluation research, and dissemination of research findings to nonresearch audiences. Moreover, we have endeavored to hold both perspectives at once and to find the complementary intersections of the needs, insights, and goals of the two enterprises. For now, it may be that the role of broker is needed to foster greater cross-fertilization. In time, however, as researchers and practitioners broaden their perspectives to incorporate what is of value from the other, the role of broker may diminish in importance. Moreover, structures and practices—such as the research and practitioner advisory boards that we have used—may continue to develop and become institutionalized to perform this vital linking role.

SUMMARY

We see the intersection of the interests, knowledge, and expertise of researchers and practitioners to be a rich and fertile ground for the promotion of both better research and program improvement. Each community has much to offer and much to learn from the other. As this case study on program archiving has shown, cooperation can facilitate the use of the best interventions and can promote their reevaluation in new settings. Moreover, additional avenues for interaction readily suggest themselves from this cooperative venture.

NOTES ◄

1. Funding for this project was provided by small-business innovation grant APR 0000964-02-1 from the U.S. Office of Population Affairs.

2. The panel members are Jeffrey D. Fisher, Ph.D., University of Connecticut; Freya Sonenstein, Ph.D., Urban Institute; Kristin Moore, Ph.D., Child Trends; Claire Brindis, Dr.P.H., University of California at San Francisco; and Brent Miller, Ph.D., Utah State University.

3. The panel members were selected from among pregnancy prevention program directors and public health professionals. Members are Larry Dickey, Maternal & Child Health Branch of the California Department of Health; Steve Gunther, Vice President for Programs, St. Anne's; Colleen K. James, Coordinator and Lead Teacher, Santa Maria Joint Union High School District; Judith MacPherson Pratt, Teen Pregnancy Prevention Strategies; and Ronda Simpson-Brown, Coordinator of Teen Pregnancy, Parenting and Prevention Programs, State of California.

4. We follow the U.S. Bureau of the Census practice of distinguishing between Hispanic ethnicity (which has to do with national and cultural origin) and race (which cuts across ethnic categories). Hispanic persons may be of any race.

5. The primary evaluation levels, in order from least to most ambitious, are a process evaluation focusing on faithfulness of implementation, an outcome evaluation focusing on short-term effects, or an impact evaluation focusing on long-term effects.

REFERENCES ◄

ARAL, S. O. (1994). Sexual behavior in sexually-transmitted disease research: An overview. *Sexually Transmitted Diseases, 21,* S59-S64.

CARD, J. J., NIEGO, S., MALLARI, A., & FARRELL, W. S. (1996). The program archive on sexuality, health & adolescence: A collection of promising prevention programs-in-a-box. *Family Planning Perspectives, 28,* 210-220.

D'ANGELO, L. J., & DiCLEMENTE, R. J. (1996). Sexually transmitted diseases including human immunodeficiency infection. In R. J. DiClemente, W. B. Hansen, & L. E. Ponton (Eds.), *Handbook of adolescent health risk behavior* (pp. 333-367). New York: Plenum.

FISHER, J. D., & FISHER, W. A. (1992). Changing AIDS-risk behavior. *Psychological Bulletin, 111,* 455-474.

FROST, J., & FORREST, J. D. (1995). Understanding the impact of effective teen pregnancy prevention programs. *Family Planning Perspectives, 27,* 188-195.

HOLTGRAVE, D. R., QUALLS, N. L., CURRAN, J. W., & VALDISERRI, R. O. (1995). An overview of the effectiveness and efficiency of HIV prevention programs. *Public Health Reports, 110,* 134-146.

INSTITUTE OF MEDICINE. (1995). *The best intentions: Unintended pregnancy and the well being of children and families.* Washington, DC: National Academy Press.

KELLY, J. A. (1994). Sexually transmitted disease prevention approaches that work: Interventions to reduce risk behavior among individuals, groups, and communities. *Sexually Transmitted Diseases, 21,* S73-S75.

KIRBY, D. (1995). *A review of educational programs designed to reduce sexual risk-taking behaviors among school-aged youth in the United States* (Pub. No. PB96108519). Springfield, VA: National Technical Information Service.

KIRBY, D. (1997). *No easy answers: Research findings on programs to reduce teen pregnancy.* Washington, DC: National Campaign to Prevent Teen Pregnancy.

KIRBY, D., SHORT, L., COLLINS, J., RUGG, D., KOLBE, L., HOWARD, M., MILLER, B., SONENSTEIN, F., & ZABIN, L. S. (1994). School-based programs to reduce sexual risk behaviors: A review of effectiveness. *Public Health Reports, 109,* 339-360.

MILLER, B. C., CARD, J. J., PAIKOFF, R., & PETERSON, J. L. (Eds.). (1992). *Preventing adolescent pregnancy: Model programs and evaluations.* Newbury Park, CA: Sage.

MOORE, K., MILLER, B. C., GLEI, D., & MORRISON, D. R. (1995). *Adolescent pregnancy prevention programs: Interventions and evaluations.* Washington, DC: Child Trends, Inc.

NIEGO, S., PARK, J., KELLEY, M., PETERSON, J. L., & CARD, J. J. (1998). *The PASHA field test: A window on the world of practitioners.* Los Altos, CA: Sociometrics Corporation.

PHILLIBER, S., & NAMEROW, P. (1995). *Trying to maximize the odds: Using what we know to prevent teen pregnancy.* Prepared for a technical assistance workshop to support the CDC Teen Pregnancy Prevention Program.

ROTHERAM-BORUS, M. J., MAHLER, K. A., & ROSARIO, M. (1995). AIDS prevention with adolescents. *AIDS Education and Prevention, 7,* 320-336.

PART III

PERCEIVED EFFICACY METHODS

CHAPTER 9

Verbal Methods in Perceived Efficacy Work

Guadalupe X. Ayala
John P. Elder

The purpose of this chapter is to introduce the reader to various verbal methods used in perceived efficacy studies (concept evaluation). It is important to note that effective verbal methods are often combined with paper-and-pencil methods, and therefore the reader is directed to Chapter 11 for an introduction to this latter type of methodology. After reading Chapters 9 and 11, the reader should have a better understanding of the various methods available to evaluate the potential efficacy of health behavior program concepts. In addition, it is hoped that the reader will appreciate the importance of assessing the perceived efficacy of program concepts before time and money are spent in its further development and full implementation. Unfortunately, it is too often the case that programs are developed without a sufficient understanding of how community members perceive a particular problem and how plausible program activities might address the issue (Brieger et al., 1996). Not only does this oversight result in the subsequent implementation of very ineffective programs that are essentially a waste of time and money, but also "intuitive" strategies heighten the distrust of the community to any future introduction of programs (Abelson, 1997).

Perceived efficacy work—a critical step in program development—until very recently either has been completely ignored or has lacked a scientifically sound set of methods (Winett, King, & Altman, 1989). We believe that this work is advancing in sophistication and will continue to gain scientific respect over the next decade. A few definitions are essential before a discussion of the various methods can begin. First, *perceived efficacy* is the process of determining how well a given program or its components might fit into an existing structure of services, how well it will be received by the target population, and the extent to which the new program or its components might meet the needs of the community (Hinkle, Fox-Cardamone, Haseleu, Brown, & Irwin, 1996). *Perceived efficacy work* refers to the phase of health behavior program development during which various program activity concepts are first evaluated for inclusion into or exclusion from a program. In perceived efficacy work, subjects are not actually provided with a completed program to evaluate (as in pilot studies) or are not actually engaged in a program activity (as in component studies). Subjects generally receive summary information about a program or program activity and make judgments regarding how successful the program or activity is likely to be if it were to be implemented, as well as perhaps whether mediators of change (see Chapter 19, this volume) are likely to have been affected by the program or program activity (Step 3 of the chain model). Generally, the process of engaging in a perceived efficacy study involves meeting with groups or individuals to determine whether program ideas, as conceptualized by the investigative team or the subjects, will be needed by and are of interest and comprehensible to the target community. This type of study permits screening among numerous potential programs or activities for testing at a subsequent stage of program development.

Second, the term *verbal methods* generally refers to the gathering of information through conversations or group discussions with members of the population of interest. For the most part, data collected using verbal methods are qualitative in nature and therefore require the identification of key themes important to the population of interest. There are several unique advantages to collecting information using verbal methods. Verbal methods provide considerable opportunity for discussing and sharing experiences and attitudes between the researcher and the community of interest. Verbal methods also allow the interviewer or facilitator to probe further on particular topics as they come up in the discussion. This type of interaction generally results in a deeper understanding of forces in a community that may impede or facilitate effective program development. Third, individuals working with low-literate populations often find it advantageous to obtain information via verbal communication (Freimuth & Mettger, 1990). Finally, by conversing with the participant, the researcher is able to assess the extent to which the participant understands the questions or needs clarification. This process increases the likelihood that questions will be understood correctly and thus responded to more accurately by participants. However, verbal methods have several limitations. Unless verbal information is obtained through one-on-one interactions, the respondent's confidentiality and anonymity are not maintained during the course of data collection. This lack of privacy may lead some respondents to inhibit self-disclosure, particularly regarding sensitive topics, and could yield less complete data compared with survey results. In addition, group verbal methods may lead to collection of data from those who monopolize the flow of interaction, rather than reflect the opinions of all target persons in the group. Finally, verbal methods are useful only for those who can express themselves well through speaking to others. Through perceived efficacy work, the investigator can determine the extent to which individuals in the target population are likely to comply with the program guidelines. If the target population views activities as inappropriate for their age group or culture, does not like the activities, or views the activities as too time-consuming, impractical, or not affecting key hypothesized mediators, these activities probably should not be retained for further testing. Perceived efficacy work can help screen out activities not likely to work.

METHODS OF PERCEIVED EFFICACY WORK

There are four basic aspects to consider when one is conducting perceived efficacy studies: (a) the basic needs of the target population, (b) available resources and services to fulfill those needs, (c) perceptions of the quality of these resources and services, and (d) implementation of and reactions to the program ideas. The first three aspects constitute the process of determining the priorities and "in-house" potential of the community as related to particular program activities. For example, homeless people may need to learn good hygiene, but they also need to learn such skills in the context of being able to locate clean places to live. Available shelters may or may not provide sanitary conditions, and homeless residents may or may not find such living conditions satisfying. The investigator would not want to assess the plausibility of using program ideas that are redundant with what is already available. However, after these first three aspects are considered, the investigator can collect ideas from theory and warehoused activities that are not redundant with currently used components. When contemplating a perceived efficacy study with the community of interest, the investigative team can consider these four aspects with the following questions (Elder, Geller, Hovell, & Mayer, 1994):

> What do we want and need to know?
> Why do we want to know this particular information?
> How will this information be used?
> Where and how can we obtain this information?

What useful data sources and archives (federal, state, and local) already exist?

Who in the community could serve as "key informants"?

Who among us should contact these individuals?

What other community agencies or entities have an interest in this issue? Should they be involved? Why or why not?

Do we need technical assistance? Where can we get it?

How much will these assessment activities cost? How much time and which resources exist to put into this program's effort?

The last aspect of perceived efficacy work is the most central feature for the purposes of program development (i.e., testing out ideas and materials with a relatively small sample of individuals who are similar to the target population) (Winett et al., 1989). It is important to present plausible program activity ideas to the target population and obtain their reactions to the ideas. For example, subjects could be asked what their reactions would be to a brochure addressing the risk of breast cancer using fear appeals versus one using similar, other role models to encourage breast cancer screening. In this way, the investigator can begin the process of screening for good program ideas. This involves testing ideas regarding program activities, products, and materials through in-depth studies (Elder et al., 1994). The parameters or purposes of the testing include the following:

- assessing the target audience's interest in and comprehension of potential program materials, logos, mission statements, themes, and so on;
- assessing desirability of channels of information for program dissemination (e.g., media, written materials, etc.);
- identifying potential specific strong and weak points of program components;
- determining the personal relevance of a message;
- measuring how controversial, sensitive, pleasant, or aversive a certain intervention may be.

Before reading further about perceived efficacy approaches and their advantages and disadvantages, be aware that perceived efficacy work should not be used as a substitute for component study or pilot testing. Small sample sizes, selection biases, and relatively high vulnerability to different interpretations of the data by different members of the research team may lead to a greater probability that erroneous conclusions are drawn from these types of studies. However, it does provide the necessary feedback to increase both the effectiveness and efficacy of a given program. In particular, many program ideas can be screened within a reasonable amount of time, taking into account the perspectives of the consumer. The following is a list of verbal methods that can be used to compose perceived efficacy studies. Tables 9.1 and 9.2 provide a concise description of each method, as well as their advantages and disadvantages.

INTERVIEWS

An interviewer generally meets privately with an interviewee and asks the interviewee a series of questions for an hour or two. It is important to start any interview by assuring the respondent of confidentiality. Next, the interviewer often will instruct the interviewee that the respondent is the expert here and that he or she is there to learn from the interviewee. The interviewer will then proceed to tell interviewees why the information they provide is important to the project and the community. Information collected includes the following: personal interviewee data, relevant to this person's status as a target person for a health behavior intervention; material relevant to prior stages of program development (e.g., perceptions of etiology of the problem or health behavior); and the interviewee's ideas on what might compose effective programming. The interviewer not only asks various questions but also may make use of stimuli on which to obtain responses. The stimuli used in an interview provide a context for responses made and can consist of a set of plausible program activity descriptions that are read to the interviewee, a set of pictures, or a list of words (also see Chapter 11, this volume). The interviewee can use this supplemental material to generate good ideas for good programming.

Structured, Unstructured, and Semistructured Interviews. Researchers have identified and used three major categories of interviews: standardized/formal/structured, unstandardized/informal/unstructured, and semistandardized/focused/semistructured (Berg, 1998). Structured interviews consist of a schedule of precise questions that are administered in a predetermined order to each participant. The objective is to provide each respondent with the same set of stimuli, thus allowing comparability of responses to the stimuli across all respondents. The technique is much more similar to the use of self-report surveys, a nonverbal approach, than other interview structures. Participants do not engage in a conversation with the researcher; instead, they respond verbally to the interviewer's questions or other stimuli as they are presented to the participant. The approach has some advantages, including comparability between participants' responses. Data coding and analysis are straightforward because an a priori coding system is part of the format of structured interviews. In other words, no new coding scheme needs to be developed. Nevertheless, the structured interview is limited in some ways for perceived efficacy work. This format generally does not allow the participant the opportunity to provide additional input into the development of the program, if the input is not directly related to a question on the interview. In addition, the selection of items to include as stimuli in the interview is based on the researcher's under-

TABLE 9.1 Types of Verbal Methods

Method	Target	Purpose	Anticipated Results
Unstructured or semistructured interviews	Community members	To assess the opinions of individuals representative of a population	Insight into how a population perceives a given problem and potential solutions to the problem
Key informant interviews	Formal and informal community leaders	To gain information on the priorities and potential of the community; to gain "buy-in" from its leaders	Insight into existing opinions and resources that may suggest modifications to the program
In-depth interviews	Community members	To assess the opinions of individuals representative of a population	Insight into how a population perceives a given problem and potential solutions to the problem
Intercept interviews	Community members	To assess the opinions of individuals representative of a population	Insight into how a population perceives a given problem and potential solutions to the problem
Community forums	Groups of community members in specially arranged or ongoing forums	Increase awareness of an issue; gain additional insight into a problem with the advantage of group dynamics and immediate feedback on ideas	Immediate information from a large group of people on the most pressing needs of the community and how these needs are discussed
Delphi technique	Group of individuals who are aware of the problem	To brainstorm new approaches to a problem; individuals never meet as a group, although each is provided feedback on his or her ideas and how they are related to the ideas of others	Creative new approaches to a problem that may not otherwise have arisen in a group setting or without feedback from others thinking about the same issue
Role-playing	Community members	To test out a situation and generate ideas based on their outcome	Salient ways of involving participants in approaching a problem and determining how other community members can become involved in the process
Focus groups	Groups of 8 to 10 community members in specially arranged gatherings	Gain additional insight into a problem with the advantage of group dynamics and immediate feedback on ideas	Information on the needs and resources of the community; insight into the strengths and weaknesses of existing programs

TABLE 9.2 Advantages and Disadvantages of Verbal Methods

Method	Advantages	Disadvantages
Unstructured interview	Provides an opportunity to build rapport with the interviewee Provides the participant with an opportunity to express his or her ideas May provide insights that were previously not considered by the investigation team Allows the interviewer the flexibility to probe as needed	Time-consuming Costly May result in tangential information
Semistructured interview	Provides the participant with an opportunity to express his or her own ideas More reliable and comparable data because an interview guide is used May be preferred by individuals who are accustomed to an efficient use of their time	Structure may not provide the respondent with the freedom to introduce new ideas
Key informant interviews	Straightforward Inexpensive Encourages broad discussion of issues among all parties involved in program development Lines of communication established between community and investigation team Unifies staff and orients them to more focused and well-defined issues	Selection or response bias may limit validity of data If key informants are not selected properly, their opinions may not be representative of or relevant to the community
In-depth interviews	Substantial information from individuals similar to the target population Good for testing sensitive issues Allows observation of person in natural setting Can be combined with a survey Good for testing a partially completed product Allows the interviewer to determine the extent to which questions are interpreted as intended	Time-consuming and expensive Accessibility to homes may be difficult Security issues should be considered
Intercept interviews	Time efficient with respect to both interview and analysis Respondents may be accessed at point where they engage in behavior	Limited time available with each respondent Sampling bias possible High refusal rates possible

(continued)

TABLE 9.2 Continued

Method	Advantages	Disadvantages
Community forums	Cost-effective and time efficient Immediate information on the opinions of a large group of people Provides an opportunity to increase awareness of an issue relevant to some community members Can be used to identify potential participants for focus groups or advisory committees	Need to find a central location in which to conduct the forum Individuals may be less likely to share information in a large group format Some individuals may not feel heard in a large group setting Participation in an ongoing forum may be inefficient use of research time
Delphi technique	Anonymous Cost-effective Guides the group toward a final decision Minimal social pressure to respond in a certain way Members are encouraged to think creatively; thus, more brainstorming may take place Maximizes members' perceived influence in the process and thus greater perceived satisfaction	Lacks a group-dynamic process Members may not be representative of the target population Somewhat time-consuming if newer technologies (e.g., e-mail) are not used Potentially poor response rate
Role-playing	Engages the participants Provides community members with an opportunity to explore new ways of looking at a problem May provide information on an intervention priority based on the respondent's behavior	May not seem relevant to the participant May be difficult to engage community members in "fake" scenarios because the problems may be perceived as far too serious for staging events Participants may be uncomfortable acting out scenarios No guarantee that participants will react realistically in the role-playing situation
Focus groups	Group interaction can enhance creativity Opportunity to observe group dynamics as it relates to the subject matter Opportunity to assess why individuals react a certain way to a particular product Economy of time, effort, and money	Individual may be intimidated or embarrassed to give opinion Higher possibility of biased responses Requires skilled facilitator

standing of the behavior. These items or activities may well reflect the researcher's bias but may not encompass all the ideas held by the target population.

The use of the unstructured interview is contingent on the assumption that the interviewer does not know in advance the exact questions that will be asked of the respondent. In essence, an interview is scheduled with a participant, the interviewer has a topic that he or she will explore with the respondent, but the interviewer does not have a well-defined set of questions prepared for the interview. The interviewer may only have developed a set of perhaps no more than five open-ended questions with which to start the interview. These and other questions come to mind based on previous literature concerning the topic, previous experience with the target population, and ongoing discussions with other members of the community. Also, unstructured interviews rely heavily on knowing how to probe effectively to stimulate an informant to provide more information. Examples of probes include (a) echoing the informant's most recent response, (b) providing verbal affirmation or approval of the subject's response, (c) asking the respondent directly for more information, (d) asking open-ended questions that work off a response (e.g., "What would that activity do for you?"), or (e) simply remaining silent and waiting for the informant to continue his or her response (e.g., Bernard, 1994). The key is to elicit more information from the respondent without injecting the interviewer's own preconceptions into the interaction. Unstructured interviews generally are characterized by a minimum of control over the respondent's information. The conversation focuses on a particular topic, but the respondent is given enough room to define the content of the discussion. The intent of the unstructured interview is to get the interviewee to open up and express himself or herself in his or her own terms and at his or her own pace (Bernard, 1994). Unstructured interviews may provide unique information about the respondent's lifestyle, adaptive and maladaptive behavioral patterns, religion, customs, and similar attributes that may affect the efficaciousness and effectiveness of a program.

The use of the semistructured interview is based on a data collection compromise. Use of an unstructured interview may give the participant too much freedom when responding to questions posed by the interviewer, leading both parties to digress during the interview. On the other hand, use of a structured interview may not allow the interviewer the freedom to probe further on issues related to program activities in question that are not part of the standard interview schedule. Thus, a semistructured interview brings the best of both alternatives to the interview process; perhaps this is why it is the most widely used type of interview in perceived efficacy studies (Higgins et al., 1996; Hubbell, Chavez, Mishra, Magana, & Valdez, 1995; Ledda, Walker, & Basch, 1997). Semistructured interviews have been used to test all three priorities in perceived efficacy studies. For example, researchers have used semistructured interviews to assess, among other health services, availability of cancer screening services and treatment (Hubbell et al., 1995) and reactions to program ideas (e.g., developing a foot self-care program for African Americans with diabetes) (Ledda et al., 1997).

Semistructured interviews also are recommended when the interviewer has only one opportunity to interview the participant. This format ensures that certain key questions will be answered and that redundant questions will be eliminated to conserve time while still providing an opportunity for additional input from the respondent (Higgins et al., 1996). During a semistructured interview, the interviewer uses an interview guide to ensure that certain topics are covered in a prescribed order. Closed-ended (one response requested), open-ended (no limit on number of responses requested), and exploratory questions are asked. In summary, semistructured interviews provide a good forum for gathering information from community members on specific issues related to the activities of the program while allowing the respondent to bring in issues about which the interviewer may not be aware.

Key Informant Interviews. Key informant interviews may be structured, unstructured, or semistructured in format. The purpose of key informant interviews is to collect information from individuals who—because of their professional training, affiliation with particular organizations, or status within a target population (e.g., spokesperson for a homeless population)—can provide important information about the target population to the investigative team. In other words, key informant interviews are conducted with people "in the know"—individuals who are very familiar with the community and its people, its needs, its behavior patterns, and intervention techniques that might be appropriate or inappropriate for that community. Religious and political leaders, business and labor representatives, and heads of service agencies and social organizations are among those typically able to provide insight into the community. However, more important and more difficult to identify are those individuals who hold informal positions of authority in the community, yet who may not have a specific title or position of authority. These individuals are often opinion leaders and may have information about the community that organized leaders may not be privy to because of structural barriers in communication.

The process of conducting key informant interviews involves the following steps:

1. With the investigative team, discuss how the key informant interviews will contribute to the process of evaluating the perceived efficacy of the program. Key informants are not representative samples of individuals; therefore, the information garnered from these individuals will not necessarily be representative of the target population as a whole. Rather, key informant interviews should be used as only one means to generate activity ideas or gauge the extent to which various existing program activities are appropriate for the target community.

2. Draw up a list of potential key informants. Key informants may be recognized leaders or experts in the community (e.g., elected officials, priests, business owners, clinic directors), or they may be individuals who are active in the community at a grassroots level. Good informants also are those individuals who may be somewhat cynical about their community because these individuals tend to be more observant and reflective about their environment (Berg, 1998). Identifying

informal opinion leaders may be more difficult to do at the onset. It may prove fruitful to first ask several community members to identify opinion leaders who are aware of the priorities and potential of the community. Overlap among these endorsements (and subsequent ones given by the initial informal leaders interviewed) should give the researchers a fairly reliable guide of lay leadership.

3. Construct an interview consisting largely of open-ended discussion questions, with direct objective questions added as needed. Open-ended questions might include items such as the following: "What activities are needed to produce a positive effect on the health behaviors of your community?" Specific questions can include assessing the perceived relevance and interest of particular activities that are being considered for inclusion into the program. Strike a balance between obtaining the information perceived as necessary, with the potential for being perceived as intrusive. Consider the time required of these busy individuals and eliminate any unnecessary information. Items also can be included to test the competence of the informants (Poggie, 1972). For example, key informants can be asked about various aspects of the community already known to the investigative team. The accuracy with which the informant answers these questions could serve as a validity check on the informant's status as a key informant. Information received from less competent informants can be either discarded or given less weight during program development.

4. Determine which members of the investigative team are going to conduct the interviews. Selection should be based on criteria such as gender, language skills, status, and experience. For example, certain key informants may perceive the program as more credible and thus provide more information about their community when they are speaking with a male researcher as opposed to a female graduate student. Other informants may be more forthcoming with information when an individual skilled in their dominant language is interviewing them. Although selection of interviewers generally is done based on availability of resources, these types of decisions could affect the collection of key data in determining the perceived efficacy of a program.

5. Decide whether the interviews will be conducted face-to-face or by phone. Face-to-face interviews are preferred over phone interviews because they allow the interviewers to record nonverbal behavior as well as present materials to the informant for review. However, both approaches provide the potential for a personal touch.

6. Schedule and conduct the interviews. It is often necessary to have well-recognized team members (e.g., established researchers) or individuals associated with the community (e.g., active members of the congregation) make the first call to the informant. Informants are generally willing to talk to a member of the investigative team if they are approached in a professional manner and if they are told that the information they provide will be valuable to program development. Key informant interviews can range from a half hour to more than

2 hours depending on the number of questions asked and how talkative the informant is. When scheduling the interview, provide the informant with an estimate of how long the interview should last with a disclaimer that it may take longer, depending on the amount of information the informant has to offer. Many interviewers prefer to audiotape the interviews, rather than simply relying on notes, because this reduces the potential for biased recall on the part of the interviewer. On some occasions, however, informants will not allow the interviewer to record the interview. In these cases, the interviewer should make notes of key points in the conversation and create a summary of the interview as soon as possible afterward. The interviewer can then ask the informant to review the summary and add any additional information not recalled by the interviewer. If informants are used to working with the media, they will be grateful for the opportunity to review their comments and ensure that they will not be misquoted or misrepresented.

7. Summarize the data, emphasizing the consistencies and inconsistencies among the respondents' answers. Information from key informants generally can be pooled together in one report. However, it is often valuable to separate information by type of organization, for example, to get a more precise assessment of the opinions of various experts. Verbatim responses can be included if they highlight a specific aspect of the program in development. Quantitative information can be included in the report, including number of interviews conducted, gender of interviewees, and number of positive responses to a particular set of materials.

By interviewing key informants, there is the potential for not only assessing their ideas and opinions on the project but also providing them an opportunity to learn about the project and what it might offer the community. Implicitly, the leader has the opportunity to "bless" the project and get in "on the ground floor." This could potentially result in a snowballing effect, wherein other members of the community become interested in the project and seek out opportunities to provide their input into the process.

In-Depth Interviews. An in-depth interview attempts to cover every possible aspect of a topic, without time limitation. Generally, an interview guide is developed so that the investigative team will ask questions that attempt to get at every aspect of the health behavior. The interviewer may begin the interview by requesting quantitative survey-type information and then continue with the qualitative in-depth interview, perhaps interspersed with additional quantitative questions. An in-depth interview can last for several hours or may extend to an additional interview session if the respondent is agreeable to that option. Respondents to the interviews should consist of individuals who are members of the target population or who are familiar with the values, beliefs, attitudes, and behaviors of this group. As with other interview data, key themes and words should be analyzed for frequency, consistency, and inconsistency.

Intercept Interviews. Intercept interviews are conducted with target population individuals at the point (time and location) they are most likely to have been exposed to promotional material or engage in health-related behavior. In general, these interception points (e.g., in a clinic waiting room, in a supermarket) should also be high-traffic areas, allowing researchers to contact large numbers of people in a short period of time. For example, intercept interviews have been used successfully to assess reactions to program components in a zoological park (Mayer, personal communication, December 4, 1998). In this example, visitors to a zoo were asked as they exited the park about the use of sunscreen and wearing a hat to protect against skin cancer. This provided additional information about the usefulness of various program activities before the intervention was fully implemented.

The purpose of the intercept interview is to assess the reaction of a targeted community member to the products and materials currently under development. To implement intercept interviews and to ensure their usefulness, one must ensure the following: (a) the interviewee must match the demographic characteristics of the target population, (b) a convenient location must be obtained from merchants or managers where the interviews can be conducted, and (c) the interviews must be brief to minimize the high refusal rate associated with this type of approach. The strength of this approach is that interviewees are approached under circumstances quite similar to those in which an intervention would be received, and hence their perceptions of activity efficacy have immediately accessible context material to draw on. The obvious weakness of the approach is that the amount of interview information that can be collected is limited by those same context considerations.

Other Considerations Related to Interviewing: Location and Mode of Interview. There are at least two other important considerations when deciding where and how to conduct interviews with members of the community. The first consideration pertains to location of the interview. Interviews that are conducted at a centralized location may not provide information as generalizable to the target population as interviews held in the respondent's home. Conducting interviews at a clinic, church, or office requires respondents to come to this location to be interviewed. This will restrict the type of person being interviewed to someone who has a certain degree of motivation, transportation, child care, and time. On the other hand, interviewers who choose instead to visit the respondent's home are more likely to achieve a representative sample of responses. The interviewer is equally likely to interview a homemaker or a semiprofessional businessperson if she or he conducts the interviews at the respondent's residence. However, home interviews are not without their limitations. It is often necessary to send two interviewers to a respondent's home for security purposes. Many people would argue that home interviews are not worth the risk of potentially endangering the safety of interviewers (Bernard, 1994). Home interviews are often plagued by numerous interruptions, especially if there are young children in the home. Last, home interviews are generally more expensive to conduct because they require a great deal of transportation costs to the project.

A consideration pertains to the mode of the interview. Interviews can be conducted face-to-face, by telephone, via an audiocassette, and, more recently, by computer (Rosenthal & Rosnow, 1991). Face-to-face interviews, although optimal in terms of developing rapport with the respondent and allowing for easy clarification of questions, also tend to be more costly, more time-consuming, and less effective for obtaining information on sensitive topics with some populations (Marín & Marín, 1989). Interviewer bias is more likely to occur in face-to-face interviews because the interviewer may adjust the wording of a question to fit the respondent or may record only a portion of their responses (Shaughnessy & Zechmeister, 1997).

Telephone interviews have some advantages over face-to-face interviews. The interviewer does not need to travel to the respondent's home. The interviewer can schedule several interviews in one day without having to consider travel time. Also, refusal rates generally are lower over the phone (Rosenthal & Rosnow, 1991). However, there are also disadvantages to conducting interviews by telephone. Phone interviews are restricted to those who have a phone and full access to it. It is more difficult to establish rapport over the phone, and the interviewee may have a more difficult time understanding only a verbal presentation of the questions. Both of these factors might lead to greater impatience on the part of the interviewee and less reliable responses.

An innovative approach to gaining information from adolescents on sensitive topics or those requiring additional privacy is the use of prerecorded questions on audiocassette (Kolbe, Kann, & Collins, 1993). Adolescents responding to the Youth Risk Behavior Survey were asked to listen to an audiocassette, which contained previously recorded questions. The adolescents were asked to mark their responses to the questions on an answer sheet, which was then returned to the interviewer in a sealed envelope. This type of approach allowed the respondent to keep completely private both the questions asked and the responses given to the questions. In addition to minimizing evaluation apprehension on the part of the respondent, such techniques also minimize experimenter expectancy effects.

Computerized interviewing is coming of age; however, most research to date on computerized interviewing has focused on the adaptation of standardized instruments to a computer format (Fowler, 1985). It is suggested that computers provide a sense of privacy for the individual to make uninhibited comments

(Conte, 1986). On the other hand, interviewing by computer requires informants to type in their responses, which may lead them to edit honest responses that are not deemed appropriate (e.g., they may be less likely to support needle exchange programs to reduce the spread of AIDS, as a current controversial example). Perhaps the future will witness the development of computer-assisted technology to assess the priorities of a community, if such a program could be made available to the general public in a centralized location. For example, a school-based computer program could be developed in which adolescents could readily access information on motor vehicle safety or the avoidance of violence. As a sound-assisted device, computer interviewing can be a full-fledged, verbal-type strategy that most persons could be trained easily to use. Much work needs to be done to determine whether computers can be used effectively in perceived efficacy work.

COMMUNITY FORUMS

Community can be defined geographically, politically, or culturally. It may refer to a single company, corporation, church, clinic, tribe, city, or particular geographic region (e.g., the East Bay of Northern California). Winett et al. (1989) defined communities as "settings in which activities take place; collections of individuals; vehicles through which interactions occur among and between individuals and institutions; and social systems that pose problems and afford opportunities to individuals and institutions within them" (p. 128), thus implying a functional set of environment-behavior relationships. As evidenced by the increasing number of town hall meetings, community forums have become very popular in the political arena. They are used to gain information about issues most salient to the community, community members' attitudes about particular topics, and possible barriers to program development and implementation.

In a community forum, leaders from different subgroups within the community unit present perspectives unique to their subgroup under the guidance of a legitimized community leader or panel. The panel or advisory board consists of persons who interact across different subgroups. There also may be subgroup leaders. Subgroup leaders may be those persons who do not bridge between subgroups but voice the opinion of their subgroup. Subgroup leaders generally are permitted to express their opinions after issues are introduced by the board. Next, individual members of subgroups may provide testimonials to advance the perspective of their subgroup. Based on the information presented, the panel, board, or all those present at the forum take a vote on the next steps needed to resolve the problem.

Community forums should generally last no more than 2 hours to maintain the attention of the participants while still providing an opportunity for input from everyone. Also, a trained facilitator should be used to pose the questions, guide the discussion, and control vocal individuals. Questions for the forum can include the level of participation, interest, and suggestions for improvement regarding current health programming. Ideas for new program activities also may be generated. It is often a good idea to use either a chalkboard or an easel to write down the questions posed to the forum, as well as the responses. Written responses can serve as a cue to elicit more information about the topic. It is rarely feasible to tape-record community forums without an extensive budget for good audio equipment. Therefore, two or three individuals should be charged with the task of writing down participant responses. These responses can then be combined to create one report. Included in the report should be information on the number of participants and demographic information (e.g., gender and ethnic breakdown, adults vs. adolescents). This information will help to make an evaluation of the representativeness of the forum participants to the target population.

Community boards often are naturally occurring. For example, within business organizations, advisory boards comprising union members and other representatives can speak about issues concerning the employees (Hunsaker & Cook, 1987). Similarly, churches often have laypersons who act as conduits between the church administration and its membership to keep abreast of the congregation's issues (Castro et al., 1995). One should make use of a naturally occurring board or form one to advance the use of community forums for the purposes of health behavior program development.

Community forums can be scheduled in schools, churches, or any other central location accessible to most community members. To maximize participation by community members, one must either advertise these forums or incorporate them into regularly scheduled meetings (e.g., parent-teacher associations). The investigator should use the media to extend the invitation to all members of the target audience and state the purpose, time, date, and location of the forum in all advertising pieces.

One example of the use of a community forum pertained to a community-wide nutrition intervention with Latinos. This forum yielded key information about conflicts between the needs of the community and school district administrators. School officials wished to modernize their menu and make cafeteria offerings more nutritious and lower in fat and sodium, whereas parents were more concerned about children having sufficient time to eat and being served hot food that they enjoyed eating. Through the use of the community forum, eventually both issues were addressed concurrently. A program development compromise was made (Elder et al., 1994).

In perceived efficacy work, community forums provide the investigative team with an opportunity to bring together a group of people to discuss the needs of the community and how a proposed program might help to address some of these needs. They also serve to prevent problems that may arise as a result of misinterpretations and miscommunications due to language barriers

(Marín & Marín, 1991). A particular advantage of community forums is that they may help to identify community members who can serve in a focus group or advisory committee. Finally, these forums provide an opportunity to increase awareness about a particular issue affecting the community that all of its members may not be familiar with. Thus, it may indirectly increase accessibility to the community by making its members aware of a particular problem and engaging them in problem-solving potential solutions. Without naturally occurring advisory boards, however, this approach may not be successfully applied.

DELPHI TECHNIQUE

The purpose of the Delphi technique is to generate ideas in a small group setting or through written or verbal communication without face-to-face interaction (Moore, 1987). It is a method of collecting, organizing, reviewing, and revising the opinions of a group of individuals through a question-feedback process (McKenna, 1994). It capitalizes on the assets and avoids the liabilities of group decision making (Hunsaker & Cook, 1987). The qualifications for a traditional Delphi are anonymity, iteration with feedback, and both qualitative and quantitative responses. The technique is most commonly used when it is not convenient or desirable for a group of individuals to come together face-to-face, although similar procedures can be used in a small group setting (Moore, 1987). It also allows for an exchange between individuals with a wide variety of experiences and backgrounds (McKenna, 1994). The technique encourages participants to think creatively about a problem and then interact with others via written judgments and suggestions, generally in the form of qualitative and quantitative responses to a questionnaire.

Suggestions can be stated verbally to a skilled mediator, who travels from participant to participant to provide iterative feedback to suggestions that are made. In a paper-and-pencil version, the participants come up with possible solutions, write them down, and then send them to a central location for recording, processing, and dissemination to other group members. In a small group setting, the questions are asked on computer terminals and synthesized immediately. In either of the processes of integrating information, this collection of ideas and responses is then used as a springboard for additional questions, which are then sent back through this feedback loop process. This process continues until a consensus has been reached or a given solution is agreed on as a priority. Often, the process can take up to 2 months to complete, although this weakness is likely to become less of a factor with the use of computer technology such as e-mail. To obtain a wide variety of responses to the questions and generate ideas based on varying opinions, individuals from several different organizations and different social strata should participate together.

Delphi techniques have been used successfully in a variety of settings (career-related decision making: Jeffery, Hache, & Lehr, 1995; outpatient treatment facility: Pruitt, Waligora-Serafin, & Besselman, 1985; job evaluations: Hornsby, Smith, & Gupta, 1994), although there is minimal evidence for their use in perceived efficacy work (McKenna, 1994). The opinions of health care providers have been assessed using the Delphi technique to set priorities for adequate patient care (Pruitt et al., 1985). The Delphi technique may prove beneficial for tailoring down a number of potentially important ideas among those who represent important actors in the delivery or receipt of health behavior programming within the community. At best, it may allow for a synthesis of several ideas into one that captures several priorities at once. And it is especially useful with topics that are somewhat controversial in nature. For example, a Delphi technique could be used to obtain creative approaches to the problem of teen pregnancy. Each member participating in the Delphi approach would be asked to relay to the mediator five creative solutions to teen pregnancy. These ideas would then be sent to a central location for synthesis and preparation of a summary. Often, ideas will overlap with one another, resulting in a more complete picture of solutions to the problem than any one individual member was able to generate on his or her own. The summary is then returned to the participants by the mediator for a second feedback process, which results in even greater specificity of potential program development ideas. Although no reported application has been found in the literature, e-mail, chat rooms, and other Internet communication formats may stimulate more widespread use of Delphi and related techniques.

ROLE-PLAYING

Even less well developed is the use of role-playing techniques in perceived efficacy work. Role-playing is a type of simulation experiment in which participants act out a given scenario by improvising, with the help of a script developed by the investigative team (Rosenthal & Rosnow, 1991). Role-playing could be used to generate ideas that are perceived as efficacious. For example, several community members might be asked to pretend they are storeowners, and several underage youth walk into the store wanting to purchase alcohol. This type of role-playing might elicit information from the participants about how to minimize the accessibility of alcohol to adolescents in their community. It may also suggest ways in which parents, storeowners, and other community members can work together to reduce alcohol consumption among their youth.

Testing the perceived efficacy of various program activities can be completed using role-playing. For example, a series of activities might be summarized in a role-play format, on which target subjects would rate their perceived efficacy. Role-playing also may provide insight into the salience and influence of various materials or products proposed for a new program. The research team may find that participants do not respond well to a particular product, even when it is pointed out to them in role-play. The use of role-play is most important when judgment of perceived efficacy includes nonverbal, behavioral data. For example, an investigator may act out refusal assertion, conversation initiation, and general assertiveness skills and ask the target subjects which of these skills are most important in the prevention of drug abuse. This behavioral data may be superior to simply telling the subjects what the different program activity ideas are.

FOCUS GROUPS

Focus groups are an excellent verbal means of linking the needs of the community with program activities. They function similarly to community forums with respect to information gathering, but they provide for more specific discussion of relevant issues. Focus groups have been used successfully to help design and develop a nutrition intervention program (Hartman, McCarthy, Park, Schuster, & Kushi, 1994) and traffic safety programs (Basch, DeCicco, & Malfetti, 1989), as well as to adapt existing interventions for a community setting (Kohler et al., 1993). Focus groups also have been used to pretest intervention materials (Freimuth & Mettger, 1990; Krueger, 1994) and develop high-quality quantitative surveys (Stewart et al., 1994).

Focus group interviewing has been used since the beginning of World War II (Berg, 1998). It has been described as "one of the most widely used qualitative research tools in the applied social sciences" (Sussman, Burton, Dent, Stacy, & Flay, 1991, p. 1773). A focus group is a type of research method in which a moderator leads approximately 8 to 10 people in an open discussion of a topic. Groups that are very small may become dominated by one or two more vocal individuals, and groups with more than 10 people are difficult to manage.

Although not always necessary or possible, focus groups generate more open dialogue if they are relatively homogeneous and the members are not familiar with each other prior to the group interaction. Often, the researcher will want to make focus groups homogeneous with respect to important characteristics, including gender, ethnicity, or the target behavior or problem to be studied. Dividing males from females or Anglos from Latinos may create a more comfortable environment for the participants, especially when sensitive topics are discussed (e.g., sexual behavior, racism/discrimination). Dividing alcoholics from occasional drinkers, clinic users from nonusers, and delinquents from "A" students allows for the application of epidemiology's "case control" logic to perceived efficacy work.

By starting with a behavioral outcome (e.g., delinquency "cases" vs. nondelinquency "controls" in socioeconomically equivalent groups), the researcher can retrospectively study "exposures" (barriers, reinforcers, modeling, etc.) that differentially affected "cases" (e.g., peer pressure, parental modeling) and possibly led them to maladaptive behavior. They also can use these case and control focus groups to evaluate specific, potential activities for a health behavior program. Evaluations of these activities provide an indication of the receptivity of programming to the general population and the target group, as well as some indication of the specificity of the programming to the target group. This type of information is likely to prove useful for program development.

The focus group has an advantage over individual interviews because it provides an assessment of the extent to which group members interact and behave toward one another on a particular issue. This process has been described as a *synergistic group effect*, in which members of the group engage in collective brainstorming of ideas, issues, and solutions to a problem (Sussman et al., 1991). For example, the extent to which social support and influential others encourage or impede the performance of healthy eating and exercise behaviors can be observed during focus groups. Focus groups are also preferred over in-depth interviews because they are more cost-effective in both time and resources expended. Many more individuals can be studied through a format that gathers 8 to 10 people at one time. Focus groups are excellent ways of generating ideas; they provide the opportunity to build and modify ideas and materials as group members present their opinions. Materials that are more salient to the audience, in terms of literacy level, content, and presentation, result in a wider distribution of the materials outside the immediate target population (Freimuth & Mettger, 1990). Focus groups are also good forums to test survey instruments to determine whether individuals similar to the target population can understand the questions presented by the investigative team (Stewart et al., 1994).

There are four steps to focus group research: setting up the group, writing the interview guide, selecting and preparing the moderator, and running the group.

1. There are a number of issues to consider when setting up a group, including determining the size of the group and deciding who should be a member of the group, where to hold the group meetings, and how many focus groups to conduct. In general, the focus groups should represent key characteristics of the target population (i.e., similar with respect to age, gender, ethnicity, socioeconomic status). Eight to 10 respondents is the maximum number of participants recommended for a focus group. The group setting should be comfortable, easily accessible, and reasonably private. As in any research, a sufficient sample size (or, in this case, number of groups) should take into account the variability between groups. The greater the variability in group responses, the greater the need to assess a larger number of groups. Although resources often dictate how many focus groups will be conducted (40—Basch et al., 1989; 4—Kohler et al., 1993), when variability in responses is low, two groups per topic should be sufficient.

2. Developing an interview guide is essential to maintaining focus on the research objectives. The guide generally consists of a general question-by-question outline, giving the moderator the flexibility to ask the questions while considering the dynamics of the group. Because a period of time might be needed to establish rapport, questions should proceed from the general and nonthreatening to the more specific and potentially controversial. This also allows the moderator to probe responses to general questions with more specific items related to the topic of interest (Basch et al., 1989). The moderator begins by introducing the rationale behind the focus group and conducting any warm-up activities as needed (e.g., having participants chat with one another for a few minutes and then introducing each other to the entire group). Questions that follow the warm-up activity should appear to naturally flow from the opening activities but should also elicit the maximum amount of information possible. In his book, Krueger (1994) suggests that there are several different types of questions, including opening questions, transition questions, key questions, and ending questions. The most important point to remember is that questions can be open-ended or closed-ended and specific or general when obtaining key information from the participants about the program. Open-ended, general questions are best used at the beginning of the focus group when the facilitator is trying to get the participants to begin thinking about the topic. For example, one successful form of an open-ended, general question is the following: "What do you think about when I say nutrition?" This type of question can elicit information ranging from "vitamins and minerals" to "knowing how to cook food without fat." Specific open-ended questions are used to gather information about particular behaviors or attitudes. For example, participants can be asked to explain what they like or do not like about various methods of birth control (Berg, 1998). Closed-ended questions, whether specific or general, are generally left until the end of the focus group (Krueger, 1994). These types of questions attempt to get at very specific information. For example, respondents could be asked how satisfied they would be with a cooking class (general question) or instruction on how to cook low-fat dinners (specific). Irrespective of the types of questions asked during the focus group, the facilitator should end the focus group by asking the participants if anything was left out in the discussion. This will provide the facilitator feedback as to whether his or her line of questioning left out an important element related to the topic of interest.

3. Selecting and preparing a facilitator are critical to ensuring functional group dynamics. The facilitator or moderator must feel comfortable interacting with others, put others at ease, be enthusiastic, have good listening skills and the ability to reflect back what is said, and generally match the personal characteristics of the respondents (e.g., dress, language, gender) (Krueger, 1994). The moderator should be thoroughly informed about the project to guide the discussion appropriately and occasionally respond to inquiries of group members. Most

important, the moderator must be able to obtain information from the respondents without biasing them in any way or leading them to give an answer they think the moderator is looking for. A skilled moderator can make a group feel comfortable enough to divulge sensitive information about themselves, which then breaks the ice for others to join in the conversation (Bernard, 1994). The focus group should be taped (either video or audio) so the content of the focus group discussion can be transcribed. If the group is relatively quiet or information is particularly sensitive, sometimes writing down information verbatim is possible (e.g., see Chapter 10, this volume). At the end of the focus group discussion, the moderator and any observers are debriefed on the session, and results of the focus groups are summarized in written form. Alternatively, some focus group material on key questions can be written down verbatim.

4. Analyzing focus group results can take several forms. First, a transcription of the focus group is made with key themes highlighted. Transcription should be performed by more than one rater to provide greater assurances that all relevant information is extracted from the tapes (Weinberger et al., 1998). In this report and in all other types of focus group reports, direct quotes can be included if they serve to emphasize a particular point. Depending on the stage of perceived efficacy work, some researchers may require a more focused analysis. This may entail looking at very specific information related to the program, essentially ignoring all other information. Alternatively, it may require an examination of the types of words used by groups, the intensity and frequency of the comments, or the specificity of the responses. In this case, responses to items may be grouped by type of response (e.g., positive or negative), gender of participant, type of organization represented (e.g., church vs. clinic), or level of involvement in the issue (e.g., participant in a cooking class vs. nonparticipant). The final report, irrespective of its level of complexity, should be distributed to all members of the investigative team who participated in the focus group to ensure that all information was recalled or transcribed accurately. A draft of the report also can be shared with the focus group participants for comment and feedback.

As noted earlier, focus groups are an excellent forum for testing out ideas, materials, and products. For example, the second author was recently asked by the U.S. Marine Corps to develop innovative interventions to reduce binge alcohol consumption among young Marines. Groups of 10 to 15 were asked to help develop or respond to a variety of program possibilities, including the following:

1. Who would be the best person to talk to you about excessive drinking—a buddy, a corporal or sergeant, a senior noncommissioned officer or officer, or someone else? What would be the best way for him to approach it?

2. Would a 3.2% light beer be acceptable to you and your buddies? What if it was priced more cheaply than other products? What can design or logo would be appealing?
3. What activities compete with drinking? How can we get more Marines to participate in these activities?
4. How does your wife or sweetheart respond to you when you get drunk or after you sober up? What could she say or do to be more effective?

Based largely on these focus group results, intervention programs, and materials, alternative activities and new (and safer) products are being developed for servicewide implementation. Another specific example of the use of focus groups can be found in Chapter 10 of this volume (Case Study 4) regarding adolescent tobacco use cessation.

SUMMARY AND CONCLUSION ◄

Perceived efficacy work in program development is essential for generating ideas that will fit within an existing community structure. When investigators attempt to bring their program ideas into the "real world," there is often a mismatch between the priorities of the community and those of the program in question. As Marín and Marín (1991) noted when discussing ways of enhancing participation by community members,

> Knowledgeable members of the community should be consulted in order to obtain information on issues of concern to the respondents, approaches to be used to announce the study properly, procedures that can be implemented to enhance participation, and methods for informing the community of the results of the study. (p. 50)

This chapter has emphasized verbal methods that can be used to evaluate the perceived quality of health behavior program activities. It is often the case that multiple sources of information yield similar results. For example, focus groups, interviews, and role-playing may yield similar information about the perceived quality of a health behavior program activity. Although some might argue against multiple sources of information because of the additional expense associated with its implementation, when these sources of information result in comparable information, then the convergent validity of the responses is more secure (Ward, Bertrand, & Brown, 1991). Grounded in basic principles of community dialogue and partnership, the philosophy underlying effective program development research is that often the greatest source of knowledge and expertise is the community and the population itself. Therefore, we do not address weaknesses without looking at strengths, needs without resources, or the community without its formal and informal leadership.

Yet, new technologies portend changes in and expansion of these research techniques. Computer-assisted interviews and data gathering in general may make it possible for greater numbers of community constituents to participate in program development in a manner, time, and place of their choosing. Using Internet chat rooms or other methods of electronic communication, as well as iterative processes such as the Delphi technique, eventually will allow researchers to more conveniently and broadly obtain this and related formative information from community gatekeepers and opinion leaders. Even role-playing eventually may be made more realistic, with digital still and video photography allowing the incorporation of the participant's image (or even perceived presence) into a virtual scenario. Nevertheless, users of these and yet-to-be-developed technologies, although revolutionizing the field, must still be careful to stay in step with the communities being served.

▶ REFERENCES

ABELSON, A. G. (1997). Managing students with behavior disorders: Perceived efficacy of interventions. *Psychological Reports, 80*(3, Pt. 2), 1167-1170.

BASCH, C. E., DeCICCO, I. M., & MALFETTI, J. L. (1989). A focus group study on decision processes of young drivers: Reasons that may support a decision to drink and drive. *Health Education Quarterly, 16,* 389-396.

BERG, B. L. (1998). *Qualitative research methods for the social sciences* (3rd ed.). Boston: Allyn & Bacon.

BERNARD, H. R. (1994). *Research methods in anthropology: Qualitative and quantitative approaches* (2nd ed.). Thousand Oaks, CA: Sage.

BRIEGER, W. R., NWANKWO, E., EZIKE, V. I., SEXTON, J. D., BREMAN, J. G., PARKER, K. A., EKANEM, O. J., & ROBINSON, T. (1996). Social and behavioral baseline for guiding implementation of an efficacy trial of insecticide impregnated bed nets for malaria control at Nsukka, Nigeria. *International Quarterly of Community Health Education, 16,* 47-61.

CASTRO, F., ELDER, J., COE, K., TAFOYA-BARRAZA, H. M., MORATTO, S., CAMPBELL, N., & TALAVERA, G. (1995). Mobilizing churches for health promotion in Latino communities: Compañeras en la Salud. *Journal of the National Cancer Institute Monographs, 18,* 127-135.

CONTE, H. R. (1986). Multivariate assessment in sexual dysfunction. *Journal of Consulting and Clinical Psychology, 54,* 149-157.

ELDER, J. P., GELLER, E. S., HOVELL, M. F., & MAYER, J. A. (1994). Assessing needs and resources and setting priorities. In J. P. Elder, E. S. Geller, M. F. Hovell, & J. A. Mayer (Eds.), *Motivating health behavior* (pp. 83-92). Albany, NY: Delmar.

FOWLER, R. D. (1985). Landmarks in computer-assisted psychological assessment. *Journal of Consulting and Clinical Psychology, 53,* 748-759.

FREIMUTH, V. S., & METTGER, W. (1990). Is there a hard-to-reach audience? *Public Health Reports, 105,* 232-238.

HARTMAN, R. J., McCARTHY, P. R., PARK, R. J., SCHUSTER, E., & KUSHI, L. H. (1994). Focus group responses of potential participants in a nutrition education program for individuals with limited literacy skills. *Journal of the American Dietetic Association, 94,* 744-748.

HIGGINS, D. L., O'REILLY, K., TASHIMA, N., CRAIN, C., BEEKER, C., GOLDBAUM, G., ELIFSON, C. S., GALAVOTTI, C., & GUENTHER-GREY, C. (1996). Using formative research to lay the foundation for community level HIV prevention efforts: An example from the AIDS community demonstration projects. *Public Health Reports, 111*(Suppl.), 28-35.

HINKLE, S., FOX-CARDAMONE, L., HASELEU, J. A., BROWN, R., & IRWIN, L. M. (1996). Grassroots political action as an intergroup phenomenon. *Journal of Social Issues, 52,* 39-51.

HORNSBY, J. S., SMITH, B. N., & GUPTA, J. N. D. (1994). The impact of decision-making methodology on job evaluation outcomes: A look at three consensus approaches. *Group & Organizational Management, 19,* 112-128.

HUBBELL, F. A., CHAVEZ, L. R., MISHRA, S. I., MAGANA, J. R., & VALDEZ, R. B. (1995). From ethnography to intervention: Developing a breast cancer control program for Latinas. *Journal of the National Cancer Institute Monographs, 18,* 109-115.

HUNSAKER, P. L., & COOK, C. W. (1987). *Managing organizational behavior.* Reading, MA: Addison-Wesley.

JEFFERY, G., HACHE, G., & LEHR, R. (1995). A group-based Delphi application: Defining rural career counseling needs. *Measurement and Evaluation in Counseling and Development, 28,* 45-90.

KOHLER, C. L., DOLCE, J. J., MANZELLA, B. A., HIGGINS, D., BROOKS, C. M., RICHARDS, J. M., & BAILEY, W. C. (1993). Use of focus group methodology to develop an asthma self-management program useful for community-based medical practices. *Health Education Quarterly, 20,* 421-429.

KOLBE, L. J., KANN, I., & COLLINS, J. L. (1993). Overview of the Youth Risk Behavior Surveillance Survey. *Public Health Reports, 108*(1, Suppl.), 1-20.

KRUEGER, R. A. (1994). *Focus groups: A practical guide for applied research* (2nd ed.). Thousand Oaks, CA: Sage.

LEDDA, M. A., WALKER, E. A., & BASCH, C. E. (1997). Development and formative evaluation of a foot self-care program for African-Americans with diabetes. *Diabetes Educator, 23,* 48-51.

MARÍN, G., & MARÍN, B. V. (1989). A comparison of three interviewing approaches to studying sensitive topics with Hispanics. *Hispanic Journal of Behavioral Sciences, 11,* 330-340.

MARÍN, G., & MARÍN, B. V. (1991). *Research with Hispanic populations.* Newbury Park, CA: Sage.

McKENNA, H. P. (1994). The Delphi technique: A worthwhile research approach for nursing? *Journal of Advanced Nursing, 19,* 1221-1225.

MOORE, C. M. (1987). *Delphi technique and mail questionnaires.* Newbury Park, CA: Sage.

POGGIE, J. (1972). Toward quality control in key informant data. *Human Organization, 31,* 23-30.

PRUITT, B. T., WALIGORA-SERAFIN, B., & BESSELMAN, L. (1985). Program development for supportive care of cancer patients: Establishing priorities with the Delphi technique. *Journal of Psychosocial Oncology, 3,* 95-100.

ROSENTHAL, R., & ROSNOW, R. L. (1991). *Essentials of behavioral research: Methods and data analysis* (2nd ed.). New York: McGraw-Hill.

SHAUGHNESSY, J. J., & ZECHMEISTER, E. B. (1997). *Research methods in psychology.* New York: McGraw-Hill.

STEWART, B., OLSON, D., GOODY, C., TINSLEY, A., AMOS, R., BETTS, N., GEORGIOU, C., HOERR, S., IVATURI, R., & VOICHICK, J. (1994). Converting focus group data on food choices into a quantitative instrument. *Journal of Nutrition Education, 26,* 34-36.

SUSSMAN, S., BURTON, D., DENT, C. W., STACY, A. W., & FLAY, B. R. (1991). Use of focus groups in developing an adolescent tobacco use cessation program: Collection of norm effects. *Journal of Applied Social Psychology, 21,* 1772-1782.

WARD, V. M., BERTRAND, J. T., & BROWN, L. F. (1991). The comparability of focus group and survey results. *Evaluation Review, 15,* 266-283.

WEINBERGER, M., FERGUSON, J. A., WESTMORELAND, G., MAMLIN, L. A., SEGAR, D. S., ECKERT, G. J., GREENE, J. Y., MARTIN, D. K., & TIEMEY, W. M. (1998). Can raters consistently evaluate the content of focus groups? *Social Science and Medicine, 46,* 929-933.

WINETT, R. A., KING, A. C., & ALTMAN, D. G. (1989). *Health psychology and public health: An integrative approach.* Elmsford, NY: Pergamon.

CHAPTER 9

Commentary

Edward G. Singleton
Jack E. Henningfield

This chapter was, frankly, one of the more enjoyable professional works we have read lately because it is intuitively and logically well written. It provides researchers and consumers of research with the tools to help address one of the fundamental issues in the use of verbal methods—namely, the fact that the content of questions as well as their means of administration can influence the answers (see discussion of these issues by Schwarz, 1999). The tools provided by Ayala and Elder include various means by which one can evaluate and control the reliability and validity of verbally based data. This chapter should prove helpful to intervention developers and many others who are not experts at evaluation but who would like to better understand these methods.

In this commentary, we will discuss further the evaluation of sensitive areas such as tobacco and other drug use and special issues that arise when evaluating culturally diverse populations—two areas where verbal methods in perceived efficacy work could be particularly relevant. Program development and evaluation rely on the provision of honest self-reports regarding perceived program concept quality estimates, behavioral intentions, or behaviors. One issue, briefly touched on by Ayala and Elder, pertains to response bias. When the testing situation involves strong social pressures to answer an item one way or another, this pressure might bring bias to the study. An important area of health in which increased sophistication in verbal methods is particularly important includes questions about tobacco and other drug use. Interestingly, one of the historical assumptions made about responses to surveys of tobacco use versus illicit drug use was that questions on tobacco use would be more likely to be truthfully and completely answered because of the relative lack of social condemnation and illegality of that behavior. The contextual basis for that assumption may be changing, however. Thus, there may be an increasing importance of using the verbal methods discussed in this chapter for the assessment of tobacco use, as well as various other aspects of teen tobacco program development.

Automated methods, despite their own novel limitations, can be useful in assessing verbal behavior because they can reduce the impact of the social forces that can influence the questions. An example of such an approach is the use of portable computerized monitoring techniques such as those used by Shiffman and colleagues to track the interrelationships between self-reported tobacco cravings, mood states, and environmental events (e.g., Shiffman et al., 1997). Another alternative, recommended by the Office on Smoking and Health of the Centers for Disease Control and Prevention, involves using tape recorders to administer questionnaires via personal headphones. Respondents record their answers on coded forms, thus reducing the socially mediated factors that can influence answers about such behaviors. For example, parents and others do not know the specifics of the questions. This approach retains the advantages of structured interviews (standardized measurement), self-report (privacy), and computer-assisted technology (automatic production of database files). Also, it can be used with participants who can hear or speak any language and allows multilingual administration of questions without requiring multilingual interviewers. The increasing social stigma associated with smoking could contribute to underreporting smoking status; self-administered questions tend to elicit more complete reporting of substance use, regardless of the drug studied.

In addition to addressing whether participants are open and honest in their responding, the verbal methods discussed in this chapter and in this commentary can provide insight into whether the target group actually understands and comprehends things in the same manner as the researcher. Often, there is considerable disagreement regarding terms typically used to evaluate program outcomes. For example, *craving* may be interpreted by users to mean any desire to use cigarettes or only a strong urge to smoke (Pickens, 1992). To further complicate the matter, reports may be substantially influenced by sociocultural factors such as age, gender, race, and level of education. For example, pretesting of craving items translated from English to standard Spanish have encountered problems in equivalency of meaning. The meaning attached to craving in the present tense (i.e., "right now") in the Spanish language depends on what time one is referring to and can be expressed in three ways: *En un instante,* or a matter of seconds, and *ahora mismo* or *en este momento,* each bound to the moment that is a little longer than an instant. This experience reinforces the significance of pretesting ideas and materials with small samples of individuals from the target population before conducting more widespread studies, as the authors contend.

The emphasis on community forums, the Delphi techniques, and focus groups underscores the significance of community participation in the program development process to ensure that programs better serve the intended audience. We know so little about the diverse populations of persons that programs are intended to reach. These verbal methods should prove useful in increasing our knowledge about drug use and other problem behaviors and assist in program development among different cultural groups. For example, a major area of concern is that most African American smokers who want to stop do not join cessation programs, and those that do seek help in breaking the habit are less successful at quitting than other populations. Recently, focus groups and other related work have been conducted with African American smokers and ex-smokers to determine if and what program improvements need to be made to increase program participation and enhance success rates. Consensus was that traditional cessation programs are targeted to a different type of population. Also, these respondents tend to report that spiritual and religious beliefs would motivate quit behavior and that the use of more nonconventional methods—such as promoting smoking cessation with other community activities in local churches and integrating ministers into the social support system—might be effective ways of encouraging more African Americans to participate (e.g., see Lopes, Sussman, Galaif, & Crippens, 1995; Manfredi, Lacy, Warnecke, & Balch, 1997).

Thus, the major task in gaining valuable program-relevant knowledge about different cultures is knowing where and how to collect that information. Unfortunately, this task often has defaulted to the media or has been vested in researchers with little or no experience with that culture. What is needed is a framework for building successful collaborations between researchers and the diverse cultures within the target communities to establish a process for sustaining cooperation and simultaneously resolving important local problems (see discussion by Segall, Lonner, & Berry, 1998). The importance of collecting valid data across populations with ethnic and cultural differences goes well beyond simply determining the effects of potential interventions in such populations. Such cross-population research can help provide insights regarding dynamics of roles served by majority populations as well as minority populations in a given geographic region. Frankly, increasing the excellence and relevance of verbally based research will require more than just using the right methods; it will require greater levels of participation of ethnically diverse populations, as discussed by Henningfield, Singleton, and Cadet (1994). Still, by appreciating the diversity and limitations of various methodological approaches, Ayala and Elder's chapter is a good start.

Overall, the information-gathering methods discussed in the chapter provide an excellent foundation on means to gather and translate perceived efficacy work (concept evaluation) into specific program activities, particularly those that matter most to persons from cultures whose priorities may differ from the researcher's own. One exciting future possibility is the potential for developing community linkages that partner researchers, faculty, graduate and undergraduate students, and staff with community members and local groups to work collaboratively on research and action projects. This notion is a derivative of the "Danish Science Shop," whose purpose is to increase access to university research in communities for those who need assistance but for whom contact with researchers and universities is not normal practice. Local problems solved through this mechanism are free of charge, and most programs are initiated by students and their mentors as part of the training. This type of approach could help "institutionalize" qualitative research into mainstream program development. The major lesson learned may be reminiscent of an important theme developed by these authors—the source of the problem often contains the solution.

▷ REFERENCES

HENNINGFIELD, J. E., SINGLETON, E. G., & CADET, J. L. (1994). Report from underrepresented populations committee. *Drug and Alcohol Dependence, 35,* 261-263.

LOPES, C., SUSSMAN, S., GALAIF, E. R., & CRIPPENS, D. L. (1995). The impact of a videotape on smoking cessation among African-American women. *American Journal of Health Promotion, 9,* 257-260.

MANFREDI, C., LACY, L., WARNECKE, R., & BALCH, G. (1997). Method effects in survey and focus group findings: Understanding smoking cessation in low-SES African American women. *Health Education & Behavior, 24,* 786-800.

PICKENS, R. W. (1992). Craving: Consensus of status and agenda for future research. *Drug and Alcohol Dependence, 30,* 127-131.

SCHWARZ, N. (1999). Self-reports: How the questions shape the answers. *American Psychologist, 54,* 93-105.

SEGALL, M. H., LONNER, W. J., & BERRY, J. W. (1998). Cross-cultural psychology as a scholarly discipline. *American Psychologist, 53,* 1101-1110.

SHIFFMAN, S., HUFFORD, M., HICKCOX, M., PATY, J. A., GNYS, M., & KASSEL, J. D. (1997). Remember that? A comparison of real-time versus retrospective recall of smoking lapses. *Journal of Consulting and Clinical Psychology, 65,* 292-300.

Case Study 4

CHAPTER 10

Use of Focus Groups for Adolescent Tobacco Use Cessation

Steve Sussman
Kara Lichtman
Clyde W. Dent

Most regular (e.g., monthly or greater) adolescent tobacco users are likely to continue to use tobacco into adulthood. For example, although only 5% of regular adolescent smokers view themselves as smoking 5 years later, 75% actually are smoking 8 years later (Charlton, Melia, & Moyer, 1990, cited in Flay, 1993). Thus, they are at particularly high risk for physical consequences of tobacco use later on, and some of these consequences begin their course in adolescence (e.g., high-density lipoprotein level changes) (Dwyer, Rieger-Ndakorerwa, Semmer, Fuchs, & Lippert, 1988). In addition, these youth are likely to become subject to negative social stereotyping by nonusers, which could perpetuate further negative behavior (e.g., other substance abuse) through a self-fulfilling prophesy (see Fishkin et al., 1993; Flay, 1993).

The prevalence of regular adolescent smoking in the United States decreased by only 1% between 1981 and 1991, and it has been increasing over the past 8 years by approximately 1% per year (Johnston, O'Malley, & Bachman, 1998). In 1997, 37% of high school seniors had smoked a cigarette in the past 30 days, and 25% of high school seniors were daily smokers (Johnston et al., 1998). Recent efforts by the Centers for Disease Control and Prevention, National Cancer Institute, American Medical Association, adolescent drug abuse inpatient facilities, schools, and numerous different research groups continue to examine the possibility that tobacco use cessation rates among adolescents can be increased (Institute of Medicine [IOM], 1994; Sussman, Lichtman, Ritt, & Pallonen, 1999; U.S. Department of Health and Human Services [DHHS], 1994).

ADOLESCENT TOBACCO USE CESSATION CLINICS: LAUDABLE NOTION BUT DISAPPOINTING RESULTS

Adolescent tobacco use cessation presents a disappointing prospect at present. Generally, 40% of adolescent smokers who have smoked in the past month report having tried to quit (mostly self-initiated cessation) at some point in the past and failed (IOM, 1994; U.S. DHHS, 1994). Although 53% of adolescent smokers report an interest in quitting tobacco use in the next 6 months, only approximately 18% of adolescent smokers are ready to take action and try to quit in the next 30 days (Pallonen, Rossi, Smith, Prochaska, & Almeida, 1993). Only 1% to 2% of heavy lifetime adolescent smokers (e.g., smoked more than 100 cigarettes; now smoke 10 cigarettes per day or more) report self-initiated quitting for at least a 30-day period (Sussman, Dent, Severson, Burton, & Flay, 1998; U.S. DHHS, 1994).

Current school-based clinic cessation program outcomes are disappointing. A variety of reports indicate that immediate postclinic smoking point prevalence cessation rates average 21%, and 3-month follow-up results have ranged from 10% to 15% (sometimes assuming that dropouts were still tobacco users) (Sussman, Dent, Burton, Stacy, & Flay, 1995; Sussman et al., 1999; U.S. DHHS, 1994). A clinic approach is likely to be well received within a school context because time is focused on those who most need it and not on those who may not need it (as in classroom-based programming), and this approach demands less self-reliance than would be entailed in the use of self-help materials. Because the school-based clinic model remains a necessary modality for the introduction of effective programming among adolescents, the means to improve such programming are needed.

REASONS FOR NOT QUITTING TOBACCO USE

Youth report several of the same reasons for difficulty quitting tobacco use as adults, including psychosocial reasons (e.g., social influences) and dependence symptoms. Several preexisting adolescent cessation interventions are built on two theoretical frameworks: psychosocial and chemical dependency counteraction. First, **psychosocial variables** are theorized to be relatively important reasons for not quitting and for relapse. In fact, those youth who report receiving more cigarette offers and who report having friends who smoke have been found to be less likely to quit smoking (Sussman, Dent, Severson, Burton, & Flay, 1998). Skills to learn how to avoid or cope with tobacco use situations have been thought to be of great importance among adolescents (Sussman et al., 1995).

Second, **tobacco use dependence** has been hypothesized as delaying attempts at quitting. More than half of adolescent smokers who try to quit report withdrawal symptoms, an indication of level of addiction or dependence on nicotine. Reports of withdrawal symptoms among adolescents include craving, irritability, insomnia, hunger, and difficulty concentrating (e.g., McNeill, West, Jarvis, Jackson, & Bryant, 1986; Sussman, Dent, Severson, et al., 1998). Information on addiction (as a shorter-term health consequence), withdrawal symptoms, strategies of quitting (e.g., tapering or abrupt withdrawal, substitutes), and coping with urges to use (e.g., "waiting it out," "seeing a slip all the way through") have been considered to be major intervention strategies to facilitate successful quit attempts (e.g., Sussman et al., 1995; Sussman, Dent, Severson, et al., 1998).

If one is motivated to quit, then learning how to counteract both psychosocial reasons to continue using and withdrawal symptoms is quite important. However, most adolescent tobacco users are motivated to quit in 6 months but not in the next 30 days (Pallonen et al., 1993). Thus, another reason that youth do not quit (or relapse) includes a general **lack of motivation** to quit now as opposed to the future.

NEED TO CONSIDER MOTIVATION

Although many theories address attitudes about tobacco use, they do not consider the importance of motivation to learn new skills and follow through with quit attempts (Aubrey, 1996; Miller & Rollnick, 1991). We posit that youth consider at least two components of motivation when they think about quitting tobacco use: **direction/goal** and **effort/energy** (see Nezami, Sussman, & Pentz, in press, for more details). First, they consider "why" they should not continue to engage in tobacco use (direction). As noted by Miller and Rollnick (1991), "A discrepancy [made explicit] between present behavior and important goals will motivate change" (p. 58). The **direction/goal** component of motivation is guided by at least three types of perceived discrepancies: (a) between one's possible or ideal social and vocational selves and one's now or real selves (desire for self-image change), (b) between environmental or informational unknowns and knowns (curiosity), and (c) between one's desired and current mood states (desire for mood enhancement). One is motivated toward an alignment between one's desired and one's subjectively real state. Thus, categories of motivational goals can be arranged as a function of self, information, and affect.

The second component of motivation that youth consider is how much **effort/energy** they are willing to expend to change their behavior. Although unobtained goals tend to reflect discrepancies between perceptions of possible and present behaviors or events, the energy component reflects sources of "pushes" or "pulls" to achieve the different goals. Three sources of energy for change include (a) matching of one's perceived response repertoire with the demands of reaching the goal (not being under- or overchallenged; capacity match), (b) one's embeddedness in a culture or lifestyle about which a comfortable end state is perceived to be reached (i.e., subjective lifestyle stability), and (c) social or intrapersonal pressure to change (subjective pressure). One is more likely to exert energy to change in some direction when one perceives that his or her capacity to change matches the challenge, does not feel embedded in a stable or comfortable lifestyle, and experiences subjective pressure to change. These three dynamic elements may operate simultaneously to affect whether one will make a movement toward change. We anticipate that manipulation of these energy elements (capacity match, subjective lifestyle stability, subjective pressure) crossed with a manipulation of each goal type (self-image, information, mood) is needed to induce a real effort to quit tobacco use among adolescents. As one example, one is more likely to seek a more positive mood state (goal), given that one perceives a discrepancy between his or her current mood state and desired (more positive) mood state and if one also feels the subjective capacity to accomplish the goal.

USE OF FOCUS GROUPS

Focus group methodology is among the most widely used qualitative research tools in the applied social sciences (Basch, 1987; Stewart & Shamdasani, 1990). This approach has been described as being applicable to various aspects of research, including exploratory or hypothesis generation, clinical uses (assessing respondents' nonverbal as well as verbal behavior), phenomenological uses (generating data within a group process-oriented setting), and confirmatory uses (interpreting results obtained through quantitative methods). This method has been proposed as a means to advance health education approaches (Basch, 1987;

Stewart & Shamdasani, 1990) and has been used fruitfully in the development of adolescent tobacco use prevention (Heimann-Ratain, Hanson, & Peregoy, 1985; Worden et al., 1988) and tobacco use or marijuana use cessation programs (Sussman, Burton, Dent, Stacy, & Flay, 1991; Weiner, Sussman, McCuller, & Lichtman, 1999), as well as a means to uncover reasons why youth drink and drive (Basch, DeCicco, & Malfetti, 1989).

Focus group procedures generally involve having a well-trained facilitator ask open-ended questions of a small group of 6 to 12 consumers. Research studies may use a standard format involving progressively more specific questions within the same group or successive groups. Although the data obtained from such groups are qualitative, it is possible that they are less fraught with response demands and can help obtain more in-depth responses, especially regarding sensitive topics, than use of a self-report questionnaire method. In addition, the experimenter has more control over group process than with some other qualitative methods such as participant observation. Furthermore, group responses can be recorded and coded into a quantitative response system, or use of pretest and posttest questionnaires can supplement information gathered from the focus group.

CONTEXT OF THE PRESENT STUDY

Continuation high schools were established in 1919 pursuant to the California Educational Code (Section 48400), which requires continued (part-time) education for all California youth until reaching 18 years of age. Usually, students who are experiencing life difficulties when beginning comprehensive high school transfer to continuation high schools where hours are more flexible and the teacher/student ratio is twice as high as that at comprehensive schools (i.e., 1:15 vs. 1:30). Every school district that has an enrollment of more than 100 students in 12th grade must have a continuation school program; there are more than 500 continuation high schools in the state of California. Continuation high school students report much higher levels of cigarette smoking (but not smokeless tobacco use) than traditional high school students (i.e., smoking at least weekly on a current use measure is approximately 47% vs. 15%, respectively, at mean age = 16.5 years) (DeMoor et al., 1994; Sussman, Dent, Stacy, & Craig, 1998). These specialized schools may provide the additional personal attention needed to help youth correct deficiencies in life skills, increase bonding with social institutions, and otherwise help them to surmount risks for tobacco or other drug abuse. However, continuation high school students also are exposed on a daily basis to numerous other students who use tobacco, and attitudes favorable to tobacco use are likely to be shaped and supported by other youth in such an environment.

In summary, there is an immediate need for the development of successful adolescent tobacco use cessation clinics for continuation high school youth. Considering that approximately 50% of these high school students are already regular smokers, tobacco use prevention efforts may not be successful, and few clinic studies have been attempted with any population (Sussman, Dent, Stacy, & Craig, 1998; Sussman et al., 1999). An iterative focus group format was used to generate information motivating youth to remain in a cessation clinic program, try to quit, and sustain a successful quit effort.

▶ METHOD

FOCUS GROUP PROTOCOL

Groups met for a 30-minute period to generate themes that might motivate youth to quit during the course of a cessation clinic. Each group of 9 to 16 ($M = 12.3$) students consisted of single classrooms of volunteers who met for one period. The participation refusal rate across these groups was less than 1%. A four-page, 30-item pretest questionnaire tapped information on demographics, tobacco use behaviors, and attitudes regarding quitting tobacco use. Open-ended questions were guided in part by the direction-energy motivation model. Verbatim notes were recorded on all strategies suggested to facilitate attempts at quitting and staying quit. A written record of focus group data was appropriate because this method protects against identification of any individuals (as opposed to use of an audiotape)—maximizing the participation rate—and this method was able to retain an exhaustive sample of responses within this population. Focus group data were compiled using qualitative analysis strategies (e.g., Dey, 1993).

The focus groups were run in an iterative style. Each set of questions in subsequent rounds was derived from responses to questions in prior rounds. Nineteen focus groups were completed, which involved 233 subjects from six schools. The first focus group study was conducted the first week of May 1997. Subjects were selected from two classes at two continuation high schools and three classes at a third school ($N = 94$, from seven classes). The Round (version) 1 focus group questionnaire consisted of a 27-item pretest self-report questionnaire, followed by focus group discussion. The focus group measure consisted of 16 general items.

The second focus group study was conducted the third week of May 1997. Subjects were selected from four classes at one continuation high school ($N = 42$). The Round 2 focus group questionnaire consisted of the same 27-item pretest self-report questionnaire, followed by focus group discussion. The focus group measure consisted of 27 general items.

The third focus group study was conducted the second week of October 1997. Subjects were selected from four classes at one continuation high school ($N = 34$). The Round 3 focus group questionnaire consisted of a 30-item pretest self-report questionnaire (which included items on daily smoking), followed by focus group discussion. The focus group measure consisted of 27 general items.

The fourth and final focus group study was conducted the last week of October 1997. Subjects were selected from four classes at one continuation high school ($N = 63$). The Round 4 focus group questionnaire consisted of the same 30-item pretest self-report questionnaire as in Round 3, followed by focus group discussion. The focus group measure consisted of 17 general items.

Two types of focus group questions were asked. The first set of questions was fairly standard and asked adolescents about reasons for smoking, reasons for quitting, and perceived efficacious activities. In addition, a few items requested information on hypothesized motivators of cessation, which were adapted from previous drug abuse prevention work among continuation high school youth (Sussman, Dent, Stacy, & Craig, 1998): (a) not being stereotyped, (b) being perceived as a moderate, and (c) placing an importance on health as a value. The second set focused on the drive-energy model of motivation. Direction variables for change include curiosity about quitting, feeling better (tobacco and mood), and self-image improvement. Energy variables for change include feeling the capacity for change (coping with withdrawal), desire for lifestyle stability (smoker's lifestyle), and feeling pressure to change (see Table 10.1).

SUBJECTS

Across groups, mean age of the subjects was 16.5 ($SD = 0.8$); 61% were male, 26% were White, 48% were Latino, 11% were African American, 4% were Asian, 4% were Native American, and 7% were of "other" ethnicity. Of the sample, 55% smoked at least once in the past 30 days ($n = 127$ current smokers), and, of these smokers, they smoked a mean of 62.2 times in the past 30 days. Also, in focus group Rounds 3 and 4, wherein it was assessed directly, 42% of the sample were daily smokers (76% of the smokers), and this subsample smoked an average of 9.6 cigarettes per day. One stages-of-change item was asked (e.g., Sussman et al., 1995). Across groups, 20% of the smokers reported being in a precontemplation stage of change, 38% reported being in a contemplation stage, 9% reported being in an action stage, and 33% reported having entered a maintenance stage (i.e., just quit and trying to stay stopped).

A total of 63% of the smokers reported that they would quit in the future, and 25% thought they might quit in the future. Also, 53% of the smokers reported having tried to quit in the past. Finally, 52% of the smokers reported that they would or might be willing to participate in a school-based quit program. In

TABLE 10.1 Evolution of Key Focus Group Questions Over Four Rounds

Topic	Round 1	Round 2	Round 3	Round 4
Obstacles to quitting	Question 1: What are obstacles to quitting cigarette smoking among adolescents?	Question 27: What are the main obstacles to quitting smoking? How would one defeat such obstacles?		
Coping with withdrawal	Question 4: How can youth be better able to tolerate cigarette withdrawal symptoms?	Question 16: How can you deal with friends who smoke when you are quitting smoking?	Question 2: What would you like to know about how ex-smokers cope with withdrawal symptoms?	Question 1: Do you think coping with withdrawal symptoms (feelings of emotional or physical discomfort an addicted person may feel when his or her body is not given nicotine) is easier when you are younger or older? Why?
Psychological addiction	Question 7: What are the emotional/ psychological dependencies teenagers have to cigarette smoking?	Question 1: How does smoking help you pass the time? Explain.		Question 4: Some students say they want a cigarette when they feel angry, stressed, or bored. How can people get through these feelings without smoking?
Improving one's image	Question 11: If youth quit smoking, will that help change their group image to others? Is this reason a motivator for quitting?	Question 7: How might quitting cigarettes possibly make you think differently about yourself as a person?	Question 10: Would quitting smoking make you feel like a more successful person? How would it make you feel about yourself?	Question 15: How would you describe someone who was successful in quitting smoking (e.g., independent)?
Motivation to quit	Question 14: What would motivate adolescents/teens to quit smoking?			

Topic	Round 1	Round 2	Round 3	Round 4
Content of quit tobacco program	Question 16: What clinic lesson material would best motivate youth to quit smoking?		Question 24: Do you think it would be helpful to involve the associated student body in planning anti-tobacco activities for the school and community? Why or why not?	Question 17: How can a school community show its support for students who decide to quit smoking?
Curiosity about quitting		Question 2: Are you curious about what quitting would be like? What is mysterious or unknown to you about quitting? Explain.	Question 2: What would you like to know about how ex-smokers cope with withdrawal symptoms?	
Tobacco and your mood		Question 6: How would quitting cigarettes possibly make you feel better emotionally (i.e., happier)?	Question 20: What are some ways people can feel more self-confident? Can quitting smoking help increase self-esteem? How?	Question 6: What do you think someone's mood would be like 1 week after quitting? What do you think someone's mood would be like 6 months after quitting?
Smoker's lifestyle		Question 12: How might quitting smoking help you to achieve a more stable lifestyle?		Question 3: In what situations do nonsmokers have more freedom than smokers (e.g., when they choose a restaurant, they don't have to worry about whether it has a smoking section)?
Social pressure to quit		Question 13: Is there any pressure for you to quit? How much pressure is there and from what sources? Explain.	Question 14: How do you feel when people tell you not to smoke?	Question 10: In what circumstances might you feel ashamed of smoking?

summary, approximately 50% of the sample were smokers (80% of whom smoked an average of half a pack a day), and 50% of them might participate in a quit program at school; that is, a maximum of 25% of a given continuation high school would be expected to become quit clinic attendees.

The focus groups were similar to each other in composition, although a few instances of interround variation were observed. In particular, the first round of focus groups was relatively larger than the others (40% of the total sample, seven vs. four groups in the other rounds). Also, in the third round of focus groups, there was a relatively greater percentage of African Americans (26% vs. an average of 7%) and Asian Americans (12% vs. an average of 2%) and a correspondingly lower percentage of Whites (12% vs. an average of 26%). Tobacco use data were quite similar across groups. The only exception to these tobacco data was that youth in the third round reported slightly lower use rates in the past 30 days compared to other groups (49% vs. an average of 55% of sample), and they were slightly more willing to attend school-based cessation programming (66% vs. an average of 49%). These findings are consistent with previous work that indicates lower smoking rates and increased willingness to quit smoking among African American and Asian American adolescents (Sussman, Dent, Severson, et al., 1998).

▶ FOCUS GROUP RESULTS

Items selected for presentation herein were those that either (a) tapped the six motivation themes, (b) were not specific-focused items (e.g., "How long do quit attempts among adolescents usually last?" [Round 1, Question 2] is too response specific to be very useful for a focus group context), or (c) succeeded in yielding responses across all groups within a round (e.g., "What are some cigarette smoking withdrawal symptoms?" [Round 1, Question 5] and "How could one better cope with each of these symptoms [list]?" [Round 1, Question 6] led to incomplete or no responses in some groups). There was, in most instances, only one response generated per question per group. This is common within this population. Interrater agreement was checked across health educators who led different groups, and it is near or at 100% within each round.

ROUND 1 FOCUS GROUPS: KEY RESPONSES (OF SEVEN GROUPS)

1. What are obstacles to quitting cigarette smoking among adolescents?

Responses: significant others smoke (six groups), addiction (five groups), availability (three groups), everybody smokes (one group), cool thing to do (one group), and stress (one group).

4. How can youth be better able to tolerate cigarette withdrawal symptoms?

   Responses: chew on things (five groups), keep busy (e.g., sports, thinking, work) (four groups), smoke marijuana (two groups), change to new friends (two groups), make the patch cheaper (one group), smoke lower-nicotine brands (one group), and seek social support (one group).

7. What are the emotional/psychological dependencies teenagers have to cigarette smoking?

   Responses: get used to smoking while engaging in other activities (drinking, after sex, after work) (five groups), get used to smoking at certain times during the day (three groups), smoke to cope with stress (three groups), smoke as a way to pass the time (two groups), smoke as a basis of friendship (one group), and get used to the smell, taste (one group).

11. If youth quit smoking, will that help change their group image to others? Explain.

    Responses: smoking is not really related to self- or social image (four groups), people will look up to you if you quit smoking (one group), and people look at continuation high school youth as losers no matter what they do (one group).

14. What would motivate adolescents/teens to quit smoking?

    Responses: money (five groups), found ways to stay busy (four groups), girlfriend/boyfriend against it (two groups), got sick from it (two groups), someone close got sick from it (two groups), and embarrassment (one group).

16. What clinic lesson material would best motivate youth to quit?

    Responses: use of small groups/sharing (two groups), listening better to smokers' problems (one group), focus on individual differences in programming (one group), make use of young ex-users (one group), provide realistic information (one group), make use of social support (one group), use of pharmacological adjuncts (one group), and make use of group pressure (one group).

The first set of focus groups revealed that both social influences and chemical dependency were relatively important reasons for tobacco use and that cues to smoke were associated with various activities and locations throughout the youths' daily lives. Also, chewing behavior and structured time were relatively important means to deal with withdrawal symptoms. It was not clear that stereotyping of continuation high school youth would be altered through quitting smoking; rather, monetary motives and means to keep busy seemed major motivators to quit. Youth showed little consensus about the composition of effective clinic material, although a trusting and intimate environment clearly is desired.

A summary of means of quitting suggestions, examined across all focus group questions, includes the following: (a) chew things such as gum; (b) keep busy, especially physical activity participation; (c) seek social support and stay away from smokers; and (d) use a pharmacological adjunct, if affordable. In terms of drug abuse prevention motives (Sussman, Dent, Stacy, & Craig, 1998), it was found that (a) quitting can result in people looking up to you, but there still are other stereotypes that continuation high school youth need to contend with; (b) conforming with a moderate self-perspective may lead only some people to quit smoking; and (c) health is viewed as an important value and is incongruent with smoking.

ROUND 2 FOCUS GROUPS: KEY RESPONSE (OF FOUR GROUPS)

The second set of focus groups yoked items more specifically to the six types of motivation themes. In addition, in two of the four classes, the focus group questions were administered to students to fill out during the discussion ($n = 7$ and $n = 9$). To equally weight across the four classes, we counted multiple, specific endorsements within a group only once.

1. How does smoking help you pass the time? Explain.

   Responses: it cures boredom (four groups), it relaxes me (three groups), takes mind off stresses (two groups), something to do with hands (one group), improves concentration (one group), and instead of eating (one group).

2. Are you curious about what quitting would be like? What is mysterious or unknown to you about quitting?

Responses: how someone could stay stopped/what discipline is about (three groups), why would someone quit when one must die sooner or later (one group), and how does one deal with boredom (one group).

6. How would quitting cigarettes possibly make you feel better emotionally (i.e., happier)?

    Responses: feel proud/accomplished that I quit (three groups), feel healthier (run farther, more energy) (two groups), happier (two groups), make others I care about feel happier/respect me (two groups), and no more mood swings (one group).

7. How might quitting cigarettes possibly make you think differently about yourself as a person?

    Responses: feel cleaner (two groups), feel more attractive (two groups), feel healthier (two groups), have more confidence in self (two groups), and feel more cool (one group).

10. Might you have the ability to quit smoking if you really wanted to? How would you get yourself to be able to endure withdrawal all day? Explain.

    Responses: keep busy (three groups), chew or eat something (candy/carrots/gum) (three groups), don't think about smoking (two groups), smoke marijuana (two groups), get help from friends (one group), stay away from smokers (one group), hang around nonsmokers (one group), and throw cigarettes away (one group).

12. How might quitting smoking help you to achieve a more stable lifestyle?

    Responses: healthier/more active (two groups), have more money (one group), better lifestyle (one group), and look younger longer (one group).

13. Is there any pressure for you to quit? How much pressure is there and from what sources? Explain.

    Responses: everyone who cares about me/family and friends (three groups), my mother (two groups), my parents (two groups), girlfriend/boyfriend/friends (two groups), sports participation demands/need physical energy (one group), and myself (one group).

27. What are the main obstacles to quitting smoking? (List). How would one defeat each obstacle?

Responses: don't hang around smokers (three groups), keep busy (two groups), replace with a better habit (two groups), get rid of advertisements (two groups), reduce accessibility at stores (two groups), get rid of all your cigarettes (one group), chew gum and keep your fingers busy (one group), tell people you want to quit (one group), be strong and pray (one group), ask smokers in family not to smoke around you (one group), get assistance for nicotine addiction (one group), and quit with a friend (one group).

This round revealed a lot more useful information. Considering all the information generated across all items, numerous suggestions were made. Regarding the direction component of motivation, suggestions were the following:

Curiosity about cessation:

1. What would one do when bored or tense? This is the major task to learn.
2. What is the quitting discipline like? How hard is it to quit and stay stopped? This is the other major task to learn.
3. Is it possible to ever smoke a little?
4. Why is it better not to smoke? What are the rewards of quitting? These include feeling good, receiving more social support, and saving money.
5. Is it possible to hang around smokers as an ex-smoker?
6. How long does nicotine stay in the body?

Feeling better:

1. Feel more respected by others/accomplished; this pride is the major perceived outcome
2. Having more energy
3. Happier
4. Less stressed
5. No more mood swings

Self-image:

1. More confidence/self-esteem
2. More self-control
3. Cleaner, more attractive, healthier

4. More positive attitude
5. More cool

Regarding the energy component of motivation, numerous suggestions were made:

Capacity match:
1. Keep busy/don't think about it; this is a main doable skill
2. Eat carrots/chew gum; this is another doable behavior
3. Be with nonusers
4. Throw cigarettes away

Lifestyle stability:
1. Live longer/be more active; this is the main endorsed response here
2. Be more serene
3. Better social life

Pressure to quit:
1. Everyone who cares about me; main response
2. Sports
3. Family
4. Friends
5. Teachers

When questions are prefaced with more specific prompts, many more responses are generated. This information provides the beginnings of motivation features that could be placed into an adolescent tobacco use cessation curriculum. One key obstacle is to figure out how not to hang around other smokers.

ROUND 3 FOCUS GROUPS: KEY RESPONSES (OF FOUR GROUPS)

The third set of focus groups also yoked items to the six types of motivation themes, as in Round 2, using some of the responses from the previous round.

2. What would you like to know about how ex-smokers cope with withdrawal symptoms?

   Responses: how do they cope (two groups).

8. What effect would quitting have on your mood in the short run? In the long run?

   Responses: more mellow in the long run (one group), shake in short run and live longer in long run (one group).

10. Would quitting smoking make you feel like a more successful person? How would it make you feel about yourself?

    Responses: more self-control/something to brag about (two groups) and more healthy (one group).

14. How do you feel when people tell you not to smoke?

    Responses: get mad (one group), offended (one group), it would bother me if my child were to tell me (one group), and I would listen to them if they used to be a smoker (one group).

20. What are some ways people can feel more self-confident? Can quitting smoking help increase self-esteem? How?

    Responses: feel good on inside and outside (one group), people who care about you would be off your case (one group), depends on what is available to replace smoking (one group), and can feel like they can accomplish goals, personal power (one group).

24. Do you think it would be helpful to involve the associated student body in planning anti-tobacco activities for the school and community? Why or why not?

    Responses: maybe, if they can find activities everybody likes (two groups); yes, they won't be smoking while they are doing it (one group); yes, adults seeing young adults doing something constructive in the community would be a good thing (one group).

This round included specific, open-ended items that apparently were too complex to complete within the focus group format. Little useful data resulted. Two groups saw quitting as being a mood-lifting, stabilizing event in the long run. It was difficult for smokers to visualize a change of mood after going through a sustained withdrawal syndrome. Also, smokers could see quitting without having something they could "take" to replace this activity with. Three groups recognized a positive impact on overall self-esteem by quitting. Most youth saw the value of using the associated student body to generate school-as-community events, with feelings that it might be a constructive thing to do even if no impact is felt on smoking.

ROUND 4 FOCUS GROUPS: KEY RESPONSES (OF FOUR GROUPS)

The fourth set of focus groups also yoked items specifically to the six types of motivation themes. This round attempted to clarify and refine questions from the third round.

1. Do you think coping with withdrawal symptoms (feelings of emotional or physical discomfort addicted persons may feel when their body is not given nicotine) is easier when you are younger or older? Why?

   Responses: younger smokers have more of an open mind, they are less cranky, and they are not as dependent on it (three groups); older smokers are more afraid of dying and they can handle more stress than younger smokers (two groups). (Note: One group was split on its perspectives here.)

3. In what situations do nonsmokers have more freedom than smokers (e.g., when they choose a restaurant, they don't have to worry about whether it has a smoking section)?

   Responses: more access to public areas such as parks/hiking (two groups), airplanes (one group), jail (one group), cigarettes are expensive (one group), hotels (one group), don't have to worry about money or going to the store (one group), and physical activity (one group).

4. Some students say that they want a cigarette when they feel angry, stressed, or bored. How can people get through these feelings without smoking?

   Responses: do something creative/keep your head busy (three groups), watch a movie (three groups), chew or eat something (two groups), go work out (two groups), get a stress toy (doll, ball) (one group), smoke marijuana (one group), go to sleep (one group), get a job (one group), talk to someone (one group), and yoga (one group).

6. What do you think someone's mood would be like 1 week after quitting? What do you think someone's mood would be like 6 months after quitting?

   Responses: from irritable, stressed, cranky, aggressive, and whiny to calm and normal (two groups); from too much energy and saying dumb things to improved breathing, relaxed, calm, and proud (two groups).

10. In what circumstances might you feel ashamed of smoking?

Responses: smoking with a disease or seeing others smoking while they are diseased (one group); dating situations (one group); when around nonsmokers, especially when they complain about it (one group); old, retired people (one group); and church (one group).

15. How would you describe someone who was successful in quitting smoking (e.g., independent)?

    Responses: strong (four groups); bad, cool (two groups); knows what they want (two groups); successful (one group); persistent (one group); patient (one group); and "on check" with others' wishes for them (one group).

17. How can a school community show its support for students who decide to quit smoking?

    Responses: give them nicotine gum or patch (two groups), congratulate them personally (two groups), throw them a party (one group), make note of it in the school newspaper (one group), give prizes (one group), help to keep them busy while quitting (one group), and provide quit-smoking classes (one group).

Generally, support was obtained for quitting while young. This information was used to develop one of the theme study activities later on in the program development sequence. Keeping one's mind on something other than smoking was considered of major importance for quitting. The mention of other activities and the mention of yoga led to the development of another theme study activity. With a clarified question on change in mood after quitting, the focus group participants did see mood as improving in a number of positive ways 6 months after quitting. This notion led to the creation of another theme study activity. Ex-smokers were looked at as strong individuals; that influenced development of yet another theme study activity (see Chapter 12, this volume).

▶ DISCUSSION

The use of the focus group is a great idea-generating device. Certainly, there is an advantage to using focus group rounds-type information (Table 10.1 shows flow of questions from round to round). Without use of this iterative protocol, information is lost. Simple, open-ended questions elicit the same old responses: One needs to prompt responding. For example, when asked what would make youth want to quit tobacco use, youth often report "if someone they knew had died" or "if a friend pushed them to quit." The same responses were derived in 1990

(Sussman et al., 1995) in a different group of youth (comprehensive high school youth). The iterative focus group approach, with use of different prompts on successive rounds, can permit a sculpting of information from groups of youth.

Of course, although very popular, focus groups are only one of a number of program development tools. It should be supplemented with other approaches to get a better assessment of the "truth" (e.g., questionnaires, theme studies). Also, the quality of any given focus group is limited by its subjects, skills of the facilitator, and domain of questions asked. Clearly, other sources of information (theory and previous work) are needed to guide the types of questions used. For example, a school-based clinic approach was addressed in the present study. However, other approaches to adolescent cessation have been attempted. The only school-based study that achieved an immediate cessation rate more than 13% was a classroom-based program (Perry, Telch, Killen, Burke, & Maccoby, 1983). However, classroom cessation programs are relatively unlikely to be acceptable to high school administrators because such programs may be perceived as being of low priority or as interfering with other course work for a large number of students who are not tobacco users (Sussman, Petosa, & Clarke, 1996). One other study of a 2-year intensive community-wide intervention for smoking and nutrition with 13- to 15-year-old students in east Finland yielded an immediate posttest cessation rate of 37% for boys and 35% for girls, compared to a spontaneous cessation rate of 0% for the no-treatment group (Pallonen, 1987). Unfortunately, such a long-term, intensive, community-wide intervention is beyond the monetary scope or priorities of many local communities (though priorities change). A school-based clinic model remains a necessary modality for the introduction of effective programming among adolescents.

REFERENCES ◄

AUBREY, L. L. (1996, February). *Motivational enhancement therapy (MET) for adolescent substance abusers.* Paper presentation for the Tobacco Cessation Project for Youth, AMA-CDC, Chicago.

BASCH, C. E. (1987). Focus group interview: An underutilized research technique for improving theory and practice in health education. *Health Education Quarterly, 14,* 411-448.

BASCH, C. E., DECICCO, I. M., & MALFETTI, J. L. (1989). A focus group study on decision processes of young drivers: Reasons that may support a decision to drink and drive. *Health Education Quarterly, 16,* 389-396.

DeMOOR, C., JOHNSTON, D. A., WERDEN, D. L., ELDER, J. P., SENN, K., & WHITEHORSE, L. (1994). Patterns and correlates of smoking and smokeless tobacco use among continuation high school students. *Addictive Behaviors, 19,* 175-184.

DEY, I. (1993). *Qualitative data analysis.* London: Routledge Kegan Paul.

DWYER, J. H., RIEGER-NDAKORERWA, G. E., SEMMER, N. K., FUCHS, R., & LIPPERT, P. (1988). Low-level cigarette smoking and longitudinal change in serum cholesterol among adolescents. *Journal of the American Medical Association, 259,* 2857-2862.

FISHKIN, S. A., SUSSMAN, S., STACY, A. W., DENT, C. W., BURTON, D., & FLAY, B. R. (1993). Ingroup versus outgroup perceptions of the characteristics of high risk youth: Negative stereotyping. *Journal of Applied Social Psychology, 23,* 1051-1058.

FLAY, B. R. (1993). Youth tobacco use: Risks, patterns, and control. In C. T. Orleans & J. Slade (Eds.), *Nicotine addiction: Principles and management* (pp. 365-384). New York: Oxford University Press.

HEIMANN-RATAIN, G., HANSON, M., & PEREGOY, S. M. (1985). The role of focus group interviews in designing a smoking prevention program. *Journal of School Health, 55,* 13-16.

INSTITUTE OF MEDICINE (IOM). (1994). *Growing up tobacco free: Preventing nicotine addiction in youth and adolescents.* Washington, DC: National Academy Press.

JOHNSTON, L. D., O'MALLEY, P. M., & BACHMAN, J. G. (1998). *National survey results on drug use from the Monitoring the Future Study, 1975-1997* (2 vols., NIH Pub. No. 98-4345/6). Rockville, MD: U.S. Department of Health and Human Services.

McNEILL, A. D., WEST, R. J., JARVIS, M., JACKSON, P., & BRYANT, A. (1986). Cigarette withdrawal symptoms in adolescent smokers. *Psychopharmacology, 90,* 533-536.

MILLER, W. R., & ROLLNICK, S. (1991). *Motivational interviewing: Preparing people to change addictive behavior.* New York: Guilford.

NEZAMI, E., SUSSMAN, S., & PENTZ, M. A. (in press). Motivation in tobacco use cessation research. *Substance Use & Misuse.*

PALLONEN, U. E. (1987, January). *Smoking cessation in adolescence.* Paper presented at the Western Area Conference on Psychosocial Research, American Cancer Society, California Division, Los Angeles.

PALLONEN, U. E., ROSSI, J. S., SMITH, N. F., PROCHASKA, J. O., & ALMEIDA, P. M. (1993, March). *Applying the stages of change and processes of change concepts to adolescent smoking cessation.* Poster presentation at the Society of Behavioral Medicine, 14th Annual Scientific Sessions, San Francisco.

PERRY, C. L., TELCH, M. J., KILLEN, J., BURKE, R., & MACCOBY, N. (1983). High school smoking prevention: The relative efficacy of varied treatments and instructions. *Adolescence, 18,* 561-566.

STEWART, D. W., & SHAMDASANI, P. M. (1990). *Focus groups: Theory and practice.* Newbury Park, CA: Sage.

SUSSMAN, S., BURTON, D., DENT, C. W., STACY, A., & FLAY, B. R. (1991). Use of focus groups in developing an adolescent tobacco use cessation program: Collective norm effects. *Journal of Applied Social Psychology, 21,* 1772-1782.

SUSSMAN, S., DENT, C. W., BURTON, D., STACY, A. W., & FLAY, B. R. (1995). *Developing school-based tobacco use prevention and cessation programs.* Thousand Oaks, CA: Sage.

SUSSMAN, S., DENT, C. W., SEVERSON, H. H., BURTON, D., & FLAY, B. R. (1998). Self-initiated quitting among adolescent smokers. *Preventive Medicine, 27,* A19-A28.

SUSSMAN, S., DENT, C. W., STACY, A. W., & CRAIG, S. (1998). One-year outcomes of Project Towards No Drug Abuse. *Preventive Medicine, 27,* 632-642, 766 (erratum).

SUSSMAN, S., LICHTMAN, K., RITT, A., & PALLONEN, U. E. (1999). Effects of thirty-four adolescent tobacco use cessation and prevention trials on regular users of tobacco products. *Substance Use & Misuse, 34,* 1469-1505.

SUSSMAN, S., PETOSA, R., & CLARKE, P. (1996). The promotion of empirical curriculum development for the prevention of substance abuse. *American Behavioral Scientist, 39,* 838-852.

U.S. DEPARTMENT OF HEALTH AND HUMAN SERVICES (DHHS). (1994). *Preventing tobacco use among young people: A report of the Surgeon General* (Government Printing Office No. 017-001-00491-0). Atlanta, GA: U.S. Department of Health and Human Services, Public Health Service, Centers of Disease Control and Prevention, National Center for Chronic Disease Prevention and Health Promotion, and Office of Smoking and Health.

WEINER, M. D., SUSSMAN, S., McCULLER, W. J., & LICHTMAN, K. (1999). Factors in marijuana cessation among high-risk youth. *Journal of Drug Education, 29*(4), 337-357.

WORDEN, J. K., FLYNN, B. S., GELLER, B. M., CHEN, M., SHELTON, L. G., SECKER-WALKER, R. H., SOLOMON, D. S., SOLOMON, L. J., COUCHEY, S., & COSTANZA, M. C. (1988). Development of a smoking prevention mass media program using diagnostic and formative research. *Preventive Medicine, 17,* 531-558.

CHAPTER 11

Nonverbal Methods of Perceived Efficacy

Elahe Nezami
Gerald C. Davison
Beth R. Hoffman

Nonverbal methods do not require an audible response; these include paper-and-pencil and object manipulation tasks. Nonverbal protocols are diverse and have been an indispensable part of assessment history, providing us with consequential knowledge in several areas. This type of measurement has been essential in intellectual, personality, educational, neuropsychological, clinical and counseling, industrial and organizational, and consumer assessments, among others. We propose that creative use of nonverbal methods can be applied productively in health behavior research and practice to measure effects on hypothesized mediators of change and the perceived quality of numerous program ideas.

Perceived efficacy studies involve a shorthand presentation of components or ideas regarding a potential program that is provided (e.g., a one-paragraph description of program activities is read to subjects) (Dent, Galaif, Sussman, & Stacy, 1996), which quickly describes or summarizes program components' contents. Judgments are made about the program components' likely short-term and long-term impacts, if they were to be delivered as written. This chapter provides a review of paper-and-pencil instruments that could be used to help construct perceived efficacy studies. More detail regarding perceived efficacy studies is provided in the next section.

PERCEIVED EFFICACY STUDIES

Sussman (1991) suggested that a scientific process should be adopted in developing programs that are intended for health behavior change. He recommended using theory as the first step in this process, followed by a second step of gathering relevant program activities. He proposed that the third step in this process should involve studies that permit the selection of the most effective activities. Finally, the selected activities would be used to produce a complete prevention program. In this scientific process, a program developer's decision making is based on the efficacy of program components in altering mediators of behavior change.

Revisiting the third step of his model, he discussed use of both perceived efficacy studies and studies of immediate impact. Regarding perceived efficacy studies, he discussed that a target sample is informed about different activity ideas, and then this sample selects a subset of activities that are perceived as most effective. The program protocol information provided to the population could include (a) viewing the activity or portions of it on videotape (e.g., Worden et al., 1988), (b) reading paragraphs about the activity (e.g., Dent et al., 1996), (c) reading one sentence or phrase descriptions about an activity (Weiner, Sussman, McCuller, & Lichtman, 1999), (d) viewing a picture that describes an activity in progress (e.g., as with the Thematic Apperception Test) (Rapaport, Gill, & Schafer, 1980), (e) hearing an audiotape or verbal description of the activity (e.g., Hops et al., 1986), or (f) watching a live demonstration of various aspects of the activity. Perceived program quality ratings are shown after delivery of an activity idea and could be of (a) perceived activity novelty or interest, (b) teaching potential or understandability, (c) believability or credibility, and (d) perceived helpfulness in preventing unhealthy behavior or promoting healthy behavior (e.g., Flay, 1981), as well as perceptions of effects on hypothesized mediators of change (likelihood to change certain attitudes or provide certain behavioral skills).

Determining the immediate impact (actual short-term efficacy) of program activities is more time-consuming and costly than use of perceived efficacy studies because, in that instance, each activity actually must be completed in total. Imagine the time it would take to try to discern the relative immediate-outcome efficacy of 50 proposed activities to compose a 15-session program. In contrast, information about the perceived quality of a program and perceptions of likely effects on mediators of change can be gathered on these many activity ideas or descriptions in a relatively brief period of time.

Previous work has shown that few differences in learning exist between activities that are read and rated versus actually engaging in the activities (e.g., knowledge item change scores), although some differences in belief change in the desired direction are found (e.g., Sussman, Dent, Simon, et al., 1995). Perceived efficacy study results have been found to be confirmed by component study results (e.g., Sussman, 1996; Sussman, Dent, Stacy, Burton, & Flay, 1995) and subsequent main trial results (e.g., Sussman, Dent, Stacy, & Craig, 1998). Thus, it would appear fruitful to include perceived efficacy studies within an arsenal of program development studies.

PERCEIVED EFFICACY METHODS ◄

Although a perceived efficacy study does not capture the internal validity and richness of immediate-impact studies, it does, however, provide an important means of screening the receptivity of various target audiences to a wide number of activities. At the very least, a perceived efficacy study will separate good approaches and programs from ones that are destined to fail due to poor receptivity (Aaker & Day, 1990; Breen & Blankenship, 1982). Measurement of a program's perceived likelihood in bringing about behavior change is in many ways similar to consumer assessment in industrial/organizational psychology. In both arenas, one assesses consumer receptivity to a product or service. Essentially, both marketing research and perceived efficacy studies are concerned with consumer attitudes to help screen among potential consumables. For example, a health behavior program activity that instructs teens in the physical consequences of drug use might use any number of different presentations of the material—a team competition, role-plays, or group interaction, as examples. The concepts could be presented to teens, and then ratings of these options might be used to select the best half of a large number of potential activities. This section of the chapter considers two important aspects of perceived efficacy studies: the subject groups that might be involved in this work and specific types of methods.

CONSIDERATION OF TARGET GROUPS

The groups involved in a perceived efficacy study should be a good fit for the target population. The study should meet two criteria to be judged appropriate for a target population. First, the task demands should match the abilities of the population. For example, paper-and-pencil types of perceived efficacy studies are especially appropriate for special groups such as deaf and mute individuals, for whom other forms of data collection such as interviews might be more challenging. On the other hand, these methods would not be suitable for illiterate populations.

Second, the study should be designed to elicit accurate and useful information from the target population. Most programs involve several participant groups—some who are the direct targets of the program, others who feel the effects of the program indirectly, and some who are asked to support implementation of the program. All such parties should be highly receptive to the program and could be involved in perceived efficacy work. For example, youth health education programs (e.g., smoking and drug abuse prevention, diet and exercise promotion, sex education) require participation from recipients or students, families, teachers and school administrators, and health educator experts or researchers. We propose that perceived program efficacy work should involve presentation of program ideas to each of these major groups.

Recipients. The most important stakeholders in any health education program are the recipients ultimately participating in the program, whose cooperation and compliance are essential for success. Intended recipients of a program ultimately are most likely to know which methods of presentation or program ideas will hold their interest and may influence their future behavior, though sometimes other groups may be more likely to know which types of information are appropriate. For example, youth might not be expected to select among program contents about which they know very little (e.g., can a 10-year-old discern the specifics of a good diet?).

Families. Families are important stakeholders in youth health education programs. Families' attitudes toward health behavior and their support of their children's behavior could provide important information for designing and refining intervention programs. For example, family involvement to support a healthy diet would play a significant role in altering children's dietary behavior. Health program components that are interesting to families are likely to be carried out and practiced more often in the home environment. In addition, if the proposed intervention is controversial (e.g., birth control information), family involvement is very important. If families are involved in the development of a program with sensitive information, they will support its implementation more than if they are not involved in the process.

Officials/Gatekeepers. Institutional settings pose unique challenges and restrictions. For example, in the school system, availability of space, distinct regulations, and classroom schedules should be considered. Health behavior programs must be acceptable and feasible to schools, particularly to the administrators approving them and the teachers implementing them. Teachers and administrators are going to be more likely to support and correctly implement a program that they consider efficacious, interesting, and memorable. Their involvement in the program's development also would help support its later implementation (Sussman, Dent, Stacy, et al., 1995). Similar restrictions operate in the worksite and other settings.

Experts. Experts in health education are another group of stakeholders whose opinions about a program component are valuable. This group of persons can provide support to a program based on their knowledge of a program's efficacy in prior research. Previous successes in health behavior programming should be used when developing or selecting components for a new program (see Chapter 7, this volume). Therefore, paper-and-pencil questionnaires could be used to assess experts' opinions about suitability of program components in altering the targeted behavior in different populations. For example, opinions of scientists with expertise in multicultural programming could be consulted when developing program curricula that one desires to be well received by individuals from several ethnic populations.

SPECIFIC METHODS

Perceived program efficacy studies involve a protocol that provides directive, semidirective, or nondirective information. Directive methods are relatively structured to address the perceived quality of an activity or activities that already have been generated through either program developer intuition or previous use of nondirective or semidirective methods. Examples of such methods include having subjects read paragraphs about different activities and then having them rate the activities using Likert ratings, line ratings, bar ratings, rankings, or polls (e.g., Dent et al., 1996).

A semidirective approach is the use of a nondirective technique (described below) along with prompting; that is, responses are cued. For example, one could be asked to write a paragraph about how an activity is likely to affect target subjects' own daily lives. The subject is not simply asked to write a paragraph about the activity but rather is asked to write about how the activity would affect her or him. Likewise, open-ended self-report questionnaire responses to generate activity possibilities to solve a specific program (e.g., "Please list a set of activities that might help teens quit smoking") involve prompting regarding the specific issue.

Nondirective methods examine responses generated spontaneously without directly prompting for such responses (e.g., Stacy, Ames, Sussman, & Dent, 1996). These methods include use of instructions to write a paragraph about an activity (e.g., using a picture or a one-sentence purpose statement as cues) or may involve use of sentence completion tasks, word association tasks, draw-a-person tasks, or activity-sorting tasks to spontaneously generate plausible activity options. Many of the nondirective methods may be adapted from earlier use in personality of diagnostic testing (Rapaport et al., 1980).

This next section presents specific paper-and-pencil presentations of perceived efficacy work. These methods are presented in order from most structured and easier to administer to less structured and requiring more administrative expertise: use of self-report questionnaires, theme studies, card sorting, memory recall, and projective techniques.

Self-Report Questionnaires. Self-report questionnaires are a popular paper-and-pencil approach. Typically, a self-report questionnaire first will gather baseline demographic and target behavior data from respondents. Next, respondents may be asked to rank or select among different activities, provided on a list, for their perceived likelihood in changing a health behavior. Alternatively, subjects may be asked to rate each activity on rating scale items such as interest, believability, and perceived helpfulness. The types of response formats used on questionnaires can vary widely, including, for example, true-false, yes-no, multiple choice (circle all that apply), forced choice (circle one best choice), ranking or numbering, or rating scale responses. Rating scales request that the subject rates how well the activity does on a dimension of perceived program quality—for example, from 0 (*not at all*) to 5 (*very well*).

Self-report questionnaires are quite convenient. Anyone can administer a questionnaire, and a questionnaire can be taken at any time (e.g., self-administration at home), unlike most of the methods discussed below, which require a trained health educator or researcher to be present and for participants to set aside a block of time to participate in the protocol. This makes the questionnaire a good method for measuring the attitudes of large groups of program recipients, gatekeepers, and experts who do not have large amounts of time available and for families, whose work schedules often conflict with data measurement sessions.

Three specific criteria have been proposed for developing questionnaires to assess perceived program quality or perceptions of effects on hypothesized mediators. The first criterion is specificity. This means that only questions that are related in some way to the target behavior should be added to the questionnaire. The second criterion is one of relevance. This criterion means that questions asked should be appropriate for the population under study. For example, relevance of questions in regard to the population's age and ethnicity should be considered (Sussman, Parker, et al., 1995). The third criterion refers to the comprehensiveness of the items. It is important to consider all of the program content domains that are relevant in perceived efficacy studies, and that, in turn, may predict future behavior. Some of the relevant components in perceived efficacy work may include assessment of program activity themes (substantive contents), program delivery modalities proposed (how the contents are likely to be delivered), cognitive abilities requested of the target population, and practicality of trying to implement certain themes or modalities.

The following guidelines are important in preventing errors in measurement. One should use simple language that is understandable to the subjects and avoid specialized words that might be unfamiliar to the audience. One also should write brief questions that thoroughly cover the content domain of the information being assessed (e.g., potential activity contents). Respondents might get bored or tired by lengthy questions, which may lead to lack of cooperation and reduced accuracy in responses. Third, one should stay away from general questions that produce vague responses, and one should try to avoid use of items that ask for more than one response. Answers to this latter type of question, referred to as "double-barreled," can become confusing and hence meaningless. Finally, one should not imply any indications for the answers in the questions. Responses to such questions may invite the participants to answer in the suggested direction and therefore would become subject to what is referred to as a "response demand" bias. (For an in-depth discussion of appropriate wording of questions, see Kalton, Collins, & Brook, 1978; Labaw, 1981; Luck & Rubin, 1987; Sudman & Bradburn, 1982.)

Questionnaires are fairly simple to analyze. Rating scale measures can be compared. For example, program aspects can be selected based on a comparison of mean ratings (e.g., use of critical values; see Chapter 12, this volume). A breakdown of the percentage of participants giving any one response is another typical method of conceptualizing the data, and chi-square analysis might be used. Qualitative measures can be analyzed by computing the frequencies of commonly given responses.

Theme Studies. In theme studies, subjects rate concise narratives (paragraphs) about health behavior change activities for their perceived interest and likelihood-to-change relevant behavior (Sussman, 1991). These activities could be generated by the health professional or by the subject population (Sussman, Dent, Stacy, et al., 1995). A theme study will allow the experimenter to consider different potential components of a prevention program for their perceived program quality (e.g., perceived helpfulness) in a short period of time.

Prior research has indicated the usefulness of theme studies for evaluating program component efficacy. The Project Towards No Tobacco Use (Project TNT) (Sussman, Dent, Stacy, et al., 1995) used different smoking prevention themes generated either by health educators or by students. In this study, there was some overlap between the student- and health educator–generated themes. But, in general, the student-generated themes were more favorably rated by students compared to the health educators' themes.

Dent et al. (1996) evaluated responses of 315 continuation (alternative) high school students to 35 written descriptions of drug abuse prevention themes. The intention of this study was to find the most preferred themes for future drug abuse prevention strategies. Orders of strategies were counterbalanced across subjects. The researchers found that novel themes were rated highly by the students, and comprehensive social influence-type strategies—preferred among lower-risk, younger youth—were least preferred by these youth. They concluded that theme studies could be used to measure desirability of different themes and that new types of programming needed to be developed for these youth.

Theme studies are quite similar in presentation format and analysis to questionnaires and therefore often can be combined with questionnaires as needed (see Chapter 12, this volume, for an example of the use of theme studies to help develop teen tobacco use cessation programming). For this reason, a theme study can be used with all the groups mentioned earlier (i.e., target subjects, significant others, gatekeepers, and experts), if not too much time for completion of the study is demanded.

Card Sorting. Card-sorting assessments historically were used as nonverbal tests of personality or cognitive functioning. The test uses a Q-sort technique in which the participants' task is to group a series of index cards into various categories. Stephenson (1953) developed this technique for a self-report measure of personality. Since then, administration guidelines and variations of design have been developed (e.g., Bem & Funder, 1978; Mischel, 1971).

For program development purposes, this technique could be used to assess interest in or desirability of program components. In this type of assessment, a series of cards depicting (a) various health messages (e.g., "smoking makes you physically unattractive to other people"), (b) alternative modes of delivering health messages (e.g., role-play, group discussion, debate), or (c) messages crossed with delivery modes (e.g., "people debate whether smoking makes one physically unattractive to others") would be developed. Each card would consist of either a picture or a few simple phrases describing the activity.

Participants would be asked to sort these cards in piles of "outstanding and memorable" to "ordinary and unremarkable." After participants complete this task, the card-sort administrator might ask participants why they had put certain cards in each category (this could be done through a nonverbal paper-and-pencil method or through use of a verbal method).

Because the content of a card is limited to a picture or a few phrases, this method is particularly useful for nonexpert groups with limited knowledge of the subject area. Card-sorting methods are particularly ideal for preliterate or illiterate populations if the information is presented in picture form; in addition, this method is ideal for mute individuals because speaking is not necessary to sort the cards. It is also suitable for young participants who easily lose interest and do not respond well to questionnaires. A picture or a phrase may not be interpreted correctly, so care must be taken to ensure that the messages presented are clear.

A card-sorting activity will elicit only ordinally ranked quantitative data (i.e., an individual's results will rank proposed activities from most to least desirable or effective) but will not tell whether one activity was judged greatly superior to another or just slightly better. Because the data collected are ordinal, a tally of the frequency of each ordinal ranking for each program is appropriate. Following the tally, a chi-square test can be used to determine if one activity was given a certain ordinal ranking more frequently than another activity. The addition of an inquiry section in which participants write down their reasoning for putting certain cards in each section can add qualitative value to the data collected.

Memory Recall. Methods for assessing short-term memory recall of program messages could be borrowed from established methods in cognitive science (e.g., neuropsychological) to assess program concepts vicariously. For program development, subjects could be instructed to read several paragraphs containing health messages in the order provided to them (message order is shuffled between each subject). Alternatively, participants could listen to audiotaped recordings of these paragraphs. Then, they could be asked to recall and write down the content of as many of the messages as they can remember. This task of recall and writing the message can be repeated after half an hour of engaging in a different activity to test memory recall following interference. Messages that are best remembered, especially after an interference period, are likely to have made more lasting impressions (note Chapter 5, this volume, on implicit cognition methods).

Although it is beneficial to use this method with the potential recipients of an activity, it is probably not important to determine which method is most memorable to parents or experts. It may be useful, though, to use this method with program gatekeepers (e.g., school staff and administrators) because they may be more eager to implement an activity that is memorable and appealing to them. However, if the task takes too long, gatekeepers may be reluctant to participate.

To analyze the memorability of activities using this method, we conducted a count of the number of people recalling each message before and after the time lapse could be collected. With these data, chi-square tests could determine if more people recalled certain messages before the time lapse, if people recalled messages at different frequencies after the time lapse, and if the memorability of certain messages stayed the same or changed between measures.

Projective Techniques. Projective techniques could be used to construct perceived efficacy studies, as well. Four methods of assessment are discussed herein: word association, sentence completion, written responses to pictures, and articulated thoughts in simulated situations (ATSS). **Word association** is a technique that was first used often by Jung (1919) in experiments on memory and learning. Continued use of this method led psychologists to believe in the utility of word association in measuring attitudes and personality characteristics (e.g., Rapaport et al., 1980; Stacy, Ames, et al., 1996). For example, word association could be used to assess cognitive and emotional reactions of the target population to specific behaviors or strategies for behavior change. Subjects could be instructed to provide the first thought or feeling that comes to mind after hearing the following phrases. In this case, the phrase "smoking cessation activities: group" can generate information about positive or negative attitudes associated with it; the first word coming to mind may be *fun* or *pressure*, for example. Another variation of word association could be to visually demonstrate pieces of a health behavior change program to the target population. Again, the target population would be asked to write down the first words that come to mind while viewing the synopses.

A second projective device for assessing perceived program quality is **sentence completion.** In the word association task, most cues are generated in the instructions to subjects, but the trunk sentence provides most of the cues in this present task. Sentence completion is used in psychological assessment as a personality inventory to reveal information about an individual's pains, desires, defense mechanisms, conflicts, fears, aspirations, and goals in life, among other issues (e.g., Mosher, 1966; Stacy, Galaif, Sussman, & Dent, 1996). Sentence completion also could be used for highly specific and direct evaluations. For example, following the description of plausible components of health behavior program change, incomplete sentences could be used to assess perceived helpfulness and attractiveness of these programs. For example, subjects could be asked to complete the following sentences: "This program activity reminds me of _____," or "This program activity makes me want to _____." Alternatively, subjects could be asked to provide plausibly effective activities by using this technique (e.g., "An activity that could help one quit smoking is by use of _____.").

Written responses to pictures is another projective technique that could be borrowed from personality assessments such as the Thematic Apperception Test (TAT) to compose a perceived efficacy study (Rapaport et al., 1980). The TAT is a projective test in which a series of pictures is presented to a participant who is asked to tell a story about each of them. Pictorial representations of some components for a health behavior change program can be used to create TAT-type pictures to be administered in a group setting similar to TAT presentations. For example, photos depicting refusal assertion training or problem solving could be used to generate evaluations about these activities within a health behavior change context. Written (or verbal) responses of individuals to these pictures could potentially provide useful information about the perceived helpfulness or desirability of the program components.

The **ATSS** method of Davison, Robins, and Johnson (1983) is used to assess immediate thoughts under controlled stimulus conditions. In this procedure, a person pretends that he or she is a participant in a situation, such as listening to a teenager argue against marijuana legalization. Presented on audiotape, the scene pauses every 10 to 15 seconds. During the ensuing 30 seconds of silence, the participant writes down (or talks aloud about) whatever is going through his or her mind in reaction to the words just heard. Then the audiotaped scene continues, stopping after a few moments so that the person can articulate his or her thoughts again. For instance, a taped scene, in which the participant overhears two pretend acquaintances criticizing him or her, could include the following segments:

First acquaintance: He certainly did make a fool of himself over what he wrote down about marijuana use. I just find that kind of opinion very closed-minded and unaware. You have to be blind to the facts of the universe to believe that. [Thirty-second pause for subject's response]

Second acquaintance: What really bugs me is the way he expresses himself. He never seems to stop and think but just writes down the first thing that comes into his head. [Thirty-second pause]

Participants readily become involved in the pretend situations, regarding them as credible and realistic. Cognitive patterns that have emerged from a few of the studies conducted thus far include the following: Socially anxious therapy patients have articulated thoughts of greater irrationality (e.g., "Oh God, I wish I were dead. I'm so embarrassed.") than have nonanxious control subjects (Bates, Campbell, & Burgess, 1990; Davison & Zighelboim, 1987); recent ex-smokers who relapsed within 3 months showed a greater tendency to think of smoking without prompting and also reported fewer negative expectations about the consequences of smoking than did those who remained abstinent 3 months later (Haaga, 1989); and men with borderline hypertension achieved significant reductions in anger, as expressed in their articulated thoughts, and experienced decreases in their blood pressure and heart rate following a program of relaxation training and medical information about diet and exercise (Davison, Williams, Nezami, Bice, & DeQuattro, 1991).

These and related findings (for a recent review of the ATSS literature, see Davison, Vogel, & Coffman, 1997) indicate that this method ferrets out people's thinking about both inherently bothersome and objectively innocuous situations. The advantages of ATSS are its unstructured production response format, resulting in a minimum of constraints on what subjects tell the facilitator about their thoughts and feelings; current rather than retrospective assessment, which minimizes distortions arising from generalized judgments for events over long periods of time; situational specificity and control, which maximize linking responses to eliciting events; and flexibility of both situation and cognitive process or product studied.

In assessing perceived quality of a program, an adaptation of ATSS can be used in which videotape or audiotape program components are shown to a group of participants in multiple brief segments. Each participant would be asked to write down what comes to mind after viewing or listening to information about each program. This written response could be scored to be analyzed readily to provide ratings of various activity concepts. Mean ratings of perceived concept quality could be averaged within segments sharing a common program component and could be compared across different components, as an example. For data analysis, responses from this method could be grouped into plausible qualitative categories, which then could be analyzed via counts of their relative frequencies and valences.

This method could be used to measure the opinions of the target population (e.g., students), as well as gatekeepers (e.g., school officials and teachers). Because a program developer must conduct this type of measure face-to-face with individuals or a small group of respondents, this method will not be useful for families, who often have complex schedules. Although experts' opinions could be measured this way, presumably they know enough about each activity to answer direct questions, so this method is not recommended for that group.

EVALUATION OF COLLECTED DATA: MULTIDIMENSIONAL SCALING

If a single method is used, data analysis is fairly straightforward. Even simple hand tabulations will suffice under circumstances in which one simply selects the most favorable half of a large set of activities. However, let us say one has the luxury of using several methods. Once data collection and initial analyses of the data have been completed, one must have a method of comparing various program components and determining the most advantageous one. Multidimensional scaling uses an attribute space to select the best program components (Torgerson, 1958). In this multidimensional perspective, one predefines the most important dimensions that should be considered in selecting a program component. For example, one may decide that memorability and interest are the most salient dimensions. If so, then one would construct the following multidimensional scale (see Figure 11.1).

Based on this figure, Activity 1 is interesting but not memorable, Activity 2 is very easy to remember and is very interesting, and Activity 3 is not particularly interesting or memorable. The program developer probably would select Activity 2.

▶ COMPUTERIZED ASSESSMENT

With the present advances in computer technology, many historically paper-and-pencil questionnaires have been adapted for computer administration and

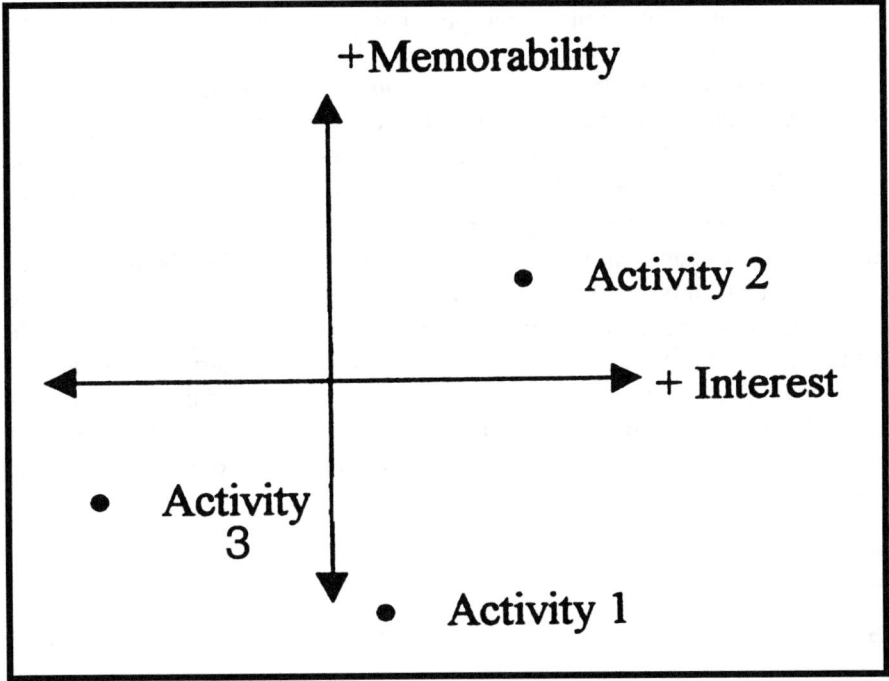

Figure 11.1. A Hypothetical Multidimensional Scaling of Two Types of Ratings of Different Concepts

scoring. Computers are easily available in various settings, including schools and workplaces, and there is a high level of computer literacy in the general population, which makes computer assessment more appealing. Many of the paper-and-pencil measurements discussed here can be adapted for computer administration.

There are many advantages of computerized assessments: They can provide more novelty in format for the assessment, they can be administered at any time when the target audience members are available, and they are easy to score. In addition, they eliminate both the data entry stage of evaluation and scoring errors, and they introduce more reliability. They are cost-effective because participants can respond to questions in an interactive computer mode without the need of a professional to administer the tests, and analysis can be completed almost instantaneously. They also introduce consistency. Different experimenters could introduce bias in assessment; however, computerized assessment eliminates this kind of bias by eliminating extraneous experimenter variables. Another benefit of computerized administration is that the same version of a test is less time-consuming when administered on a computer compared to paper-and-pencil versions (Butcher, 1987).

This is not to imply that computer administrations are always preferable to paper-and-pencil forms of assessments. There are drawbacks to computer assessments, as well. Participants may fill out items incorrectly if questions arise that affect their responses and there is no professional present to answer them. In addition, no body of research has yet proven that computer forms of assessments are equivalent to paper-and-pencil measures (Butcher, 1987). The use of computers in perceived program efficacy work certainly bears watching, but any use of computers for this task should be approached with knowledge of possible problems. Certainly, though, images or sentences that summarize potential program activities could be projected on a computer screen, serially or in parallel, and could be rated on the computer as well by the target sample. The means in which activities could be summarized for presentation and means of collecting response data are limitless through this modality.

▶ CONCLUSIONS

In summary, different methods can be used to construct perceived efficacy studies. The strengths and weaknesses of these methods are summarized in Table 11.1.

Although many methods can be used for more than one type of participant pool, researchers should be careful to match the type of measure with the population to be tested. A program component can be presented to the target population via written vignettes, TAT-type pictures, audiotape or videotape presentation, computer simulation, or live demonstration. These presentations, regardless of mode of presentation, should be followed by an assessment to evaluate program concepts. Regarding use of any of these methods, confidentiality of responses is important to ensure cooperation of subjects and improve validity.

Perceived efficacy studies can be successfully used to screen among plausible program components, compare more established program components with new and innovative ones, and generate new concepts and models for program development. It also can be of assistance in the study of the feasibility of program components with various ethnic populations before implementation. Verbal and nonverbal perceived program efficacy studies are valuable techniques to enhance our success in program development for health behavior change.

TABLE 11.1 Characteristics of Nonverbal Assessment Methods

	Resources	Target Group	Expertise	Pros	Cons
Card sorting	Card with picture or a few phrases for each activity	Participants	Explanation of task necessary	Ideal for low reading level populations, easy to administer, many applications possible	Limited quantitative data unless rationale is measured
Questionnaire	Series of scaled or open-ended questions	Participants Families Gatekeepers Experts	No expertise necessary	Convenient, less time-consuming analysis with large groups	Structured responses may limit feedback
Memory recall	Paragraphs containing health messages	Participants Gatekeepers	Explanation of task necessary	Direct measure of memorability of activities	Time-consuming to conduct, done by individuals or small groups
Projective technique	List of pertinent words, phrases, sentences, or pictures	Participants Gatekeepers	Explanation of task necessary; knowledge of analysis techniques	Elicits unstructured feedback from respondents	Done by individuals or small groups
Theme study	Narratives describing each activity; ratings sheet	Participants Gatekeepers Experts	No expertise necessary	Similar to questionnaire; can be used in conjunction	Similar to questionnaire

REFERENCES ◄

AAKER, D. A., & DAY, G. S. (1990). *Marketing research* (4th ed.). New York: John Wiley.

BATES, G. W., CAMPBELL, I. M., & BURGESS, P. M. (1990). Assessment of articulated thoughts in social anxiety: Modification of the ATSS procedure. *British Journal of Clinical Psychology, 29,* 91-98.

BEM, D. J., & FUNDER, D. C. (1978). Predicting more of the people more of the time: Assessing the personality of situations. *Psychological Review, 85,* 485-501.

BREEN, G. E., & BLANKENSHIP, A. B. (1982). *Do-it-yourself marketing research.* New York: McGraw-Hill.

BUTCHER, J. N. (1987). *Computerized psychological assessment: A practitioner's guide.* New York: Basic Books.

DAVISON, G. C., ROBINS, C., & JOHNSON, M. (1983). Articulated thoughts during simulated situations: A paradigm for studying cognition in emotion and behavior. *Cognitive Therapy and Research, 7,* 17-40.

DAVISON, G. C., VOGEL, R. S., & COFFMAN, S. G. (1997). Think-aloud approaches to cognitive assessment and the Articulated Thoughts in Simulated Situations paradigm. *Journal of Consulting and Clinical Psychology, 65,* 950-958.

DAVISON, G. C., WILLIAMS, M. E., NEZAMI, E., BICE, T. L., & DeQUATTRO, V. L. (1991). Relaxation, reduction in angry articulated thoughts, and improvements in borderline essential hypertension. *Journal of Behavioral Medicine, 14,* 453-469.

DAVISON, G. C., & ZIGHELBOIM, V. (1987). Irrational beliefs in the articulated thoughts of college students with social anxiety. *Journal of Rational-Emotive Therapy, 5,* 238-254.

DENT, C. W., GALAIF, E. R., SUSSMAN, S., & STACY, A. W. (1996). Use of the "theme study." *Journal of Drug Education, 26,* 377-393.

FLAY, B. R. (1981). Evaluation of mass media prevention campaigns. In R. R. Rice & W. J. Paisley (Eds.), *Public communication campaigns* (pp. 239-313). Beverly Hills, CA: Sage.

HAAGA, D. A. F. (1989). Articulated thoughts and endorsement procedures for cognitive assessment in the prediction of smoking relapse. *Psychological Assessment, 1,* 112-117.

HOPS, H., WEISSMAN, W., BIGLAN, A., THOMPSON, R., FALLER, C., & SEVERSON, H. H. (1986). A taped situation test of cigarette refusal skill among adolescents. *Behavioral Assessment, 8,* 145-154.

JUNG, C. G. (1919). *Studies in word association.* New York: Moffat, Yard.

KALTON, G., COLLINS, M., & BROOK, L. (1978). Experiments in wording opinion questions. *Applied Statistics, 27,* 149-161.

LABAW, P. (1981). *Advanced questionnaire design.* Cambridge, MA: Brooks.

LUCK, D. J., & RUBIN, R. S. (1987). *Marketing research.* Englewood Cliffs, NJ: Prentice Hall.

MISCHEL, W. (1971). *Introduction to personality.* New York: Holt, Rinehart.

MOSHER, D. L. (1966). The development and multitrait-multimethod matrix analysis of the measures of three aspects of guilt. *Journal of Consulting Psychology, 30,* 25-29.

RAPAPORT, D., GILL, M. M., & SCHAFER, R. (1980). *Diagnostic psychological testing.* New York: International Universities Press.

STACY, A. W., AMES, S. L., SUSSMAN, S., & DENT, C. W. (1996). Implicit cognition in adolescent drug use. *Psychology of Addictive Behaviors, 10,* 190-203.

STACY, A. W., GALAIF, E. R., SUSSMAN, S., & DENT, C. W. (1996). Self-generated drug outcomes in high-risk adolescents. *Psychology of Addictive Behaviors, 10,* 18-27.

STEPHENSON, W. (1953). *The study of behavior.* Chicago: University of Chicago Press.

SUDMAN, S., & BRADBURN, M. (1982). *A practical guide to questionnaire design.* San Francisco: Jossey-Bass.

SUSSMAN, S. (1991). Curriculum development in school-based prevention research. *Health Education Research, 6,* 339-351.

SUSSMAN, S. (1996). Development of a school-based drug abuse prevention curriculum for high-risk youths. *Journal of Psychoactive Drugs, 28,* 169-182.

SUSSMAN, S., DENT, C. W., SIMON, T. R., STACY, A. W., GALAIF, E. R., MOSS, M. A., CRAIG, S., & JOHNSON, C. A. (1995). Immediate impact of social influence-oriented substance abuse prevention curricula in traditional and continuation high schools. *Drugs and Society, 8,* 65-81.

SUSSMAN, S., DENT, C. W., STACY, A. W., BURTON, D., & FLAY, B. R. (1995). *Developing school-based tobacco use prevention and cessation programs.* Thousand Oaks, CA: Sage.

SUSSMAN, S., DENT, C. W., STACY, A. W., & CRAIG, S. (1998). One-year outcomes of Project Towards No Drug Abuse. *Preventive Medicine, 27,* 632-642.

SUSSMAN, S., PARKER, V. C., LOPES, C., CRIPPENS, D. L., ELDER, P., & SCHOLL, D. (1995). Empirical development of brief smoking prevention videotapes which target African-American adolescents. *International Journal of the Addictions, 30,* 1141-1164.

TORGERSON, W. S. (1958). *Theory and methods of scaling.* New York: John Wiley.

WEINER, M. D., SUSSMAN, S., McCULLER, W. J., & LICHTMAN, K. (1999). Factors in marijuana cessation among high-risk youth. *Journal of Drug Education, 29*(1), 337-357.

WORDEN, J. K., FLYNN, B. S., GELLER, B. M., CHEN, M., SHELTON, L., SECKER-WALKER, R. H., SOLOMON, D. S., SOLOMON, L. J., COUCHEY, S., & COSTANZA, M. C. (1988). Development of a smoking prevention mass media program using diagnostic and formative research. *Preventive Medicine, 17,* 531-558.

CHAPTER 11

Commentary

Jeffrey L. Kibler
Ronald S. Drabman

It is generally agreed among health care providers that there is a particularly serious behavioral health problem in the United States. Too many individuals engage in behaviors that greatly increase the risk of adverse health consequences. High-fat diets, excessive alcohol use, and tobacco use are just some of the behaviors that contribute to lower life expectancy and this nation's expensive health care burden. Large-scale costly projects are needed to help ameliorate these problems. Which of these projects will work and which will be the most cost-effective are still in question. Agencies are reluctant to allocate large expenditures for projects unless everything possible has been done to reduce the risk of failure. This is due to limited funds and the possibility that inefficient efforts will perpetuate the poor health behaviors. One way of attempting to increase the likelihood that programs will be successful before enormous sums of money, time, and effort are spent is to measure the perceived program quality of the project or its constituents (perceived efficacy studies/concept evaluation).

This chapter by Nezami, Davison, and Hoffman provides a comprehensive background of perceived efficacy studies, which may be used for the assessment of health behavior programs before actually conducting an intervention. These studies are essentially the prestudy psychometrics that can aid a health care provider in designing better health behavior interventions. Providers may efficiently gather data about the expected efficacy of certain program component ideas from a representative sample of the target group, as well as from other individuals with direct or indirect interest in the program (participants' families, experts, administrative personnel). Perceived efficacy studies have the advantage of cost and time effectiveness, relative to direct immediate-impact measures of program efficacy that typically follow the completion of a program. This advantage may create opportunities for health care professionals to do program assessments that might not have been feasible with other methods. The authors of the preceding chapter survey a multitude of paper-and-pencil instruments that could be used to assess perceived program quality or mediation of change. Many issues, insightfully presented in this chapter, have widespread application in the field of health behavior change but are too often overlooked. We briefly touch on some of the issues that appeared especially interesting and that may have important implications for providers considering perceived efficacy studies in their own work.

Perhaps the clearest point from this chapter is the applicability of numerous types of perceived efficacy studies to a wide array of common behavior change programs (e.g., exercise, weight management, smoking cessation, chemical abuse or dependence, multicomponent heart disease interventions). The development of any health care program that derives outcome from changes in the participants' behaviors toward a healthier lifestyle would presumably benefit from structured data pertaining to the program components that would predict these behaviors. In addition, because there is often considerable comorbidity among certain chronic illnesses in terms of behavioral risk factors, investigators using perceived efficacy studies may find that certain program components perceived as efficacious for a particular patient population will generalize to other behavioral disorders. Although this type of generalization is often assumed, measures of perceived efficacy can provide empirical evidence to either support or refute the generalizability of specific program component ideas shown to work in specific contexts.

Differences in quality ratings when perceived efficacy studies involve a comparison of various settings or environments also may prove to be an important distinction. An intervention that is successful and well accepted in one clinical setting might be perceived as less useful in another. For example, stress management interventions might be appreciated and rated as an efficacious technique to be used with a chronic pain patient presenting to an outpatient mental health clinic. However, the same intervention might not be as well received by the same type of patient being seen during a visit to the family physician. Results of perceived efficacy studies may help differentiate what subjects are likely to be receptive to in one setting versus another and may have implications for the need to provide extra rationale in the setting where novel techniques are not well received.

Discussion of the implications of perceived efficacy work for assessing potential health behavior change as a function of population variance (e.g., cultural beliefs and practices, physical or cognitive limitations) shows a critical sensitivity to this issue. A hypothetical example that comes to mind is perceived efficacy work that assesses the likely receptivity of a low-fat dietary intervention being proposed in a community where there are already strong societal cues to eat more healthfully (e.g., California and other more metropolitan areas of the United States) versus geographical areas such as the southern states, where cues to eat healthfully are not as common, and fried or other high-fat foods are more abundant. In fact, ratings of both regions could be made by subjects from both regions. Clearly, the way in which this type of intervention is presented may affect how it is received in these two regions. The authors also point out that including experts with backgrounds in multicultural programming in perceived efficacy studies will likely result in more widely accepted health behavior programs. Because it is important to be able to engage all potential participants in perceived efficacy work, there is a need for methods of assessment that will suit each population. The authors skillfully illustrate this point in the section of the chapter focusing on specific perceived efficacy study methods (e.g., description of the card-sorting task for illiterate populations). Considering the receptivity of planned interventions for various target audiences has direct implications for compliance and motivation.

The authors clearly illustrate the advantages of screening program concepts among all groups of individuals who are potentially invested in the success of a health behavior program (recipients, family members, administrators, experts). An important distinction is made between actual program participants and those who are more indirectly involved. This discussion illustrates insight into the influences of others' perspectives on the program outcome. Perhaps the importance of involving family when planning an intervention is best portrayed by two common statements that most health behavior professionals would recall hearing from their patients: (a) "My spouse doesn't see any good in this group, so we've decided it is better if I don't participate," or (b) "It is just so hard to quit smoking with others smoking in the house." These statements highlight the impact that the family's understanding, involvement, or lack thereof may have on a patient's success in a program. Administrators also are discussed as an important nonrecipient population that is invested in programs. The use of memory recall for those in administrative positions is an excellent idea. These individuals represent a mechanism for conveying information about the program to others in the community. However, the authors thoughtfully note the importance of sensitivity to time when engaging in perceived efficacy work among administrators.

The multidimensional nature of perceived efficacy work should not be overlooked. The authors list a number of different aspects of perceived efficacy work that could be considered. Certainly more exist, depending on the type of program, and it seems likely that measuring as many different dimensions in as many ways as possible will result in the best overall representation of a potential program. Perhaps perceived efficacy work in a provider's respective specialty could result in a weighted multidimensional model. This seems especially important in areas of health behavior change in which certain perceived quality variables might be known to predict an outcome.

The authors describe the efficiency and consistency gained by using computer assessment while also touching on some of the limitations (less direct supervision during questionnaire administration). The point is made that there is little support for the equivalency of computer and paper-and-pencil measures. Although this may be true, there may be differences between computer assessment and paper-and-pencil methods that make computer techniques advantageous. In comparison to other self-report measures, which are criticized for being inaccurate representations of historical data (with desirability often being identified as the reason for distortion), automated data collection may be perceived as more confidential and less susceptible to participant-experimenter interaction effects. Recently, Romer et al. (1997) showed that interviews delivered by "talking computers" elicited more reports of sexual experience and positive feelings toward sex than face-to-face interviews among 396 Black children ages 9 to 15. Furthermore, a subsample of the children ($n = 31$) who completed both types of interviews reported more favorable feelings toward sex in the computer interview. It is also notable that the computer interviews did not result in more missing data than the face-to-face method. For interested readers, other papers focus on the issue of computer assessment versus other self-report techniques (Johnston & Walton, 1995; Paperny, Aono, Lehman, Hammar, & Risser, 1990; Tourangeau & Smith, 1996). With computerized assessments becoming more commonplace, researchers also are turning to the Internet for access to a wider audience and a greater number of research participants. Although these assessment procedures are in their infancy, the advent of the Internet II (or "academia-only" Web system) will provide researchers with an arena for development and testing of Internet-based assessment protocols and easier standardization of collaborative efforts. Obviously, the computer is a great mechanism for presenting activity ideas for which ratings can be made. Visual depictions of activities can be provided as a cartoon or movielike sequence, in addition to providing activity ideas through written displays on the screen.

As with any scientific endeavor, the implications that can be drawn from perceived efficacy work are limited. Just as "face validity" is not necessary for predictive validity, perceived efficacy study outcomes are not necessary for programmatic efficacy. Thus, there is a great need for research to measure (and increase whenever possible) the variance in programmatic efficacy that is accounted for by prior perceived efficacy work. In this way, not only will programs become more cost-efficient, but so will the perceived efficacy studies that precede them. Those conducting future research in the area of perceived efficacy studies also might investigate the relative utility of different types of measurement scales for these studies. Figure 11.1 in the chapter provides an interesting illustration of the multidimensional framework of perceived quality. Further examination of the most important program development factors for specific areas of health behavior research might help determine which dimensions should be emphasized.

In sum, this chapter is very interesting and provides insight into a mechanism of improved program development for health behavior change. The need for perceived efficacy studies is presented with the understanding that not all programs work the same way for all persons. Persons bring a varying array of cultural beliefs and personal expectations into a clinical or other treatment setting, and a person's appraisal of an intervention will affect outcome in most cases. As alluded to in this chapter, the applicability of perceived efficacy work is widespread, and its measurement allows providers to address issues pertaining to a given population's interests and needs.

REFERENCES

JOHNSTON, J., & WALTON, C. (1995). Reducing response effects for sensitive questions: A computer-assisted self interview with audio. *Social Science Computer Review, 13,* 304-319.

PAPERNY, D. M., AONO, J. Y., LEHMAN, R. M., HAMMAR, S. L., & RISSER, J. (1990). Computer-assisted detection and intervention in adolescent high-risk health behaviors. *Journal of Pediatrics, 116,* 456-462.

ROMER, D., HORNIK, R., STANTON, B., BLACK, M., LI, X., RICARDO, I., & FEIGELMAN, S. (1997). "Talking" computers: A reliable and private method to conduct interviews on sensitive topics with children. *Journal of Sex Research, 34,* 3-9.

TOURANGEAU, R., & SMITH, T. W. (1996). Asking sensitive questions: The impact of data collection mode, question format, and question context. *Public Opinion Quarterly, 60,* 275-304.

Case Study 5

CHAPTER 12

Use of a Theme Study for Adolescent Tobacco Use Cessation

Clyde W. Dent
Kara Lichtman
Steve Sussman

A theme study consists of brief written descriptions of several hypothetical activities that are rated by students in the target population for the purpose of determining their potential interest, likability, and perceived helpfulness (Dent, Galaif, Sussman, & Stacy, 1996; Sussman, Petosa, & Clarke, 1996). This type of study varies from component or pilot studies (see Chapters 13 and 16, this volume), as the latter assess activities for logistical aspects and student reactions during actual participation in activities. The strengths of the theme study approach are that (a) standardization of material presentation can be maintained across classrooms, (b) many more activities can be assessed per unit of time, and (c) an empirical evaluation of hypothetical activities can be obtained. Theme studies can help screen out activities that are of particularly low or high interest and perceived helpfulness through use of a time-effective protocol.

The theme study is an important step in the process of empirical program development because it allows the a priori ascertainment of subject preferences regarding potentially applicable activities. Theme studies elicit information regarding the appropriateness of using certain topics in specific populations. The activities that yield high subject preference may then confidently be developed further into complete activities or sessions for immediate-impact testing through component and pilot studies.

GOALS OF PRESENT STUDY

In the present case study, the goals were twofold. First, there was an interest to determine which among two alternative presentation modalities—"game" or "talk show"—of nine "traditional motivation-enhanced" smoking cessation themes (Nezami, Sussman, & Pentz, in press) was most acceptable to continuation high school (CHS) students. Second, there was an interest to determine which in a set of eight "novel" activities, derived from eight unique alternative medicine-related themes (e.g., Benson, 1984), were as or more acceptable to CHS students than the best activities derived from traditional motivation themes. Thus, written paragraph descriptions of 26 activities, built on 17 themes (9 traditional and 8 novel), were used in a theme study format to determine those activities that were of the most interest and applicability to CHS students. Retained activity paragraphs would be developed into full activities, eventually leading to the creation of a motivation-enhanced tobacco use cessation program for high-risk adolescents.

THEORY

To understand and control the effectiveness of smoking cessation programs, one must have a conceptual framework of behavior change. Each strategy in a proposed curriculum should have a theoretical or quasi-theoretical assumption about the mechanisms by which activities affect behavior. Sussman (1996) and Nezami et al. (in press) have described several theoretical concepts and mechanisms that underlie the motivation to change, relevant to tobacco use prevention and cessation. In the theme activity paragraph development process, the following concepts were adopted as conceptual guides.

Motivation can be said to lie in two conceptual dimensions. The first is *direction*. Direction motivation elucidates a discrepancy between what is and what could be to motivate a change. In this study, the categories of self-image, affect, and curiosity were used as direction motivation themes. The second theoretical dimension is *energy*. Energy motivation describes the impetus that drives an individual toward the direction indicated. Lifestyle stability, capacity match, and social pressure were used in this study as key motivation energy themes. Crossing the three key concepts from each dimension, we derived nine specific motivation themes used in this study (e.g., improved affect directed-capacity match energy).

In addition to the motivation concepts used earlier, the *novel* concepts of body awareness and social awareness were used. One's increased awareness of his or her external and internal environments may provide motivation for health change (e.g., Benson, 1984; Duval & Wicklund, 1972; Sussman, Nezami, & Mishra, 1997). These alternative concepts were not a priori connected to the motivation concepts of energy and direction and so were defined as novel.

Within each of the general theoretical concept areas outlined earlier, a number of possible types of activities could be generated to address the specific goal. These activity variations generally are variations in teaching method or group process. For the purposes of this study, we define variation in concept focus as a theme, variations in teaching methods as modalities for a theme, and activity as a particular theme or teaching method combination. We included two modalities popular among these teens: (a) the talk show, which is formatted like a daytime talk show such as *Oprah*, and (b) a game, which demands group participation, competition, and cooperation toward learning a point (Dent et al., 1998).

METHOD ◄

ACTIVITY POOL

We began activity pool generation by defining concept focus areas within the motivation and novel conceptual dimensions to produce themes. We then defined a teaching goal for each theme. Following the generation of the theme goals, we generated paragraphs describing two teaching alternatives for each of the nine traditional motivation themes. Each pair of alternative activities maintained the same theme and teaching goal but varied in teaching method (modality).

We then generated eight novel activities that consisted of five body awareness and three social awareness themes. The novel activities were generated from a variety of sources, including suggestions from school staff and students, a review of the health behavior literature (e.g., Benson, 1984), adaptation of clinical behavior therapy techniques, and analyses of focus group data previously obtained from CHS students (e.g., see Chapter 10, this volume). We included them in this study to explore their utility for further investigation. Table 12.1 lists a summary of the activity paragraphs used in this study.

TABLE 12.1 The Theme Paragraphs

Title	Motivational Category	Modality	Goal
Smoking and Stress Poster Contest	Affect/lifestyle stability	Game	To present information to students about how cigarettes affect your body in a way that increases your overall feeling of stress, even though you may immediately and temporarily feel calmed by a cigarette.
Is Smoking on the Menu?	Curiosity/social pressure	Game	To inform students about the dangers of second-hand smoke and get smokers to think about how their smoking affects others and how other people feel about it.
The Age Game	Curiosity/capacity match	Game	To inform students that it is much easier to quit smoking when they are young.
Family Portrait	Affect/social pressure	Game	To show students that many people in their lives may wish they would quit smoking. Also, to show that when smokers say, "I don't care what people say about my smoking," they may not be entirely honest about their feelings.
Pin the Blame on the Tobacco Industry	Self-image/social pressure	Game	To reveal how the tobacco industry uses lies to pressure people into smoking although they may not even be aware of it. Smokers may think they are making an independent decision, but they are actually being controlled.
Romantic Match or Mismatch	Curiosity/lifestyle stability	Game	To show students how nonsmokers have more freedom to make choices, which increases their enjoyment of life.
Musical Chairs	Self-image/capacity match	Game	To show students that they will feel many different ways about themselves during the several-week period they are quitting smoking, but ultimately they will feel centered and confident. Feeling like they cannot do it or feeling bad about themselves is part of the process, but it does not mean that they actually cannot do it.
Quitting for Life	Self-image/lifestyle stability	Game	To show students that quitting smoking can have many positive effects on their lives that are not necessarily directly related to tobacco.
Coping Without Smokes	Affect/capacity match	Game	To show students that often our worst fears about what would happen if we let our emotions get out of control are not really so bad after all. Many smokers say they use cigarettes to control their moods, but maybe those moods do not need to be so heavily controlled after all. Students learn to trust their abilities to handle different moods and also learn that these moods pass in time.

Best Friends: One Smokes, the Other Doesn't	Curiosity/lifestyle stability	Talk show	To show students how nonsmokers have more freedom to make choices, which increases their enjoyment of life.
Second-Hand Smoke in Restaurants	Curiosity/social pressure	Talk show	To inform students about the dangers of second-hand smoke and get smokers to think about how their smoking affects others and how other people feel about it.
Warning: Waiting to Quit Smoking May Be Hazardous to Your Peace of Mind	Curiosity/capacity match	Talk show	To inform students that it is much easier to quit smoking when they are young.
Quitting Smoking Changed My Life	Self-image/lifestyle stability	Talk show	To show students that quitting smoking can have many positive effects on their lives that are not necessarily directly related to tobacco.
Are You a Sucker for the Tobacco Industry's Lies?	Self-image/social pressure	Talk show	To reveal how the tobacco industry uses lies to pressure people into smoking, although they may not even be aware of it. Smokers may think they are making an independent decision, but they are actually being controlled.
Quitting Smoking: I've Been There and It Does Get Better	Self-image/capacity match	Talk show	To show students that they will feel many different ways about themselves during the several-week period they are quitting smoking, but ultimately they will feel centered and confident. Feeling like they cannot do it or feeling bad about themselves is part of the process, but it does not mean that they actually cannot do it.
Your Cigarettes May Be Stressing You Out	Affect/lifestyle stability	Talk show	To present information to students about how cigarettes affect their bodies in a way that increases their overall feeling of stress, even though they may immediately and temporarily feel calmed by a cigarette.
Family and Friends Confront Smokers About Their Habit	Affect/social pressure	Talk show	To show students that many people in their lives may wish they would quit smoking. Also, to show that when smokers say, "I don't care what people say about my smoking," they may not be entirely honest about their feelings.
Smokers Talk About What Would Really Happen If They Let Their Emotions Go	Affect/capacity match	Talk show	To show students that often our worst fears about what would happen if we let our emotions get out of control are not really so bad after all. Many smokers say they use cigarettes to control their moods, but maybe those moods do not need to be so heavily controlled after all. Students learn to trust their abilities to handle different moods and also learn that these moods pass in time.

(continued)

TABLE 12.1 Continued

Title	Motivational Category	Modality	Goal
Peer Motivational Counseling		Novel	To involve other students as motivational counselors in the Project EX clinic. Counselors can share their experiences and motivate their peers and friends.
Media Outreach		Novel	To celebrate the success of quitters at the end of the clinic by creating a media announcement such as a poster or a newspaper article.
Quitting Smoking and Your Body		Novel	To help students prepare for the changes in their bodies that happen when they quit smoking.
Healthy Breathing Exercise		Novel	To encourage students to think about their own breathing patterns and to learn an exercise that promotes healthy breathing that can help ease withdrawal symptoms and promote relaxation and well-being.
Movement and the Body-Mind Connection		Novel	To inform students of the connections between their physical state and their mental, emotional, and spiritual states. Students explore these connections through movement and role-play. Students are encouraged to consider everything they do to their bodies as messages being sent to their spirits and minds as well. Appreciating the mind-body connection will make them feel better about quitting and help to prevent relapse.
Letting Feelings Pass		Novel	To instruct students in the principles of meditation so they can learn simply to let their feelings pass. Sometimes people get upset about being upset, and quitters may be especially susceptible to this when they are dealing with withdrawal symptoms. Meditation offers a strategy for letting go of things to increase peace of mind and state of health.
Yoga		Novel	To teach students some exercises that get the blood moving, increase body awareness, and reduce stress. Yoga exercises can help students lessen withdrawal symptoms.
Social Support		Novel	To inform other students at the school about what they can do to most effectively support students who have decided to quit smoking.

NOTE: The Motivational Category column applies only to the direction-energy motivation model constituents; it is blank for all novel themes.

DESIGN

A total of 17 themes, expressed in 26 written activity paragraphs, were to be evaluated. Themes were arbitrarily grouped into two sets of 13, such that all the traditional motivation themes in one modality were randomly paired with 4 novel themes. Activity sets were then randomized within classrooms at four participating schools in a systematically rotated order.

SAMPLE

A total of 391 students from four continuation high schools participated in this study. Within this sample, 51% reported weekly use of cigarettes (43% daily), 43% reported weekly marijuana use, and 39% reported weekly alcohol use. Monthly self-reported use of illegal drugs was 15% for stimulants, 11% for hallucinogens, 8% for cocaine and inhalants, and 4% for "other" substances. Because the focus of this study was on smokers, weekly smokers ($n = 201$) are the sample used in all subsequent analysis. They were 60% male, 38% Latino, 37% White, 11% Black, and 14% reporting "other" ethnicity; 16% were in 10th grade, 49% in 11th grade, and 30% in 12th grade. Approximately half (51%) had been at a CHS for 1 year, 38% for 2 years, and 9% for 3 years. Their mean age was 17 years ($SD = 1.6$ years). Approximately 55% reported that they live with both parents, 22% live with only their mother, and 10% live with their father or another person. Approximately 30% of the students reported that their mothers, fathers, or both had completed high school. Twelve percent of the sample reported being a parent.

PROCEDURE

The study procedure was completed during regularly scheduled, 50-minute classroom periods. Two trained health educators who were unknown to the students conducted the study in classrooms. Participation was completely voluntary—at any time during the procedure, students could refuse or decline from participation, although none chose to do so. All data collected were anonymous.

Sessions took place over 3 consecutive days. On the first day, students were administered a general psychosocial pretest survey. On the second day, students were administered a package of materials containing a brief demographic survey, the 9 traditional motivation activity descriptions using the talk show modality, 4 (of 8) novel activity disciplines, and 13 brief posttest activity evaluation forms. On the third day, students were given a package similar to the second day. However, the 9 motivation themes were presented in a game modality, along with the remaining 4 novel activities. Within each classroom, activity order was randomized, except that the novel activities were always the last 4 to be evaluated.

Each activity description was in a standardized format that included an activity title, the activity goal, and a brief (half-page) description of what the activity entailed. All activity descriptions were approximately the same length, detail, and reading level. Titles varied for each activity. The goals were presented in a concise and understandable manner. The statement of activity goal was the same for the game and talk show modalities of the same theme.

Prior to evaluating the activities, students were asked to complete the brief demographic survey. Students were then asked to read along, as a health educator read each activity description. After reading each description of the activities, students were asked to answer the questions on an evaluation form regarding the quality of the activity. One evaluation form was provided for each activity paragraph evaluated.

MEASUREMENT

The evaluation questionnaire administered to the students elicited pertinent demographic information, such as age, grade, gender, ethnic identification, parental education (as a proxy for socioeconomic status), and drug use behavior. The activity paragraph evaluations assessed (a) how interesting it would be to do the activity, (b) how understandable the activity would be, (c) how much the students could learn from doing the activity, (d) how likely the activity would help to not increase or to not start drug use, and (e) the ability of the activity to meet the stated goal it was intended to accomplish. These items were all rated on a 4-point response scale: 1 = *very*, 2 = *moderately*, 3 = *a little*, and 4 = *not at all*. A factor analysis of the five items produced a single factor, and the items were averaged to form a single activity "quality" rating. Cronbach's alpha for the scale was .84. The raw scale mean was 2.45, and the standard deviation was 0.76.

ANALYSIS

A mixed-model analysis of variance model was used to analyze quality score ratings using each rating of an activity as the unit of analysis. Schools, classes nested within schools, and students nested within classes were included as random factors. Activities nested within sets were fixed factors. Demographic factors of gender and age were included as covariates.

TABLE 12.2 Project EX Theme Study Smokers' Paragraph Ratings

Rank	Paragraph	Mode	N Raters	Mean	SEM
1	Warning	Talk[a]	123	2.33	0.076
2	Romantic	Game[a]	119	2.40	0.075
3	Sucker	Talk[a]	124	2.41	0.073
4	Confront	Talk[a]	123	2.44	0.070
5	Peer	Novel	104	2.46	0.093
6	Yoga	Novel	127	2.48	0.081
7	Stress	Talk[a]	124	2.49	0.074
8	Feelings	Novel	113	2.49	0.081
9	Better	Talk[a]	122	2.51	0.074
10	Social	Novel	109	2.51	0.084
11	Body	Novel	115	2.52	0.080
12	Movement	Novel	125	2.52	0.081
13	Breath	Novel	113	2.54	0.079
14	Romantic	Talk	129	2.54	0.074
15	Media	Novel	133	2.57	0.080
16	Menu	Game[a]	117	2.58	0.073
17	Menu	Talk	126	2.58	0.069
18	Coping	Game[a]	87	2.59	0.083
19	Coping	Talk	88	2.60	0.087
20	Warning	Game	116	2.61	0.076
21	Confront	Game	116	2.61	0.074
22	Sucker	Game	119	2.62	0.076
23	Life	Game[a]	116	2.63	0.073
24	Life	Talk	126	2.63	0.078
25	Stress	Game	120	2.63	0.068
26	Better	Game	119	2.63	0.078

a. Teaching method with the highest rating (between 2 for a given theme).

RESULTS

Table 12.2 lists all 26 paragraphs, rank ordered by their raw quality score rating. That table also shows the number of students who rated the paragraph and indicated which, between the two teaching modes, received the highest (best) rating for a given theme. The rating scores ranged from 2.33 (best) to 2.63 (worst), with standard errors of the mean (*SEM*) averaging about .08. The formal test of rating differences across all paragraphs was significant ($F = 6.88, p = .01$), indicating that at least one paragraph was significantly different from the grand mean. As a rule of thumb, paragraphs that differ by more than two standard errors (difference score = at least .16) could be considered statistically different from each other.

Of primary interest was which teaching mode would be considered best for a given theme within the theory-driven set of themes. Formal testing revealed that the talk show mode was best for the warning paragraph ($F = 5.78, p = .01$) and almost significantly so for the sucker paragraph ($F = 3.36, p = .06$). All other mode comparisons were not significant, and the judgment of which was best was made based simply on the absolute values of the rating scores (i.e., their rank).

As can be seen in Table 12.2, no real pattern for teaching mode preference (game or talk show) was apparent—the best theory-based paragraphs were composed of 5 talk show mode paragraphs and 4 game mode paragraphs. A formal test of teaching mode (across all paragraphs) revealed no statistical differences between modes, although it is interesting to note that the talk show mode did appear more often in the higher-ranked paragraphs. Also of interest, the novel mode appeared in 7 of the top 13 paragraphs (but not significantly more often than chance).

▶ DISCUSSION

One goal of the present case study was to determine which among two alternative presentation modalities—game or talk show—of nine motivation-enhanced smoking cessation themes was most acceptable to CHS students. The use of the written paragraphs enabled us to select a preferred teaching mode for each theory-based theme by ranking the paragraphs by student ratings. Although only one theme showed statistically significant differences in teaching mode, all paragraphs could be judged for which teaching method for a given content was rated higher.

Similarly, the second goal of the study was to determine which, among a set of eight "novel" activities, were as or more acceptable to CHS students than the "best" activities based on traditional motivation themes. In general, these novel themes ranked quite highly; seven of the eight were rated in the top half of all paragraphs. Although the formal test for differences failed to reveal a reliable pattern, a pattern is evident nonetheless in these data.

All activities were rated as moderately good. The warning talk show was rated as best, significantly lower (better rating) than all activities ranked 7 or higher. The essence of this activity was that it is better to quit tobacco use when one is young (curiosity-capacity match). The next two lowest-ranked (best) activities tap romantic choices when being tobacco free and not being a victim of tobacco company advertisements. These activities were rated significantly lower than all activities ranked 15 or higher. Interestingly, practice of yoga also was a preferred novel activity to assist in motivating one to quit tobacco. Essentially, the top half among the activities was retained for component study testing.

The utility of the paper-and-pencil method helped this study achieve its goals in an efficient manner. The screening of such a large number of potential activities and the assessment of the best teaching method could not have been completed in such a short time frame or with such a large number of student raters without the use of a method such as the theme study.

REFERENCES ◄

BENSON, H. (1984). The relaxation response and stress. In J. D. Matarazzo, S. M. Weiss, J. A. Herd, N. E. Miller, & S. M. Weiss (Eds.), *Behavioral health: A handbook of health enhancement and disease prevention* (pp. 710-718). New York: John Wiley.

DENT, C. W., GALAIF, E. R., SUSSMAN, S., & STACY, A. W. (1996). Use of the "theme study" as a means of curriculum development in continuation high schools. *Journal of Drug Education, 26,* 377-393.

DENT, C. W., SUSSMAN, S., HENNESY, M., GALAIF, E. R., STACY, A. W., MOSS, M. A., & CRAIG, S. (1998). Implementation and process evaluation of a school-based drug abuse prevention program: Project Towards No Drug Abuse. *Journal of Drug Education, 28,* 361-375.

DUVAL, S., & WICKLUND, R. A. (1972). *A theory of objective self awareness.* New York: Academic Press.

NEZAMI, E., SUSSMAN, S., & PENTZ, M. A. (in press). Motivation in tobacco use cessation research. *Substance Use & Misuse.*

SUSSMAN, S. (1996). Development of a school-based drug abuse prevention curriculum for high-risk youths. *Journal of Psychoactive Drugs, 28,* 169-182.

SUSSMAN, S., NEZAMI, E., & MISHRA, S. I. (1997). On operationalizing spiritual experience for health research and practice. *Alternative Therapies in Clinical Practice, 4,* 120-125.

SUSSMAN, S., PETOSA, R., & CLARKE, P. (1996). The use of empirical curriculum development to improve prevention research. *American Behavioral Scientist, 39,* 838-852.

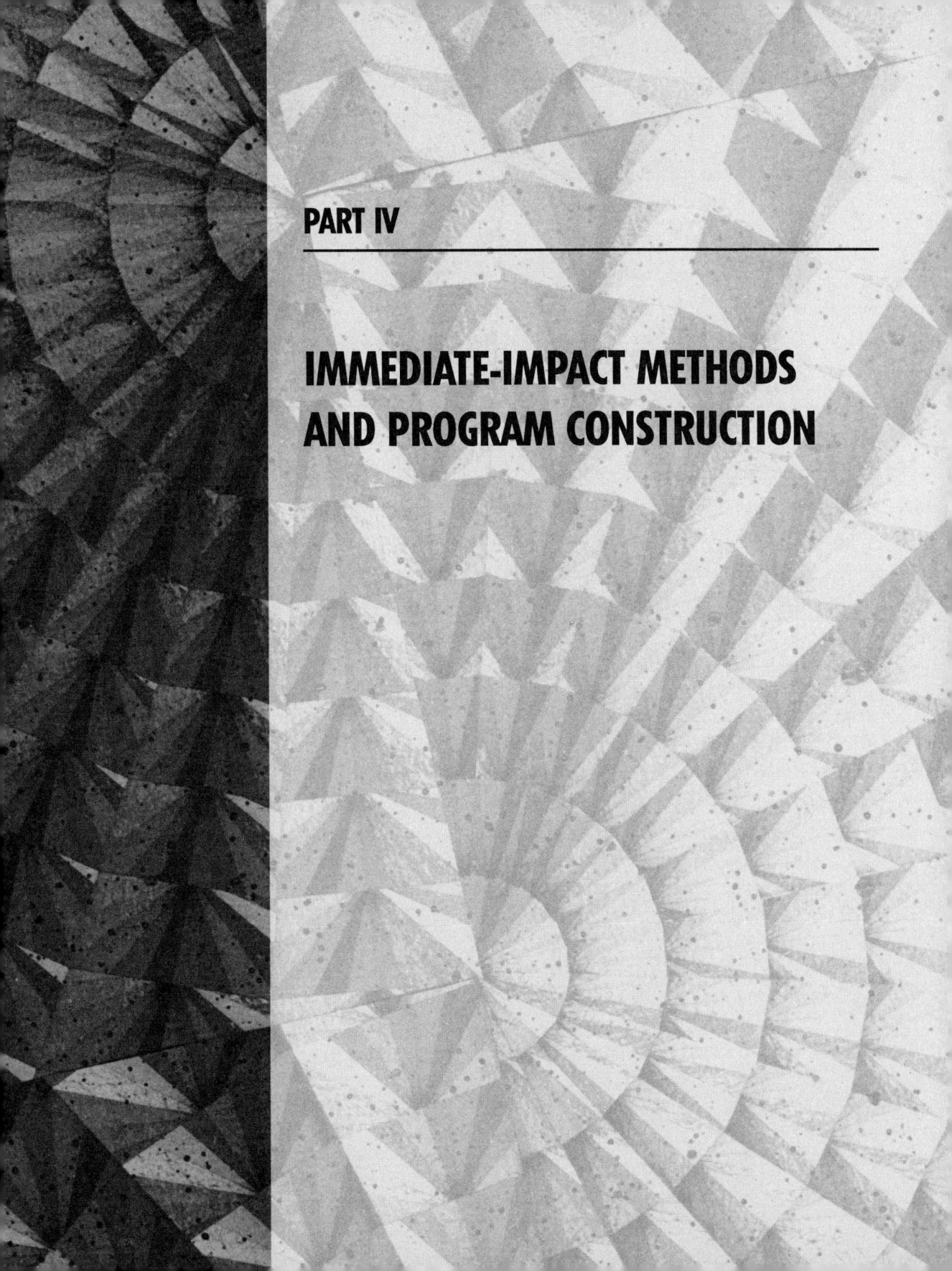

PART IV

IMMEDIATE-IMPACT METHODS AND PROGRAM CONSTRUCTION

CHAPTER 13

Component Studies

Thomas R. Simon
Kris Bosworth
Jennifer B. Unger

As anyone who has developed a health promotion or disease prevention program can attest, it is a complicated process involving many important decisions. Fortunately, there are some useful tools to help program developers make informed decisions. The component study is one such program development tool. In this chapter, we address two questions: (a) What are component studies? and (b) How are component studies conducted? We answer the first question by providing definitions, descriptions of component study types, and a list of typical questions addressed by component studies. To answer the second question, we describe component study evaluation issues such as the types of constructs measured, sampling, study design, and interpretation of results.

WHAT ARE COMPONENT STUDIES? ◄

DEFINITIONS

Health promotion and disease prevention programs generally are composed of multiple components. Components are the smallest identifiable content unit (material theme) or process unit (instructional method) of an intervention, generally consisting of one or two activities of a 15-minute to 40-minute duration.

The term *component studies* refers to the systematic testing and improvement of the components of a health promotion program. Component studies involve the examination of individual components of an intervention independently or in some combination to determine the contribution of each to the goals of the intervention. These studies provide a way to identify and enhance the most promising aspects of a health promotion and disease prevention program and to change or eliminate those components that are not useful. Later, the most promising components are put together for feasibility and pilot testing (see Chapters 15 and 16, this volume). Thus, component studies are often used as an aid to program developers as they transition from an idea for a prevention component to development of the actual program content. For example, in the course of developing a substance abuse prevention curriculum for high-risk youth, Sussman, Simon, et al. (1997) exposed students to 32 different activities (i.e., 16 different activity contents crossed with two instructional methods, self-instruction or health educator-led instruction) and compared posttest knowledge scores and process ratings on interest, helpfulness, and likability collected after participation in each activity. The three process ratings were combined to create a perceived program quality index. A ranking of the activities on this index was used to decide which activities to include in the pilot testing of the complete curriculum. Consistent with prior theoretical assumptions and theme study work, motivation, social skill, and decision-making-type components were favored and were later combined to produce an effective program for high-risk youth (Sussman, Dent, Stacy, & Craig, 1998).

Because most health-related behaviors are multidetermined, health promotion and disease prevention programs typically require multiple components (Dryfoos, 1991). For example, a recent program designed to influence HIV risk sexual behaviors among African American men included components to address self-identity, social support, AIDS education, assertiveness training, and behavioral commitment (Peterson, Coates, Catania, & Hauck, 1996). Gone are the days when a single component or theory such as an inspirational speaker was the epitome of prevention efforts. Recognizing that later behavior change requires a variety of proximal changes in knowledge, beliefs, attitudes, skills, social norms, and intentions, developers of modern health promotion programs typically incorporate multiple activities designed specifically to achieve these diverse objectives.

COMPONENT STUDY EVALUATION VERSUS OUTCOMES EVALUATION

Although several of the same methods may be used, a component study evaluation is fundamentally different from a (main trial) outcomes evaluation. In the former, the goal is to determine which components of a health promotion or disease prevention program are most promising and how they can be enhanced. The component study evaluation is focused on the factors that mediate the effect of the program on behavior (e.g., knowledge, attitudes, beliefs, social norms, intentions) rather than on behavior change itself.

In an outcomes evaluation, the goal is to determine if the health promotion program (usually involving a combination of components) had a significant effect on the intended outcomes (e.g., smoking, condom use, diet). Because the intended outcomes usually include a sustained change in behavior, outcomes evaluations generally focus on the longer-term follow-up of participants. Thorough outcome evaluations also assess the implementation process as well as the effects of the program on the mediators and the association between the mediators and the behavioral outcomes.

TYPES OF RELATIONS AMONG COMPONENTS ◄

Each component has its own theoretical relevance and objective (e.g., see Chapter 4, this volume), and these components relate to each other in several different ways. To examine how component studies can be used effectively to enhance program development, one should identify four general relationships that can exist among components: similar goals, building blocks, complementarity, and constellation.

SIMILAR GOALS

In the first kind of relationship, two or more components are intended to have the same immediate effect. They generally consist of different instructional strategies yet have the same goal. For example, as part of a violence prevention program, Self-Enhancement, Inc., a community-service organization, provides middle school students with multiple classroom-based activities designed to improve conflict resolution skills (Gabriel, Haskins, Hopson, & Powell, 1996). The conflict resolution techniques taught in school also are reinforced by mentors in an after-school program. The rationale for this approach is that exposure to multiple activities delivered by multiple presenters with a common theme will reinforce the critical message. Effective component study work can help program developers to maximize the level of reinforcement while avoiding excessive redundancy when designing multiple components to achieve the same immediate goal.

BUILDING BLOCKS

The second type of relationship can be called *building blocks* because one component provides the foundation for the next. Within a health promotion program, two or more components may be related to each other sequentially in that Component A is necessary for the effectiveness of Component B. The building-blocks relationship is often found in skills-building curricula; to learn a skill, students must first learn the steps involved in the new skill (Component A) before they can practice it by role-playing (Component B). Component studies can test relationships between different building-block sequences.

COMPLEMENTARITY

The third type of relationship among components is *complementary*. Two or more components present different types of material, and these components enhance the effects of each other. By enhancing each other's effects, they may achieve a greater impact than either might when provided alone (i.e., a synergistic effect pattern results). For example, drug abuse prevention programs that focus on normative education have been shown to be relatively effective (Hansen, 1992). The impact of the prevention program is enhanced when both normative education and resistance skills training are included. These are not building blocks because learning one within the classroom setting does not help the student to learn the other. However, programs that provide students with the skills to resist offers of drugs and with the antidrug beliefs engendered in normative education can equip students with the tools and motivation to avoid substance use. Effective component study work can help to identify important complementary activities.

CONSTELLATION

The fourth type of relationship is the *constellation*. Many prevention interventions have multiple components, with each addressing the needs of a different audience (e.g., parents, adolescents, teachers, school administration, community members, police, etc.). The component for each of these audiences is designed to address the role each plays in disease prevention and health promotion. Each component may be entirely different, even though the developers hope that they will work in concert to modify the same end points. For example, in the Midwestern Prevention Project, five distinct components are involved with the intervention: mass media, a school program, a parent program, community organization, and policy change (Pentz et al., 1989). These components were implemented sequentially to determine the incremental impact of each. These components varied in both activity contents and instructional methods. Component studies can help the program developer to select appropriate constellations of components.

TYPES OF COMPONENT STUDIES

It is useful to group component studies into categories according to their goals. Three common types of component studies are substantive component contrasts, order-based studies, and group comparison evaluations.

SUBSTANTIVE COMPONENT CONTRASTS

In the substantive component contrasts, the program developer evaluates the immediate effectiveness of the various components of a health promotion strategy. This can be done in at least two ways. First, the components can be compared with each other. When two or more components are designed to achieve the same objective within a health promotion program, it may be desirable to compare their effectiveness so that only the most successful component will be included in the final program. For example, their scores on a perceived program quality index could be compared using standardized critical values as a measure of difference. Second, the effect of a component may be compared to an external standard. The standard may be the strategy currently implemented in the target population (including no strategy at all), or it may be the best-known existing program components. For example, ratings completed by subjects not exposed to the component (standard care control) or participant pretest ratings of the efficacy of other activities the participant has been exposed to could be used as the external standard against which component study posttest ratings could be compared.

ORDER-BASED STUDIES

The order-based component study involves testing different sequences of two or more components to determine the most effective building-block sequence. Only small segments of a program are compared. All participants in order-based component studies are exposed to the same component content and delivery format; only the sequence is varied. These studies often will lead to elimination of unnecessary material (e.g., if a skill deficit is due primarily to a need to practice the skill, as opposed to a lack of knowledge and practice) (see Sussman, Dent, Burton, Stacy, & Flay, 1995). (Chapter 15, this volume, discusses the sequencing of program material in more detail.)

GROUP COMPARISON EVALUATION

Finally, in the group comparison evaluation, the immediate impact of the components of a health promotion program is compared across different target groups or across different subgroups within a target group. Group comparison evaluations provide an opportunity to identify components of a health promotion program that are relevant and feasible across different audiences, giving health researchers and practitioners a sense of the generalizability of program effects. For example, a recent group comparison evaluation compared the immediate effects of nine social influence activities on drug-related knowledge and beliefs for students enrolled in traditional high schools versus students enrolled in alternative high schools. This study determined that several activities were more effective in producing knowledge and belief change for students in traditional high schools, and this study identified potential limitations of social influences-oriented activities for students in alternative high schools (Sussman, Dent, Simon, et al., 1995).

The three types of component studies are not necessarily independent. Ideally, the information obtained through one type will inform and build on the other. For example, a substantive component study could be used to identify the most promising components of an alcohol use prevention program for members of a fraternity. A group comparison evaluation study might then be used to determine how well the components of the program function for sorority members. If the results indicate that the original components were less effective for the second subgroup, another substantive component study might be needed to identify more appropriate components. Order-based component studies also may be completed to determine whether a different order of two or three components should be offered across comparison groups. Combinations of component study types often are needed when examining constellation-type components because multiple audiences may be addressed with different combinations of components.

▶ TYPES OF GENERAL QUESTIONS ASKED IN COMPONENT STUDIES

Once the components of a health promotion program are developed and the intended associations among these components are understood, a new set of questions emerges about the effectiveness of the components, analyzed separately and in combination. Although theoretical and perceived efficacy work presented in Chapter 4 and Chapters 9 through 12 provides information about components that might be successful, component studies are the means by which subjects are actually run through the activity. The outcome data collected are measures of immediate impact. Component studies yield information about how the components of a health promotion program may actually function when provided to the target population. The immediate impact of a component can be stronger (or weaker) when included in a total program package; however, if a component cannot produce the intended immediate impact when examined separately, its contribution when later nested within a program is likely to be minimal as well.

Component studies save time, money, and effort because components that are unpopular, impractical, or ineffective can be eliminated or revised before they are included in an expensive effectiveness trial or, worse yet, disseminated as part of a larger untested program. Component studies are intended to help the program developer answer the following types of questions:

1. *To what extent does a component have the intended effect?* This is the most important question for a program developer to ask about each component. The component study provides an opportunity for the program developer to determine whether a particular component can produce the intended effect (e.g., change knowledge, attitudes, skills, social norms).

2. *What is the relative impact of each component?* When provided with an opportunity to choose from among a set of component(s) which component(s) to include in a program, it is helpful to determine which components have the greatest immediate effect. Components that are relatively more effective at producing an immediate impact can be given preference over other components that target the same specific immediate effects.

3. *Is a particular combination of components more effective than the individual components implemented alone?* This question is important when determining whether the addition of a new component can increase the impact of another component or set of components and whether it is worth the resources required to make the addition.

4. *To what extent is a component that has been found to be effective for one subgroup of the target population effective for another subgroup?* This question pertains to the generalizability of a program. When adapting an intervention for use in a new target group, it can be beneficial to examine the immediate effects of each component to determine whether effectiveness differs in the new target group.

▶ HOW ARE COMPONENT STUDIES CONDUCTED?

All evaluation studies should include the following elements:

- Identifying constructs
- Determining the target group
- Deciding how to expose participants to the component
- Choosing a study design
- Selecting measurement strategies
- Interpreting the results

The next section of the chapter will examine each of these elements as they pertain to the composition of a component study.

IDENTIFYING CONSTRUCTS

The first step in conducting a component study is to decide on the criteria for evaluating components. These criteria can be determined in a variety of ways. They can be guided by theory (see Chapter 4), based on previous research (e.g., assessment studies; see Chapter 6), or suggested by the target audience (i.e., perceived efficacy studies; see Chapters 9 or 11) who will ultimately benefit from the programs (Loue, Lloyd, & Loh, 1996). For example, a program developer may believe that students and teachers are bored with traditional health programs that use a didactic (lecture) instructional method and provide health consequences information (activity content). A review of the literature also may suggest that an interactive program that aims at change in peer social norms may more strongly affect the target behavior. Hence, the program developer may determine that to be included in a program, a component should be rated as enjoyable to students, involve interaction among students (e.g., through use of group discussions and games), and have an immediate effect on perceived norms (e.g., Sussman, Dent, Burton, et al., 1995). The developer could then develop questions to assess these basic criteria.

Some characteristics examined in component studies apply across components, but others are specific to the particular component studied. For example, all components included in health promotion programs should be acceptable and accessible to the target audience (Aspen Reference Group, 1997; Timmreck, 1995). Other evidence of the immediate effectiveness of the component, such as acquiring a particular skill, understanding a set of facts, or adopting a particular belief, depends on the focus of the specific component studied.

Acceptability and Accessibility. The criteria of acceptability and accessibility are vital to any successful health promotion program. These are general concepts that include a variety of measures. As examples, for a component to be acceptable to the target population, it should be rated as novel, interesting, or enjoyable; relevant, providing a learning experience, or thought provoking; believable, credible, or realistic; and useful, helpful, or capable of providing a direct effect on the target behavior. These 12 adjectives tend to be highly correlated and provide a very good assessment of acceptability (also called "perceived program quality") when placed on a 4-point rating scale (*not at all, a little, somewhat, very much*).

Accessibility pertains to parameters of the component that facilitate ("tailoring") or deter ("barriers") participation in that component, such as whether the component has been tailored to be linguistically and culturally compatible with the target population, the level of comprehensibility of the component as measured through objective measures (e.g., reading level), and socioenvironmental factors (e.g., cost, transportation, child care) (Aspen Reference Group, 1997). Potential barriers range from the concrete, such as the inability to participate in a component because of transportation or child care obstacles, to the more abstract, such as individuals' psychological preparedness for behavioral change (Prochaska, DiClemente, & Norcross, 1992) and cultural norms inconsistent with the intervention component (e.g., portraying tobacco use as evil among many Native American tribes).

Acceptability and accessibility are determined not only by the content of a component but also by the means of instruction. For example, a component study that compares students' acceptability or perceived program quality responses following exposure to a classroom lesson led by a health educator versus exposure to an independent study (self-instruction) lesson examines the acceptability of delivery mode (Sussman, Dent, Simon, et al., 1995). Interestingly, the percentage of subjects who make spontaneous comments regarding the means of instruction during delivery can provide an anecdotal but potentially useful means of assessing acceptability. Similarly, health promotion messages provided via either health educator or written materials will be inaccessible if they are not verbalized or written at the appropriate language or reading level for the target audience. The program developer should consider soliciting participants' reports of any additional barriers they encountered themselves or that they might anticipate others encountering when trying to participate in the component. Perceptions of barriers can be assessed with open-ended questions included in the posttest survey or interview.

Specific Characteristics. Acceptability and accessibility are necessary but insufficient qualities of an effective health promotion program component. The immediate specific effects of a component provide the hypothesized mechanism through

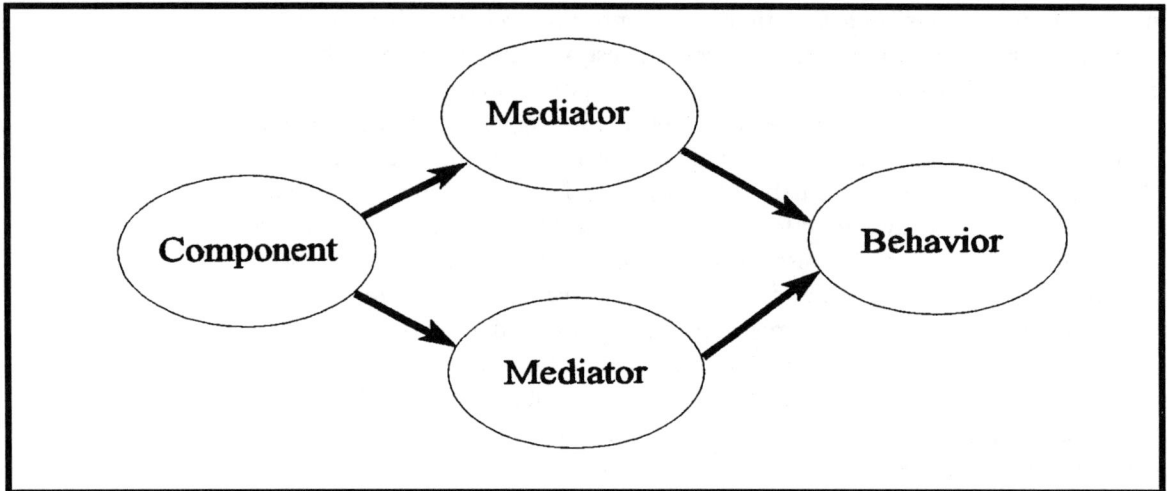

Figure 13.1. Mediation of Component Effects

which the component can influence behavior. As shown in Figure 13.1, mediators are the factors directly influenced by the component. The mediators, in turn, influence behavior. Therefore, the effect of the component on behavior can be described as "working through" the mediators or as being "mediated by" these factors.

Even programs with the goal of long-term behavioral change have immediate objectives for the specific components. Attitudinal change, for example, is an immediate goal for many prevention components and has been found to mediate program effects (Tobler & Stratton, 1997). Therefore, although the ultimate goal of a program may be to prevent initiation of cigarette smoking, for example, the goal of a particular component in the program may be to create changes in attitudes that are thought to influence risk for initiating cigarette smoking (e.g., attitudes toward smokers, attitudes toward enforcement of anti-tobacco policies, or attitudes toward the tobacco industry) (Independent Evaluation Consortium, 1998). In this case, the component study can examine the extent to which exposure to that component produces a change in these specific attitudes. Ultimately, outcome studies are used to confirm whether the changes in hypothesized mediating variables actually result in behavior change.

In addition to attitudes, a variety of other mediator effects can be assessed in component studies. These include increased recognition of the problem; changes in specific knowledge, beliefs, values, norms, or intentions; commitment to change behavior; and behaviors that can be measured immediately, such as the ability to demonstrate the skills taught or immediate initiation or cessation of a behavior. A longer period of time is required to assess change for most behaviors. Therefore, long-term behavior change is typically assessed with outcome trials (see Chapter 19 for a more detailed presentation of mediation and moderation of program effects, and see Chapter 20 for a summary of potentially important mediators of health behavior programming).

If the immediate evaluation goals for the components of a health promotion program have not been clarified previously, the component study process provides an opportunity to make these explicit. Program developers should specify the process through which they expect the component to change behavior and then try to identify one or more mediators in this process. They can then focus on measuring the extent to which the component has an impact on those mediators. For example, a school-based alcohol prevention study (Donaldson, Graham, & Hansen, 1994) included a resistance-skills component and a social-norms component. The researchers hypothesized that exposure to the social-norms component would result in decreased perceptions regarding the acceptability of alcohol use, whereas exposure to the resistance-skills component would result in improved ability to resist alcohol offers. After the mechanisms of program effects had been postulated, the components were evaluated to determine whether they indeed influenced students' perceptions regarding the acceptability of alcohol use and their ability to resist alcohol offers. This change in the mediators was observed, and a corresponding later change in actual alcohol use was noted.

DETERMINING THE TARGET GROUP AND COLLECTING INFORMATION FROM SUPPLEMENTAL GROUPS

Several groups can provide useful information when conducting component studies. Obviously, a primary source of information is the population for whom the program is being designed (i.e., the target audience). Members of the target audience for the program usually can provide the most useful information on the acceptability, accessibility, and specific impact of a component, and samples from this audience should be recruited for component studies (Sussman, Dent, Burton, et al., 1995). The better the audience can be specified and the more similar the samples are to the audience, the more relevant a component study is likely to be to later stages of program development and the main trial.

In addition to the target audience, other supplemental groups may help to provide a more complete perspective on the relevance and likely immediate impact of the components on the target sample. Such groups include those who control access to the target population (e.g., gatekeepers such as school board members, health maintenance organization administrators, scout leaders, employers), those who ultimately will administer the component (e.g., health educators, facilitators, nurses, social workers, elementary school teachers), those who have completed similar health promotion programs with the target audience (i.e., other experts), and the target audience's family members. These groups can read verbal descriptions or observe the components being delivered, and they can provide comments in an interview or a focus group or as part of a theme study (see Chapters 9 and 11, this volume).

These supplemental groups can provide valuable information about the likely acceptability and accessibility of the components. For example, gatekeepers can help the program developer determine whether the implementation of a component is logistically possible, and family members can provide their perspectives on the target audience's ability to participate in and comprehend the component. Also, the perceptions of the larger community are particularly important when trying to garner support and resources for a program. As a corollary, it is important to recognize the potential for a particular component to encounter resistance within a community. Health behavior activities such as sex education, condom distribution, methadone clinics, needle exchange programs, suicide awareness activities, and midnight basketball may be perceived as acceptable, accessible, and effective by the target audience but may meet with considerable opposition from some members of the larger community. Earlier stages of program development (e.g., theme studies; see Chapter 12, this volume) can and should involve ratings of numerous plausible activities by supplemental parties. However, the component study stage of program development can give the supplemental parties a chance to observe each component in action and voice concerns that might not be anticipated when only imagining what implementation of a component might be like. For example, actually watching a 12-year-old refuse role-played sexual advances in a classroom may provoke a very different reaction than just reading about that activity component.

Statistical Power Issues. The power to detect statistically significant differences in immediate impact (effectiveness) between groups is determined, to a large extent, by the size of the sample studied. Small differences between groups require a larger sample to statistically differentiate effects—that is, to make an accurate decision regarding whether the difference is due to chance. Because component studies are only one stage in the program development process, and because resources tend to be very limited for this type of evaluation, the size of the sample is likely to be small. Therefore, the power to detect a significant difference may be lower than what will be available in the final outcome evaluation. On the other hand, because component studies focus on the immediate effects of a component, such as changes in knowledge, beliefs, or attitudes, the magnitude of the differences between groups might be larger than what is expected for behavior in the final outcome evaluation. Therefore, the component study sample does not need to be very large (see discussion of statistical power in Chapter 16).

If possible, a program developer should use samples large enough to ensure adequate statistical power. Several software programs are available that can aid in determining the sample size necessary to detect a small, medium, or large effect with a particular design and analytic strategy (Borenstein & Cohen, 1988; Dean et al., 1995; SPSS, Inc., 1997). When it is not possible to enroll a large enough sample to permit tests of statistical significance, the program developer may choose to adopt another criterion for selecting components, such as ranking the components according to posttest scores, percentage change from baseline, or a combination of strategies. For example, Sussman, Dent, Burton, et al. (1995) used a series of component studies to determine which activities, from an initial set of 43, to include in a tobacco use prevention curriculum. They focused on change in intentions to start smoking, knowledge change, and the percentage of participants reporting that the activity was interesting. After the initial component study, any activity was dropped if it was associated with an increased intention to use tobacco, less than a 3% average increase in knowledge, or less than 40% of participants reporting interest.

EXPOSING PARTICIPANTS TO THE PROGRAM COMPONENT

If feasible, each component should be delivered in the manner that it might be used in the final program. The components of a health promotion program ultimately are delivered as a set, and the effectiveness of any one component may be enhanced (or possibly negated) when combined with the other components (e.g., complementary components). For example, one might speculate that those exposed to a social-norms component of a breast cancer prevention program might be convinced that breast self-exam is appropriate for them to do. Therefore, they would be more motivated to acquire the skills necessary for an effective breast self-exam during a skills-training component. Thus, one might want to include such components in an order-based component study. However, in most such cases, there is still much value in providing separate implementation and evaluation of the components. In the example given, even marginally motivated participants should be able to understand the instructions and acquire the skills taught in the skill-building component without first completing the norms or motivation component. If each component is effective when delivered independently, the cumulative multicomponent effect should be maximized. At the component study stage of program development, the most important issue to address is the evidence that each component is as effective as possible at achieving its specific goal.

Nonetheless, there may be times when it is impossible to evaluate one component without having participants first complete another component (i.e., very strong building-block relationship). For example, suicide prevention programs often incorporate a screening component to identify those at great risk for suicide so that these persons can receive additional intervention components (Centers for Disease Control and Prevention, 1992). Because the interventions are effective only if the screening is sensitive enough to identify those at risk, the validity of the screening component should be confirmed before testing the treatment components.

Similarly, an activity in which students create anti-tobacco posters designed to counteract the positive images of smokers in pro-tobacco advertisements (*activism activity*) may build on information learned in an activity in which students identify the positive images of smokers in the advertisements (*information activity*). If components build on each other very tightly, perhaps they should be evaluated together. In the present example, the program developer might want to ensure that participants learn a sufficient number of advertising techniques in an information activity (e.g., smoking as being sophisticated, attractive, exciting, sexy, independent) to be able to apply one or more of them in the activism activity. Here, the developer may be interested in determining whether the second component contributes to the desired outcome above and beyond the effects of the earlier delivered component. Conversely, the program developer may wonder whether the informational component is necessary to conduct the second component successfully. In that case, only the second component would be tested. Alternatively, the program developer may wonder whether the two components should be combined into one general activity (informational introduction followed by the activism activity). A quasi- or true experimental design (see the next section) can be used to compare the immediate effects observed in groups that receive both components to those observed in groups that receive only the one component or a combined component of the same delivery duration.

One caveat is in order. Although the ideal strategy is to expose participants to the complete component directly, practical limitations in terms of cost, time, subject cooperation, or other resources may make it impossible to have participants complete each component in its entirety. If so, abridged activities could be completed. Although less desirable, even minimal exposure to program components permits some means of avoiding problems later on when piloting a complete program.

CHOOSING A STUDY DESIGN

Most of the evaluation study designs described in any research methodology text can be used for component study work. The choice of study design will depend on the evaluation question and resources available. Whenever feasible, the randomization of subjects to component conditions provides the most rigorous evaluation. However, to compare the strength of immediate effectiveness across components, the quasi-experimental design is generally adequate. To determine whether a specific component is accessible, acceptable, and capable of influencing the desired mediators (e.g., knowledge, attitudes, and behavior), one may find that a single-group pretest-posttest design is also sufficient. The most common designs used in component studies are the single-group pretest-posttest and the quasi-experimental designs.

Single-Group Pretest-Posttest Study Design. For the purposes of component studies, the pretest-posttest design can provide a great deal of information with minimal cost and planning. The basic design involves recruiting a representative group of participants from the target audience, measuring the initial or baseline levels of the specific characteristics the component is expected to influence, exposing the participants to the component, and then measuring the levels of the characteristics again as well as the accessibility and acceptability of the component (the latter measures being addressed at posttest only). Change in the characteristics between baseline and immediate posttest levels generally can be attributed to exposure to the component. Descriptive statistics such as percentages or mean levels can be used to quantify the impact of the program on posttest-only measures, and inferential statistics such as chi-square or t-tests can be used to determine if the difference observed between baseline and posttest is significantly different from zero. In this way, each component's success in achieving the intended goals can be examined.

For example, the pretest-posttest design was used to develop the curriculum used in the Television, School, and Family Project's smoking prevention and cessation programs. Students' pretest-posttest knowledge gains and the perceived helpfulness of 10 smoking prevention curriculum components were used to revise the content of the components and the sequence in which they were presented (Flay et al., 1988). The relative ease of implementation of the single-group pretest-posttest design permits the use of multiple-component studies, providing an opportunity to make changes in the components and reevaluate their effects (see Sussman, Craig, Simon, & Galaif, 1997). Replications of this design across different subject groups permit an iterative means of refining the contents and instructional methods of a component (Sussman, Dent, Burton, et al., 1995).

Quasi-Experimental Design. The disadvantage of the single-group pretest- posttest design is that all subjects receive the component. Therefore, one cannot rule out the possibility that pretest-posttest differences might be due to something else that happened at the same time or that the differences are a result of the increased attention and measurements given to the group studied. Having multiple groups can be preferable in situations such as the following: (a) when one desires to compare the effectiveness of one component against that of another, (b) when a component's effects are compared across subgroups of the target population, and (c) when one component's effects may or may not be dependent on implementation of another component. Quasi- and true experimental designs allow the program developer to compare the magnitude of effects observed in a group that receives one component to those observed in a group that receives another component or series of components. Each group would serve as the control or comparison for the other. Alternatively, one comparison group may be provided with no treatment and serve as the no-treatment control for the other groups.

In a quasi-experimental design, the program developer is able to control the when and where of measurement but not always the when and where of exposure to the component material. In quasi-experiments that compare different components, the goal is to identify several groups of participants who are presumed to be similar (e.g., comparable distribution for basic background characteristics such as age, sex, race/ethnicity, and education, as well as pretest levels on the target behaviors of interest). Ideally, baseline data on the demographic characteristics and outcomes of interest can be collected. These data can be used to assess whether the two groups truly are similar, and, if not, these data may be used to statistically control for differences. The groups are assigned or self-select to receive different components or a no-treatment control component. The scores on measures of immediate effects can then be collected after the participants are exposed to the component activities.

For example, the effects of a bicycle-riding safety education program can be tested among subjects who live in regions where helmet use is mandatory and where helmet use is not required. Through use of this comparison evaluation-type component study, the effects of the program with or without a legal support can be assessed among subjects who self-select their place of residence (e.g., see Dannenberg et al., 1993, who present this type of design as a trial, not a component study).

In quasi-experimental designs, if baseline data for groups are similar, the program developer can have some confidence attributing differences observed at posttest to the component exposure (Cook & Campbell, 1979). Descriptive and inferential statistics can then be used to compare the immediate effects across conditions. If the groups differ at baseline on some measurable characteristic (e.g., demographics), the program developer should control for these differences in the statistical analyses.

True Experimental Design. Although quasi-experimental designs are valuable for addressing most component study questions, they are considered not as good as true experimental designs. Quasi-experimental designs can be flawed because even if baseline data are collected and groups are found to be comparable on all characteristics measured, groups may still differ on other unmeasured factors that will influence participants' response to the components studied. For a detailed discussion of other threats to validity that can influence the interpretability of results from quasi-experimental designs, see Cook and Campbell's (1979) text.

In a true experimental design, a sample of individuals from the target population is randomly assigned to component conditions. Thus, the program developer controls both the when and where of measurement and exposure to the component (see also Chapter 16, this volume). This strategy ensures that the variation within the sample of participants will be dispersed equally across exposure conditions. Therefore, a program developer can be confident that any differences observed at posttest are due to exposure to the component condition. For example, a randomized experimental design was used to compare the immediate effects of a health-based (skin cancer) message to an appearance-based (skin-aging) message on intentions to use sunscreen. Both messages resulted in greater intentions to use sunscreen relative to a control message for older participants, and neither message influenced intentions for younger participants (Mahler, Fitzpatrick, Parker, & Lapin, 1997). Because participants were randomized to experimental conditions before the intervention, the program developer can infer that any postintervention differences between the groups are a result of the intervention, rather than an artifact of preintervention differences between the groups. Of course, to develop a maximally effective message for young people, program developers need to conduct additional component study work. These three designs are discussed again regarding their relevance to pilot study work in Chapter 16.

SELECTING MEASUREMENT STRATEGIES

Qualitative or quantitative methods can be used effectively in component studies. Qualitative methods are open-ended and permit greater flexibility in the responses. Such methods also allow the program developer to identify unknown issues related to a program component that may affect its implementation. The participants might recognize potential barriers to effective implementation that the program developer did not anticipate. For example, participants from the target audience may associate some aspect of an intervention component with an event from the local news or a popular television show. The event may influence the immediate effectiveness of a treatment in ways that the program developer cannot anticipate. In component studies, qualitative techniques are especially useful when debriefing subjects to elicit such additional information.

Quantitative methods are useful for assessing levels of a particular construct and assigning a numerical value to that construct. Such methods permit the use of descriptive or inferential statistics. Descriptive statistics characterize the outcome by providing a value such as a percentage, rate, mean, or change score. Descriptive statistics make it possible to rank activities on the various dimensions of acceptability, accessibility, and degree of manipulation of specific mediators. Inferential statistics are used to determine whether comparisons are statistically significant (i.e., whether differences observed across groups or over time are due to chance or to a real difference). Descriptive and inferential statistics can facilitate decision making when one is forced to choose from among a set of competing components. For example, one can choose the component with the maximum average score on the outcomes or the component that resulted in a statistically significant increase in knowledge between pretest and posttest.

Quantitative and qualitative methods are not mutually exclusive. When used together, the two strategies often can provide a more complete understanding of the immediate effects of a program. For example, when developing the multimedia component of a comprehensive adolescent health promotion program, Bosworth (1997) used both quantitative and qualitative methods to examine students' perceptions of the characters, script, information, and technical quality of the component. The quantitative ratings suggested a potential problem with technical quality. The source of the problem was identified from several subjects' comments expressed during the qualitative evaluation, which indicated that the verbal message from one of the characters was difficult to understand. This problem was relatively easy to correct and might not have been pinpointed without the use of both quantitative and qualitative strategies.

INTERPRETING THE RESULTS

Component studies provide the program developer with some unique challenges when trying to interpret the results. Because component studies often have a small number of participants, provide preliminary findings, and usually test several components using several measures, it is important for the program developer to consider the following: statistical versus clinical significance, balance between results and theory, and criteria for choosing which components to implement.

Statistical Versus Clinical Significance. When interpreting the results of a component study, the program developer must be careful not to confuse statistical significance with clinical or "real-world" significance. If the results of a component study indicate that target subjects prefer one component over another and this difference is statistically significant, it is tempting to conclude that the component rated more highly is better. However, with large samples (e.g., $n = 1,000$), even small differences can be statistically significant. For example, if two activities are rated 4.8 and 4.9 on a 5-point scale of likability, the difference may not be meaningful. In this case, the program developer may choose between the two activities by using a criterion other than likability, such as ease of implementation (i.e., pragmatics).

Conversely, the program developer should not interpret a lack of statistical significance as an indication that two activities are equivalent. If the sample size is small (e.g., $n = 20$), meaningful differences between activities may not achieve statistical significance. If the program developer finds, for example, that the mean likability ratings of two components (on the same 5-point scale) are 2.0 and 4.0, the program developer may decide to choose the more highly rated component, even if the difference in the ratings was not statistically significant. Statistical significance (or a lack thereof) should not take the place of good judgment. As in any evaluation, results are not always definitive. As mentioned earlier, it is often helpful, before making the final decisions, to include representatives of the target group and the people who implement the program to assist in the deliberations.

Balance Between Results and Theory. The program developer should consider the results of component studies in the context of the current body of knowledge about behavior change. Even if subjects or staff indicate that they prefer a particular component, this component should not be implemented if it has been shown in previous studies to be ineffective in producing behavior change. For example, teens may say they prefer a substance use prevention program consisting of scare tactics and fear appeals (they may also enjoy going to horror movies), but previous research has shown that these tactics are ineffective in changing behavior (Brotman & Suffet, 1973; Orleans, 1985; Witte & Morrison, 1995), at least as currently developed for teens (e.g., they may not produce fear, which is the mediator here). The program developer should not be too quick to abandon well-established disease prevention and health promotion strategies based on one result from a single-component study.

Criteria for Choosing Which Components to Implement. Time constraints and budgetary limitations frequently limit the number of components that can be included in a health promotion program. After conducting a component study, the program developer can make an informed decision as to which components to include in the program. As shown in Figure 13.2, a reasonable strategy is to drop

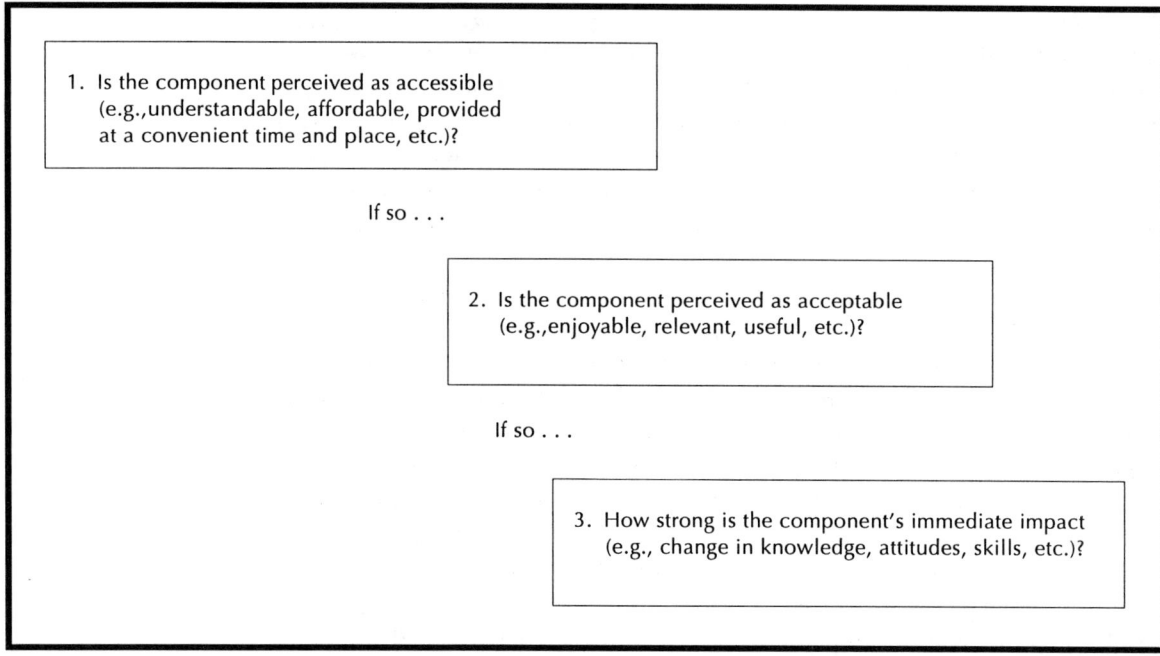

Figure 13.2. Steps for Deciding Which Components to Retain

those components that fail to meet a minimum level of accessibility and acceptability. One easy rule of thumb is the three-quarters rule. Components should be able to be accessed by at least 75% of the target population to be worthwhile to distribute. Aside from logistical problems suffered by the target population, there also may be logistic concerns suffered by the deliverers. Thus, for example, it is preferable to choose the activities presenting the fewest delivery context challenges, such as the need for special rooms or equipment. The reason is that any logistic concerns suffered by the deliverers are likely to "trickle down" to the consumer. In addition, if the logistical barriers to program implementation are too large, the people who deliver the program may choose not to deliver the inconvenient components at all. One should be quite careful when making judgments of accessibility. One might hope that such logistic problems are considered in earlier stages of program development, but, if not, the three-quarters rule, considered carefully, is a good one to follow.

Likewise, components should receive mean acceptability ratings on at least a "somewhat high" level on a 4-point scale of acceptability (*not at all, a little, somewhat, very*) to be retained. The three-quarters rule, as applied here, means that an average score that is three-quarters of the highest possible value should be obtained to retain the component. Components that are both accessible and acceptable may then be considered with regard to the strength of the immediate effects they elicit on specific mediators. For example, suppose a developer is planning a seven-component program that will best mesh with the time demands of a busy clinic environment. The developer begins with 20 promising components derived from earlier perceived efficacy work. A component study may show that 14 of 20 activities were reasonably accessible and acceptable, using the three-quarters rule. From these 14 activities, the developer may then choose the 7 activities with the strongest effects on mediating variables while considering relationships among the components. As a second rule of thumb, it is wise to test at least twice as many components as one expects to retain for the next step of producing a full-draft program. This may be referred to as the "keep-half" rule.

After selecting a set of activities to include in a comprehensive program, it may be helpful to solicit evaluations of the entire proposed program. When viewing the program as a whole, it is important to identify logistical barriers to implementation (e.g., the need to move participants repeatedly to different rooms for different activities). It is also necessary to identify potential problems in the transition between components (e.g., it may not be advisable to follow a humorous component with a serious activity because students may remain in facetious moods during the serious component and thereby undermine its effectiveness). Building-block components likely will be retained as a set and will need to fit along with other components or sets of components. The components of a prevention program should be consistent and avoid redundancy. For details on constructing a complete program, see Chapter 15 (this volume).

CONCLUSIONS ◄

Most health promotion programs incorporate multiple components to address the various factors that influence health-related behaviors. Component studies can be used to evaluate the extent to which each component considered for inclusion in a program "measures up." Each component in the program should show reasonable accessibility and acceptability as well as demonstrate an immediate impact on participants such as changes in knowledge, attitudes, skills, or social norms. These changes are the mechanisms through which the health promotion program ultimately influences behavior and health. To maximize program effectiveness and reduce the cost of program implementation, only the best components should be included in the final program.

Evaluation of a program component requires conceptualization of the factors that the component is expected to influence immediately. The components then are provided to participants who represent the larger target group, and the immediate impact is assessed. Immediate impact can be examined within a single subgroup, compared across groups receiving different components, or compared across different subgroups (representing different target audiences) that evaluate the same components. All components should be acceptable and accessible to the targeted group, and the components should be successful at producing the intended specific immediate effects. The "three-quarters" (minimum standards) and "keep-half" (retaining components) rules are quite handy rules of thumb to consider regarding component retention for later program construction.

Successful component studies require the collaboration of research and practitioner minds. Research expertise is useful for developing the study design, selecting a sampling strategy, and analyzing and interpreting the results. Practitioners' skills are helpful for providing a focus for qualitative studies; determining the most important indicators of accessibility, acceptability, and immediate effectiveness; and deciding how to change components to improve their immediate effects. (If barriers between practitioners and researchers, expressed in Chapter 3, can be overcome, much cooperative productivity can result.)

Component studies that are systematically completed and well documented aid in the development of effective health promotion programs. Unfortunately, health professionals often complete component studies without documenting their contributions to the process leading to the final program product. Documentation of information about the components that were rejected, as well as information about program components that were retained, may provide invaluable information to other professionals who might want to either (a) capitalize on time savings or (b) review all components previously tested for their potential inclusion in a program to be applied to a new setting or population. Also, for the benefit of the field of health promotion, it is just as important for the cumulative knowledge base to know why a particular component may be ineffective under certain circumstances as it is to know why a component is effective.

▶ REFERENCES

ASPEN REFERENCE GROUP. (1997). *Community health education and promotion: A guide to program design and evaluation.* Gaithersburg, MD: Author.

BORENSTEIN, M., & COHEN, J. (1988). *Statistical power analysis: A computer program.* Hillsdale, NJ: Lawrence Erlbaum.

BOSWORTH, K. (1997). *NCI technical report*. Bloomington: Indiana University.
BROTMAN, R., & SUFFET, F. (1973). Illicit drug use: Prevention education in the school. *Psychiatric Annals, 34,* 48-69.
CENTERS FOR DISEASE CONTROL AND PREVENTION. (1992). *Youth suicide prevention programs: A resource guide.* Atlanta, GA: Author.
COOK, T. D., & CAMPBELL, D. T. (1979). *Quasi-experimentation: Design and analysis issues for field settings.* Boston: Houghton Mifflin.
DANNENBERG, A. L., GIELEN, A. C., BEILENSON, P. L., WILSON, M., & JOFFE, A. (1993). Bicycle helmet laws and educational campaigns: An evaluation of strategies to increase children's helmet use. *American Journal of Public Health, 83,* 667-674.
DEAN, A. G., DEAN, J. A., COULOMBIER, D., BRENDEL, K. A., SMITH, D. C., BURTON, A. H., DICKER, R. C., SULLIVAN, K., FAGAN, R. F., & ARNER, T. G. (1995). *Epi Info, version 6: A word processing, databases, and statistics program for public health on IBM compatible microcomputers.* Atlanta, GA: Centers for Disease Control and Prevention.
DONALDSON, S. I., GRAHAM, J. W., & HANSEN, W. B. (1994). Testing the generalizability of intervening mechanism theories: Understanding the effects of adolescent drug use prevention interventions. *Journal of Behavioral Medicine, 17,* 195-216.
DRYFOOS, J. G. (1991). Adolescents at risk: A summation of work in the field: Programs and policies. *Journal of Adolescent Health, 12,* 630-637.
FLAY, B. R., BRANNON, B. R., JOHNSON, C. A., HANSEN, W. B., ULENE, A. L., WHITNEY-SALTIEL, D. A., GLEASON, L. R., SUSSMAN, S., GAVIN, M. D., GLOWACZ, K. M., SOBOL, D. F., & SPIEGEL, D. C. (1988). The Television School and Family Smoking Prevention and Cessation Project: I. Theoretical basis and program development. *Preventive Medicine, 17,* 585-607.
GABRIEL, R. M., HASKINS, M., HOPSON, T., & POWELL, K. E. (1996). Building relationships and resilience in the prevention of youth violence. *American Journal of Preventive Medicine, 12*(Suppl. 2), 48-55.
HANSEN, W. (1992). School-based substance abuse prevention: A review of the state of the art in curriculum, 1980-1990. *Health Education Research: Theory and Practice, 7,* 403-430.
INDEPENDENT EVALUATION CONSORTIUM. (1998). *Final report of the independent evaluation of the California Tobacco Control Prevention and Education Program: Wave I data, 1996-1997.* Rockville, MD: Gallup Organization.
LOUE, S., LLOYD, L., & LOH, L. (1996). HIV prevention in U.S. Asian Pacific Islander communities: An innovative approach. *Journal of Health Care for the Poor and Underserved, 7,* 364-376.
MAHLER, H. I. M., FITZPATRICK, B., PARKER, P., & LAPIN, A. (1997). The relative effects of a health-based versus an appearance-based intervention designed to increase sunscreen use. *American Journal of Health Promotion, 11,* 426-429.
ORLEANS, C. T. (1985). Understanding and promoting smoking cessation: Overview and guidelines for physician intervention. *Annual Review of Medicine, 36,* 51-61.
PENTZ, M. A., DWYER, J. H., MACKINNON, D. P., FLAY, B. R., HANSEN, W. B., WANG, E. Y., & JOHNSON, C. A. (1989). A multicommunity trial for primary prevention of adolescent drug abuse: Effects on drug use prevalence. *JAMA, 261,* 3259-3266.
PETERSON, J. L., COATES, T. J., CATANIA, J., & HAUCK, W. W. (1996). Evaluation of an HIV risk reduction intervention among African-American homosexual and bisexual men. *AIDS, 10,* 319-325.
PROCHASKA, J. O., DiCLEMENTE, C. C., & NORCROSS, J. C. (1992). In search of how people change: Applications to addictive behaviors. *American Psychologist, 47,* 1102-1114.
SPSS, INC. (1997). *SPSS advanced statistics 7.5.* Chicago: Author.
SUSSMAN, S., CRAIG, S., SIMON, T. R., & GALAIF, E. R. (1997). School-as-community activity selection at continuation high schools. *Substance Use & Misuse, 32,* 113-131.
SUSSMAN, S., DENT, C. W., BURTON, D., STACY, A. W., & FLAY, B. R. (1995). *Developing school-based tobacco use prevention and cessation programs.* Thousand Oaks, CA: Sage.
SUSSMAN, S., DENT, C. W., SIMON, T. R., STACY, A. W., GALAIF, E. R., MOSS, M. A., CRAIG, S., & JOHNSON, C. A. (1995). Immediate impact of social influence-oriented substance abuse prevention curricula in traditional and continuation high schools. *Drugs & Society, 8,* 65-81.

SUSSMAN, S., DENT, C. W., STACY, A. W., & CRAIG, S. (1998). One-year outcomes of Project Towards No Drug Abuse. *Preventive Medicine, 27*, 632-642.

SUSSMAN, S., SIMON, T. R., DENT, C. W., STACY, A. W., GALAIF, E. R., MOSS, M. A., CRAIG, S., & JOHNSON, C. A. (1997). Immediate impact of thirty-two drug use prevention activities among students at continuation high schools. *Substance Use & Misuse, 23*, 265-281.

TIMMRECK, T. C. (1995). *Planning, program development and evaluation: A handbook for health promotion, aging and health services.* Boston: Jones & Bartlett.

TOBLER, N. S., & STRATTON, H. H. (1997). Effectiveness of school-based drug prevention programs: A meta-analysis of the research. *Journal of Primary Prevention, 18*, 71-128.

WITTE, K., & MORRISON, K. (1995). Using scare tactics to promote safer sex among juvenile detention and high school youth. *Journal of Applied Communication Research, 23*, 128-142.

CHAPTER 13

Commentary

Brian R. Flay

Simon, Bosworth, and Unger have done a fine job of describing component studies. As they have defined them, component studies are small-scale studies of the feasibility, acceptability, and likely effectiveness of small components of a proposed larger intervention before compiling them into the larger intervention. Component studies are part of the developmental research that should be conducted before testing full-scale interventions.

Simon and colleagues provide a nice explanation of why we need component studies, what they are, and how to conduct them. I will comment directly on their chapter only briefly. I will first discuss the place of component studies in the broader scheme of the development of health promotion interventions. I will then address Simon et al.'s focus on proximal determinants of behavior. Finally, I will discuss how component studies may have to be conceptualized more broadly to accommodate changes in the types of interventions being developed for the future.

PHASES OF RESEARCH

In terms of phase models of health promotion or prevention research, this work should occur before efficacy trials (i.e., main, large-scale trials of a program or programs). In other words, component studies fall into Phase II work in the National Cancer Institute or National Heart, Lung, and Blood Institute schemes (methods development), Phase III in my scheme (Flay, 1986), and Phase II of one scheme recently developed for alcohol problem prevention research (Holder et al., 1999). I characterized this Phase III of research in the development of health promotion programs as "pilot-applied research." The idea was to conduct "preliminary tests of new approaches toward using basic research results to achieve specific immediate effects related to specific health promotion goals" (Flay, 1986, p. 459). Note that I emphasized the use of basic research results as the starting point. By this, I meant that the ideas for new approaches should come from or be supported by basic research in health promotion or some other discipline that addresses behavior change such as education, psychology, sociology, or communications research (theory and assessment studies).

I suggested that Phase III studies be "pilot (pre- or quasi-experimental) [tests of] innovative manipulations; very small scale (few individuals or aggregated units per condition)" (Flay, 1986, p. 459). The suggestions by Simon et al. in their chapter are all very consistent with these recommendations. They do emphasize attempting experimental and quasi-experimental tests and avoiding single-group pretest-posttest-only designs, and I agree with this emphasis.

Unfortunately, examples of formal component studies are few and far between, or at least they are rarely reported. The two sets of work by Sussman and his colleagues (Sussman, 1996; Sussman, Dent, Burton, Stacy, & Flay, 1995) provide examples that, together with this chapter and this volume, should motivate more such work. Sussman et al. focused on immediate outcomes that are presumed to be mediators of behavioral outcomes, just as advocated by Simon et al.

Simon et al.'s focus on proximal determinants of behavior seems to make sense from both theoretical and practical points of view. From the practical point of view, component studies must produce an immediate change in some variable related to future behavior. The theoretical view supports this, suggesting that intervention components should each change something immediately that is a proximal determinant of the behavior of interest. For example, an activity designed to alter students' normative beliefs about peer smoking should do so immediately, and then, in the longer term, the changed normative perceptions should influence their own behavior. In this example, normative beliefs are proximal cognitive or affective determinants of behavior, as are knowledge, attitudes, self-efficacy, and intentions.

LOOKING TO THE FUTURE

The importance of many distal and ultimate influences on behavior (Flay & Petraitis, 1994; Petraitis, Flay, & Miller, 1995) means that it is also necessary to develop intervention components to alter such influences. The importance of addressing more distal influences also is being underlined by increasing recognition that changes in proximal influences will not be maintained if distal influences are not also altered. For example, changes in normative beliefs (which are really perceptions of what others are doing and what you think they want you to do) will not be maintained if the behaviors and attitudes (approval/disapproval) of others in the school, family, and community environments are not also changed.

The question becomes, How adaptable are component studies to testing activities designed to alter others' behavioral modeling, parental bonding, worksite, or school policy changes, as well as other more distal determinants of behavior? Can component studies be used for such large-scale interventions, or must we be satisfied with suggestive data from naturally occurring variations?

The future of health promotion will emphasize programs that (a) change multiple behaviors rather than only one, (b) influence distal determinants of behavior in addition to or instead of proximal influences, and (c) will be ongoing rather than short term. The latter two projections are not controversial, although we do not necessarily know how to achieve them. The first projection is recognized by many, particularly practice and policy people, but current science does not support this approach. Current science says that to change a particular behavior, such as smoking, one must have a domain-specific program that targets smoking (or tobacco use) exclusively. Some research suggests that programs that attempt to address multiple domains are not as successful. This seems to be less true for closely related behaviors, such as tobacco, alcohol, and drug use, but more true the less related the behaviors are (e.g., smoking, violence, and sexual behavior).

Fortunately, recent evidence suggests that programs can successfully target a range of behaviors. Such programs attempt to exert effects on a broad set of intrapersonal (e.g., self-esteem and personal and social skills), interpersonal (e.g., building relationships and bonds with positive peers, parents, and community), and sociocultural (e.g., media literacy, advocacy, policy change, social services) domains. By changing such distal as well as proximal influences on behavior, the hope is to alter multiple attitudes, normative beliefs, and intentions and, thereby, the course of multiple behaviors (Johnson, MacKinnon, & Pentz, 1996).

Again, the question is, Can the component study methodology described by Simon et al. be adapted for interventions that address multiple behaviors and distal influences? For some interventions, the answer is clearly yes. The school-based programs each have components that address certain microlevel skills, attitudes, beliefs, or behaviors. The effectiveness of these components can be tested for their immediate effects in the ways described by Simon et al. Obviously, the various component activities of family-based interventions can be tested in the same ways. However, the linkage from changes in parenting styles or behavior and child behavior involves a much longer causal chain, many links of which will be changed by many outside influences such as relatives, peers, schools, neighbors, media, politics, and the biological development of the child. Thus, the ultimate evaluation of complex or early interventions faces the same conundrums faced in the evaluations of mass media campaigns (Flay & Cook, 1981). In essence, component studies that are sensitive to small effects on immediate outcomes may be of low practice, policy, or theoretical relevance to the outcomes or impact of ultimate value. The outcomes achieved most quickly occur for variables that are also easily changed by other events in the environment. Thus, they may not have large effects on the target behavior of interest, or they may not last. Future program developers will have to contend with this conundrum and explore ways of reducing or overcoming it. This may or may not be accomplished, in part, by creative component study work.

SUMMARY

Simon et al. and the other authors of this volume have done a great service to the field. Following the advice laid out in these pages will improve future health promotion and disease prevention efforts. Such improvement is greatly needed. Too many programs are developed without careful formative research and evaluation, of which component testing is one important phase. Dismal failures and a great deal of wasted public funds are the result. Unfortunately, too many programs, even ones of known efficacy (i.e., they can work if implemented fully), are implemented on a wide scale without evaluations of their development, implementation, and eventual effectiveness—with the result that the expected changes are not obtained, and many more millions of public funds are wasted. Researchers, program developers, program adopters and implementers, and public decision makers would do well to heed the advice in this volume.

REFERENCES

FLAY, B. R. (1986). Efficacy and effectiveness trials (and other phases of research) in the development of health promotion programs. *Preventive Medicine, 15,* 451-474.

FLAY, B. R., & COOK, T. D. (1981). Evaluation of mass media prevention campaigns. In R. R. Rice & W. Paisley (Eds.), *Public communication campaigns* (pp. 239-313). Beverly Hills, CA: Sage.

FLAY, B. R., & PETRAITIS, J. (1994). The theory of triadic influence: A new theory of health behavior with implications for preventive interventions. In G. S. Albrecht (Ed.), *Advances in medical sociology: Vol. 4. A reconsideration of models of health behavior change* (pp. 19-44). Greenwich, CT: JAI.

HOLDER, H., FLAY, B. R., HOWARD, J., BOYD, G., VOAS, R., & GROSSMAN, M. (1999). Phases of alcohol problem prevention research. *Journal of Alcoholism: Clinical and Experimental Research, 23,* 183-194.

JOHNSON, C. A., MACKINNON, D. P., & PENTZ, M. A. (1996). Breadth of program and outcome effectiveness in drug abuse prevention. *American Behavioral Scientist, 39,* 884-896.

PETRAITIS, J., FLAY, B. R., & MILLER, T. Q. (1995). Reviewing theories of adolescent substance abuse: Organizing pieces of the puzzle. *Psychological Bulletin, 117,* 67-86.

SUSSMAN, S. (1996). Development of a school-based drug abuse prevention curriculum for high-risk youths. *Journal of Psychoactive Drugs, 28,* 169-182.

SUSSMAN, S., DENT, C. W., BURTON, D., STACY, A. W., & FLAY, B. R. (1995). *Developing school-based tobacco use prevention and cessation programs.* Thousand Oaks, CA: Sage.

Case Study 6

CHAPTER 14

Project EX Component Study

Kara Lichtman
Clyde W. Dent
Brian Colwell
Dennis W. Smith
Steve Sussman

Quality curricula result from a careful design process, not from good luck, pure intentions, or happenstance. Program development should be driven by data related to the problem to be addressed and sound underlying behavioral theories, from which a menu of possible activities is generated and tested (the first 12 chapters of this text). At that point, the component study is used by researchers to develop the parts of a program or curriculum and to select various individual components for inclusion in a multicomponent health behavior change program. Each component represents a single activity or session that generally differs from other activities or sessions in content or mode of delivery (e.g., method of instruction). Selection of activities is based on feasibility (e.g., time constraints, ease of implementation), theoretical compatibility with materials composing the rest of the curriculum (Rogers, 1995), and relative effectiveness on immediate outcomes (e.g., attitudes or knowledge), often assessed through a pretest activity/posttest design (Sussman, 1991). Some of the immediate-impact variables that have been examined include changes in beliefs and knowledge, self-efficacy, behavioral intent, skill improvement, facilitator likability, and ability to motivate behavior change (Sussman, 1991). These variables are assessed in the same type of population that will receive the future program, to tailor the material for that group. Comparing these variables both before and after a program can help explain the relative effects of different components. Assessing these components separately allows for greater precision in curriculum design. Program developers are able to make decisions systematically regarding which components will provide the desired benefits in the target population, thus ensuring a combination of effective activities in the final program.

Youth tobacco use rates have shown continuous increases throughout the 1990s (Johnston, O'Malley, & Bachman, 1998). Legislators, health providers, and researchers are currently taking a distinct interest in youth tobacco use, its prevention, and its cessation. Although tobacco cessation studies in the past have demonstrated moderate success, there is a great need for tobacco use cessation programs, tested using advanced research designs, that increase cessation and reduction rates over spontaneous cessation and reduction rates among adolescents (Sussman, Lichtman, Ritt, & Pallonen, 1999). Such a program is needed most among at-risk youth whose tobacco use rates are higher than the rest of the youth population and who typically receive fewer resources and programs directed toward tobacco prevention and cessation.

The component study that follows was used in the development of a motivation-enhanced adolescent tobacco cessation curriculum for high-risk youth within an alternative high school setting. In California, continuation high schools are alternatives to the regular, comprehensive high school setting. Students attend continuation high school when they are unable to achieve their school credits in a timely manner due to social, emotional, or learning difficulties. Project EX builds on the work of an earlier tobacco cessation project, Project Towards No Tobacco Use (Project TNT). Project TNT provided a model, standard curriculum that was used as the basis of the Project EX curriculum. Our objective was to enhance the standard curriculum by producing a program specifically tailored to motivate continuation high school youth to quit smoking now rather than waiting until later (Sussman, Dent, Burton, Stacy, & Flay, 1995).

Project TNT was funded by the National Cancer Institute from 1987 to 1992. The project tested the efficacy of two tobacco use cessation clinic programs within comprehensive high school settings. The two curricula were similar in format (type of session order, several quit strategies), but one focused on the chemical dependency aspects of tobacco use, and the other focused on psychosocial dependency associated with tobacco use. The project used an experimental design, multiple measures of cessation, multiple types of control groups, and multiple measurement time points. A control group was created by recruiting a group of would-be clinic participants and placing them on a wait list for the duration of the first clinic round. These students represent a motivated group of people who are very similar to the program group. Three months after the conclusion of the program, no differences were found between groups experiencing either curriculum, with both groups achieving an 8% to 10% cessation rate for cigarette smoking. This cessation rate was not found to be significantly different from that obtained for the motivated wait list control group. An enduring differential effect, however, was found for smokeless tobacco use of 13% for each program versus 0% for the motivated wait list control (see Sussman et al., 1995, for details).

After Project TNT ended, the two single-component programs were combined, with the assumption that a combination of the separate interventions would be more effective or do no worse than either component. The programs were linked easily because of the similarity of formatting. Minor updating was completed to improve the ability of developers to disseminate it (e.g., videos and quit package materials were removed) and to enhance coverage of withdrawal symptoms (e.g., more information on anger management was provided). The final product of this process is the Project TNT comprehensive adolescent tobacco use cessation guide. This curriculum is now a five-session combined curriculum, including both the psychosocial- and chemical dependency-oriented programs.

This combined program became the foundation for building a motivation-enhanced curriculum known as Project EX. Project TNT includes most standard tobacco cessation material, including information on reasons for using tobacco, physiological effects of tobacco use, nicotine withdrawal symptoms and strategies for managing them, and psychological coping such as anger management and relaxation, avoiding weight gain, relapse prevention, and maintenance. Starting with this base from Project TNT, Project EX contains additional motivation components. These components were tested in the continuation high school context for likability, relevance, and ability to motivate students to try to quit tobacco use. The additional motivational activities have the dual purpose of motivating students to keep coming back to the clinic (i.e., maximize retention) and to quit tobacco use immediately rather than waiting until an indefinite later time.

COMPONENT DEVELOPMENT AND TESTING

Before components can be tested in the component study format, various research tools and behavior theories are used to generate potential activities likely to be motivating and likable to the target audience. In the case of Project EX, previous case studies in this text presented initial focus group work to learn potential motivation themes (Chapter 10) and theme study work to select plausible activities for testing (Chapter 12). Focus groups were the first step in assessing what concerns and opinions these students have about tobacco. Focus groups were conducted in four stages, with each stage delving deeper into the topics covered in the previous stage.

On the basis of the results of the focus groups, a pool of ideas was developed for activities that may be motivating to continuation high school youth. Twenty-six paragraphs, each describing a possible activity, were presented to students in the theme study to assess which of these were found to be the most motivating and likable. On the basis of this previous research, 14 activities were chosen to be fully developed and tested in a component study format (Table 14.1 lists these activities, modalities, and a brief description).

The component study was the final step before the initial piloting of a complete motivation-enhanced curriculum. The primary purpose of this study was to allow students to determine the activities they found most relevant and motivating, after actually experiencing the activities. The highest-rated activities were then added to the standard five-session curriculum.

DETAILS ON TESTS LEADING UP TO THE PRESENT STUDY

The 14 Project EX components varied from each other in lesson content and modality. Lesson contents were developed considering nine motivational categories that were derived from combinations of two different types of motivation (three direction and three energy motivation categories) (e.g., see Miller & Rollnick, 1991; Nezami, Sussman, & Pentz, in press). Self-image, affect, and curiosity represent "direction" motivation. Direction motivation creates a discrepancy between what is and what could be to motivate the subject to change. Lifestyle stability, capacity match, and social pressure represent "energy" motivation, which provides the impetus to drive an individual toward the direction indicated. The nine new motivation categories were created by crossing the direction and energy categories with each other, resulting in categories that each address a single direction category as well as a single energy category (e.g., self-image/lifestyle stability, self-image/capacity match, self-image/social pressure, affect/lifestyle stability). These categories provided the lesson contents for nine of the activities tested in the component study. The remaining five activities were based on a novel format that incorporated discussion and exercises (see Chapter 12).

Three modalities were tested, including a talk show format, a game format, and a novel format. Four of the components tested were in a game format, and five were in a talk show format. The talk show format, in which students actually

TABLE 14.1 Component Study Activities and Descriptions

Name of Activity	Modality	Motivation Category (Direction/Energy)	Brief Description
"WARNING"—Warning: Waiting to quit smoking may be hazardous to your peace of mind	Talk show	Curiosity/capacity match	Talk show guests of varying ages talk about quitting smoking. Students learn that younger quitters have a much easier time. Older quitters have begun to suffer negative consequences and are more addicted.
"ROMANTIC"—Romantic match or mismatch	Game	Curiosity/lifestyle stability	Students role-play a "dating game." Students learn how smoking limits your freedom to enjoy yourself.
"SUCKER"—Are you a sucker for the tobacco industry's lies?	Talk show	Self-image/social pressure	Talk show guests include a tobacco company executive, a smoker, and an expert on the tobacco industry. Students learn how tobacco companies use manipulative techniques to confuse you about the risks of tobacco.
"CONFRONT"—Family and friends confront smokers about their habit	Talk show	Affect/social pressure	Talk show guests include a young smoker, his or her mother, and his or her grandfather. The smoker talks about how he or she feels nagged all the time, and the family members talk about their worries for the smoker and how they have noticed the smoker has changed (irritable, doesn't want to spend time with them, etc.).
"PEER"—Peer motivational counseling	Novel	Affect/capacity match	A student ex-smoker describes how he or she quit smoking and how quitting changed his or her life (particularly in regard to lifestyle stability, self-image, and affect).
"YOGA"—Yoga	Novel		Students learn several easy yoga postures and learn that they can use yoga to feel more relaxed, strong, and flexible.
"COPING"—Coping without smokes	Game	Affect/capacity match	Students play a board game that contains squares directing them to draw an "anger," "anxiety," or "boredom" card. The cards either describe a coping technique and tell them to move forward or say, "Oops, you smoked a cigarette; move back two spaces."
"FEELINGS"—Letting feelings pass	Novel	Affect/lifestyle stability	Students discuss how they react to feelings such as anger or stress. They learn that they may react in a way that makes them feel worse. Sometimes just letting the feeling pass can be the most effective coping technique. Students learn relaxation and breathing meditations to help them feel calm.

"BODY"—Quitting smoking and your body	Novel		Students talk about how their body will change when they quit smoking (increased taste and smell; more oxygen) and the benefits of increased body awareness for health and well-being. Several exercises encourage students to pay attention to their bodies and the messages they may be sending them (stressed out, tight shoulders, etc.).
"BREATHING"—Healthy breathing exercise	Novel		Students discuss breathing and how different things may affect their breathing for the worse (e.g., smoking). Students participate in exercises that promote healthier breathing.
"STRESS"—Your cigarettes may be stressing you out	Talk show	Affect/lifestyle stability	Talk show guests include an ex-smoker, a physician, and a psychologist. Guests discuss the common myth that smoking helps relieve stress. The guest doctors tell how tobacco actually increases stress both physically and psychologically.
"BETTER"—Quitting smoking: I've been there and it does get better	Talk show	Self-image/capacity match	Talk show guests are smokers who are at different stages in the quitting process. One has not yet decided to quit, one just decided to quit, one quit a week ago, and one quit a month ago. They illustrate how doubts and rationalizations are part of the process of quitting and do not mean you will fail. You do not need to wait until you are completely confident about quitting because that day may never come.
"MENU"—Is smoking on the menu?	Game	Curiosity/social pressure	Students break up into teams and compete to answer questions about second-hand smoke. They receive a "menu" of possible categories and "order" a question from the health educator.
"LIFE"—Quitting for life	Game	Self-image/lifestyle stability	Students play a board game that contains squares directing them to draw a "relationship," "health," or "career" card. The cards either describe how quitting smoking may benefit these areas of their lives and tell them to move forward, or they say, "Oops, you smoked a cigarette; move back two spaces."

NOTE: The Motivational Category column applies only to the direction-energy motivation model constituents; it is blank for all novel themes.

role-play guests and the audience of a talk show, was shown to be highly popular with continuation high school students in the Project Towards No Drug Abuse (TND), an indicated drug prevention program for continuation high school students (Sussman, 1996). The game format was chosen because the added aspect of competition may increase enjoyment and encourage students to pay attention (Sussman et al., 1995). Nine of the 14 activities fit into one of these two modalities. The remaining 5 used novel modalities that were mainly oriented toward discussion and completing brief experiential exercises. The results of the theme study incidentally led to selection of 1 activity for each of the nine crossed motivation categories. Coincidentally, the 14 activities chosen maintained a fairly even balance of modalities, with 5 talk shows, 4 games, and 5 novel activities being selected.

▶ METHOD

SUBJECTS

The component study was conducted in three continuation high schools of approximately equal size. Students' parents were sent home letters about the study at least 1 week prior to participating, whereby they could refuse their child's participation. A total of 327 students, in 35 classrooms, Grades 10 through 12, participated in the study. About half (51%, $n = 168$) of the surveyed students were self-reported smokers, and these students are the focus of the current analysis (similar to DeMoor et al., 1994). Mean age of the student smokers was 16.9 years ($SD = .68$), which was slightly older than the mean age of 16.7 years for student nonsmokers, $t(327) = 1.94, p < .05$. A total of 68% and 55% of the student smokers and nonsmokers were male, respectively; $\chi^2(1) = 5.5, p < .01$.

STUDY MEASURES AND PROCEDURES

The study protocol was completed in each classroom over a 3-day period. On the first day, students completed a baseline general survey gathering information that included school, smoking status, age, and gender. The students then participated in a single activity, after which they completed an evaluation of that activity. On the second and third days, students participated in two more activities each day, completing an activity evaluation immediately after each activity. Five activities were evaluated by all participants over the 3-day period.

Each set of activity evaluation forms for a given day had a cover sheet on which the students indicated their age and sex. They also indicated on the cover sheet if they were a smoker by answering a simple yes/no question: "smoker?" No other identifying information was requested or recorded on the evaluation forms, ensuring anonymity of participants.

Each activity evaluation form contained a blank space at the top where students were asked to write in the name of the activity they were evaluating. Study staff also wrote the names of the activities conducted on the board and on the front of a collection envelope to eliminate the chances of error by participants. The activity evaluations consisted of 11 questions about the activity, all of which were rated on a 4-point response scale: *very, moderately, a little,* and *not at all.* The first 5 questions were perceived quality rating items and assessed the following: (a) how interesting it would be to do the activity, (b) how understandable the activity would be, (c) how much the students could learn from doing the activity, (d) how likely the activity would help to not increase or to not start drug use, and (e) the ability of the activity to meet the stated goal it was intended to accomplish. The remaining 6 items were directed at a potential motivation manipulation. These included 2 questions that measured "general" motivation (lead you to change something about yourself, see how you could have a better life), 2 that measured whether the activity provided direction motivation (how much would the activity motivate someone to try to quit, stay quit), and 2 that measured whether the activity provided energy motivation (activity gives you sense of enthusiasm, energy).

The complete set of 14 activities was scheduled at each school, and activity set combinations were randomly composed and then balanced for number of presentations across classrooms. In a few instances, scheduled activities could not be completed because of small class attendance or because there were too many students present who had already participated in another class. Overall, an average of 36 students rated each activity. Ten of the 14 activities were completed in all three schools. Two activities ("coping" and "life") were completed at two schools, and 1 ("menu") was completed only in one school because of these class size-related reasons.

Another activity, related to peer motivational counseling, was dropped from the menu of activities after testing at the first school because it required recruiting student volunteers. The activity was rated highly on the theme study but was not considered feasible for the component study because it involved a presentation followed by a question-and-answer period led by a student who had quit smoking and could share his or her experiences with peers. Recruitment of ex-smokers was supposed to occur on the day consents were delivered, and the volunteers would then meet with a project staff liaison the week before the activity was scheduled to review the presentation. A peer motivation counseling booklet was provided to volunteers to aid them in developing a presentation. Although six students volunteered on the day of consents, only two were able to meet with the liaison because the others were either absent or no longer attending school, and on the day of the activity, none of the volunteers agreed to do their presentation. This activity was therefore conducted at only one school with a project staff person acting as the peer motivation counselor, after which it was dropped.

ANALYSIS

A factor analysis of the 11 evaluation items (5 perceived quality and 6 motivation) produced a single factor, and the items were standardized ($M = 0$, $SD = 1$) and averaged to form a single-activity "quality" rating. Cronbach's alpha for the scale was .93. The raw scale mean was 2.50, and the standard deviation was 0.06. Negative z scores indicate quality scores higher than the overall mean, and positive z scores indicate poorer relative ratings.

The principal analytic strategy was to determine the ordering of the activities, best liked to least, using the quality score index. Formal statistical testing to determine which activities differed from each other in quality rating was completed using a mixed-model analysis of variance, using each rating of an activity as the unit of analysis. Schools, classes nested within schools, and students nested within classes were included as random factors to control for possible interdependence effects. Students also were considered as a repeated factor because they each rated multiple activities. Activities were considered fixed factors. Demographic factors of age and sex were included as covariates. In addition, two-way interaction terms between activity with age, sex, school, and smoking status were examined to formally test whether subgroups formed by those factors varied in perceived activity quality ordering.

▶ RESULTS

The focus of this analysis was on student smokers because they are the ultimate target of the program being developed. However, it is interesting to note that, overall, smokers generally rated all the activities as of lower perceived quality than did nonsmokers; mean smokers = 2.54, nonsmoker mean = 2.28, $F(1, 310) = 22.70$, $p < .001$. However, smokers and nonsmokers did not vary in the ordering of activities; $F(1, 310) = 1.11$, $p = .35$. That is, although smokers may like an activity less than nonsmokers, they did so by a consistent increment across all activities.

Among smokers, girls also rated all the activities more favorably than did boys; mean males = 2.48, mean girls = 2.34, $F(1, 149) = 7.54$, $p = .006$. But boys and girls did not differ in their ordering of the activities, as indicated by a nonsignificant interaction between sex and activity, $F(1, 149) = 1.12$, $p = .33$. We also found no evidence for differential acceptance of activities at different

TABLE 14.2 Component Study Activities in Order of Likability

Name of Activity	Number of Raters	Mean (SD)	z Score	Different Set[a]
1. Is smoking on the menu? (MENU)	12	2.17 (0.17)	−.44	a
2. Peer motivational counseling (PEER)	21	2.25 (0.18)	−.44	a
3. Quitting smoking: I've been there and it does get better (BETTER)	39	2.41 (0.10)	−.21	b
4. Yoga (YOGA)	26	2.48 (0.14)	−.12	b
5. Family and friends confront smokers about their habit (CONFRONT)	46	2.52 (0.11)	−.09	bc
6. Letting feelings pass (FEELINGS)	33	2.52 (0.11)	−.09	bc
7. Warning: Quitting smoking may be hazardous to your peace of mind (WARNING)	47	2.54 (0.11)	−.08	bc
8. Your cigarettes may be stressing you out (STRESS)	45	2.59 (0.12)	−.02	bc
9. Healthy breathing (BREATHING)	34	2.67 (0.13)	0.01	bc
10. Romantic match or mismatch (ROMANTIC)	55	2.67 (0.10)	0.01	bc
11. Are you a sucker for the tobacco industry's lies? (SUCKER)	31	2.67 (0.15)	0.03	bc
12. Quitting smoking and your body (BODY)	57	2.69 (0.10)	0.09	c
13. Quitting for life (LIFE)	33	2.76 (0.14)	0.16	c
14. Coping without smokes (COPING)	31	3.11 (0.15)	0.72	d
All (1-14)	168	2.50 (0.06)	0.00	bc

a. Same letters denote activities that belong to the same set.

schools, $F(2, 149) = 1.81$, $p = .17$; for different orderings among smokers at each school, $F(1, 149) = 1.01$, $p = .93$; or by age, main effect, $F(1, 149) = 1.19$, $p = .30$, and interaction with activity, $F(1, 149) = 1.02$, $p = .88$.

The main results are presented in Table 14.2, which lists the activities ranked by perceived quality rating (from most to least favorable). It also displays the number of students who rated the activity, raw scale means, standard deviations, and standardized (z) scores equivalent to the mean ratings. A grouping of activities that are statistically the same or different from each other, with common letters signifying same group membership, is also shown in Table 14.2. The activities "menu" and "peer" were the two most favorably rated activities, and "coping," "life," and "body" were the least favorably rated. Others follow the order presented but are less distinguishable statistically from each other and from an overall rating (grand mean).

▶ DISCUSSION

There are several benefits as well as a few limitations to conducting a component study such as the one described earlier for the purpose of tobacco cessation curriculum development. Regarding benefits, the component study is an excellent tool for determining subjects' preferences and reactions—which may vary from the curriculum writers' subjective opinions about what is most appealing or effective. Furthermore, the component study provides a means of providing convergent validation with previous perceived efficacy work (see Chapters 9 and 11, this volume) by actually testing promising activities on immediate impact. Although one has better confidence in the efficacy of an activity if it is rated favorably in different types of studies (convergence of results), some activities that sound good on paper (e.g., use of a theme study) are not as successful when they are fully developed and carried out. Besides providing an assessment of immediate impact, the component study also is a good opportunity for health educators and curriculum developers to gauge the feasibility of the activities so that they can be fine-tuned before engaging in a pilot study. For example, we established that "peer motivational counseling" was not a feasible activity. Generally, the component study is an excellent opportunity to trim away nonfeasible parts of a curriculum and to ensure that the remaining components are producing the proper immediate impact on students.

The component study described earlier does have a few limitations in terms of providing the most accurate feedback on each activity. First, there may be a slight difference in how subjects react to activities in the study compared to how they would actually react if enrolled in the future cessation program. Circumstances are different. The component study was conducted in preexisting classrooms with both smokers and nonsmokers participating. Project EX would be implemented in a counseling atmosphere in a classroom designated specifically for clinic use by smokers only. Also, Project EX would be taught to a group of tobacco users motivated to enter a school clinic program, whereas the component study assessment included tobacco users who would not be willing to enter a clinic program. Although we considered only the ratings of tobacco users in our analysis, the participation of nontobacco users and (perhaps) unmotivated tobacco users may have affected some of the tobacco users' ratings of the activities. For example, activities tested in a regular school classroom may receive imprecise ratings because potential clinic subjects do not feel as comfortable as they would in an alternate location where confidentiality is ensured and a therapeutic atmosphere already has been established. This possibility may have particularly affected the ratings of some of the more unconventional activities such as meditation and yoga. Cessation studies may perhaps benefit from implementing component studies in preexisting cessation programs that are in place in many high schools. Alternately, in future work, tobacco users who might be interested in a clinic program could be removed to another location in the school as part of the component study protocol. The easiest option is for health educators simply to fully explain and emphasize to the students the importance of taking into consideration the future context of the activities when rating them. However, such instructions do not necessarily control for potential differential social mix effects.

A second limitation to the component study is that each activity is tested as a separate and stand-alone activity. In the final curriculum, activities will be embedded in a cohesive curriculum package. Some activities may suffer more than others for lack of introductory material. Activities should be made to stand on their own as much as possible to prevent this possibility. Also, it is unclear how activities would interact with each other placed in the same program. Such activities could potentially either attenuate other activities or potentiate them. This is a matter for future research, but it is certainly worthy of the consideration of program developers, and sequencing of components must be considered (see Chapters 13 and 15, this volume). Thus, further program development testing, including pilot studies of the curriculum, is still important.

An objective basis for selecting the activities for the pilot study and the main intervention trial was established. Following removal of the "peer motivation counseling" activity, it was determined that the eight top-ranked activities would be retained and added to the standard five-session TNT program. These activities were found to be quite easy to implement, and it seemed clear to the developers where to place each activity into the TNT program, which resulted in an eight-session clinic program. Clearly, though, at least three other activities not included (e.g., romantic match or mismatch activity; see Table 14.2) could have been placed into this or a longer program. Nevertheless, a cutoff point for inclusion of materials was made, and health educator judgment was used to break the tie scores at this point.

Although careful component study work was completed, the developers could not, in this instance, totally escape using implementer judgment. Perhaps iterative component studies would help make better discriminations among previously equally favored activities, or perhaps larger subject samples would have made the results more discriminable. It is possible, though, that the use of health educator judgments, if well grounded in health behavior and communication theory, would yield similar results at a potentially much lower cost. All of these possibilities could be tested through additional component study work.

Despite these few limitations, the classroom-based component study still provides an excellent opportunity for shaping and testing components considered for an adolescent tobacco cessation curriculum. Conducting this study helped ensure that Project EX was sound and acceptable to the target audience. It helped us address the difficult task of trying to guess or predict which activities would be most acceptable, and it contributed significantly to the overall curriculum development process by incorporating the perspectives of the adolescent target audience. The two pilot clinics smoothed out sequencing and feasibility of these activities. Continued component study research will help us advance the scientific approach to program development, especially the validation of material by target audiences. Significant research effort also needs to focus on linking theory and implementation among various user groups such as program directors (teachers, clinicians, etc.) and social support groups to augment the program development process.

▶ REFERENCES

DeMOOR, C., JOHNSTON, D. A., WERDEN, D. L., ELDER, J. P., SENN, K., & WHITEHORSE, L. (1994). Patterns and correlates of smoking and smokeless tobacco use among continuation high school students. *Addictive Behaviors, 19,* 175-184.

JOHNSTON, L. D., O'MALLEY, P. M., & BACHMAN, J. G. (1998). *National survey results on drug use from the Monitoring the Future Study, 1975-1997* (2 vols., NIH Pub. No. 98-4345/6). Rockville, MD: U.S. Department of Health and Human Services.

MILLER, W. R., & ROLLNICK, S. (1991). *Motivational interviewing: Preparing people to change addictive behavior.* New York: Guilford.

NEZAMI, E., SUSSMAN, S., & PENTZ, M. A. (in press). Motivation in tobacco use cessation research. *Substance Use & Misuse.*

ROGERS, E. M. (1995). *Diffusion of innovations* (4th ed.). New York: Free Press.

SUSSMAN, S. (1991). Curriculum development in school-based prevention research. *Health Education Research: Theory and Practice, 6,* 339-351.

SUSSMAN, S. (1996). Development of a school-based drug abuse prevention curriculum for high-risk youths. *Journal of Psychoactive Drugs, 28,* 169-182.

SUSSMAN, S., DENT, C. W., BURTON, D., STACY, A. W., & FLAY, B. R. (1995). *Developing school-based tobacco use prevention and cessation programs.* Thousand Oaks, CA: Sage.

SUSSMAN, S., LICHTMAN, K., RITT, A., & PALLONEN, U. E. (1999). Effects of thirty-four adolescent tobacco use cessation and prevention trials on regular users of tobacco products. *Substance Use & Misuse, 34*(11), 1469-1505.

CHAPTER 15

Sequencing Issues in Health Behavior Program Development

William B. Hansen
David G. Altman

"There is timing in the whole life of the warrior, in his thriving and declining, in his harmony and discord. Similarly, there is timing in the Way of the merchant, in the rise and fall of capital. All things entail rising and falling timing. You must be able to discern this."

—Miyamoto Musashi (1584-1645)

Temporal order is important to just about everything in the universe. Many processes, both organic and inorganic, as well as those sociological and psychological, have an order to them. This order may be appear chaotic and complex (Waldrop, 1992). Nonetheless, one development generally precedes another, and one instruction often precedes the next. Often, we think of temporal order as being linked with causation, although that is often debated. However, our experience has shown that when intervention activities are completed without consideration of the timing of the introduction of different activities (i.e., sequencing), disastrous (or, sometimes, humorous) outcomes result. Yet, with all the common sense about and scientific appreciation for this inherently important issue, there is relatively little written about temporal order and sequence that is available to intervention program developers. There is a growing recognition that a consideration of order is important, and there also exist some loose rules of thumb regarding sequencing of whole programs for a target population at different developmental levels, sequencing of whole sessions within a program, and sequencing of activities within a session.

The purpose of this chapter is to begin the task of putting forth the basics for a science of sequencing within the arena of health behavior program development. We define *sequencing* as the ordering of programming events to maximize the potential for those events to have a desired outcome. In our experience, the failure to adequately consider sequence issues has unnecessarily limited the effectiveness of many programs. As a result, the design, implementation, and evaluation of interventions have been compromised.

We have taken a broad approach to this topic. We discuss sequencing issues from three perspectives: sequencing interventions within life course development and environmental contexts, sequencing intervention components over multiple points of intervention, and sequencing elements within a single point of intervention. Life course and environmental issues reflect a need to time and sequence interventions to fit within developmental levels of the target population—designing interventions that are appropriate to different ages and stages of biological, psychological, cognitive, social, and emotional development and establishing the readiness of the target setting to receive different types of program information. Multiple points of intervention issues pertain to sequencing the components of interventions, typically across days, weeks, and months. Sequencing intervention components within a single intervention requires an understanding of how to structure the moment-to-moment flow of the intervention within each component.

▶ IMPORTANCE OF SEQUENCING

Part of the reason sequencing issues are rarely addressed may be due to two facts. First, sequencing is often divorced from content. Many program developers place primary concern on the content of interventions without considering content within a temporal context. Content issues are typically embodied in the selection of modifiable mediating variables (Hansen & McNeal, 1997). Clearly, which mediators to target has been the primary focus of debate among program developers during the past two decades (Hansen, 1992; Hawkins, Catalano, & Miller, 1992; Tobler & Stratton, 1997). In some fields, such as drug abuse, the debate is approaching resolution, but debate continues regarding development of new approaches and contradictory findings of programs across different target populations; divergent opinions are still being expressed by leaders in the field. Mediating variable analysis (MacKinnon, 1994; MacKinnon & Dwyer, 1993) provides a tool that is well grounded theoretically and may help resolve content of intervention issues. However, sequencing is not now addressed by mediation analysis; it should be considered simultaneously with content in program design. For example, normative beliefs about drug use recently have been identified as a modifiable mediating variable worthy of intervention. We recently have found that normative beliefs exist within a developmental context that must be considered to maximize intervention effectiveness (McNeal & Hansen, in press). Specifically, normative beliefs start by being very conventional and only become deviant once youth have begun participating in deviant behaviors. Different referent norms require different interventions. Identifying what should be the focus of intervention cannot be considered independently of considering how, in temporal sequence terms, an intervention should be structured and when it should be delivered.

The second fact that has limited research on sequence issues has to do with basic methodological concerns related to the challenge of advancing knowledge in this arena. Without theories on which to base tests of sequence, the possible order of interventions becomes unmanageably large methodologically. For example, suppose a program developer has been requested to create a program for a specific age group and has decided that it should contain three intact content elements. These content elements may be sequenced in six possible ways. If each were to be included in a randomized experimental test, the number of test cases needed would be unreasonably large. Such a study would have academic interest but would have relatively little value from a policy perspective. Furthermore, those who have been heavily involved in program development would point out that even though it might be possible to create six orders, an intuitive analysis of the specific content of interest will render at least several of the possible orders implausible. The circumstance that program developers are left with is an understanding that sequencing is important but without systematic rules of sequence and supportive empirical work. This chapter will address topics of importance insofar as sequencing programmatic events is concerned.

CONCEPTUAL APPROACHES TO SEQUENCING ◄

Sequencing is not an issue that will be subjected to extensive experimental design-type evaluations. Without such tests, a science of program development that speaks to sequencing issues must look elsewhere for the crucial information needed for putting a maximizing order on program components. We must concern ourselves with learning about sequencing issues using other conceptual or empirical tools. Our concern is with assembling principles of sequence that underlie a science of program development. Intuition has played a prominent role in how program developers resolve sequence. To move beyond intuition, which is valuable but can be erroneous, program developers need to learn to rely increasingly on scientific theory and data. We hope to provide insights that will allow sequencing issues to be resolved using theoretical and empirical approaches.

Medical science has paid extensive attention to biological development, documenting the order, rate, and age at which developmental changes occur. Such sequences have been important to the development of medical diagnosis and intervention protocols. The degree to which medicine is theoretically informed and data driven has evolved significantly over the past century. The information that exists for describing the course (sequence) of disease has become voluminous. The social sciences have similarly paid extensive attention to developmental phenomena, at least at the general level. However, the application of theory and data to solving program development problems remains less scientific than it might become.

We have not yet arrived at a science of sequence in health behavior program development. We suspect that developers will continue to intuit the best orders of different programs for different populations, orders of components within a program, and orders of activities within a component (the "art" of program development). However, we hope a program of research will be built in this arena, and, even now, information about sequence can be useful to program developers. We believe that basic principles of sequencing currently can be outlined and defined.[1]

We have identified several specific models related to human behavior that can provide useful information to sequencing program material for a population at different points in time. We review these in an attempt to provide some additional grounding beyond intuition for a discussion about our topic.

STAGES OF CHANGE MODELS

A sizable body of research, notably from social psychology, has identified precursors to change. Among theories currently referenced in intervention research is the transtheoretical model (TTM) (Prochaska, DiClemente, & Norcross, 1992) of change. This model specifies a number of stages that define a diagnostic of likelihood of voluntary change on the part of a target group. From this perspective, individuals as well as groups inclusive of communities go through sequential stages prior to attempting behavior change. These include a *precontemplation stage*, during which a minimal awareness of a problem and consequently no intent to invest in change exists; a *contemplation stage*, during which there is an awareness of a problem but no commitment to action; a *preparation stage*, during which there is a clear recognition of the problem and exploration of options; an *action stage*, during which there is an active attempt to institute voluntary changes in behavior; and a *maintenance stage*, during which there is an active attempt to maintain changes in behavior that have been achieved. TTM has been applied successfully to smoking cessation in which individuals clearly pass through each of the stages, as well as to other health areas.

Interventions should be matched with stage of readiness to change. However, there are several limitations to the current applications of TTM. Most important, the model provides a general framework for developing motivation but does not specifically address how to achieve movement of people from one stage to another or how to institute effective change during the action stage. There are situations, particularly in prevention, in which the primary goal is the maintenance of a nonbehavior (e.g., not smoking, not fighting, not having sex), which this model does not directly address. An adaptation of TTM to smoking acquisition among adolescents has been suggested (Stern, Prochaska, Velicer, & Elder, 1987). In this model, everything becomes reversed. That is, precontemplators are those who have not yet begun to think about smoking. Contemplators are those who are considering starting to smoke. Youths in the action stage are those who are actively experimenting with smoking. Finally, those who have established habits are considered to be in a maintenance stage.

TTM was by no means the first theory that addressed stages of development or change. Piaget (1952, 1970, 1977) observed general stages of cognitive and intellectual developmental change that occurred during the life course of children. These include a sensorimotor stage (development of motor coordination), a preoperational stage (development of representational capacities), a concrete operational stage (development of an understanding of logical principles as applied to concrete and specific objects), and a formal operational stage (development of the ability to generalize, think abstractly, and test hypotheses). Similarly, Kohlberg (1969) studied the development of moral reasoning patterns. These include a preconventional stage (during which emphasis is placed on getting rewards and avoiding punishments), conventional stage (during which emphasis is placed on social rules), and a postconventional or moral stage (during which there is an emphasis on moral principles and conscience).

These theorists' primary postulate is that there are definable stages through which children pass as they mature. Individuals enter into any given stage and exit from one stage into another stage at highly individualistic rates that are related to age but not determined by it. Indeed, individuals do not necessarily transition into higher stages. In the case of both Piaget's and Kohlberg's theories, the transition from one stage to another is thought to be determined by a variety of secondary developments that bring the individual to a state of readiness for change. Because of the complexity of the interactions between biological, psychological, and other systems that account for readiness, neither theorist projected that stage changes could be induced through interventions. Changes from one stage to another cannot be hastened. Rather, both suggested tailoring any educational or other interventions to fit with the natural patterns that accompany the stage the person is at. The implications of these models are that different programming is going to be differentially relevant to a person at different stages of development, and windows of learning opportunity can be used to develop the most effective programming at different life development time points.

GUTTMAN MODELS

Research, originally conducted with attitude development and subsequently expanded to include the development of behavior, has discussed the linking of sequences of behavior. Drug use behaviors are known to be sequenced. For example, research by Denise Kandel and her colleagues (Kandel, Yamaguchi, & Chen, 1992) has shown that beer and wine use typically precedes cigarette smoking, which precedes the use of hard liquor and marijuana. This sequence may be pushed back even further than this. Collins, Graham, Rousculp, and Hansen (1997) have shown that heavy caffeine use (cola drinks and coffee) temporally precedes the initial use of beer and wine.

Similarly, sexual activity is known to be sequenced. Several studies (Hansen, Paskett, & Carter, in press; Hansen, Wolkenstein, & Hahn, 1992) have identified several precoital behaviors that are ordered and scalable using Guttman techniques. In order, these behaviors include hugging, spending time together, holding hands, kissing, cuddling, lying down together, and being undressed together, all of which precede sexual intercourse for both males and females.

The results of Guttman-type modeling analyses provide information that may be useful for the program developer. One can know which behaviors to target for intervention at different points in the development of a potentially problematic set of behaviors. This information is most useful for correctly targeting interventions to groups of similar individuals from a life course perspective. Such information also may prove useful in terms of sequencing multiple components within a program or sequencing moment-to-moment events, if information and skills being taught are stochastic in structure (e.g., follow a building-block principle; see Chapter 13, this volume).

SEQUENCING LEVEL 1: ENVIRONMENT AND LIFE COURSE DEVELOPMENT

In deciding when to deliver programming and what type of programming to deliver, one must be concerned with the context that life course development offers and with the readiness of the environmental context. In this section, we address sequencing at these levels.

DEFINITION OF ENVIRONMENTAL AND LIFE COURSE CONCERNS

Increasingly, policymakers are calling for interventions to be applied throughout the life course. Because there are insufficient resources to deliver comprehensive interventions throughout the life course, interventionists need to be judicious in the allocation of resources. There are never unlimited resources, and all possible goals cannot be achieved. By circumstance, interventions need to select limited numbers of target ages. Who the targets of intervention are, when they will receive the intervention, and the context in which the targets live need to be systematically considered by policymakers, program developers, and implementers. We have growing information about development and environmental context. This information should be used as one considers sequence issues in interventions.

DEVELOPMENTAL PATTERNS

Human development is manifested in processes such as biology, cognitive ability, social ability, and motivation, as well as psychological identity. The intervention must account for and be appropriate for each of these. The complexity of development is such that simple rules cannot be stated. However, two guiding principles that apply to program development can be defined. First, the intervention must target behaviors during developmental periods when behaviors naturally emerge or change. Second, the program must be developed and delivered so that its components match the developmental capabilities and readiness of the target individuals.

Information about psychosocial development is often available from the research literature. In the broadest sense, information provided by research such as that of Piaget (1953, 1970, 1977) and Kohlberg (1969), which were discussed briefly earlier in this chapter, needs to be understood and considered. However, it

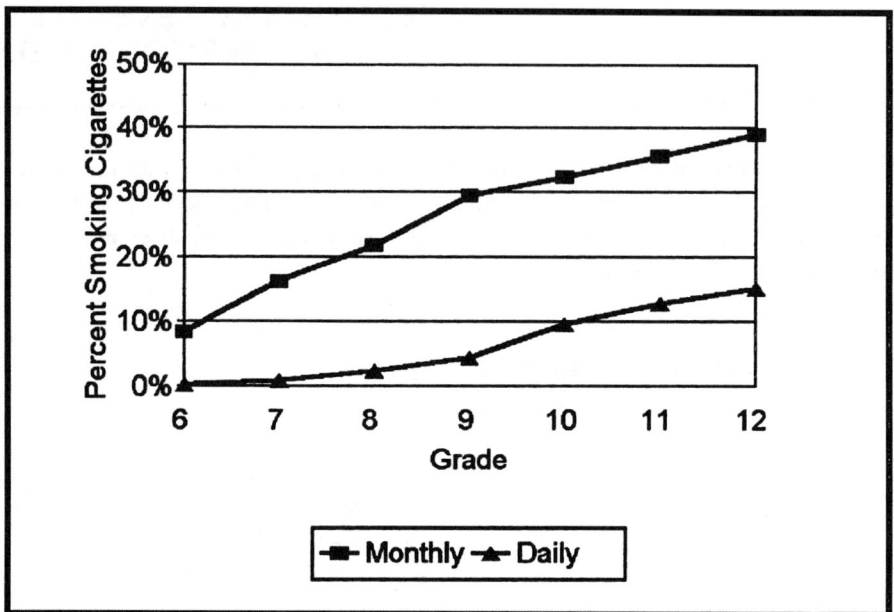

Figure 15.1. Percentage of Cigarette Smoking as a Function of Grade

is likely that specific information about the behavior of interest also will be known. For example, in reference to developing tobacco intervention programs, we observed that the period of onset of initial smoking and the subsequent process of development that transformed experimental smokers into regular smokers were highly related to age. Figure 15.1 depicts data from surveys conducted in Forsyth County, North Carolina ($N = 31,148$), that reveal the patterns of smoking onset and development. More than 50% of the experimentation with cigarettes (monthly smoking) occurs in the 3-year period of sixth, seventh, and eighth grades. Twenty percent occurs prior to sixth grade, and 25% occurs after eighth grade. (The rate of increase during elementary school years is not shown in our data but is slight during fourth- and fifth-grade years.) Increases in monthly smoking during the high school years are half what they were during middle school. Therefore, it is clear that the middle school years are crucial for interventions that target suppressing experimentation. (This same pattern has been replicated by many others in different locations and time points; e.g., see Sussman, Dent, Burton, Stacy, & Flay, 1995.)

At the same time, the greatest increases in daily smoking occur among 9th- and 10th-grade students. By 11th and 12th grades, the percentage of daily smokers has become relatively stable. Early smoking cessation is clearly most economically targeted at this age group.

The data themselves speak to issues of appropriate programming for different ages. One might reasonably ask several questions about this approach. Is there any potential payoff for prevention that occurs prior to sixth grade or after ninth grade? Is there any potential payoff for attempting programs of smoking cessation before ninth grade? Perhaps. However, if principles of economy of force are applied, it becomes clear that there will be wasted effort in trying to accomplish goals outside these basic time frames. A wiser strategy may be to target programs when they are most likely to have a large payoff first and then add support programs that target other age groups if resources are available.

Each targeted behavior, whether it be sex, drugs, violence, or reckless driving, is likely to have similar patterns of either onset or development that should figure prominently in the strategic targeting of interventions. Different forms of drug use have similar, although not identical, onset patterns. For example, marijuana use closely parallels tobacco use but usually occurs somewhat later. Alcohol use parallels tobacco use and usually precedes its occurrence. The use of inhalants tends to occur early and then, unlike other substances, nearly disappears in high school (Collins, Graham, Long, & Hansen, 1994; Hansen & Rose, 1995).

The onset patterns seen in these examples are similar to a phenomenon widely referred to under the topic of diffusion of innovations. Diffusion of innovations was first systematically studied in the 1940s (Ryan & Gross, 1943). Rogers (1962/1983) provided the earliest and broadest theoretical conceptualization and review of the literature on diffusion. According to Rogers's description, not everyone adopts new practices at the same rate. Rather, people adopt in a time sequence that classifies them into five categories: innovators (the first 2%-3%), early adopters (the next 12%-13%), early majority (the next 20%), late majority (the next 20%), and laggards (the remaining 10%). When depicted as a cumulative response curve that reflects the proportion of people who have adopted an innovation by a given time (see Figure 15.2), diffusion of innovations has an S shape. The adoption of new practices is at first very slow. Innovators and early adopters of innovations are clearly in the minority and are often thought of as being either elite or eccentric. The area of the diffusion curve after about 15% and up to 20% to 25% adoption is the heart of the diffusion process. After that point, the rate of adoption becomes rapid and often appears to take on a life of its own. There are those who either do not adopt an innovation or do so only with external pressure.

The same sequence of diffusion is expected with regard to all innovations, including the adoption of high-risk health behaviors. Innovators are the very first set of individuals within a target group who adopt a high-risk behavior. These individuals are expected to be different in radical ways from mainstream youth in many respects. They may be prone to adopt high-risk behaviors irrespective of programmatic intervention. They also may experience multiple underlying characteristics or environmental stresses that may defy economical program devel-

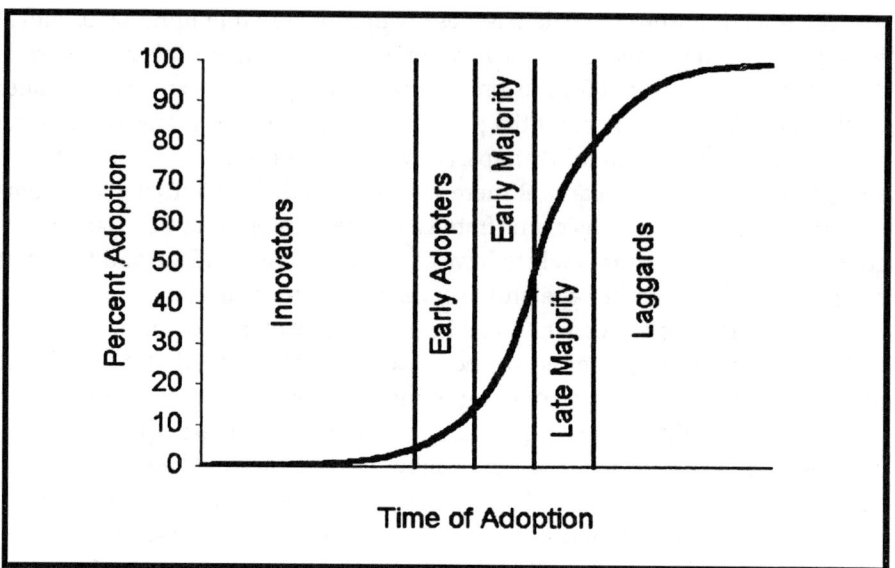

Figure 15.2. Percentage of Adoption of an Innovation as a Function of Time of Adoption

opment. Instead, the program intervention may be best timed to address the appearance of early adopters and the early majority.

Once behavioral patterns are understood, a key to program design is developing intervention methods that fit with the biological, cognitive, social, and psychological characteristics of the target populations. Across ages, there are clearly differences in people's ability to pay attention to and process information; simplistically stated, older youth generally have the ability and temperament to deal with more complex information. However, even within students in a given age or grade, there are marked differences in ability and motivation. Understanding clearly who the target group is and where it is in terms of development becomes crucial to the success of a program. In this chapter, we can provide only examples. The details that must guide the program developer require extensive examination, study, and, often, experimentation.

ENVIRONMENTAL OPPORTUNITIES AND CONSTRAINTS

There are institutional issues that program developers must consider. That is, institutions (schools, agencies, community groups, etc.) in which interventions can be launched are, themselves, likely to be at different levels of readiness for hosting, adopting, or implementing different programs. In addition to considering the impact of life course development on the sequencing of interventions, program developers also must consider the context of intervention delivery. An intervention could be designed perfectly for the developmental stage of program targets but fail because the context of intervention was less than ideal.

For example, take the case of a school-based substance abuse prevention curriculum. If the curriculum were delivered under any of the following circumstances, consider how achieving program goals might be affected by circumstance, even if the curriculum were designed with developmental principles in mind: (a) in a community that had not yet decided that substance abuse prevention was important, (b) just before or after lunch, (c) by a teacher who had not yet gone through training, (d) in a school that had recently experienced a death related to drugs or violence, (e) in a city in which laws about the sale of tobacco and alcohol to minors was recently passed, or (f) in a city in which local politicians just defeated proposed legislation to reduce tobacco and alcohol advertising near schools. In each case, the quality of the program might be augmented or diminished because of recent events that had transpired in the community. Physical and social environments are constantly changing. Interventionists should be aware of such changes and strive to take advantage of current or recent changes in the physical and social environment in which it is being delivered. Strategic doctrines, such as maneuver, economy of force (applying force only when victory can be achieved with surety), taking the offensive, and surprise (Dupuy, 1990) may be useful guides for taking advantage of such developing situations.

Like individuals, communities exist at different stages of development. Indeed, from this perspective, it is reasonable to adapt the TTM described earlier with respect to individual stages of change to contextual stages of change. By considering readiness to change both from the perspective of individuals and from the context in which individuals reside, interventions have a better chance of achieving desired effects. From this perspective, the context in which interventions are launched is likely to be at different levels of readiness for hosting, adopting, or implementing programs. At the organizational level, some institutions are mature in that they have well-established means of accomplishing their goals. They have published formats and a defined structure for going about their business. Without a clear threat from without or within, many of these mature institutions resist change and innovation. Within established institutions, there may be a premium placed on working through sources of power. On the other hand, there are institutions that embrace new methods and actively seek out innovation. Often, these institutions are new, growing, and seeking to establish themselves as different from their predecessors or competitors. The state of an institution reflects its history as much as its resources.

At Tanglewood Research, we have recent experience with two cases that underscore this dilemma. In the first case, we developed an innovative program for high schools that was to use peer opinion leaders, identified by a social network analysis of social groups, to serve as norm change agents about alcohol within the school. We quickly found that the structure and operation of the group were unacceptable to the high school administrators, who had no desire to empower students to accomplish what they perceived to be their own role and responsibility. The principal had been struggling with political issues of control with his district and was in a position of trying to gain additional control. This program was abandoned before it could be pilot tested.

Our second case yielded a much more satisfactory outcome. For this program, we were asked to develop innovative materials for elementary school drug and violence education. We were aware that state mandates required the development of new programming. Knowing this, we found it easy to obtain a complete list of math, science, language art, and other teaching requirements for these schools. We developed a program that could be easily adopted because it met a pressing new need within the schools. We built the program around emerging goals and used methods familiar to teachers, including innovation in method only when necessary. This program was much more readily adopted and implemented.

Several researchers (e.g., Oetting et al., 1995; Plested, Smitham, Jumper-Thurman, Oetting, & Edwards, 1999) have recently developed a scale for measuring institutional readiness for change. Like the scales that measure personal readiness, institution scores are postulated to be predictive of whether the institution will adopt an innovative program. In this schema, the earliest stage of community readiness for intervention is characterized as apathy and hopelessness. Communities then move into a stage of denial. The next level of readiness is vague awareness, which is followed in turn by a preplanning stage, a planning and preparation stage, and an initiation of action stage. This stage may be followed by three subsequent stages: stabilization, confirmation and expansion, and professionalization. One way of approaching this from a program development perspective may be to consider what type of program could be developed that would move an institution from an existing stage to the next stage. There also may be differential readiness to deviate from past practice that is embedded in this characterization of communities. That is, some groups may be ready to adopt only conventionally framed programs that operate using methods that are accepted within the organization. On the other hand, there may be groups that are ready to experiment with programs that embody methods that are a radical departure from a conventional approach.

There may well be means for moving an institution along in terms of its readiness to adopt innovative programs. For example, research (Gingiss, Gottlieb, & Brink, 1994) demonstrates that training can increase the likelihood of adopting innovative teaching methods. However, other research (Rohrbach, Graham, & Hansen, 1993) concludes that training to implement innovative interventions among teachers who previously have been taught established methods is most likely to fail.

Similar constraints may influence the suitability of individually targeted interventions. Maslow (1943) proposed a hierarchy of needs that also may be thought of as sequential and that may reflect environmental constraints on the individual. The first level of need is physiological and biological, such as oxygen, food, water, clothes, and protection. Safety needs, such as those felt by adults during emergencies or periods of disorganization in the social structure, are second in this order. Social needs, such as the need to escape loneliness and alienation and give and receive love, affection, and the sense of belonging, are third in this sequence. At the fourth level are esteem needs, including the need for a high level of self-respect and respect from others. Finally, Maslow proposed a set of needs described as self-actualization needs. These include a person's need to be and do that which the person was born to do. AIDS researchers, for example, have found that until basic human needs such as food, shelter, and child care are taken care of, targeted participants may not be willing or ready to be engaged in programs that address psychosocial issues.

GUIDING PRINCIPLES

We suggest several principles that program developers should consider adopting, based on this discussion of Level 1 sequencing. First, programs should be developed to fit within the existing psychosocial developmental level of the average person who will be the target of intervention. This implies that such diverse issues as reading level, complexity of concepts (abstract vs. concrete), emphasis on independent study of program material, the salience of peer group versus authority figures as instructors, and the importance of style and fashion be considered and defined prior to beginning program development activities. If needed, pilot data on the unique characteristics of a particular target group should be considered (see Chapter 16, this volume).

Second, programs that address behaviors that have a natural sequence of development associated with age or other markers of maturity should target implementation primarily during the initial periods of increasing prevalence (referred to as "inflection" points). We specifically suggest avoiding targeting interventions before the inflection point (e.g., before the behavior is engaged in by at least 5% of target students). However, once engaged, programs need to have sufficient resources so that they can reach an entire population for an extended period of time. Thus, we strongly recommend making the intervention sufficiently powerful and of sufficient duration to ensure that the period of risk is covered. For example, this might include systematic boosters, which have been found to be crucial to the long-term success of programs (Botvin, Baker, Dusenbury, Botvin, & Diaz, 1995) long after the inflection point has been crossed.

Third, programs should be designed to fit within the structure, goals, and methods of the host institution. Innovative methods that may be most effective overall may not be adopted by institutions that are well established and have predefined ways of accomplishing their goals and objectives. Program methods may need to be constructed that mimic or conform to existing patterns. When only innovative methods can be expected to accomplish the desired goals, program developers may need to think and plan beyond program design itself and also concern themselves with the environment and ecology into which the program will be placed.

Fourth, programs should take into account the environmental context in which implementation occurs. That is, it is important to recognize that individuals both influence and are influenced by the environments in which they live. Thus, sequencing issues raised by considering life span development are best viewed as interactions among individuals and environments. For example, designing a developmentally appropriate school-based tobacco intervention in North Carolina would require attending to the historical role of tobacco production; the fact that many children come from families that depend on tobacco as a source of family income; the social acceptance, if not desirability, of tobacco use; and the many civic contributions that tobacco money has provided. Along similar lines, it is important to monitor and take advantage of social, political, cultural, and economic opportunities that the environment affords.

▶ SEQUENCING LEVEL 2: SEQUENCING COMPLEX PROGRAM ELEMENTS

DEFINITION OF PROGRAM SEQUENCING CONCERNS

Programmatic interventions are almost always based on attempts to change mediating variables that, in turn, change behaviors whether or not the program is driven by intuition, theory, or data (see Chapter 19, this volume). In nearly every instance, program developers target multiple mediators simultaneously. For example, drug abuse prevention programs may try to deter the development of drug use by teaching skills for coping with peer pressure or by establishing conventional norms within the group. By virtue of the fact that multiple variables are addressed and because the characteristics that programs often attempt to change are complex and resistant to change, multiple sessions of intervention often are devised.

Beyond having multiple objectives, is there a need to order program components? Or can any component occur at any time with equal effectiveness? We need to consider the devil's advocate position that order is not important and that sequence is irrelevant. Certainly, programs would be easier to bind together if that position were true. A Tanglewood Research case study is worth considering. The Nebraska Council to Prevent Alcohol and Drug Abuse requested that we develop a multicomponent version of All Stars (Hansen, 1996) that could be delivered without order. That is, they wished for a set of lessons, a menu from which the implementer could select material as desired. To meet this need, we crafted a program that addressed four mediating variables (multiple sessions and multiple activities per variable).

The original structure of the program that we were asked to adapt, All Stars, had a relatively definable sequence to it. The sequence was embedded in the detailed flow of sessions in which a later session would often refer to topics discussed in an earlier one. To comply with the request of the Nebraska Council, we removed references to earlier topics. In as many ways as possible, we created a program that provided implementers with stand-alone components. We were able to create such a program, yet the program was never implemented. After thinking about what we had created and a careful consideration of sequencing issues, the Nebraska Council recommended that the original sequence be adopted.

This case report does not constitute scientific evidence that a necessary and effective sequencing of sessions is inherent in health behavior programming. However, this example is typical of many effective programs that have been developed over the years. That is, a sequence eventually emerges that appears to maximize potential for implementation. The principles that can guide how an intervention sequence should be organized have not heretofore been defined. We believe that, at a minimum, several issues should be identified and addressed as part of determining a sequence of intervention.

INTERPERSONAL DYNAMICS

The first principle that guides sequencing of events in a program has to do with the development of interpersonal relationships between implementer and target. We have found that a sequence to the development of interpersonal relationships contributes to strong program design and implementation. A trusting attachment needs to form between implementer and target, and interaction needs to reach targets at an emotional level. Issues of attachment and exerting an emotional impact often are discussed in clinical (psychological) treatments and improving organizational behavior (e.g., see Miller & Rollnick, 1991). As we consider the mediating variables that matter for health behavior change—accepting conventional norms, developing and maintaining values that are incongruent with high-risk behaviors, and making voluntary commitments—we realize that these variables tap an emotional domain that require the target of intervention to be willing to trust the implementer.

In many cases, programs are delivered by individuals who begin the intervention without the benefit of having first established a relationship of trust and the ability to deal with a participant on an emotional level. Program developers need to provide a means of developing trust between teacher and participants and among participants themselves. Developing trust and the ability to communicate ultimately depends on more than the design of a program. However, it is clear that a program can be designed to maximize these features.

As a case in point, Tanglewood Research's goal in All Stars was to have, as the last session of the prevention program, participants making deep and serious commitments to avoid drug use, violence, and premature or high-risk sexual activity. Specific commitments were not prescribed. Instead, they were encouraged to make commitments that reflect a personal understanding of what is healthy and realistic. We met with participants one-on-one to discuss their commitments and challenged them to be clear, precise, and truly committed to what they had written.

From our perspective, the emotional demands of the commitment meeting required that we lay groundwork from the beginning that would allow a relative stranger to ask highly personal questions. We therefore orchestrated the program so that it began with activities that were enjoyable and not emotionally threatening and that allowed the teacher to diffuse mistrust. During the initial phase, the target topics of drugs, violence, and sex were not discussed at all. Indeed, in the second and third sessions, participants often questioned the purpose of the program. The initial phase of teaching addressed topics that included an emotional component to them but that avoided the potential for confrontation. Standards of open interaction were established, consistently encouraging students to express their thoughts. At first, discussions focused on nonthreatening topics. Subsequently, once acceptance of opinions was ensured, topics that have potential to arouse strong opinions were included. Throughout the program, opportunities to provoke and challenge students increased in frequency.

Programs that are intended to systematically change characteristics that have an emotional root need to craft the development of interpersonal relationships. We would not exclude programs that are intellectual (knowledge dissemination) or competency based (skills development) from this requirement. It is likely that even these programs require trust and emotional acceptance of the messages of the program before effects can be observed. The goal of sequencing should be, from our perspective, focused on allowing the program implementers to demonstrate through word and deed that they can be trusted, which is a logical prerequisite to providing them with opportunities to engage in emotional challenges.

TIMING AND LOGICAL SEQUENCE ISSUES

The second set of issues to be addressed is the general ordering of topics and the speed with which they are addressed. When multiple mediators are addressed, multiple possibilities for ordering topics exist. Depending on the nature of the mediators selected, it may be possible to address several either simultaneously or in an interwoven style. On the other hand, it may be necessary to deal with one topic, bring it to a conclusion, and then move on to a second topic (see Chapter 13, this volume).

There are other fields in which sequence among topics is clearly expressed. For example, education gradually has evolved a sequence to teaching topics such as mathematics and language. Indeed, a major theme of current educational practice is that students must learn topics in order. Skipping fundamental or prerequisite knowledge is debilitating when trying to learn more complex or abstract material.

There are several means one could use to establish a potential best sequence of sessions in a program. For example, health educators or other experts could provide their own order of the best sequence of first to last sessions. A matrix could be created in which preferred order (rows) by raters (columns) is formed. Average rankings could be used to determine overall preference of order. The degree to which this association is stable could even be tested using methods such as Kendall's coefficient of concordance (Hays, 1973). This statistic was found to be useful in assisting with determining sequence in at least one health program (Sussman et al., 1995).

It also might be possible to create a limited number of competing sequences that reflect different theoretical assumptions about conceptual progression. Teachers might teach a program in each of the orders and then repeat the above rating procedures to see if a preferred order emerges as a result of such an experimental manipulation. A more limited version of this method might be to consider pairs of sessions, flipping selected small numbers of sessions to see whether this reveals information regarding preferred ordering of paired sessions.

RECURSIVENESS

Recursiveness refers to repetition using systematic variations in approach. People need to have multiple exposures to programs but often tire when the same approach is reused over and over. Yet, one issue that drug prevention research has yielded information about is the need for multiple points of reinforcement (i.e., repetition and integration of material concepts into daily living). Programs without boosters are almost always inferior to programs that have boosters. The programs with the longest observable successes have included boosters (Botvin et al., 1995) or other forms of reinforcement.

The major challenge facing program developers is developing booster programs that are not simply the original program all over again. We conducted observations of a pilot test of the Drug Abuse Resistance Education (DARE) middle school program as part of a study of normal teaching practices about drug abuse prevention (Hansen & McNeal, 1999). The version of the middle school program we observed was amazingly similar to the earlier fifth-grade program. The most common unsolicited comment from students was that they had done these activities before.

Booster programs need to accommodate changes in how participants will act and react based on changes in their development. Some adolescents, particularly those who are prone to sensation seeking (Donohew, Palmgreen, & Lorch, 1998), are unwilling to repeat some experiences more than once. As they grow older, adolescents increasingly strive for independence. They have additional experiences that must be accounted for and that influence relevance of program contents. Most important, as youth grow older, they are increasingly likely to have engaged in some form of high-risk behavior. It appears that the very experience of having engaged in such behaviors, even experimentally, alters a variety of propensities (the key issue is no longer prevention of use, for example, but differentiating use from abuse). Well-designed booster programs need to anticipate such changes and build these changes into the program while reinforcing concepts and other attributes that are appropriate for the target population.

GUIDING PRINCIPLES

Our first principle of sequencing is to identify logical components of order. Typically, optimal sequences move from simple to complex and from definition and knowledge to application. Program developers are encouraged to organize the concepts they intend to address through their programming so that the logically simplest components occur first. Sometimes, basic vocabulary and simple concepts are needed before class discussion can occur. For example, in designing an intervention that addressed building idealism among fourth-grade students, Tanglewood Research created a number of activities. The goal was to encourage students to think deeply about their own ideals. However, a pilot test with one child revealed that the language of idealism was not understood. We therefore broke elements into ordered skills (spelling, identifying meaning, using words in sentences, identifying concepts in literature) that were then followed by more advanced activities, including completing stories about characters who have similar ideals on an interactive CD.

Our second principle is to order events according to their natural occurrence in the social world. Of primary importance, we believe that developing a relationship naturally occurs before engaging in a change process. We believe that a key to successful intervention is developing emotional openness between teacher and student. Relationship development often occurs prior to accomplishment of major instrumental goals. One might hypothesize that the degree of trust between students and their teachers would depend on a sequence of events that includes learning names, giving informal greetings, discussing topics of mutual interest, providing opportunities to tease and banter, discussing friends and family, and feeling free to ask about personal behaviors. Guttman scaling information can be particularly helpful in understanding these issues. A survey of students about these topics should quickly reveal which are most common (and therefore earliest in sequence) and which are more rare (and therefore latest in sequence).

Our third principle for ordering events is to gather data by means of observing interventions in progress and periodically assessing mastery of concepts and skills to determine the degree to which the intervention can keep up with expectations. The proof of an intervention is found in its execution. It is often the case that an expert can identify simply from observing the delivery of an intervention whether recipients are confused rather than enlightened. If a program is designed around the idea of mastery prior to progressing to the next steps, tests of mastery can reveal essentially the same facts. Such data are especially useful in refining intervention approaches.

Our fourth principle is to develop systematic recursiveness. Nearly all programs need some form of booster to reinforce concepts and skills. Program developers should strive to include novelty in the format of booster programs. Furthermore, booster programs need to be adaptive to developmental issues that require adjustments in format and content.

SEQUENCING LEVEL 3: SEQUENCING WITHIN SINGLE POINTS OF AN INTERVENTION

DEFINITION OF CONCERNS FOR SEQUENCING WITHIN SINGLE TOPICS

Many adults have become used to a form of working and interacting that could be considered psychological time-sharing. That is, we begin one task, get interrupted to work on a second task, and then fail to complete both the first and second tasks to start working on a third task. We pick up the telephone and have a brief conversation that is an extension of previous conversations and experiences. Somehow, these all become connected, but it appears at first glance that we experience a set of disjointed events that are without order. One may refer to this phenomenon as psychological time-sharing. Psychological time-sharing does not work when one is trying to influence the course of psychological and social development among people. Once engaged in the interactive process of the intervention, the effectiveness of intervention benefits from a flow that allows people to become and remain engaged in the process itself.

FLOW

We are used to having events flow so that there is a definable progression from one moment to the next. The clearest examples of this flow can be found in music and drama. Each will serve as initial examples.

Two elements of music relate to moment-to-moment sequencing: form and harmony. Classical music evolved several different forms. The most notable and identifiable is the sonata-allegro form (Eakle, 1998). Movements composed in the sonata-allegro form are divided into three broad sections: the exposition, the development, and the recapitulation. The exposition begins with the presentation of a theme in the tonic key. The piece then transitions to a second theme, which is presented in the dominant key (a fifth higher than the tonic). During the development section, one or more themes from the exposition are developed by taking thematic elements and altering them by changing key or creating variations. In the final section, the recapitulation, both themes are again presented, usually in the tonic key. Sometimes, a coda section appended at the end allows the composer to finish things off.

Drama, including everything from cartoon shorts and stand-up comedy to dramatic stage productions and movies, relies on sequence in the presentation. Classical Greek plays provided a similar structure of form (Kastel, 1998), although it is likely that this structure emerged as a postproduction analysis rather than as a guiding form employed by Greek playwrights. The sections of this structure include a prologue during which the situation is explained, a development during which various competing elements emerge, a climax during which the competing elements clash, a reconciliation during which the various actors respond to the climax, and an epilogue during which the moral lesson from the play is summarized and the playwright brings the play to closure. Modern drama often uses a similar flow of events to maintain interest and deliver its message to the audience.

The key elements from both music and drama that have allowed both to be successful in terms of bringing audiences into the event are related to flow characteristics. Using music and drama as a springboard, we present an example from All Stars (Hansen, 1996) as a case study. Many sessions required a series of iterations before the flow was optimized. One particular session introduces students to debates as a means of establishing conventional norms within the class. In the first version of the program, the instructor was directed to jump quite quickly into a debate activity. Preparing and motivating students to participate were not considered. We learned that students had little prior experience with debate and that teachers actively suppressed the open expression of opinions by students. We also experienced a number of unexpected outcomes in which students as a group took unconventional stands, reinforcing antithetical goals and potentially causing the norm within the group to shift in an undesired direction. In particular, to foster debate on topics about which there was nearly uniform agreement, we encouraged students to adopt a "devil's advocate" position. An unintended consequence was that students fought for the opportunity to be the devil's advocate and took great liberty in acting out their roles. This session originally had a single theme, jumped directly to the point, but then became discordant and diffuse. Too many performance demands were made too soon, and the flow was lost or directed toward divergent thinking.

The flow of the revised session differed in definable ways that essentially restructured the flow of events, although the theme of the session itself was not changed. Before the session, we made sure the teacher understood what was going to happen and begged for indulgence. We introduced the purpose of the activity with a structured discussion that related to citizenship, constitutional rights, conscience, and other topics that allowed students to get their motivations set. The open debate itself was shortened and moved to the end of this session and carried forward into the next session. We now asked students to first simply express their opinions by standing under signs that expressed those opinions. When a clear majority opinion emerged, conclusions were drawn about what composed existing group norms. When there was disagreement, the issue was set aside for debate. Devil's advocates were not needed because only those with sincere differences in opinions were involved in the debate.

The form of the session now reflected an interplay of themes, similar to both musical and dramatic elements of form. Multiple themes were introduced (the constitutional rights of free speech, the role of conscience, declaring opinions, and defending opinions). There was a period of development that allowed competing opinions to emerge. The change in flow provided for outcomes that were much more likely to reinforce conventional norms. Students were allowed time to develop skills and become emotionally engaged in the activity.

TAILORED MODIFICATIONS

It has been the common experience of many teachers that knowledge and skills emerge and attitudes are formed only after repeated exposure to a topic. Current research (Gardner, Kornhaber, & Wake, 1996) suggests that people differ from one another in the senses they use to learn. Some individuals are highly visual, others are highly verbal, and others are tactile. Some learn through introspection, others through the help of social input. Some learn and form opinions quickly, but others do so slowly. Some learn by study, others by experience. We believe that within single periods of instruction, building recursiveness into intervention strengthens the potential of the intervention to yield positive and desired outcomes. The same message can be repeated through use of multiple senses within the course of delivery of a single topic to provide both repetition and variation.

GUIDING PRINCIPLES

Two principles emerge from our consideration of how to sequence events at this level. First, we encourage program developers to consider the flow of events. Moment-to-moment needs include a means for ensuring attentiveness, comprehension, and acceptance of messages. We recommend applying techniques from music (introduction of themes, development, contrast, counterpoint, etc.) and drama (prologue, development, climax, reconciliation) to ensure that an order that maintains interest and develops understanding is attained. For example, programs may start by introducing a topic to participants. The development may rely on having participants gather contextual information that may be essential to a broad comprehension of issues and that allows competing issues to emerge. Climax elements may encourage participants to find resolution of conflicting thoughts. Such a lesson format is very different from simply presenting facts in one area, followed immediately by presenting new facts in a different area.

The second principle is to develop multiple activities that use a variety of sensory dimensions within and over multiple points in time. Providing variety, appropriately paced, allows those with different learning styles and those who have different thresholds for attentiveness to maximize their chances of success. This is true for gaining understanding as well as for successfully making attitude adjustments.

▶ CONCLUSIONS

Sequencing plays an important role in the design of successful programs. We have outlined three levels at which programming plays an important role. A fully developed, empirically based theory that provides program developers with guidance about how to address sequence issues does not yet exist. Nonetheless, we believe the principles outlined in this chapter can be useful to those who wish to improve their ability to develop effective interventions. Program developers should carefully consider sequence issues that may influence effectiveness, including those issues within the individual, the group, and the organization.

Researchers in the field need to develop a literature in which sequence variables are at least elaborated if not tested. Unlike the experimental methods that use systematic controlled variation to determine attributable cause, observational methods are more likely to predominate. Traditions of social science render nonexperimental findings to a lesser role. Nonetheless, for advancing understanding about sequence issues, these methods may be all that are available and should be used wisely.

To summarize, we have suggested a number of principles to guide program developers. These include the following:

Sequencing Level 1: Environment and life course development

Programs should be developed to fit within the existing psychosocial developmental level of the average young person who will be the target of intervention.

Programs that address behaviors that have a natural pattern of development associated with age or other markers of maturity should target implementation primarily during the initial periods of rapid increase.

Programs should be designed to fit within the structure, goals, and methods of the host institution.

Sequencing Level 2: Sequencing complex program elements

Identify the logical components of order.

Order events according to their natural occurrence as determined empirically through Guttman scaling or other techniques, if possible.

Gather data by means of observing interventions in progress and periodically assessing mastery of concepts and skills to determine the degree to which the intervention can keep up with expectations.

Develop systematic recursiveness, including developmentally appropriate booster programs.

Sequencing Level 3: Sequencing within single topics

Program developers should consider the moment-to-moment flow of events to ensure attentiveness, comprehension, and acceptance of messages.

Develop multiple activities that use a variety of sensory dimensions within and over points in time. Providing variety allows those with different learning styles and those who have different thresholds for attentiveness to maximize their chances of success. This is true for gaining understanding as well as for successfully making attitude adjustments.

▶ NOTE

1. Sequencing comes up as an important research consideration in a lot of different areas. For example, military science and business literatures contribute to a conceptual understanding of sequence in behavior, particularly at the campaign development level. In issues of peace and warfare, as well as issues of marketing and management, sequencing events becomes an important issue that must be addressed if success is to be achieved. In military terms, there are issues related to order of battle, gaining surprise through the timing of attacks and setting and closing traps, which frequently come into play in the strategists' decision making. Similarly, marketing must be coordinated with production and distribution in business to gain market share and advantage over competitors. General principles of sequencing can be adapted from this literature, although specific applications may fail to translate into health behavior intervention development. Nonetheless, the literature of military (Clausewitz, 1833/1976; Dupuy, 1990; Tzu, 1983) and marketing strategy (Michaelson, 1987; Peacock, 1984, provides a rich source of ideas and constructs that communicate well about sequencing issues that we may want to consider in future work.

▶ REFERENCES

BOTVIN, G. J., BAKER, E., DUSENBURY, L., BOTVIN, E. M., & DIAZ, T. (1995). Long-term follow-up results of a randomized drug abuse prevention trial in a white middle-class population. *Journal of the American Medical Association, 273,* 1106-1112.

CLAUSEWITZ, C. V. (1976). *On war* (3 vols.). Princeton, NJ: Princeton University Press. (Original publication 1833)

COLLINS, L. M., GRAHAM, J. W., LONG, J. D., & HANSEN, W. B. (1994). Cross validation of latent class models of early substance use onset. *Multivariate Behavioral Research, 29,* 165-183.

COLLINS, L. M., GRAHAM, J. W., ROUSCULP, S. S., & HANSEN, W. B. (1997). Heavy caffeine use and the beginning of the substance use onset process: An illustration of latent transition analysis. In K. J. Bryant, M. Windle, & S. G. West (Eds.), *The science of prevention: Methodological advances from alcohol and substance abuse research* (pp. 79-99). Washington, DC: American Psychological Association.

DONOHEW, L., PALMGREEN, P., & LORCH, E. (1998). Applications of a theoretic model of information exposure to health interventions. *Human Communication Research, 24,* 454-468.

DUPUY, T. N. (1990). *Understanding defeat.* New York: Paragon.

EAKLE, K. (1998). *Mr. E's virtual music classroom: Sonata-allegro form* [Online]. Available: http://cnet.unb.ca/achn/kodaly/koteach/resources/son-allegro.html.

GARDNER, H., KORNHABER, M. L., & WAKE, W. K. (1996). *Intelligence: Multiple perspectives.* New York: Harcourt Brace.

GINGISS, P. L., GOTTLIEB, N. H., & BRINK, S. G. (1994). Increasing teacher receptivity toward use of tobacco prevention education programs. *Journal of Drug Education, 24,* 163-176.

HANSEN, W. B. (1992). School-based substance abuse prevention: A review of the state of the art in curriculum 1980-1990. *Health Education Research, 7,* 403-430.

HANSEN, W. B. (1996). Pilot test results comparing the All Stars program with seventh grade D.A.R.E.: Program integrity and mediating variable analysis. *Substance Use & Misuse, 31,* 1359-1377.

HANSEN, W. B., & McNEAL, R. B., Jr. (1997). How DARE works: An examination of program effects on mediating variables. *Health Education & Behavior, 24,* 165-176.

HANSEN, W. B., & McNEAL, R. B., Jr. (1999). Drug education practice: Results of an observational study. *Health Education Research, 14,* 85-97.

HANSEN, W. B., PASKETT, E. D., & CARTER, L. J. (1999). The Adolescent Sexual Activity Index (ASAI): A standardized strategy for measuring interpersonal heterosexual behaviors among youth. *Health Education Research, 14*(4), 485-490.

HANSEN, W. B., & ROSE, L. A. (1995). Recreational use of inhalant drugs by adolescents: A challenge for family physicians. *Family Medicine, 27,* 383-387.

HANSEN, W. B., WOLKENSTEIN, B. H., & HAHN, G. L. (1992). Young adult sexual behavior: Issues in programming and evaluation. *Health Education Research, 7,* 305-312.

HAWKINS, J. D., CATALANO, R. F., & MILLER, J. Y. (1992). Factors for alcohol and other drug problems in adolescence and early adulthood: Implications for substance abuse prevention. *Psychological Bulletin, 112,* 64-105.

HAYS, W. L. (1973). *Statistics for the social sciences.* New York: Holt, Rinehart.

KANDEL, D. B., YAMAGUCHI, K., & CHEN, K. (1992). Stages of progression in drug involvement from adolescence to adulthood: Further evidence for the gateway theory. *Journal of Studies on Alcohol, 53,* 447-457.

KASTEL, S. (1998). *5 parts and 10 types: A simplified rhetoric of Greek tragedy* [Online]. Available: http://www.slip.net/~stepx/greek/index.html.

KOHLBERG, L. (1969). Stage and sequence: The cognitive-developmental approach to socialization. In D. Goslin (Ed.), *Handbook of socialization theory and research.* Chicago: Rand McNally.

MacKINNON, D. P. (1994). Analysis of mediating variables in prevention and intervention research. In A. Cázares & L. A. Beatty (Eds.), *Scientific methods for prevention intervention research* (NIDA Research Monograph No. 139, pp. 127-154). Rockville, MD: National Institutes of Health.

MacKINNON, D. P., & DWYER, J. H. (1993). Estimating mediated effects in prevention studies. *Evaluation Review, 17,* 144-158.

MASLOW, A. (1943). A theory of human motivation. *Psychological Review, 50,* 370-396.

McNEAL, R. B., Jr., & HANSEN, W. B. (1999). Developmental patterns associated with the onset of drug use: Changes in postulated mediators during adolescence. *Journal of Drug Issues, 29*(2), 381-400.

MICHAELSON, G. A. (1987). *Winning the marketing war: A field manual for business leaders.* Knoxville, TN: Pressmark International.

MILLER, W. R., & ROLLNICK, S. (1991). *Motivational interviewing: Preparing people to change addictive behavior.* New York: Guilford.

OETTING, E. R., DONNERMEYER, J. F., PLESTED, B. A., EDWARDS, R. W., KELLY, K. J., & BEAUVAIS, F. (1995). Assessing community readiness for prevention. *International Journal of the Addictions, 30,* 659-683.

PEACOCK, W. E. (1984). *Corporate combat: Military strategies that win business wars.* New York: Berkley.

PIAGET, J. (1952). *The origins of intelligence in children.* New York: International University Press.

PIAGET, J. (1970). Piaget's theory. In P. H. Mussen (Ed.), *Carmichael's manual of child psychology* (Vol. 1). New York: John Wiley.

PIAGET, J. (1977). *The development of thought: Equilibrium of cognitive structures.* New York: Viking.

PLESTED, B., SMITHAM, D. M., JUMPER-THURMAN, P., OETTING, E. R., & EDWARDS, R. W. (1999). Readiness for drug use prevention in rural minority communities. *Substance Use and Misuse, 34,* 521-544.

PROCHASKA, J. A., DICLEMENTE, C. C., & NORCROSS, J. C. (1992). In search of how people change: Applications to addictive behaviors. *American Psychologist, 47,* 1102.

ROGERS, E. M. (1983). *Diffusion of innovations* (3rd ed.). New York: Free Press. (Original publication 1962)

ROHRBACH, L. A., GRAHAM, J. W., & HANSEN, W. B. (1993). Diffusion of a school-based substance abuse prevention program: Predictors of program implementation. *Preventive Medicine, 22,* 237-260.

RYAN, B., & GROSS, N. C. (1943). The diffusion of hybrid seed corn in two Iowa communities. *Rural Sociology, 8,* 15-24.

STERN, R. A., PROCHASKA, J. A., VELICER, W. F., & ELDER, J. P. (1987). Stages of adolescent cigarette smoking acquisition: Measurement and sample profiles. *Addictive Behaviors, 12,* 319-329.

SUSSMAN, S., DENT, C. W., BURTON, D., STACY, A. W., & FLAY, B. R. (1995). *Developing school-based tobacco use prevention and cessation programs.* Thousand Oaks, CA: Sage.

TOBLER, N. S., & STRATTON, H. (1997). Effectiveness of school-based drug prevention programs: A meta-analysis of the research. *Journal of Primary Prevention, 18,* 71-128.

TZU, SUN. (1983). *The art of war.* New York: Dell.

WALDROP, M. M. (1992). *Complexity: The emerging science at the edge of order and chaos.* New York: Simon & Schuster.

CHAPTER 15

Commentary

Douglas Longshore

This far-ranging, provocative chapter offers much insight and useful guidance on the sequencing of program content and the design of programs to match the readiness of a target population and its environment. In my commentary, I develop the sequencing theme further by describing interventions based on stage models of behavior change. In view of favorable evidence of their effects, I suggest a corollary to one of the guiding principles proposed by Hansen and Altman.

The authors argue convincingly that programs should be designed "to fit within the existing psychosocial developmental level of the average young person who will be the target of the intervention" (first principle under Sequencing Level 1). Their underlying logic is twofold. First, programs are likely to be more effective if they call on cognitive, behavioral, and ethical capabilities already possessed by the audience and if they target needs most relevant to that audience. Second, it is wiser to meet an audience "where they are" in a developmental sequence than to try to induce forward movement in the sequence. The authors attribute to moral development theorists Kohlberg and Piaget the view that change from one stage to another cannot be hastened. This may be too pessimistic. I will discuss three stage-based interventions that can be used to hasten change: motivational intervention based on the transtheoretical model, moral reconation therapy, and node link mapping.

Transtheoretical studies have identified five discrete stages in behavior change: precontemplation, contemplation, preparation, action, and maintenance. Recent studies based on the transtheoretical model (e.g., Prochaska & Norcross, 1994) have also focused on *how* people change (i.e., what they think, feel, and do as they move across stages). Are particular cognitions, emotions, and behaviors more salient in some stage transitions than in others? The answer is yes. Change processes known as consciousness raising, dramatic relief, and environmental reevaluation are associated with moving from precontemplation to contemplation. These processes all involve raising one's awareness of a problem and assessing its impact on oneself and others. At later stages, change processes appear to be more behavioral (e.g., reinforcement management, counterconditioning, and stimulus control). Such processes are geared toward actively managing one's environment to facilitate and maintain the change that one has started to make.

Findings on the processes of change have been applied in the development of motivational interventions that assess a person's stage of change and apply counseling techniques likely to trigger the processes that move a person forward in the stage sequence (Miller & Rollnick, 1991). Such interventions, delivered one-on-one or in small-group formats, rely on five techniques: (a) expressing empathy (counselor accepts clients' feelings without judging, criticizing, or blaming), (b) developing discrepancy (counselor leads clients to see the discrepancy between their values/concerns and current behavior), (c) avoiding argument (clients are not directly confronted about negative aspects of their behavior), (d) rolling with resistance (counselor uses the clients' own words to guide them to appropriate insights and decisions), and (e) supporting self-efficacy (counselor encourages clients to take steps that they view as achievable).

Social scientists at the UCLA Drug Abuse Research Center and Imoyase, in collaboration with Surviving in Recovery (a community-based self-help organization in Los Angeles), have developed a motivational intervention to promote recovery among drug and alcohol users recruited from street settings. Expecting most clients of the intervention to be at the precontemplation and contemplation stages of change, we trained counselors to work on the change processes most relevant at those early stages (i.e., consciousness raising and dramatic relief). Accordingly, counselors used the clients' own words to trigger new insights and decisions and sought to develop discrepancies between clients' stated values or concerns and their substance use. Counselors also expressed empathy and, especially with clients in the contemplation stage, supported self-efficacy for taking initial steps toward recovery. In a randomized field trial, we assigned clients either to one session of motivational intervention or to one session of generic counseling. Those in the motivational intervention were, by self-report and counselor rating taken immediately after the intervention, more involved in the session, more willing to self-disclose, and more motivated to change (Longshore, Grills, & Annon, 1999). At a 1-year follow-up, these clients were also more likely to be drug or alcohol abstinent, as indicated by self-report and urine test results (Longshore, 1998). We recently adapted the intervention for use in multisession, group-based counseling to promote HIV risk reduction (Longshore, Grills, Annon, & Grady, 1998). Additional evidence for the potential impact of motivational interviewing has emerged in the fields of alcohol treatment for adults (Bein, Miller, & Boroughs, 1993; Brown & Miller, 1993), HIV education for adults (Carey et al., 1998; Prochaska, Redding, Harlow, & Rossi, 1994), and secondary prevention of smoking and problem drinking among adolescents and young adults (Baer, 1993; Colby et al., 1998; Lawendowski, 1998).

With obvious implications for primary prevention, Pallonen, Prochaska, Velicer, Prokhorov, and Smith (1998) have expanded the stage-of-change continuum to cover smoking acquisition as well as cessation among adolescents. For example, the precontemplation stage of smoking acquisition is, "I am not thinking about trying smoking," whereas the preparation stage is, "I am thinking about trying smoking in the next 30 days." The goal in primary prevention would be to move people backward in the stage sequence. An important task for future research is to identify the change processes that underlie health-enhancing backward movement and to determine how those processes are similar to or different from the processes that underlie health-enhancing forward movement (e.g., "I am thinking about quitting smoking") and health-threatening backward movement (e.g., "I sure would like a cigarette after this meal").

Another stage-based intervention is moral reconation therapy, which seeks to rehabilitate criminal offenders by moving them from lower to higher stages in Kohlberg's moral development sequence. Offenders complete a series of exercises in which they examine their past behavior from a pleasure-seeking and pain-avoiding perspective while also learning to view their behavior from higher-level perspectives of adherence to social norms and dictates of conscience. Greater emphasis is placed on higher levels of moral reasoning as offenders meet the criteria for success in each exercise. Research indicates that moral reconation therapy promotes favorable change in moral reasoning and reduces recidivism (Little & Robinson, 1989; Little, Robinson, & Burnette, 1991; National Institute of Justice, 1998).

A Texas Christian University (TCU) treatment protocol featuring node link mapping serves as a final example of stage-based intervention and, in other ways as well, reflects the concept of sequencing (Dansereau, Joe, Dees, & Simpson, 1996; Simpson, Chatham, & Joe, 1993). At the outset of treatment, counselors focus on developing trust and rapport and on stabilizing the client's motivation for behavior change. This emphasis is in keeping with Hansen and Altman's assertion that "a trusting relationship needs to form between implementer and target" early in their relationship. TCU's counseling techniques include node link mapping, which helps clients define their goals (i.e., changes in thoughts, feelings, or behavior) and visualize the interrelationships among goals. In this way, clients are met "where they are," and their competing concerns (e.g., hunger, income, and interpersonal relationships) are dealt with in the proper sequence. Note also that therapeutic community protocols recently have been conceptualized as a stage-based effort to promote development of prosocial behaviors and higher-level moral reasoning among drug and alcohol users (De Leon, 1996).

The interventions described here are in some ways a mixed bag. Some are in the domain of prevention; others are part of an extended treatment protocol. Most have targeted adults, although adolescents and young adults have been the audience for some. They all share two features, however. Clients are met "where they are" (i.e., at their existing stage of awareness and motivation). More important, the interventions do not stop there; they attempt to hasten behavior change by triggering cognitive and behavioral processes thought to underlie movement toward later stages and by gauging clients' progress through the stage sequence. The success of stage-based interventions suggests a corollary to the Sequencing Level 1 principle that programs should be designed "to fit within the existing psychosocial developmental level of the average young person who will be the target of the intervention." That corollary is the following: "Programs designed to change behavior by promoting psychosocial or moral development should focus on the cognitive and behavioral processes underlying forward movement from the existing level of the average person who will be the target of the intervention."

A final comment on intervention "dose." Under the topic of recursiveness, Hansen and Altman cite the importance of booster lessons or other reinforcement as a means of sustaining behavior change over the long term. It is tempting to speculate that multiple boosters may actually be more important than the amount of intervention delivered initially. That is, the eventual dose may matter more than the first dose. In defense of this speculation, I cite mental health and other programs that have come to be known as "brief interventions" inasmuch as brevity is their defining characteristic. (These are sometimes but not always based explicitly on the transtheoretical model.) As in the motivational intervention described earlier, brief intervention clients typically receive a single session of counseling, view an educational video, and/or read a self-help manual. Such programs have shown success (Heather, 1995; Miller & Taylor, 1980), perhaps because they have a "kindling" effect; that is, they trigger small changes in behavior, thoughts, or feelings that culminate in clear recognition of the problem and acceptance of the need for change (De Leon, 1994). In short, I am suggesting that intervention planners consider *how much* program content is actually needed to produce effects worth the investment and how much of this content needs to be front-loaded if boosters will occur later and if the overall amount of time available for delivering a recursive program is, as will often be the case, very limited.

REFERENCES

BAER, J. S. (1993). Etiology and secondary prevention of alcohol problems with young adults. In J. S. Baer, A. Marlatt, & R. J. McMahon (Eds.), *Addictive behaviors across the life span* (pp. 111-137). Newbury Park, CA: Sage.

BEIN, T. H., MILLER, W. R., & BOROUGHS, J. M. (1993). Motivational interviewing with alcohol outpatients. *Behavioral and Cognitive Psychotherapy, 21,* 347-356.

BROWN, J. M., & MILLER, W. R. (1993). Impact of motivational interviewing on participation and outcome in residential alcoholism treatment. *Psychology of Addictive Behaviors, 7,* 211-218.

CAREY, M. P., MAISTO, S. A., BRAATEN, L. S., DURANT, L. E., FORSYTH, A. D., JAWORSKI, B. C., WEINHARDT, L. S., WRIGHT-WILLIAMS, M., & GLEASON, J. R. (1998, June). *Reducing HIV risk among low-income women using motivational enhancement and behavioral skills training.* Paper presented at the 12th World AIDS Conference, Geneva, Switzerland.

COLBY, S. M., MONTI, P. M., BARNETT, N. P., ROHSENOW, D. J., WEISSMAN, K., SPIRITO, A., WOOLARD, R. H., & LEWANDER, W. J. (1998). Brief motivational interviewing in a hospital setting for adolescent smoking: A preliminary study. *Journal of Consulting and Clinical Psychology, 66,* 574-578.

DANSEREAU, D. F., JOE, G. W., DEES, S. M., & SIMPSON, D. D. (1996). Ethnicity and the effects of mapping-enhanced drug abuse counseling. *Addictive Behaviors, 21,* 363-376.

DE LEON, G. (1994). The therapeutic community: Toward a general theory and model. In F. M. Tims, G. De Leon, & J. Jainchill (Eds.), *Therapeutic community: Advances in research and application* (pp. 16-53). Rockville, MD: National Institute on Drug Abuse.

DE LEON, G. (1996). Integrative recovery: A stage paradigm. *Substance Abuse, 17,* 51-63.

HEATHER, N. (1995). Brief intervention strategies. In R. K. Hester & W. R. Miller (Eds.), *Handbook of alcoholism treatment approaches: Effective alternatives* (pp. 105-122). Boston: Allyn & Bacon.

LAWENDOWSKI, L. A. (1998). A motivational intervention for adolescent smokers. *Preventive Medicine, 27,* A39-A46.

LITTLE, G. L., & ROBINSON, K. D. (1989). The effects of moral reconation therapy upon moral reasoning, life purpose, and recidivism among drug and alcohol offenders. *Psychological Reports, 64,* 83-90.

LITTLE, G. L., ROBINSON, K. D., & BURNETTE, K. D. (1991). Treating drug offenders with moral reconation therapy: A three-year recidivism report. *Psychological Reports, 69,* 1151-1154.

LONGSHORE, D., & GRILLS, C. (2000). Motivating recovery from illegal drug use: Evidence for a culturally congruent intervention. *Journal of Black Psychology, 26,* 288-301.

LONGSHORE, D., GRILLS, C., & ANNON, K. (1999). Effects of a culturally congruent intervention on cognitive factors related to recovery. *Substance Use and Misuse, 34*(9), 1223-1241.

LONGSHORE, D., GRILLS, C., ANNON, K., & GRADY, R. (1998). Promoting recovery from drug abuse: An Africentric intervention. *Journal of Black Studies, 28,* 319-333.

MILLER, W. R., & ROLLNICK, S. (1991). *Motivational interviewing: Preparing people to change addictive behavior.* New York: Guilford.

MILLER, W. R., & TAYLOR, C. A. (1980). Relative effectiveness of bibliotherapy, individual and group self-control training in the treatment of problem drinkers. *Addictive Behaviors, 5,* 13-24.

NATIONAL INSTITUTE OF JUSTICE. (1998). *The Delaware Department of Corrections Life Skills Program* (NCJ 169589). Washington, DC: U.S. Department of Justice.

PALLONEN, U. E., PROCHASKA, J. O., VELICER, W. F., PROKHOROV, A. V., & SMITH, N. F. (1998). Stages of acquisition and cessation for adolescent smoking: An empirical investigation. *Addictive Behaviors, 23,* 303-324.

PROCHASKA, J. O., & NORCROSS, J. C. (1994). *Systems of psychotherapy: A transtheoretical analysis* (3rd ed.). Pacific Grove, CA: Brooks/Cole.

PROCHASKA, J. O., REDDING, C. A., HARLOW, L. L., & ROSSI, J. S. (1994). The transtheoretical model of change and HIV prevention: A review. *Health Education Quarterly, 21,* 471-486.

SIMPSON, D. D., CHATHAM, L. R., & JOE, G. W. (1993). Cognitive enhancements to treatment in DATAR: Drug Abuse Treatment for AIDS Risk Reduction. In J. A. Inciardi, F. M. Tims, & B. W. Fletcher (Eds.), *Innovative approaches in the treatment of drug abuse: Program models and strategies* (pp. 161-177). Westport, CT: Greenwood.

CHAPTER 16

Pilot Studies

Michael Lynskey
Steve Sussman

The baby begins to walk. At this point in program development, a complete draft program has been constructed with previously tested components. Next the complete package needs testing. This chapter discusses the use of pilot studies to establish the integrity of a newly developed program. A pilot study may be defined as a test of a complete draft program that involves a relatively small sample size. Any bugs in the program can be detected, some further refinements can be made, and then the program is ready to run. (This is Step 5 of the chain model.) There are a number of benefits to implementing a pilot project before proceeding to full-scale implementation of a health intervention. First, the pilot program provides an opportunity to examine and test the ease of implementing the program. Second, such programs give an opportunity to assess the acceptability of the program to participants. Third, pilot programs provide a vehicle for the preliminary testing of a program's likely effectiveness. Fourth, in a pilot study, one can manipulate potential mediators of change of the complete program. Finally, and most important, pilot programs provide an empirical basis for making program changes and refinements before large-scale implementation of a program.

Pilot studies differ from main, large trials of an intervention in a number of ways. Specifically, they generally are considerably smaller in scale and involve more in-depth consideration of factors affecting the process of program implementation, whereas full-scale trials are often more concerned with outcome evaluation rather than the process of program implementation. A weakness of the pilot-testing approach is that one is only conducting an immediate-outcomes evaluation, and therefore effects on longer-term outcomes are less certain. Pilot testing is the single most popular program development method (see Chapter 1, this volume).

Table 16.1 provides a brief description and summary of a number of pilot studies that have been conducted in the area of health promotion. The studies in this table were identified through a search of MedINFO and PsycINFO, using the terms *formative research* and *program development* for the period from 1984 to 1998. This search assessed aspects of program development in a range of diverse areas and identified 37 separate pilot studies. Please note that the focus of the search was on program development per se (a search that simply uses the key words *pilot study* will reveal a hundred times more articles). These areas include prevention of substance use among adolescents (Flay et al., 1988; Sussman, 1996), pain management among the chronically ill (Ferrell, Rhiner, & Ferell, 1993; Torrestad, Hakanson, & Axelli, 1992), asthma self-management (Mesters, Meertens, Kok, & Parcel, 1994; Snyder, Winder, & Creer, 1987), sexually transmitted disease (STD) and HIV prevention (Guthrie et al., 1996; Sikkema, Winett, & Lombard, 1995), cancer screening (Dignan et al., 1995; Herity et al., 1997; Ostwald & Rothenberger, 1985; Tatum, Wilson, Dignan, Paskett, & Velez, 1997), and programs for the chronically mentally ill (Kaufmann, Ward-Colasante, & Farmer, 1993; McFarland & Blair, 1995; Schramski, Harvey, & Bennetti, 1985).

The mean reported sample size (based on data reported in 19 of the search abstracts) was 309; the sample size for half of the pilot studies was less than 100, for 25% of the studies was less than 500, and for the remaining 25% was more than 500. There also was wide variation in the sample size across pilot studies. This variation is due, at least in part, to the wide variety of interventions and the scope and intensity of these interventions. Some studies examined relatively simple interventions that required minimal resources to implement, but others involved more extensive and time-consuming interventions that were spread over several months. Clearly, one determinant of the sample size included in a pilot study will be the nature and intensity of the intervention being piloted: Programs that are relatively quick and easy to implement may include a relatively large number of subjects, but other, more intensive interventions may have relatively fewer subjects in their pilots.

The studies presented in Table 16.1 have been divided into a number of broad categories based on the experimental design (single-group, quasi-experimental, and experimental designs). Each of these types of design is discussed in more detail below.

(text continues on page 397)

TABLE 16.1 Pilot Studies Literature Review

Context	Authors	Design Description	Outcome Measures
Single-group designs			
Cervical screening—inner city	Herity et al. (1997)	One method, multiple-target group deliveries	Pap smears response rate
Outreach for breast and cervical cancer prevention, African American women	Tatum, Wilson, Digman, Paskett, and Velez (1997)	Five strategies: combined classes, media, church, information center, and community-wide events for women in public housing	Feasibility of program
Health education against parasites in rural Mexico	Sarti et al. (1997)	Education program development	Knowledge, behavior, percentage of pigs with parasite
Foot care program for diabetic African Americans	Ledda, Walker, and Basch (1997)	Brief one-on-one orientation session and a take-home foot self-care program, Afrocentric	Program likability
Cervical cancer education for Native Americans, North Carolina	Dignan et al. (1995)	Development and implementation of an individualized health education program	Pap smears response rate
Coalition-based drug abuse prevention	Desjardins, Kishchuk, and Lamoureux (1994)	Development, implementation, and process evaluation of a health promotion program	Implementation and perceived efficacy
Delivering services to homeless mentally ill	McFarland and Blair (1995)	Development of comprehensive residential program	Acceptance, entry, and graduation rate
Wellness education for chronic mentally ill patients	Byrne, Brown, Voorberg, and Schofield (1994)	Lodging home involvement in wellness education, exercise, and smoking reduction	Activities participation rate
Health education for parents of preschool children with asthma	Mesters, Meertens, Kok, and Parcel (1994)	Development of asthma self-management program for parents of children with asthma	Pretest-posttest knowledge, attitude, self-efficacy, and self-management behaviors
Monitoring health care professionals	Buxton (1990)	Clinical observations of reentry of chemically dependent health care professionals	Resource assessment

(continued)

TABLE 16.1 Continued

Context	Authors	Design Description	Outcome Measures
Yoga program for geriatric clinic	Allen and Steinkohl (1987)	Development of a yoga program for geriatric clients of a community mental health center	Frequencies of complaints and social interactions
Group home for dual diagnosis	Schramski, Harvey, and Bennetti (1985)	Describes program development for individuals with a dual diagnosis (developmentally disabled/mental health)	Program feasibility
Health education for a life care community	Barbaro and Noyes (1984)	Describes assumptions, content, and planning of a health education program	Program feasibility to reduce effects of aging on lives
Community mental health center	Ehrlich, Broskowski, and Wood (1983)	Reports the experiences of a community mental health center in establishing employee assistance and health promotion programs	Resource assessment
Audio/visual testicular self-examination (TSE) program	Ostwald and Rothenberger (1985)	Several different age samples, mostly college students	Program likability; intent to use TSE and behavior change
Comprehensive obesity prevention programs	Broussard et al. (1995)	Two single-group programs mentioned; Native American communities	Program feasibility; effects on rate of excess weight gain
Home-based intervention to reduce passive smoking	Strecher et al. (1989)	Home-based program for mothers of infants (< 6 months old)	Mothers use of tobacco around infants
Palliative care program for cancer patients	Didich and Weick (1989)	Palliative care team approach	Standards assessment (Joint Commission on Accreditation of Hospitals—hospice)
Unit for mentally retarded and mentally ill patients on the grounds of a state hospital	Gold, Wolfson, Lester, Ratey, and Chmielinski (1989)	Massachusetts State Psychiatric Facility, 40-bed unit, specialized habilitative and rehabilitative environment program	Number of patients in day programming, setting restrictiveness, drug dosage
Adolescent smokeless tobacco cessation progra	Eakin, Severson, and Glasgow (1989)	Cognitive-behavioral intervention for males	Quit rates at posttest and 3-month follow-up

Mental health drop-in centers	Kaufmann, Ward-Colasante, and Farmer (1993)	Demonstration project	Attendance; satisfaction; desire for more services
After-school community intergenerational program	Poole and Gooding (1993)	Elementary school students integrated with isolated seniors at nearby apartment complex	Program likability; treatment agent importance
Oncology health management program	Grassman (1993)	Involves social support, stress management, and laughter therapy at Bay Pines VAMC-FL	Program components usefulness and likability
Treatment of chronic pain	Torrestad, Hakanson, and Axelli (1992)	Demonstration project; action research	Symptoms and self-confidence assessment
People affected with occupational hearing loss	Getty and Hetu (1991)	Male workers; one group meeting with spouses; rehabilitative program	Perceptions of severity and manageability of hearing loss
Literary clinic for children at risk (6 to 60 months old) at Children's Hospital–LA	Needlman, Fried, Morley, Taylor, and Zuckerman (1991)	Waiting room readers, provision of children's books, and guidance about literacy development for parents	Number of books taken and looked at with child
Skin care program for male and female patients	Van Etten, Sexton, and Smith (1990)	Education of nursing staff, provision of skin care products; patients 60 to 69 years old	Incidence of nosocomial pressure ulcers
Drug abuse prevention for high-risk youth	Sussman (1996)	One iteration delivering school-based drug abuse prevention curriculum	Program feasibility, receptivity; knowledge, novelty; drug commitment
Quasi-experimental designs			
Inpatient hospital-based immunization program	Scarbrough and Landis (1997)	Two methods compared 3 months later; part of job of nurses and physicians versus family nurse practitioner	Immunization rate
Sexually transmitted disease (STD) prevention in adolescent females	Guthrie et al. (1996)	Peer-led, adult-led, quasi-experimental control	Program feasibility

(continued)

TABLE 16.1 Continued

Context	Authors	Design Description	Outcome Measures
Chemical health education for high school coaches	Corcoran and Feltz (1993)	Education and control groups; three 1-hour sessions	Knowledge and confidence to teach drug dependence
School-based primary prevention of heart disease	Walter and Wynder (1989)	Classroom instruction in diet, exercise, and smoking; "Know Your Body" program	Strong effects relative to no treatment
Smoking prevention for middle school youth	Flay et al. (1988)	Delivered social influences versus physical consequences programming	Knowledge, attitudes, homework process
Experimental designs			
HIV—user reduction for female college students	Sikkema, Winett, and Lombard (1995)	Cognitive behavior (C-B) skills versus education only, 1-month follow-up	Knowledge, self-efficacy, and skills assessment
Multicomponent smoking relapse prevention at a public health clinic	Lowe et al. (1997)	Randomly assigned to treatment or control; 10-minute counseling; pick stay-quit buddy; staff reinforcement	Percentage remaining abstinent
Adult asthma self-management program	Snyder, Winder, and Creer (1987)	Random assignment to treatment or wait list control; 3-month follow-up	Knowledge and number of attacks
Pain management education for the elderly	Ferrell, Rhiner, and Ferrell (1993)	Two conditions; random assignment to program or control	Program feasibility for patients and their caregivers

METHODS OF PILOT STUDIES

In much the same way as there is large variation in types of health promotion activities, there also is large variation in the methods used to conduct a pilot study. Before discussing types of pilot studies, it should be emphasized that there is no one best method for conducting a pilot study. Thus, the type of pilot study best suited for a particular intervention will be determined by a number of factors, including (a) the time and resources available for the pilot study, (b) the aims of the pilot study (outcome measures), and (c) the type of program being piloted (e.g., health promotion or disease prevention, clinic or worksite).

Due to a perceived need or urgency to move to the large-scale implementation of a program, the time and resources available to complete a pilot program often may be quite limited. Others may perceive that a more careful use of pilot testing yields worthwhile later benefits, particularly those working in novel research arenas. Similarly, there may be quite large variation in the aims of a pilot study. Some pilot studies aim to examine the issue of whether it is even possible to implement a given program within a specific setting (feasibility). Other studies may wish to examine the extent to which the program is acceptable to participants, whereas other programs may wish to examine whether the program leads to immediate changes in a variety of outcomes, including knowledge, attitudes, and behavior. The extent of variation in the aims of specific pilot programs is illustrated by the range of different programs identified in Table 16.1. These include large-scale, community-based interventions targeting healthy lifestyles within communities (Broussard et al., 1995); individual-oriented interventions targeting specific groups of people, such as those with chronic illnesses (Ferrell et al., 1993; Ledda, Walker, & Basch, 1997; Mesters et al., 1994; Snyder et al., 1987); and school-based interventions aiming to reduce substance use and abuse (Flay et al., 1988; Sussman, 1996), risky sexual behaviors (Guthrie et al., 1996), and other health-compromising behaviors (Walter & Wynder, 1989).

The construction of pilot programs to be implemented often will be determined by a combination of these factors (resources available, aims, type of program). For example, a program with a lot of resources and few time constraints, which aims to increase self-care among a targeted group of individuals with a chronic illness, may choose to implement an experimental design. Outcomes (e.g., knowledge of self-care practices, actual behavior) are assessed in two groups of people: one group that receives the intervention and an identically composed control group that does not receive the intervention. Conversely, a study with relatively few resources and tight time constraints, which wishes to examine the practicality and acceptability of a school-based program to reduce or delay the onset of potentially health-compromising behaviors, may conduct a single-group design. The intervention is implemented in a number of schools, and problems with implementation and the reactions of participants to the program are studied intensively. However, it also should be noted that the various forms of pilot study are not mutually exclusive, and it is possible and perhaps even desirable to conduct a number of separate pilot studies.

Consideration of the literature on research design suggests that the gold standard for conducting a pilot study would involve the implementation of an experimental design. In an experimental design, the program developer is able to control both the "when" and "to whom" of exposure and is able to randomize exposure (e.g., flipping a fair coin to determine which of two conditions a subject is assigned to). An experimental design provides the clearest interpretability of results obtained, that is, the greatest validity. Unfortunately, however, it is not always possible within the context of applied health promotion research to control these exposures (see also the discussion in Chapter 13 on component study designs).

In discussing potential threats to the validity of experimental results, Campbell and Stanley (1963) draw a distinction between internal validity and external validity. Internal validity refers to the extent to which treatments make a difference within the specific context of the experiment, whereas external validity refers to whether the results of the experiment are likely to generalize to other settings outside the specific experiment. Campbell and Stanley then discuss a number of factors that may influence or jeopardize either internal or external validity of experimental results. Factors influencing internal validity include (a) events occurring between repeated testing, (b) maturation or natural change in the subjects, (c) the effects of testing per se, (d) changes in the methods used to assess outcomes, (e) regression to the mean (selection of subjects on the extreme of a behavioral dimension will tend to result in a behavioral change toward the middle as a function of time, regardless of the treatment), (f) preexisting differences between experimental and control subjects, (g) differential subject attrition from control and experimental groups, and (h) in some complex quasi-experimental designs, there may be an interaction between sample selection factors and naturally occurring maturation.

Factors that may potentially jeopardize the external validity of an experiment (i.e., the extent to which experimental findings can be generalized to the wider population) include (a) effects of pretesting; (b) interaction effects between subject selection factors and the experimental manipulation; (c) effects of experimental participation per se, which would be absent in those exposed to the intervention in a nonexperimental setting; and (d) the effects of exposure of the same individuals to multiple interventions that may occur in some experiments.

The next section of this chapter discusses a variety of different methods used to conduct pilot studies. In discussing these methods, studies presented in Table 16.1 are used to illustrate the different methodologies and the types of studies that have been conducted. Issues of internal and external validity are discussed.

Although the methods described below encompass those methods used most commonly for pilot studies, it should be noted that they do not provide an exhaustive list of all possible means for conducting a pilot study. For a more comprehensive discussion of research design and experimental methodology, see Campbell and Stanley (1963) or Cook and Campbell (1979).

SINGLE-GROUP DESIGNS

Table 16.1 shows that most pilot studies identified in the literature search used a single-group design in which the process of implementation, participants' reactions to the program, and program outcomes were intensively studied for a single group of people exposed to the intervention. For example, Broussard et al. (1995) described two single-group studies of the acceptability and efficacy of school-based programs to prevent obesity in Native American communities. Their results indicated that potential participants were receptive to the program, and, furthermore, evidence suggested that the programs might have slowed the rate of excess weight gain. Similarly, Ostwald and Rothenberger (1985) evaluated a pilot program to teach and encourage testicular self-examination among men and found that the participants enjoyed the program and that they intended to use the protocol in the future. Further follow-up 1 to 2 years after the intervention also suggested an increased rate of testicular self-examination.

Single-group designs can be used to assess a number of outcomes, including the extent to which it is possible to implement the program as designed, the acceptability of the program to participants, and the extent to which the program may have an effect on the desired outcomes. In particular, a pretest-posttest design, in which a range of measures (e.g., knowledge, intentions, behavior) are assessed prior to and after program implementation, enables the researcher to examine the effects of the program. Any change in these measures before and after the program implementation may be due to the program itself and provides a preliminary indication of program effectiveness.

However, in the absence of control groups that have not been exposed to the program, it is not possible to conclude that any observed changes are entirely due to the program. Instead, it could be argued that such changes reflect natural changes that would have occurred even in the absence of the intervention. For example, any changes in schoolchildren's knowledge of health risks could be due to maturation factors, the effects of other programs (including normal classroom teaching), or even simply the effects of repeated testing.

Similarly, single-group designs cannot be used to address issues of whether one specific intervention or presentation format is superior to another. To conduct such comparisons and provide increased confidence that any observed changes in the knowledge, attitudes, and behavior of the target group are due to the intervention per se rather than to other factors, one must implement experimental designs. A brief discussion of these designs is provided below.

EXPERIMENTAL DESIGNS

One of the most important features of an experimental design centers on the random allocation of subjects to control and intervention conditions. Random assignment is necessary to ensure that the various groups are similar on a number of measures and that any changes in the behavior (or other outcomes) observed between the two groups after program implementation are not simply due to preexisting differences between the groups.

Two-Group Experimental Designs. Perhaps the most rigorous means for conducting a pilot study involve experimental designs in which outcome measures are compared between two or more groups. The simplest experimental design is a two-group design in which one group receives the pilot intervention and a second group (the control group) does not receive the intervention. Comparisons can then be made between the groups on a variety of measures—including attitudes, intentions, and behavior—and, provided that rigorous experimental controls have been used, any observed differences between the groups can be confidently attributed to the intervention.

Examples of pilot studies that have implemented a rigorous experimental design include the study of pain management education reported by Ferrell et al. (1993), the self-management program for adults with asthma reported by Snyder et al. (1987), and the smoking relapse prevention program reported by Lowe, Windsor, Balanda, and Woodby (1997). All three of these studies compared outcomes between a group exposed to a specific intervention and a control group that did not receive the intervention. For ease of presentation, we have based the above discussion on the simple two-group design, but this design easily generalizes to cases in which there are more than two groups. A brief discussion of such studies is provided below.

Comparisons Between Multiple Different Program Formats. A pilot program also may be used to test the extent to which different ways of implementing the program affect a number of factors, including cost, acceptability to the target population, recall and identification of the aims of the program, knowledge, beliefs and intentions regarding health behaviors targeted by the program, and subsequent behavior. For example, Weeks et al. (1997) examined the effects of parental involvement in a school-based AIDS education pilot program on a variety of outcomes, including knowledge, attitudes, intentions, and behavior. They employed an experimental design in which school districts were randomly assigned to one of three groups: classroom curricula, classroom curricula and parent-interactive component, and a control group that received no intervention. Longitudinal evaluations indicated that although both intervention groups showed improvements on a range of outcomes relative to the control group, there were few differences between the two intervention groups on these measures. Although these findings may have been due, in part, to a relatively low rate of parental participation in the program, they suggest that parental involvement in AIDS prevention programs may be relatively less important than implementation of school-based curricula.

Reeder, Pryor, and Harsh (1997) also conducted an experimental evaluation of different formats (information based vs. activity based) and different levels of perceived similarity (high or low) of peer educators in pilot workshops designed to encourage safer sex among college students. In the activity-based conditions, peer leaders acted as facilitators who lead the participants through a series of small-group exercises. In the information-based conditions, there were no small-group activities, and the peer leaders, instead, addressed the group on a range of topics. Perceived similarity of the peer leaders was manipulated by having leaders describe themselves either as students from the same college who shared similar beliefs to those of the participants or as students from another college who held beliefs dissimilar to those thought to be typical of program participants. Results of this four-condition study, in which subjects were randomly assigned to conditions, indicated that the activity format resulted in higher levels of condom use in the month following the workshop, and participants in the workshops led by high-similarity peers expressed more positive intentions toward condom use. Although the authors caution that their results are only preliminary, they point to the superiority of activity-based interventions led by peers similar to the target group in altering safer-sex intentions and behaviors.

Both of these studies illustrate the potential benefits in conducting a pilot study of different methods for implementing an intervention. Both used experimental designs—which protected the interpretability of the results obtained. Clearly, it is valuable to learn this information prior to large-scale implementation of the program.

QUASI-EXPERIMENTAL DESIGNS

One of the most important distinguishing features of a true experimental design is the random allocation of subjects to different conditions (e.g., intervention vs. nonintervention or control). As discussed earlier, such random assignment has a number of advantages. However, it may not always be practically feasible to implement random allocation of subjects to groups. For example, due to scarce resources, the intervention may be available only for a select group or only a few groups. Randomization is meaningless when only a few groups are assigned to conditions because baseline comparability on all relevant variables is unlikely. As a second example, participation in a program may be voluntary. In other words, groups may self-select the condition they want to be in. Perhaps a clinic is so busy that potential participants will agree only to be in the control condition of a pilot study. In such circumstances, it still may be possible to compare outcomes between the groups to examine intervention efficacy using a quasi-experimental design (Kenny, 1975). Such a design is broadly similar to the experimental design in which the outcomes of two or more groups (e.g., those who receive the pilot intervention and the control group) are compared after the pilot has been implemented. The program developer still controls the when and where of measurement but not the when and where of exposure to the program. In the quasi-experimental design, preexisting differences between the groups (assessed prior to the implementation of the project) are controlled for during the statistical analysis of outcome data. Such methods have been discussed by a number of authors (Kenny, 1975; Snow & Tebes, 1991) and involve the use of methods of analysis such as analysis of covariance or multiple-regression analysis to take account of any preexisting differences between the two groups due to nonrandom group assignment.

Quasi-experimental designs can control for internal validity confounds such as time effects and effects of repeated testing simply by having multiple conditions that are measured at the same times and in the same ways. Furthermore, through use of repeated pretest and posttest measurement, some control can be gained over external validity confounds as well (e.g., error variance can be minimized). For example, Scarbrough and Landis (1997) compared the efficacy on achieving patient immunization of nurses or physicians who worked on three hospital units versus family nurse practitioners who entered three other hospital units (there were a total of six units, three units composed each condition, with 250 patients per unit). They found that family nurse practitioners achieved a 16% immunization rate, whereas the others achieved only a 1% rate (compared to no immunizations prior to the effort). Because the patients across units were similar, it is not likely that differences in results were due to patient factors. Because the units were similar, it is not likely that differences in results were due to differences in the units per se. However, perhaps unit workloads limited the unit physician and nurse participation; that is, the treatment agent manipulation may not have been successful (internal validity confound). Study participation could have been measured through a formalized immunization plan that was either implemented or not. In this way, some protection against this internal validity confound would have been provided. Alternatively, possibly, the effects of experimental participation (this special, extra effort) led to the results, as opposed to differences in the treatment agents (external validity confound). Subject expectancies of treatment success could have been used as measures to provide some protection for this confound.

DESIGN ISSUES ◄

RECRUITMENT AND STRATIFICATION OF SUBJECTS

Regardless of the design of the pilot study, a number of issues need to be considered in the selection of subjects. First, it is important that subjects included in a pilot study are similar to the wider population that is to be the target of the health promotion intervention. If the pilot study is conducted with subjects who differ from the intended targets of the intervention, any results obtained during the pilot study may not be applicable to the wider population.

Second, if a program is being developed for widespread applicability, it is desirable to make sure that there are an adequate number of program participants across sociodemographic strata (age, gender, ethnicity, socioeconomic status). If so, it will be possible to test the relative efficacy of the intervention across different groups. For example, within the context of a single-group pilot study, one may find that the program is easily implemented and acceptable to participants who share particular characteristics (e.g., male gender, White ethnicity). Additional pilot studies will need to be completed to establish that the program is easy to implement or acceptable to participants who do not share these characteristics. It should be noted that pilot interventions might find that a program is differentially effective with participants of different sociodemographic characteristics. For example, there is growing recognition that programs that have been shown to be successful for middle-class participants may not be as effective for individuals from minority or underprivileged groups (Marin et al., 1995; Sussman, Dent, Stacy, Burton, & Flay, 1995). Unfortunately, given the time and budget constraints that are often placed on pilot studies, it may not always be possible to include a large enough sample in the pilot phase of a program to be able to address these issues.

SELECTION OF CONTROL AND COMPARISON GROUPS

In conducting an experimental or quasi-experimental study, it is also important to consider the type of control group to be used and, in particular, how members of the control group will be recruited. Again, this will be largely determined by the nature of the program being piloted, and there are many different ways in which a control group might be recruited. For example, in a study testing an intervention with individuals who are seeking treatment, it may be possible to construct a control group from potential program participants who are on a waiting list to receive the intervention. Ideally, the control group should have an identical range of characteristics to those receiving the intervention. Then, if the study finds significant differences between the two groups on a range of outcome measures, these differences cannot be attributed to preexisting differences between the groups (e.g., motivation to change).

SAMPLE SIZE AND STATISTICAL POWER

A further issue that needs to be considered in the design and implementation of pilot programs concerns the size of the pilot program and the number of people (or groups) who will receive the pilot intervention. The trial has to be conducted on a large enough group so that a good sense of the likely outcome can be obtained. At the same time, obvious cost and logistic considerations limit the size and scope of a pilot program.

An important design consideration concerns the power of a study to detect an expected effect size (i.e., the amount of change the investigator expects the intervention to achieve). Thus, for example, investigators implementing a program to reduce the uptake of smoking among children might hope, based on the findings of previous studies, that children who receive the intervention will be 40% less likely to initiate smoking than children who do not receive the intervention. In some instances, expected effect sizes might be quite large, but there are likely to be very few interventions that would be expected to obtain a 100% success rate. Thus, those evaluating an intervention should be aware that an intervention that achieves less than a 100% success rate may still be a beneficial and worthwhile program. However, at the same time, if the expected effect size is very small, policymakers might question the utility of implementing a particular intervention (note the discussion in Chapter 13, this volume, on clinical significance).

Statistical power refers to the capacity of a study to detect a given effect size and is proportional to the number of subjects studied. In evaluating a specific intervention, it is important that the pilot program has the statistical power to detect an effect size of the expected magnitude. As sample size increases, the power of a study to detect a given effect size also increases. In conducting interventions, therefore, it is important that samples are large enough to be able to detect the expected effect size. Otherwise, a study that finds no difference between intervention and control groups on a range of outcomes may inappropriately conclude that the intervention had no effect when, in fact, the intervention did lead to the desired changes, yet the size of the sample was too small to be able to detect them.

To demonstrate the application of effect size estimates and the calculation of statistical power, one should consider an example. In a recent meta-analysis of the effectiveness of school-based substance use prevention programs (large-scale main trials), Tobler and Stratton (1997) estimated that interactive programs (those that involved a high degree of student participation) reported a median effect size of .20. Let us assume this effect size is accepted as the minimum desired effect size expected from a new program. It can be estimated from standard power tables (Cohen, 1977) that a two-group experimental design (intervention group and control group) would need a minimum sample size in each group of 309 to have 80% power to detect this effect size of .20 as significant at alpha = .05, two-tailed, or a sample size of around 190 in each group for a one-tailed test (because it would be expected that the intervention group would do better than the control but not the converse).

Within the context of pilot studies, however, it will not always be necessary to consider issues of statistical power. Specifically, statistical power is relevant only to those studies that test for the presence of an effect of an intervention of some type, such as in single-group designs that involve a pretest-posttest comparison or in true experimental designs. Pilot studies that primarily examine issues of implementation, in which only one group is assessed and in which participants' reactions to the program are extensively studied, will not generally have to consider issues of effect size and statistical power.

In pilot studies that do consider statistical power, oftentimes changes in knowledge or attitudes are the primary outcome variables. Such measures tend to show large effects, necessitating much smaller sample sizes. In addition, adequate statistical power is only a matter of convention. The value of an 80% chance of detecting a true alternative effect was originally established by multiplying the value of rejecting a true null hypothesis by 4 (i.e., .05 × 4). Certainly, one could be more liberal when engaging in a pilot study for the purposes of program development (e.g., see Turner et al., 1993). Arguably, at least a 50% chance of detecting a true alternative would seem to be a minimum acceptable power. The needed sample size for each group in a comparison, for different effect sizes, is shown in Table 16.2. Effect sizes are .2 (small difference between conditions at posttest), .4 (moderate difference), and .6 (large difference) and are shown for two-tailed (nondirectional) and one-tailed (directional) tests at $p < .05$.

THE UNIT OF ANALYSIS

A further (and highly controversial) area in the field of health behavior research concerns the appropriate unit of analysis. Although many studies will analyze individuals, it has been argued that the correct unit of analysis should be the unit of randomization and intervention, rather than the individual. Thus, for example, a study that randomizes communities either to receive an intervention or to act as a control should not analyze individual-level data. Instead, the data should be aggregated and analyzed at the community level. Such procedures are

TABLE 16.2 Statistical Power for Pilot Studies: Needed Sample Size for Different Effect Size and Power Estimates

		Power		
		.50	.70	.90
Two-tailed	$p < .05$			
$d' = .2$		97	155	63
$d' = .4$		25	39	66
$d' = .6$		11	18	30
One-tailed	$p < .05$			
$d' = .2$		68	118	215
$d' = .4$		17	30	54
$d' = .6$		8	14	24

important because individuals within a cluster probably will resemble each other more than individuals in other clusters, so their responses to the intervention will not be statistically independent (i.e., one must consider the intraclass correlation coefficient). Failure to take account of clustering in the statistical analysis of data will lead to an overestimation of the statistical significance of an effect (Donner, 1982).

Clearly, there are instances, such as when a pilot study is implemented on a community-wide basis, when the aggregation of data is not only appropriate but also the optimal analytic strategy. Analysis of aggregated data also raises a number of technical issues. These have been discussed in detail and include issues of statistical power, data analysis, and interpretation (Diehr, Martin, Koepsell, & Cheadle, 1995; Diwan, Eriksson, Sterky, & Tomson, 1992; Sahai & Khurshid, 1996; Simpson, Klar, & Donner, 1995).

Although the analysis of aggregate-level data may be the optimal research strategy for the evaluation of outcomes in a large-scale trial, it is not always feasible to conduct such analyses within the context of a pilot program. Specifically, the analysis of aggregate-level data results in a loss of effective sample size and a corresponding loss of statistical power. For example, if analyses are conducted at an individual level, a pilot program that compares outcomes among students in two classes (one of which receives the intervention and another control group that does not receive the intervention) has an effective sample size of 60 (assuming 30 students in each class). However, if the same program is evaluated using aggregate (classroom) level analyses, then the effective sample size is only 2. Thus, although the analysis of aggregate-level data may be considered optimal, it often may be more practical to analyze individual-level data collected as part of a small-scale pilot study.

Another consideration when engaging in pilot studies is that the nested sample size usually is small. For example, when a nested sample size is below 30, the intraclass correlation is likely to be quite small (e.g., < .05). A nested design would not be necessary (see Murray, Moskowitz, & Dent, 1996). Conversely, a sample size of 100 or more for a subunit is likely to be correlated with its supraunit. To minimize this issue, the program developer would do better to select few subunits from many supraunits (e.g., two classes from each of six schools) than to select many subunits from few supraunits (e.g., six classes from each of two schools).

EVALUATION MEASURES IN PILOT PROGRAMS

A number of different measures or classes of measures may be assessed in the course of a pilot study. These range from evaluations of the extent to which it is possible to implement the program to evaluations of the extent to which the program results in behavior change. A brief description and discussion of the main types of immediate-impact measures that are typically assessed in pilot programs are provided in Table 16.1 and below. The following discussion has been divided into four separate evaluation subsections: (a) implementation evaluation, which examines aspects of program delivery; (b) process evaluation, which examines how well a program is accepted by participants; (c) outcome measures, which typically are the primary intervention measures and include effects on knowledge, attitudes, beliefs, intentions, and behaviors; and (d) cost-effectiveness analysis, which provides an assessment of the monetary impact of a program on health.

IMPLEMENTATION EVALUATION

An important issue to be considered in evaluating a pilot program concerns the extent to which it is possible to implement the program as intended and the extent to which the implementation matches the original plans. Pentz and Trebow (1991) suggest that at least three specific issues need to be addressed when considering the implementation of a health intervention:

1. *Adherence.* Did the program, as implemented, match or adhere to the original design? There are two distinct components to adherence. The first component refers to whether the program was administered or implemented as planned (e.g., in a classroom intervention, it may be necessary to ask whether all

planned lessons were presented to the target students and whether the lesson plans adhered to those devised by the program developers). Second, for experimental designs, it is important to consider whether the experimental manipulation was successfully implemented. In particular, experimental crossover, contamination, or unplanned diffusion of the intervention to control groups may occur. Similarly, control groups may have adopted or been exposed to other similar health promotion programs (Cook & Campbell, 1979).

2. *Exposure.* How much of the program did the target population receive? This question may refer both to whether the program was fully implemented as planned (e.g., were all components of a classroom-based intervention presented to the students?) and whether the program was received or recognized by the target group (e.g., in the case of media campaigns, was the target group exposed to and was it able to recall program materials?).

3. *Reinvention.* Was the program changed during implementation? Pentz and Trebow (1991) suggest that the major difference between adherence, exposure, and reinvention is that reinvention reflects planned or intentional changes to the program ("Was the program implemented as written?" "Did you find a need to alter the program somewhat during your delivery of it?"), whereas exposure refers to the reach of the program ("Were all activities completed with all target persons?"), and adherence refers more simply to whether the program was fully implemented ("Were all activities delivered?").

Sussman et al. (1995) similarly define implementation using these terms. However, they clarify differences by suggesting that these terms refer to departures from ideal delivery (actual delivery is 100% of that intended). According to them, adherence refers to whether the program was delivered at all as planned (did the manipulation take place), exposure refers to how much of the program was delivered to whom, and reinvention indicates, given that the whole program was implemented, whether the program was delivered as written. Sussman et al. (1995) also included an additional smaller departure from ideal delivery, regarding smoothness of delivery, which refers to whether there were interruptions in the delivery of material.

There are a number of methods for evaluating the quality of implementing a program, including use of self-report questionnaires, interviews, and focus group discussions with those implementing the program; similar data collections with the targets of the program; and direct observational studies of the program's implementation. Regarding assessment of social skills development, role-play observational assessments may be relevant (e.g., Turner et al., 1993). Again, the nature of any implementation evaluation is likely to be heavily dependent on the nature of the intervention itself. Classroom or small-group interventions may be easily amenable to direct observational studies of their implementation. On the other hand, large-scale, community-wide interventions that involve media campaigns might be evaluated using questionnaires and interviews with people within the community to determine the extent to which they were aware of and exposed to the intervention material. Generally, program implementers (treatment agents) are the best sources of implementation information, at least if they do not try to provide an overly favorable report (halo effect).

A detailed discussion of issues needed to be addressed when conducting implementation evaluations has been provided by Lytle et al. (1994) in their evaluation of the Child and Adolescent Trial for Cardiovascular Health (CATCH). Although this was a large-scale intervention (96 schools across four different sites) rather than a pilot program, the authors' recommendations concerning evaluations include a number of points that are likely to be relevant to the evaluation of pilot studies. These issues include designing measures that assess important questions, establishing priorities for data collection, scheduling activities and data collection within the established timetables of the target institutions, gaining the trust and cooperation of the target institutions and their staff, addressing unique problems as they arise, and ensuring the quality of any data collected.

The importance of conducting an implementation evaluation has been highlighted by Dobson and Cook (1980). They suggest that program integrity may moderate program effectiveness. More recently, Hansen, Graham, Wolkenstein, and Rohrbach (1991) reported that the quality of program delivery played a significant moderating role in program effectiveness of their alcohol use prevention study. Similarly, Taggart, Bush, Zuckerman, and Theiss (1990) reported considerable variation in the effectiveness of teachers' implementation of a program designed to reduce coronary heart disease risk factors among elementary and junior high school students. Furthermore, they reported that ratings of the effectiveness of program implementation were significantly associated with more favorable student outcomes.

PROCESS EVALUATION

Unlike implementation evaluation, which focuses on the extent to which a program has been implemented as planned, process evaluation is concerned primarily with the reaction and response to the program by the program participants (including those conducting the intervention). Thus, process evaluations will focus primarily on the acceptability and attractiveness of the program to both the program participants (or targets) and those running the program. Methods used in process evaluation typically include intensive questioning and discussion with the participants to gauge their perceptions of the program. Issues addressed in a process evaluation may include the extent to which the participants found the program interesting or enjoyable—one they believe they learned something from and was credible, worthwhile, or helpful. Such items tend to be highly correlated and can be combined to form a perceived quality index (e.g., Sussman et al., 1993). For example, in an evaluation of a teacher-administered program to increase young children's awareness of sun precautions, Hughes (1994) reported that teachers were able to present the material without special training and, importantly, that both teachers and students responded to the program enthusiastically.

OUTCOMES EVALUATION

In addition to evaluating the ease of implementing a program and the acceptability of a program to participants, those evaluating a pilot program also may wish to examine the extent to which an intervention may change specific outcomes. These outcomes may include (a) knowledge, (b) attitudes, beliefs, and intentions, and (c) behaviors and are discussed below. Of importance, the outcomes evaluation focuses on the extent to which the theoretical processes underlying an intervention (hypothesized mediators of program effects) are manipulated. (Process ratings also may mediate program effects but may reflect relationship with the teacher or unexplained factors.)

Knowledge. One of the important goals of many health promotion programs is to increase participants' awareness and knowledge of the dangers associated with certain activities, means for avoiding these potential dangers, benefits of certain alternative activities, and means for completing healthy activities. Knowledge changes have been found to mediate program impact on later behavior in some studies but not others (Tobler & Stratton, 1997). Thus, for example, one component of antismoking campaigns often has focused on aims such as increasing young people's knowledge of the physical health dangers associated with tobacco use. Similarly, health and lifestyle programs, although teaching about the health risks associated with improper diet (among other things), also have attempted to impart knowledge about the nutritional content of different foods and the components of a healthy diet. For programs such as these, one legitimate means of evaluating a program's efficacy may be to assess participants' knowledge of a core set of constructs that are addressed in the program.

As another example, Snyder et al. (1987) demonstrated that an intervention for chronic asthma sufferers increased knowledge about asthma and self-management practices for preventing or limiting symptoms. Similarly, Sikkema et al. (1995) showed that a program combining education with teaching cognitive-behavioral skills was successful in increasing female college students' knowledge about prevention of HIV infection. Importantly, both these studies demonstrated that increased knowledge was accompanied by changes in behavior. The experimental group in the study reported by Snyder et al. (1987) experienced fewer asthma attacks over a 3-month period, whereas Sikkema et al. (1995) reported that the increase in knowledge observed in their intervention group was accompanied by a decrease in risky sexual behaviors.

Attitudes, Beliefs, and Intentions. A further target for evaluation may include the extent to which a program has resulted in a change in participants' attitudes, beliefs, and intentions toward a particular behavior. Attitudes are judgments of goodness or badness regarding a behavior, whereas beliefs are judgments of whether a behavior is associated with certain positive or negative outcomes and why the behavior is associated with these outcomes. Intentions are subjective judgments regarding the likelihood that a subject will engage in the target behavior in the future. Some meta-analytic work suggests that program effects on later behavior are mediated by changes in these types of variables—that is, if subjects' reports become more unfavorable toward an unhealthy behavior or more favorable toward a healthy behavior (Tobler & Stratton, 1997). Thus, for example, a number of programs aiming to prevent or delay the onset of substance use behaviors among youth have evaluated whether program participation has led to a more negative attitude toward substance use or reduced intentions to use drugs in the future.

Although an alteration in participants' attitudes, beliefs, and intentions toward a certain behavior is a desirable goal, there is continuing debate in the social-psychological literature about the extent to which it is possible to predict future behavior on the basis of these attitudes, beliefs, and intentions. According to the theory of reasoned action (Fishbein & Ajzen, 1975), attitudes and subjective norms combine to determine intentions that, in turn, influence behavior. This theory and more recent elaborations of it (e.g., the theory of planned behavior) (Ajzen, 1985) have remained controversial (Olson & Zanna, 1993), as a number of authors have argued that there is often little correspondence between attitudes and behavior (Eagly & Chaiken, 1992).

Nonetheless, there is increasing recognition that attitudes do predict and influence behavior. For example, several studies have demonstrated that children's perceptions of the desirability of smoking predict subsequent smoking behavior (e.g., Dinh, Sarason, Peterson, & Onstad, 1995). These authors conducted a 4-year longitudinal study and found that positive perceptions of smokers in fifth grade were significant predictors of weekly smoking in ninth grade. Similarly, MacKinnon et al. (1991) conducted a study in which they examined the effects of a social influences-based drug abuse prevention program on drug use. At 1-year follow-up, students who received the program were less likely to report drug use, and, importantly, the most substantial mediator of program effects on drug use was change in perceptions of friends' tolerance of drug use. In addition, there was evidence that intentions to use and beliefs about the positive consequences of use also mediated program effects.

Such findings illustrate both that changing children's perceptions of the desirability of smoking is an appropriate goal for intervention and that such intervention efforts could or should begin at young ages. Clearly, resolution of the extent to which changes in knowledge, attitudes, beliefs, and intentions may predict changes in future behavior is pivotal to a consideration of the utility of evaluating such beliefs. If a program is successful in changing participants' beliefs about certain behavior but these altered beliefs do not translate into behavior change, then the utility of the program is open to debate. The most robust method for addressing these concerns clearly would be to assess the extent to which the program leads to behavior change. Such evaluations are described briefly below.

Behavioral Outcomes. The clearest indication that a program has been successful would be a demonstration that program implementation led to a reduction in health-compromising behavior and an increase in health-enhancing behavior. An example of an evaluation of the effectiveness of a pilot program that examined behavioral outcomes has been provided by Mesters et al. (1994), who described the results of an asthma self-management protocol delivered to parents of preschool children who had asthma. The intervention consisted of 16 educational modules provided by general practitioners. The efficacy of this program was assessed using a two-group experimental design. Results of the evaluation showed that, among a range of other positive outcomes, parents in the experimental group reported performing appropriate management behaviors significantly more often than parents in the control group. Importantly, a follow-up study of the experimental group at 1 year indicated that these changes had been sustained and that these behavioral changes had translated into significant reductions in the experimental group's use of medical services.

This finding raises the further issue of the extent to which any short-term behavioral change will persist and the extent to which any such apparent changes may decay over time. Although the Mesters et al. (1994) study found that behavioral changes persisted over a 1-year period, other studies have reported that intervention effects may decay over time. For example, repeated evaluations of project Drug Abuse Resistance Education (DARE) have indicated that although this program may have modest short-term effects on students' attitudes toward drug use and ability to resist peer pressure, these effects are likely to diminish or decay over time (Clayton, Cattarello, & Johnstone, 1996; Ennett et al., 1994). Findings such as these have led to suggestions that it may be necessary to conduct booster sessions over a number of years for substance use prevention programs to be successful (Clayton et al., 1996; Ellickson, Bell, & McGuigan, 1993; Ennett et al., 1994). These findings also raise the issue, discussed below, of the extent to which it may be necessary to conduct longer-term follow-ups to assess the long-term benefits of an intervention.

IS IT NECESSARY TO CONSIDER LONG-TERM OUTCOMES?

Thus far, the program evaluations we have discussed have involved the evaluation of processes or outcomes assessed immediately after cessation of the program. However, in the case of knowledge, beliefs, intentions, and behavior, the extent to which any short-term changes may be maintained over time is open to question. Clearly, to justify large-scale implementation of a health promotion campaign, it is important that any initial changes observed immediately after the implementation of a program be maintained over a protracted period of time.

To address this issue, it may be possible to assess participants' beliefs and behaviors over a longer period following program participation and determine the extent to which any initial benefits of the program are retained or wash out over time. In conducting such studies, a number of important issues need to be considered, including the length of follow-up, the selection of an appropriate control group, and methods for retaining contact with the sample and minimizing sample attrition. The issue of sample attrition may be particularly problematic in conducting longitudinal research because loss of sample numbers will affect statistical power, and the differential loss of subjects may directly impugn the validity of conclusions. Regarding the latter problem, if those lost to follow-up are different in some way from those who are followed up, it may be the case that the results obtained by the study will not hold for all program participants. The results of the study may hold only for those with whom the study was able to maintain contact (typically those who are least at risk for adverse outcomes in the first place). Although sophisticated methods are available to adjust parameter estimates for the effects of nonrandom sample loss (e.g., Berk, 1983; Kessler, Little, & Groves, 1995), it is clearly desirable that as high a percentage of the sample be retained as possible.

However, the extent to which it may be feasible to conduct long-term follow-ups as part of an initial pilot study is open to debate. In particular, both cost and logistical considerations preclude conducting longitudinal studies as part of the initial evaluation of a health promotion intervention. In addition, as will be discussed in the final section of this chapter, there are often considerable pressures to finalize a program's content and move to full-scale implementation of the program. Under these conditions, it is not always possible to delay full-scale implementation of a program while waiting for the results of a long-term follow-up of a pilot study.

Despite these difficulties, a number of pilot programs have conducted longer-term follow-ups to assess outcomes. For example, Snyder et al. (1987) conducted a 3-month follow-up of adults enrolled in an asthma management program. Similarly, Ostwald and Rothenberger (1985) conducted a 2-year follow-up of a testicular self-examination pilot program. Both these examples were able to demonstrate that the pilot programs had achieved some success in affecting target behaviors and were thus able to argue for the implementation and evaluation of larger-scale trials based on the initial pilot program.

In summary, although a consideration of the long-term effects of a health intervention may be desirable, it may not be possible to conduct such an evaluation within the context of a pilot program. Such evaluations may be delayed until the implementation of a full-scale trial.

COST-EFFECTIVENESS ANALYSIS

One area that is receiving increasing research and policy attention in recent years concerns the extent to which programs provide value for money or are cost-effective. Given increasing competition for scarce financial resources, it is increasingly necessary for programs to demonstrate benefits. Similarly, when considering the results of a pilot study, it may be necessary to ask, before moving to large-scale implementation of a program, what the costs of implementing the program would be and whether the program, if implemented, would provide value for money. Although it may not be necessary for an intervention to be able to demonstrate that it saves money (compared to standard treatment), it should be able to demonstrate that it is cost-effective (i.e., benefits are greater than costs). However, a number of authors have suggested that preventive interventions are often held to a higher standard than other interventions, such as treatments, because not only are they expected to demonstrate cost-effectiveness, but they are also expected to demonstrate that they save money (Elixhauser, Luce, Taylor, & Reblando, 1993; Phillips & Holtgrave, 1997).

Within the area of health promotion, there are a number of difficulties with attempting to implement cost-benefit analyses. In particular, although the costs of implementing a program may be comparatively easy to determine, how does one quantify the benefits of these programs? In other words, can one place a monetary value on good health? When one considers all the variables that might be considered in such an evaluation, the list of variables can become quite long, and the mathematics involved can become quite complex. Still, several pilot studies or trials have attempted to engage in cost-effectiveness testing.

An evaluation of the costs and cost-effectiveness of a mass media campaign to prevent smoking among adolescents was recently reported by Secker-Walker, Worden, Holland, Flynn, and Detsky (1997), who examined the cost-effectiveness of a 4-year mass media campaign that previously had been shown to prevent the onset of smoking. They used a matched control design and found that the cost per life year gained for young smokers was $696. The authors concluded that their results indicated both that the media intervention was cost-effective and that it compared favorably with other preventive and therapeutic interventions. Similarly, Baxter et al. (1997) examined the cost-effectiveness of a community-based coronary heart disease health promotion project using a prospective study of changes in health behaviors in two communities: one receiving the intervention and a matched control community. Outcomes were assessed through the use of individual questionnaires sent to members of each community. Although the intervention achieved only modest changes in health behaviors (a statistically significant reduction in smoking and an increase in the proportion drinking low-fat milk), the authors concluded that the intervention was cost-effective (the estimated cost per life year gained was only 31 British pounds).

In terms of informing policy and advocating for the large-scale implementation of a health promotion program that has been piloted successfully, it clearly is desirable to be able to demonstrate that the program is cost-effective. The extent to which it is possible to achieve such an assessment within the context of a small-scale pilot program is, however, open to debate. Much of the evaluation in a pilot program involves either evaluation of the process of program implementation or the evaluation of short-term outcomes such as knowledge, beliefs, or intentions. Although, as discussed earlier, there is solid evidence to indicate that changes in these short-term outcomes are likely to translate into longer-term behavioral changes, the nature of this link is difficult to quantify. Thus, it becomes difficult to quantify the amount of behavioral change that may be achieved by a program when only short-term outcomes are evaluated. This clearly indicates the need for longitudinal data to be used in an analysis of the cost-effectiveness of a program, and, as discussed earlier, it is often not possible to collect such data within the context of a small-scale pilot study.

Certainly, though, it is possible to calculate the monetary cost of implementing a program completely. In addition, one can gauge the degree of change in benefits, in terms of reduction in health costs or increased productivity, that would need to be elicited to balance out costs. Then, one could also gauge the degree of behavioral change that may be needed to result in that minimal change in benefits. Finally, one could at least make a rough estimate regarding how much behavior change is expected given the degree of change in program mediators. Thus, although a program targeting self-management practices for people with asthma may have neither the time nor the resources to assess the impact of the program on health care use, it may be possible to assess the extent of immediate behavior change. Given prior information about the associations between behavior and subsequent health care use, it may then be possible to estimate the expected impact of the intervention on health care use and thus the potential cost-benefits of the program. Thus, by taking such estimates, some calculation of cost-effectiveness of a program is possible through use of a pilot study.

▶ DISCUSSION

This chapter has detailed a number of methodological issues in the conduct and implementation of pilot programs. Pilot programs form a vital stage between initial feasibility studies and large-scale implementation of initiatives in health promotion. There are at least four advantages of such programs, as discussed earlier. First, they provide an opportunity to examine and test the ease of implementing the program. Second, they provide an opportunity to assess the acceptability of the program to participants. Third, they provide a vehicle for the preliminary testing of a program's likely effectiveness. Finally, pilot programs provide an empirical basis for making program changes and refinements before large-scale implementation of a program.

Despite these advantages, implementation of pilot programs sometimes is overlooked in the development of health promotion activities. The reasons for this are likely to be varied but may include a perception on the part of policymakers that action is urgently needed in a particular area of health promotion and that large-scale implementation of a project should be fast-tracked to ensure that an identified problem is addressed immediately. Although such sentiments are understandable, they are also somewhat shortsighted because large-scale implementation of a program that is not fully developed or tested may, in the long term, be counterproductive.

Given the identified need for pilot programs, it is relevant to turn to the issue of how best to conduct such programs. A number of aspects of the proper design and conduct of pilot programs were discussed earlier and include a need for such programs to be implemented in a manner that is as close as possible to how it is envisaged that the final program will be implemented (e.g., ensuring that the participants in the pilot will be broadly representative of the target group for the large-scale project) while ensuring rigorous control of the implementation (e.g., adequate control group). There have been instances in the past when apparently favorable outcomes achieved in a pilot phase of a project's development have not been replicated in the large-scale implementation of the intervention. There are at least three reasons for this apparent discrepancy in findings. First, the pilot program was tested on a group of individuals that is not representative of the target group for the intervention. Second, the skill, enthusiasm, and dedication of staff involved in the implementation of the pilot program were not being matched by comparable levels of skill and dedication in those who are involved in the implementation of the final program. Finally, an effect, labeled the Hawthorne effect, may occur. The Hawthorne effect may be defined as the tendency for participants in an experimental program and evaluation to change because they are the targets of special attention in the study (Fletcher, Fletcher, & Wagner, 1984). Such an effect may occur regardless of the nature of the intervention but is unlikely to be replicated in the large-scale implementation of the project. Although this effect has been most thoroughly studied within the field of industrial psychology, Bouchet, Guillemin, and Briancon (1996) demonstrated that quality-of-life measures were sensitive to such an effect; that is, inclusion in a study without any intervention was associated with significant changes in quality-of-life measures over time. Items that measure the likelihood that the program being delivered will be successful (baseline success expectancies) provide a means to statistically control for the operation of Hawthorne effects (Sussman et al., 1995).

Although careful design and implementation of pilot programs can reduce or eliminate many of these potential problems, it will not invariably be the case that favorable results obtained in the pilot phase of a project will be replicated in subsequent large-scale implementation. Thus, the evaluation of pilot programs should not be seen as the final step in program evaluation but should instead be viewed as the first important step in the formal evaluation of a program's effectiveness. Although it is an important step in program development, a pilot program is, after all, a pilot.

REFERENCES

AJZEN, I. (1985). From intentions to actions: A theory of planned behavior. In J. Kuhl & J. Beckmann (Eds.), *Action control: From cognition to behavior* (pp. 11-39). Heidelberg, Germany: Springer-Verlag.

ALLEN, K. S., & STEINKOHL, R. P. (1987). Yoga in a geriatric mental clinic. *Activities, Adaptation and Aging, 9,* 61-68.

BARBARO, E. L., & NOYES, L. E. (1984). A wellness program for a life care community. *The Gerontologist, 24,* 569-571.

BAXTER, T., MILNER, P., WILSON, K., LEAF, M., NICHOLL, J., FREEMAN, J., & COOPER, N. (1997). A cost effective, community based heart health promotion project in England: Prospective comparative study. *British Medical Journal, 315,* 582-585.

BERK, R. A. (1983). An introduction to sample selection bias in sociological data. *American Sociological Review, 48,* 386-398.

BOUCHET, C., GUILLEMIN, F., & BRIANCON, S. (1996). Nonspecific effects in longitudinal studies: Impact on quality of life measures. *Journal of Clinical Epidemiology, 49,* 15-20.

BROUSSARD, B. A., SUGARMAN, J. R., BACHMAN-CARTER, K., BOOTH, K., STEPHENSON, L., STRAUSS, K., & GOHDES, D. (1995). Toward comprehensive obesity prevention programs in Native American communities. *Obesity Research, 3*(Suppl. 2), 289S-297S.

BUXTON, M. (1990). Monitoring, reentry, and relapse prevention for chemically dependent health care professionals. *Journal of Psychoactive Drugs, 22,* 447-450.

BYRNE, C., BROWN, B., VOORBERG, N., & SCHOFIELD, R. (1994). Wellness education for individuals with chronic mental illness living in the community. *Issues in Mental Health Nursing, 15,* 239-252.

CAMPBELL, D. T., & STANLEY, J. C. (1963). *Experimental and quasi-experimental designs for research.* Chicago: Rand McNally.

CLAYTON, R. R., CATTARELLO, A. M., & JOHNSTONE, B. M. (1996). The effectiveness of Drug Abuse Resistance Education (project DARE): 5-year follow-up results. *Preventive Medicine, 25,* 307-318.

COHEN, J. (1977). *Statistical power for the behavioral sciences.* New York: Academic Press.

COOK, T. D., & CAMPBELL, D. T. (1979). *Quasi-experimentation: Design and analysis issues for field settings.* Chicago: Rand McNally.

CORCORAN, J. P., & FELTZ, D. L. (1993). Evaluation of chemical health education for high school athletic coaches. *Sport Psychologist, 7,* 298-308.

DESJARDINS, N., KISHCHUK, N., & LAMOUREUX, M. (1994). Youth and drug abuse: Evaluation of the rationale and implementation of a community coalition-based prevention program. *Canadian Journal of Community Mental Health, 13,* 145-161.

DIDICH, J., & WEICK, J. K. (1989). The development of a palliative care program. *Cleveland Clinic Journal of Medicine, 56,* 762-764.

DIEHR, P., MARTIN, D. C., KOEPSELL, T., & CHEADLE, A. (1995). Breaking the matches in a paired *t*-test for community interventions when the number of pairs is small. *Statistics in Medicine, 14,* 1491-1504.

DIGNAN, M. B., SHARP, P., BLINSON, K., MICHIELUTTE, R., KONEN, J., BELL, R., & LANE, C. (1995). Development of a cervical cancer education program for Native American women in North Carolina. *Journal of Cancer Education, 9,* 235-242.

DINH, K. T., SARASON, I. G., PETERSON, A. V., & ONSTAD, L. E. (1995). Children's perceptions of smokers and nonsmokers: A longitudinal study. *Health Psychology, 14,* 32-40.

DIWAN, V. K., ERIKSSON, B., STERKY, G., & TOMSON, G. (1992). Randomization by group in studying the effect of drug information in primary care. *International Journal of Epidemiology, 21,* 124-130.

DOBSON, D., & COOK, T. J. (1980). Avoiding Type III error in program evaluation: Results from a field experiment. *Evaluation and Program Planning, 3,* 269-276.

DONNER, A. (1982). An empirical study of cluster randomization. *International Journal of Epidemiology, 11,* 537-543.

EAGLY, A. H., & CHAIKEN, S. (1992). *The psychology of attitudes.* San Diego, CA: Harcourt Brace.

EAKIN, E., SEVERSON, H., & GLASGOW, R. E. (1989). Development and evaluation of a smokeless tobacco cessation program: A pilot study. *NCI Monographs, 8,* 95-100.

EHRLICH, R. P., BROSKOWSKI, A., & WOOD, G. L. (1983). The development of a community mental health program for occupational settings. *New Directions for Mental Health Services, 20,* 37-48.

ELIXHAUSER, A., LUCE, B. R., TAYLOR, W. R., & REBLANDO, J. (1993). Health care CBA/CEA: An update on the growth and composition of the literature. *Medical Care, 31,* JS1-JS11.

ELLICKSON, P. L., BELL, R. M., & McGUIGAN, K. (1993). Preventing adolescent drug use: Long-term results of a junior high program. *American Journal of Public Health, 83,* 856-861.

ENNETT, S. T., ROSENBAUM, D. P., FLEWELLING, R. L., BIELER, G. S., RINGWALT, C. L., & BAILEY, S. L. (1994). Long-term evaluation of drug abuse resistance education. *Addictive Behaviors, 19,* 113-125.

FERRELL, B. R., RHINER, M., & FERRELL, B. A. (1993). Development and implementation of a pain education program. *Cancer, 72*(11, Suppl.), 3426-3432.

FISHBEIN, M., & AJZEN, I. (1975). *Belief, attitude, intention and behavior: An introduction to theory and research.* Reading, MA: Addison-Wesley.

FLAY, B. R., BRANNON, B. R., JOHNSON, C. A., HANSEN, W. B., ULENE, A. L., WHITNEY-SALTIEL, D. A., GLEASON, L. R., SUSSMAN, S., GAVIN, M. D., GLOWACZ, K. M., SOBOL, D. F., & SPIEGEL, D. C. (1988). The television school and family smoking prevention and cessation project: 1. Theoretical basis and program development. *Preventive Medicine, 17,* 585-607.

FLETCHER, R. H., FLETCHER, S. W., & WAGNER, E. H. (1984). *Clinical epidemiology: The essentials.* Baltimore: Williams & Wilkins.

GETTY, L., & HETU, R. (1991). Development of a rehabilitation program for people affected with occupational hearing loss: 2. Results from group intervention with 48 workers and their spouses. *Audiology, 30,* 317-329.

GOLD, I. M., WOLFSON, E. S., LESTER, C. M., RATEY, J. J., & CHMIELINSKI, H. E. (1989). Developing a unit for mentally retarded-mentally ill patients on the grounds of a state hospital. *Hospital and Community Psychiatry, 40,* 836-840.

GRASSMAN, D. (1993). Development of inpatient oncology educational and support programs. *Oncology Nursing Forum, 20,* 669-676.

GUTHRIE, B. J., WALLACE, J., DOERR, K., JANZ, N., SCHOTTENFELD, D., & SELIG, S. (1996). Girl talk: Development of an intervention for prevention of HIV/AIDS and other sexually transmitted diseases in adolescent females. *Public Health Nursing, 13,* 318-330.

HANSEN, W. B., GRAHAM, J. W., WOLKENSTEIN, B. H., & ROHRBACH, L. A. (1991). Program integrity as a moderator of prevention program effectiveness: Results for fifth-grade students in the adolescent alcohol prevention trial. *Journal of Studies on Alcohol, 52,* 568-579.

HERITY, B., McDONALD, P., JOHNSON, Z., CARROLL, B., CODY, M., DUIGNAN, N., McGEE, D., O'KELLY, F., & HURLEY, M. (1997). A pilot study of cervical screening in an inner city area—lessons for a national programme. *Cytopathology, 8,* 161-170.

HUGHES, A. S. (1994). Sun protection and younger children: Lessons from the Living With Sunshine program. *Journal of School Health, 64,* 201-204.

KAUFMANN, C. L., WARD-COLASANTE, C., & FARMER, J. (1993). Development and evaluation of drop-in centers operated by mental health consumers. *Hospital & Community Psychiatry, 44,* 675-678.

KENNY, D. A. (1975). A quasi-experimental approach to assessing treatment effects in the nonequivalent control group design. *Psychological Bulletin, 82,* 345-362.

KESSLER, R. C., LITTLE, R. J., & GROVES, R. M. (1995). Advances in strategies for minimizing and adjusting for survey nonresponse. *Epidemiologic Reviews, 17,* 192-204.

LEDDA, M. A., WALKER, E. A., & BASCH, C. E. (1997). Development and formative evaluation of a foot self-care program for African Americans with diabetes. *Diabetes Educator, 23,* 48-51.

LOWE, J. B., WINDSOR, R. A., BALANDA, K. P., & WOODBY, L. (1997). Smoking relapse prevention methods for pregnant women: A formative evaluation. *American Journal of Health Promotion, 11,* 244-246.

LYTLE, L. A., DAVIDANN, B. Z., BACHMAN, K., EDMUNDSON, E. W., JOHNSON, C. C., REEDS, J. N., WAMBSGANS, K. C., & BUDMAN, S. (1994). CATCH: Challenges of conducting process evaluation in a multicenter trial. *Health Education Quarterly, 21*(Suppl. 2), S129-S141.

MACKINNON, D. P., JOHNSON, C. A., PENTZ, M. A., DWYER, J. H., HANSEN, W. B., FLAY, B. R., & WANG, E. Y. (1991). Mediating mechanisms in a school-based drug prevention program: First-year effects of the Midwestern Prevention Project. *Health Psychology, 10,* 164-172.

MARIN, G., BURHANSSTIPANOV, L., CONNELL, C. M., GIELEN, A. C., HELITZER-ALLEN, D., LORIG, K., MORISKY, D. E., TENNEY, M., & THOMAS, S. (1995). A research agenda for health education among underserved populations. *Health Education Quarterly, 22,* 346-363.

McFARLAND, B. H., & BLAIR, G. (1995). Delivering comprehensive services to homeless mentally ill offenders. *Psychiatric Services, 46,* 179-181.

MESTERS, I., MEERTENS, R., KOK, G., & PARCEL, G. S. (1994). Effectiveness of a multidisciplinary education protocol in children with asthma (0-4 years) in primary health care. *Journal of Asthma, 31,* 347-359.

MURRAY, D. M., MOSKOWITZ, J., & DENT, C. W. (1996). Design and analysis issues in community-based drug abuse prevention. *American Behavioral Scientist, 39,* 853-867.

NEEDLMAN, R., FRIED, L. E., MORLEY, D. S., TAYLOR, S., & ZUCKERMAN, B. (1991). Clinic-based intervention to promote literacy. A pilot study. *American Journal of Diseases of Children, 145,* 881-884.

OLSON, J. M., & ZANNA, M. P. (1993). Attitudes and attitude change. *Annual Review of Psychology, 44,* 117-154.

OSTWALD, S. K., & ROTHENBERGER, J. (1985). Development of a testicular self-examination program for college men. *Journal of American College Health, 33,* 234-239.

PENTZ, M. A., & TREBOW, E. (1991). Implementation issues in drug abuse prevention research. In C. G. Leukefeld & W. J. Bukoski (Eds.), *Drug abuse prevention intervention research: Methodological issues* (NIDA Research Monograph No. 107, pp. 123-139). Rockville, MD: National Institute on Drug Abuse.

PHILLIPS, K. A., & HOLTGRAVE, D. R. (1997). Using cost-effectiveness/cost-benefit analysis to allocate health resources: A level playing field for prevention? *American Journal of Preventive Medicine, 13,* 18-25.

POOLE, G. G., & GOODING, B. A. (1993). Developing and implementing a community intergenerational program. *Journal of Community Health Nursing, 10,* 77-85.

REEDER, G. D., PRYOR, J. B., & HARSH, L. (1997). Activity and similarity in safer sex workshops led by peer educators. *AIDS Education and Prevention, 9*(Suppl. A), 77-89.

SAHAI, H., & KHURSHID, A. (1996). Formulae and tables for the determination of sample sizes and power in clinical trials for testing differences in proportions for the two-sample design: A review. *Statistics in Medicine, 15,* 1-21.

SARTI, E., FLISSER, A., SCHANTZ, P. M., GLEIZER, M., LOYA, M., PLANCARTE, A., AVILA, G., ALLAN, J., CRAIG, P., BRONFMAN, M., & WIJEYARATNE, P. (1997). Development and evaluation of a health education intervention against Taenia solium in a rural community in Mexico. *American Journal of Tropical Medicine & Hygiene, 56,* 127-132.

SCARBROUGH, M. L., & LANDIS, S. E. (1997). A pilot study for the development of a hospital based immunization program. *Clinical Nurse Specialist, 11,* 70-75.

SCHRAMSKI, T. G., HARVEY, D. R., & BENNETTI, R. (1985). Deinstitutionalizing a residential environment for individuals with dual diagnosis. *Psychosocial Rehabilitation Journal, 8,* 60-66.

SECKER-WALKER, R. H., WORDEN, J. K., HOLLAND, R. R., FLYNN, B. S., & DETSKY, A. S. (1997). A mass media programme to prevent smoking among adolescents: Costs and cost effectiveness. *Tobacco Control, 6,* 207-212.

SIKKEMA, K. J., WINETT, R. A., & LOMBARD, D. N. (1995). Development and evaluation of an HIV-risk reduction program for female college students. *AIDS Education & Prevention, 7,* 145-159.

SIMPSON, J. M., KLAR, N., & DONNER, A. (1995). Accounting for cluster randomization: A review of primary prevention trials, 1990 through 1993. *American Journal of Public Health, 85,* 1378-1383.

SNOW, D. L., & TEBES, T. K. (1991). Experimental and quasi-experimental designs in prevention research. In C. G. Leukefeld & W. J. Bukoski (Eds.), *Drug abuse prevention intervention research: Methodological issues* (NIDA Research Monograph No. 107, pp. 140-158). Rockville, MD: National Institute on Drug Abuse.

SNYDER, S. E., WINDER, J. A., & CREER, T. J. (1987). Development and evaluation of an adult asthma self-management program: Wheezers Anonymous. *Journal of Asthma, 24,* 153-158.

STRECHER, V. J., BAUMAN, K. E., BOAT, B., FOWLER, M., GREENBERG, R. A., & STEDMAN, H. (1989). The development and formative evaluation of a home-based intervention to reduce passive smoking by infants. *Health Education Research, 4,* 225-232.

SUSSMAN, S. (1996). Development of a school-based drug abuse prevention curriculum for high-risk youths. *Journal of Psychoactive Drugs, 28,* 169-182.

SUSSMAN, S., DENT, C. W., STACY, A. W., BURTON, D., & FLAY, B. R. (1995). *Developing school-based tobacco use prevention and cessation programs.* Thousand Oaks, CA: Sage.

SUSSMAN, S., DENT, C. W., STACY, A. W., HODGSON, C., BURTON, D., & FLAY, B. R. (1993). Project Towards No Tobacco Use: Implementation, process and post-test knowledge evaluation. *Health Education Research, 8,* 109-123.

TAGGART, V. S., BUSH, P. J., ZUCKERMAN, A. E., & THEISS, P. K. (1990). A process evaluation of the District of Columbia "know your body" project. *Journal of School Health, 60,* 60-66.

TATUM, C., WILSON, A., DIGNAN, M. B., PASKETT, E. D., & VELEZ, R. (1997). Development and implementation of outreach strategies for breast and cervical cancer prevention among African American women: FoCaS Project. Forsyth County Cancer Screening. *Journal of Cancer Education, 12,* 43-50.

TOBLER, N. S., & STRATTON, H. H. (1997). Effectiveness of school-based drug prevention programs: A meta-analysis of the research. *Journal of Primary Prevention, 18,* 71-128.

TORRESTAD, A., HAKANSON, M., & AXELLI, T. (1992). Development of a program for the treatment of chronic pain and anxiety: A learning process leading from unsound to sound assessment. *International Journal of Technology Assessment in Health Care, 8,* 85-92.

TURNER, G. E., BURCIAGA, C., SUSSMAN, S., KLEIN-SELSKI, E., CRAIG, S., DENT, C. W., MASON, H. R. C., BURTON, D., & FLAY, B. R. (1993). Which lesson components mediate refusal assertion skill improvement in school-based adolescent tobacco use prevention? *International Journal of the Addictions, 28,* 749-766.

VAN ETTEN, N. K., SEXTON, P., & SMITH, R. (1990). Development and implementation of a skin care program. *Ostomy Wound Management, 27,* 40-54.

WALTER, H. J., & WYNDER, E. L. (1989). The development, implementation, evaluation, and future directions of a chronic disease prevention program for children: The "Know Your Body" studies. *Preventive Medicine, 18,* 59-71.

WEEKS, K., LEVY, S. R., GORDON, A. K., HANDLER, A., PERHATS, C., & FLAY, B. R. (1997). Does parental involvement make a difference? The impact of parent interactive activities on students in a school-based AIDS prevention program. *AIDS Education and Prevention, 9*(Suppl. A), 90-106.

CHAPTER 16

Commentary

Shirley M. Glynn

With research and health program funding becoming increasingly competitive, it is imperative to scientists, clinicians, educators, policymakers, and the general public that the available resources be well used. Careful, thorough project planning and preparation of health interventions are essential. As Lynskey and Sussman accurately observe, a well-conducted pilot can provide a wealth of information on ease of implementation, program acceptability, immediate effectiveness, and possible modifications to strengthen a subsequent larger project. Pilots can provide invaluable data on probable benefits of participation (program effectiveness) in the larger project and the likely strength of those benefits (e.g., effect sizes). Even weighed against the urgency of implementing a larger project quickly, the period spent conducting an informative pilot is usually time very well spent.

Nevertheless, a pilot study will be informative only in direct relation to the extent that it is well considered. That is, a pilot is useful to the extent the program developer or investigator has carefully considered all of the available research in an area, made a considered choice about the components of a proposed intervention, integrated them in the sequence he or she believes is most likely to be effective, identified and secured a place to conduct a trial run that approximates the setting that will be used in the subsequent final project, and selected a design that will permit the investigator to draw some preliminary conclusions about the implementation feasibility and effectiveness of the final intervention. The review on internal and external threats to valid interpretation of pilot results offered in Lynskey and Sussman's chapter is particularly pertinent here.

This commentary will expand on a number of points made by Lynskey and Sussman. First, the implications of the different time frames for final interventions and pilot studies will be outlined, followed by a discussion of the importance of attending to process variables in pilot implementation. Then, issues related to defining a pilot as a trial run of a composite intervention—recognizing the importance of the dynamic, interactive process between those responsible for developing the project and those responsible for implementing it—and the role of facilitator competence are presented. In the final section, the topic of sample sizes in pilot studies is revisited.

Developing programs or conducting systematic research to prevent or treat physical or mental health problems can be a long, arduous task. Pilot studies are a refreshing antidote to this enduring wait for outcomes. A program or research design may take 6 months to develop, and a subsequent grant proposal may require 12 to 18 months to obtain funding. After 2 years of planning and preparation, it will likely require another 3 to 4 years to implement the project and evaluate its effects and perhaps another year to analyze and write up the results. Developing, implementing, and systematically evaluating the outcomes of a health intervention is clearly an exercise in delayed gratification.

Pilots are faster. As the chapter by Lynskey and Sussman aptly illustrates, the collection of pilot data is perhaps the one time when the investigator or developer is well advised to micromanage the work and examine the results as frequently as he or she desires—on a daily basis, should one wish. In contrast to waiting years for information, the wait can be only days, and it is to the investigator's benefit to observe the implementation of the intervention closely, talk with the participants frequently, examine the data quickly, and make procedural modifications as needed in the intervention.

In pilot studies, attention to *process*, rather than outcomes, is especially critical. Most large-scale investigations involve tests of hypotheses, and it is the results of those tests that are most scientifically compelling. However, a pilot test necessarily involves a complementary set of goals. Rather than focusing narrowly on the results of tests of hypotheses, the investigator's emphasis is on the broader implementation effort: Which components of this intervention are being delivered well? Which components are being criticized by participants? What should be changed before the full program is "set in stone" in the project manual? Are components redundant or confusing? In short, the investigator must be continually mindful of the work and proactively engaged in identifying intervention strengths and weaknesses with an eye to making necessary changes.

In addition to an emphasis on process evaluation, a good pilot study also addresses another issue—is the totality of the intervention greater than the sum of its parts? That is, a pilot study typically involves an integration of many components or therapeutic tasks into a single program or course of therapy. Issues related to the selection, evaluation, and sequencing of these single components have been discussed in detail in prior chapters in this volume (see Chapters 13 and 15, this volume). However, the pilot typically provides the first opportunity to see how these individual components actually meld together, for good or ill. The investigator must be alert to the possibility that therapeutic activities or program components that are exemplary as "stand-alone" pieces may feel repetitive or off-point when offered as a later exercise in a program (e.g., as in the seventh or eighth exercise in a 10-week intervention). Alternatively, the investigator may find that group cohesion and increased self-efficacy effects may make a later activity or therapeutic task even more effective than when it was initially evaluated as a single component of the intervention. In short, the best pilots permit developers to create programs that are the strongest amalgams of their individual components.

A critical aspect of the piloting process is intense, ongoing dialogue between research investigators or program developers, who often work in academic or administrative environments, and those who will be implementing the intervention, who typically work in school, clinic, or community settings. Interventions may have the advantage of being grounded in strong theory but be unworkable in a real-world setting. For example, if an educational intervention relies heavily on written materials, it is imperative that the project developer know whether the proposed participant population is literate and comfortable with that mode of information exchange. Obtaining this information will typically necessitate conversation with individuals who are likely actually to implement the intervention in the target setting.

Lynskey and Sussman observe that the implementation of a pilot can be evaluated on at least three domains: adherence, exposure, and reinvention. It seems clear that a fourth issue is equally relevant: competence or skill level in administering the intervention. Facilitator competence involves both knowledge and skill. That is, the individual implementing the intervention must both know the protocol material and be able to convey it in a way that others can absorb with ease. Two teachers or clinicians may each conduct an intervention with a high level of adherence to a protocol or manual but differ dramatically in their skill level (e.g., ability to respond to unexpected obstacles while remaining consistent with the overarching principles of the intervention) or in those nonspecific factors (e.g., enthusiasm, warmth) that are likely to be related to better project effects. In evaluating a pilot outcome, it is critical to discern whether only very skillful implementation of the intervention will yield benefits or if any reasonably trained individual can administer the intervention to good effect.

A note on pilot sample size is in order. Pilots are typically conducted with modest resources, and they are often contrasted with final projects by their sample size. Lynskey and Sussman note that, in their comprehensive review of published program development and pilot studies, the mean number of subjects was 309. For those working in mental health settings, this number is daunting—it is almost as large as or larger than most of the rigorously implemented U.S. multisite collaborative psychosocial intervention studies ever conducted—for example, the collaborative depression study ($n = 239$; Elkin et al., 1989), the treatment strategies for schizophrenia study ($n = 313$; Schooler et al., 1997), or the ongoing Veterans Administration Cooperative Study No. 420—Group Treatment for Posttraumatic Stress Disorder ($n = 360$) (Friedman & Schnurr, 1996).

Obviously, in the field of mental health, pilots are likely to be much smaller than large school- or community-based intervention projects; in part, this is due to the higher costs (in face-to-face contact hours) of case identification, screening, and outcome assessment in mental health research. In determining adequate pilot size, the investigator or program developer has few guidelines. A feasible rule of thumb for adequate sample size might be that the pilot should match 5% to 10% of the proposed final project sample. In some research areas (e.g., school-based programs), this sample size will still permit some determination of likely intervention effect sizes; in other arenas (e.g., mental health research), this sample size may be too small to yield reliable effect size estimates but will at least reveal critical information of implementation feasibility.

In summary, Lynskey and Sussman offer a thoughtful and practical guide to the role of pilots in program development and intervention efforts. A pilot can provide critical data on program implementation, acceptability, and effectiveness to strengthen a subsequent larger project. Paying close attention to the implementation process, investigating the totality of the intervention (in contrast to its single components), keeping information networks open among key stakeholders, examining the effects of competence in program implementation, and ensuring that the pilot size is large enough to be informative but small enough to be feasible are all important. Although the optimal conduct of pilot studies is a too often underemphasized topic in many training programs for health professionals, it is probably not an exaggeration to say that the knowledge gained in a well-done pilot can make or break the outcome of the final project. In the life of a project, time spent conducting a useful pilot is time well spent.

▷ REFERENCES

ELKIN, I., SHEA, M. T., WATKINS, J. T., IMBER, S. D., SOTSKY, S. M., COLLINS, J. F., GLASS, D. R., PILKONIS, P. A., LEBER, W. R., DOCHERTY, J. P., FIESTER, S. J., & PARLOFF, M. B. (1989). National Institute of Mental Health Treatment of Depression Collaborative Research Program: General effectiveness of treatments. *Archives of General Psychiatry, 46,* 971-982.

FRIEDMAN, M. J., & SCHNURR, P. P. (Coprincipal proponents). (1996). *Department of Veterans Affairs VA Cooperative Study 420: Group treatment of PTSD* (2 vols.). White River Junction, VT: National Center for PTSD.

SCHOOLER, N. R., KEITH, S. J., SEVERE, J. B., MATTHEWS, S. M., BELLACK, A. S., GLICK, I. D., HARGREAVES, W. A., KANE, J. M., NINA, P. T., FRANCES, A., JACOBS, M., LIEBERMAN, J. A., MANCE, R., SIMPSON, G. M., & WOERNER, M. G. (1997). Relapse and rehospitalization during maintenance treatment of schizophrenia: The effects of dose reduction and family treatment. *Archives of General Psychiatry, 54,* 453-463.

Case Study 7

CHAPTER 17

Development and Pilot Testing of Project SMART

Louise Ann Rohrbach
Jill English
William B. Hansen
C. Anderson Johnson

Project SMART (Self-Management and Resistance Training) was a school-based trial of the relative efficacy of two approaches to the prevention of tobacco, alcohol, and marijuana use among adolescents (Graham, Johnson, Hansen, Flay, & Gee, 1990; Hansen, Johnson, Flay, Graham, & Sobel, 1988). One aim of the study was to compare a social-influences approach, focused on peer pressure resistance training and correction of normative expectations, to an affective education approach focused on person-centered influences to use drugs, such as stress management and poor self-image enhancement. Both prevention program approaches were developed and tested during the 1970s. When the Project SMART trial began in 1982, the social-influences model had been shown to be successful in reducing the onset of regular tobacco use (e.g., Botvin & Eng, 1982; Botvin, Eng, & Williams, 1980; Evans et al., 1978; Leupker, Johnson, Murray, & Pechacek, 1983). In contrast, evaluations of the affective education approach had been few and generally of poor quality, and they had not provided evidence of effectiveness for substance abuse prevention (Schaps, DiBartolo, Moskowitz, Palley, & Churgin, 1981).

Most of the early substance abuse prevention research focused on a single "gateway" substance, usually cigarettes. Tobacco, alcohol, and marijuana are considered gateway drugs because they are the most widely used by young people and typically precede initiation of harder drugs such as cocaine (Kandel, 1975). When Project SMART was initially proposed, there was only preliminary evidence that a social-influences approach might reduce the onset of alcohol and marijuana use in addition to tobacco use (McAlister, Perry, Killen, Slinkard, & Maccoby, 1980). Thus, a second aim of the Project SMART study was to determine whether a program that specifically targeted all three gateway substances, using a social-influences approach, would be successful.

Project SMART was the first systematic investigation of one drug abuse prevention approach versus another. It was one of the first prevention trials conducted in a large metropolitan school district with students from diverse socioeconomic backgrounds. As such, it charted new ground in the drug abuse prevention field. It was the "parent" of two nationally recognized prevention programs that were developed later: Students Taught Awareness and Resistance (STAR) (Pentz et al., 1989) and Drug Abuse Resistance Education (DARE) (Bureau of Justice Assistance, 1988).

This chapter describes the program development and pilot-testing process that was used in Project SMART. It focuses on the challenges of developing two distinct curricula simultaneously—the ways that pilot-test data were collected and used to refine the curricula and the implications of the pilot-test process for future program development efforts.

▶ PROGRAM DEVELOPMENT

The two Project SMART curricula were developed by a team of five White female health educators, four who were in their late 20s and early 30s and one who was in her 40s. Collectively, they had backgrounds in primary and secondary education, public health, social services, and curriculum development. Two of the women had a master's degree in public health, one had a bachelor's degree in education and was a certified science teacher, and two had bachelor's degrees in health education, with a concentration in school health. Except for the health educator who had been a science teacher for 10 years and a district administrator for 5 years, on average, the health educators had been in the workforce for about 4 years.

The health educators worked as a team of peers, each of whom was at the same level in the research project's organizational structure. They reached consensus on curriculum issues through discussion, negotiation, and compromise. Although technically, the principal investigators supervised the health education team, all worked on an equal level with regard to program development. Constructive criticism was freely given and received by all.

During the curriculum development phases, the health educator team met once or twice a week. After implementation began, the team met weekly, generally on Fridays, which were not scheduled for program implementation. The meetings lasted from 1 to 4 hours and were quite lively in the discussions about what worked, suggestions for improvement, anecdotal stories, and the provision of support for each other. More often than not, everyone agreed that a particular activity worked or did not work. The recommendations primarily concerned (a) refining discussion questions, (b) clarifying written directions, and (c) providing clear examples of student responses. Occasionally, there were portions of the lesson that all agreed did not work but for which there was little consensus on improvement. These issues required intense negotiation and brainstorming on the part of the health educators. Although there were few substantive disagreements, the principal investigators made the final decision regarding changes. Occasionally, these decisions were grounded more in theory than practice. However, as a general rule, the recommendations of the health educators were accepted by the principal investigators.

The program development process began with a review of the theoretical foundations for the social-influences and affective education approaches. The social-influences approach was based on social learning theory (Bandura, 1977), the theory of reasoned action (Ajzen & Fishbein, 1980), and other social psychological theories of influence and comparison (e.g., Asch, 1955; Festinger, 1954), as well as available epidemiological evidence on psychosocial predictors of drug abuse (e.g., Flay, D'Avernas, Best, Kersell, & Ryan, 1983). The affective education approach drew on theories of personal well-being based on in-vogue educational themes such as values clarification, decision-making training, and self-esteem building (Goodstadt, 1980; Goodstadt & Sheppard, 1983; Goodstadt, Sheppard, & Chan, 1982; Schaps et al., 1981).

The next step of the development process was to identify the primary components of the new curricula, based on the review of theory and previous intervention trials. The components of the social-influences ("social") program would include peer pressure resistance training, information about parental and other adult influences, inoculation against mass media messages that glamorize drug use, and correction of normative expectations (i.e., students' beliefs about the prevalence of drug use among their peers). The affective program would include goal setting, decision making, self-esteem building, and assertiveness. In addition, four components were included in both curricula: information about the consequences of drug use (with an emphasis on immediate consequences), motivations to use and not use drugs, alternatives to drug use, and a public commitment to not use drugs. Although the activities for each of the shared components were similar, each included a different emphasis. For example, in the social curriculum, follow-up discussion questions written into the consequences activity emphasized social consequences (e.g., losing friends when one begins smoking), and discussion in the affective curriculum emphasized personal consequences (e.g., the ways that drugs exacerbate problems and interfere with the achievement of personal goals).

Each of the curriculum components addressed at least one hypothesized mechanism of behavior change. For example, building students' self-efficacy to refuse drug offers and resistance skills was hypothesized to be a mediator of reductions in substance use for the social-influences program. Therefore, peer pressure resistance training was a key component of the social curriculum. Skills to achieve personal goals were hypothesized to mediate reductions in substance use for the affective program, so it focused on personal goal setting and decision making.

The health educator team also identified teaching strategies that were felt to be important in the delivery of effective substance abuse prevention programs, which would be incorporated throughout each curriculum, particularly use of demonstration, skills practice, role-playing, small-group exercises, Socratic discussions, and the use of same-age peer opinion leaders (Johnson, 1982; Sussman, 1991). These teaching strategies were identified through the review of existing social-influences smoking prevention curriculum guides (e.g., Leupker et al., 1983) and the scientific literature on effective school health education approaches.

The primary objective of the development process was to produce two curricula that had distinct content yet were balanced in regard to number of sessions, curriculum format, use of effective teaching strategies, and enjoyability on the part of students. To generate a pool of possible activities to address each curriculum component, the health educators reviewed existing curricula and brainstormed new ideas. The team organized the proposed activities into curriculum sessions that would be the length of a typical classroom session (45 minutes). They decided that each session would include several activities, begin with a review of the previous lesson, and end with a summary.

Under the direction of the project investigators, each health educator took primary responsibility for developing several social and affective curriculum sessions. Because the project was an efficacy trial of the two curricula, standardization of lesson delivery was a primary goal. Thus, the lesson plans were structured such that they outlined a specific order of presentation, discussion questions, and specific language the teacher would use. After the draft sessions were written, the project investigators reviewed and commented on the draft. On the basis of these comments, the sessions were revised. Once the draft curricula were typed, they were ready for pilot testing. Table 17.1 summarizes the set of lessons that were developed for each curriculum.

Some comment is appropriate on the process of program development. The craft of program development during this period was very different from the craft as currently employed or endorsed for the future in other places within this text. The program text was produced using a typewriter, the only method that existed prior to the availability of personal computers and word-processing programs. That is, the approach was almost solely focused on the development of theoretically appropriate messages put into the format of a written protocol that was judged by the expert staff to have potential to convey the intended messages. Prior to pilot testing, no focus group meetings were held. During pilot testing, no data were collected to estimate the magnitude of effects on mediating variables. Data analysis at the time required keypunching to cards, analysis on mainframes, and then waiting for the job to be printed and going to a centralized site to pick up the job; this was too time-consuming and cumbersome to be considered as a method for checking immediate outcomes. Most data on potential for program impact came from subjective reports of teachers and the observation of health educators and investigators.

It is also important to describe the context for school-based drug abuse prevention education when Project SMART was developed and tested. In the 1980s, the science of drug abuse prevention was evolving rapidly. The curriculum components that we developed, including stress management, clarifying normative beliefs, refusal skills, social influences, and others, were innovative at the time. In fact, one of the factors that made the implementation of Project SMART possible was that drug education was virtually nonexistent in schools. Although some of these approaches had been tried in schools before, most of them had not been implemented in the context of a theory-based drug education program. Thus, as we presented local schools with the opportunity to be a testing site for our experimental approaches, we were to encounter receptivity and excitement, as well as some skepticism on the part of school administrators and teachers.

FIRST PHASE OF PILOT TESTING ◄

Five months were built into the Project SMART timeline for the development and pilot testing of both curricula. There were several objectives for the pilot testing. First, we wanted to assess the general workability of the curriculum sessions in terms of message coherence, length of time required for delivery, transitions between activities, and the extent to which the activities accomplished the objectives of the session. Second, we wanted to assess students' receptivity to the ses-

TABLE 17.1 Summary of Lessons for Two Substance Abuse Prevention Curricula, First Year of Implementation

Session	Social-Influences Curriculum	Affective Curriculum
1	Introduction 　Program format 　Group identification exercise	Introduction 　Program format 　Self-esteem enhancement exercise
2	Motivations 　Motivators for using and not using drugs 　The nature of peer pressure	Motivations 　Motivators for using and not using drugs 　Sources of stress
3	Normative expectations 　Clarifying misperceptions regarding the prevalence of peer drug use 　The nature of friends' influences	Alternatives 　Alternative solutions to problems 　Deep breathing (skills introduction) 　Self-monitoring
4	Consequences 　Consequences of using and not using drugs 　Using consequences to resist peer pressure	Goal setting—Part I 　Goal-setting essentials 　The interference of drug use in achieving personal goals 　Deep breathing (practice)
5	Peer pressure resistance skills 　Techniques to say no 　Scripting resistance to offers to use drugs	Goal setting—Part II 　Setting a personal goal 　Deep breathing (practice)
6	Role-playing peer pressure resistance 　Social situations that encourage drug use 　Role-playing techniques 　Role-playing resisting peer pressure to use drugs	Consequences 　Monitoring personal goals 　Consequences of using and not using drugs 　Deep breathing (practice)
7	Adult influences 　Role-playing resisting peer pressure to use drugs 　The nature of modeling 　Positive and negative parental influences 　Talking to adults about drugs	Decision-making skills 　Monitoring personal goals 　The decision-making process 　Deciding about drug use
8	Media influences 　Media awareness 　Advertising techniques 　Evaluating advertising influences 　Resisting media influences	Self-esteem 　The value of self-esteem 　Building self-esteem 　Complimenting others
9	Entertainment influences 　Influences to use and not use drugs in entertainment venues 　Social activism on behalf of nondrug use in entertainment	Assertiveness—Part I 　Defining assertive behavior 　Making assertive statements 　Muscle tension relaxation (skills introduction)
10	Alternatives 　The concept of alternatives 　Alternatives to drug use 　Saying no (practice)	Assertiveness—Part II 　Introduction to role-playing 　Role-playing assertiveness 　Muscle tension relaxation (skills practice)

Session	Social-Influences Curriculum	Affective Curriculum

11	Positive friendships
	  Qualities of good friends
	  Techniques to develop and keep good friends
	  Saying no (practice)
		Summary
		  Achieving goals
		  Role-playing assertiveness
		  Alternatives

12	Public commitment
	  Videotaping of students' commitment to say no to pressure to use drugs
		Public commitment
		  Videotaping of students' commitment to engage in alternatives instead of using drugs

sions. In particular, we wanted to make sure that the social and affective curriculum approaches appeared equally enjoyable to students. Third, we wanted to make sure that the activities were appropriate for the age group (seventh grade) and diverse ethnic groups of the target population (approximately 40% White, 35% Latino, 20% African American, and 5% Asian/Pacific Islander).

One middle school with student demographic characteristics similar to those of the intervention schools was recruited for the pilot testing. Arrangements were made with the school principal and classroom teacher to pilot test all 12 curriculum sessions for each curriculum with three classrooms of students (i.e., a total of six classes were involved). Pilot testing each lesson more than once allowed the health educators to observe how well the activities worked with different groups of students. For each curriculum, all three classes (usually three periods in a row) received the same lesson. Then, the health educators went back to the office and discussed the lessons and revised them. In only two instances—the norm lesson and the goal-setting lesson—they engaged in additional pilot testing at an additional class for each lesson before finalizing the lesson. Most major changes were made between the pilot test and the trial, not during the pilot test.

Two health educators conducted the pilot test. One taught the lessons, and the other observed. With the second classroom of students, the health educators switched roles. The health educator-observer documented when each activity began and ended, what the health educator-implementer said, how what she said varied from the lesson plan, and how students responded to discussion questions. She also noted her impressions of student receptivity to the lesson —for example, the degree of participation by students and the proportion who paid attention to the discussion or focused on the task. Lessons were rated as well received when students were willing to share their opinions and personal experiences with the class and when they showed enthusiasm for the activities. The health educators also assessed the appropriateness of the lessons for the grade level and cultural groups represented in the pilot classrooms (i.e., through their consensual subjective perceptions).

The health education team compared observation notes and student worksheets to determine which activities and lessons needed revision. For example, pilot testing indicated that some activities were too long. In the pilot version of the consequences activity, students were placed in small groups and instructed to brainstorm the consequences of using and not using the three gateway drugs. The health educator then asked each group to report its results, and she recorded them on the blackboard. Not only did it take the groups longer to brainstorm than was expected, but asking each group to report all of their consequences was also time-consuming and repetitive. We expected the entire activity to take 20 minutes, but in the pilot it took at least 35 minutes. In the revision process, this lesson was adjusted to make it effective. We decided to assign each group one gateway substance only, asking students to brainstorm the consequences of both using and not using that substance. Each class would be divided into six groups, and two would address each substance (tobacco, alcohol, and marijuana). After the brainstorming, the teacher would review the students' findings for each substance. The first group would report their lists of consequences, and the second group would report only those consequences that had not been listed by the first group. This process was repeated for the other substances. The revision of this activity reduced its length and improved its pace.

Pilot testing also showed that some revisions to student materials and verbal instructions for activities were needed. For example, students told us that written instructions on one of the homework assignments, in which they were asked to monitor how television programs depicted drug use, were confusing. They were not sure how many programs we wanted them to monitor and which behaviors they were to record on the monitoring sheet. Based on the students' feedback, the instructions were made more explicit.

In other instances, the pilot test indicated that written information added to the students' workbooks would facilitate their learning of specific concepts. For example, in the assertiveness lesson in the social curriculum, we demonstrated and discussed the differences between assertive, aggressive, and passive behavior styles. The primary objective of the activity was to teach students the verbal and nonverbal elements of assertive responses to drug offers. The pilot suggested that the students were having trouble remembering these elements. Thus, we developed a handout called "Being Assertive," which listed aspects of an assertive response to a drug offer. In the revised version of the lesson, we encouraged the students to consult the handout frequently.

We also found that our verbal instructions for activities such as role-playing could be improved. In the pilot, we asked the students to observe the role-plays and be prepared to provide the actors with specific feedback regarding their behaviors. Before beginning their role-plays, we provided a demonstration role-play, after which the health educator modeled the type of feedback we were seeking (e.g., commenting on how the student said no to the drug offer, how he or she gained control of the situation, etc.). Despite this modeling, when small groups of students performed their role-plays for the class, we found that the students generally were not able to provide explicit feedback. Therefore, we revised the lesson so that the health educator would not only model how to give feedback after a role-play but also write specific questions on the blackboard that she wanted the class to be prepared to answer (e.g., What technique did the student use to say no? Was he or she assertive? How would this work if it were a real-life situation?).

In some cases, pilot testing revealed a need to restructure an entire activity. For example, the health educators were in agreement that the activity designed to correct students' misperceptions about the prevalence of peer substance use was not well received by students and did not appear to achieve its objectives. In the pilot test, we asked students to estimate the prevalence of peer use of each gateway substance, averaged their estimates, and presented data about prevalence rates from recent local surveys. The lesson did not work as well as planned for several reasons. First, even though it was interesting to ask students to estimate prevalence before presenting actual prevalence rates (because it demonstrated the extent to which they overestimate prevalence), it took too much time to average their estimates. Second, some students questioned the validity of the actual prevalence rates that we presented, stating the belief that "our school is different." We concluded from the pilot that the pace of the lesson needed improvement, and we needed to find a way to present prevalence data that would be credible to these students. Thus, we revised the lesson to include a brief survey of gateway drug use prevalence at their school. This anonymous survey was to be distributed during the prior lesson, and the results were to be tallied by the health educator before a normative expectations lesson (see Table 17.1). If the health educator had more than one classroom period in which she taught the program, she was encouraged to average the survey responses across classes. The presentation of the results was improved in several ways. The health educator asked the class to estimate peer drug use prevalence first, but she allowed only some of the students, rather than the whole class, to share their estimates. This was followed by a presentation of the actual prevalence rates of the class (or combination of classes) based on the survey, a discussion of why students may have overestimated the rates, and a concluding statement that most of their peers did not use drugs.

Another example of an activity that needed to be restructured was goal setting in the affective curriculum. The activity was designed to have students identify several goals they wanted to achieve in their lives, list steps they could take in the next few months to work toward achieving those goals, and list ways in which using drugs might preclude them from achieving them. In the pilot test, we found that most of the goals identified by students were long term or nonspecific (e.g., become a doctor, be a good citizen, etc.), and this resulted in difficulty in identifying short-term steps that could be taken to achieve the goals. Because we wanted to monitor students' progress toward reaching their goals throughout the curriculum implementation period, we decided to restructure the activity to emphasize short-term goals (e.g., getting good grades that year) rather than longer-term goals (e.g., graduate from high school). Before we asked the students to identify short-term goals that they wanted to achieve in the next few months, we built in a preliminary lecturette and demonstration of how goals could be achieved in 2 months, what steps one would take to achieve those goals, and how they were related to longer-term goals. We also modified the worksheets for this activity to include several examples of short-term goals, steps toward achieving goals, and ways that drug use could interfere with achieving short- and long-term goals.

Finally, other data from the pilot testing were used to refine the draft lesson plans. When the lessons were delivered under real-world pilot test conditions, the health educators sometimes posed new discussion questions that came to mind as a result of a teachable moment. For example, after reviewing the consequences of gateway drug use that students listed in their small groups, discussing whether these were mostly negative or positive outcomes, and finding that the students believed they were primarily negative, the health educator asked the students, "If most of the consequences of drug use are negative, why do people use them?" This teachable moment-type discussion question allowed her to review briefly the discussion from the prior lesson about motivations for using and not using drugs. We found that when health educators wrote lesson plans, they did not always think of all important discussion questions ahead of time. Some questions came to mind as they led discussions for the first time. Our revised lesson plans incorporated as many of these additional questions as were appropriate to enhance interaction in the classroom within the allotted time. Pilot testing also helped to identify language that the teacher could use to make smooth transitions from one activity to another. Such comments were written into the final curriculum when appropriate.

By the end of the first phase of pilot testing, the revised versions of the social and affective programs were judged to be equally balanced in terms of effectiveness of teaching methods, student receptivity, and potential for meeting educational objectives. This judgment represented a consensus of the health educators and project investigators.

▶ FIRST-YEAR IMPLEMENTATION OF PROJECT SMART

The two Project SMART curriculum approaches were tested on the first of three cohorts of seventh-grade students in 16 junior high schools in the Los Angeles metropolitan area, beginning in the 1982-1983 school year (Hansen et al., 1988).

Curriculum lessons were implemented once a week over a 12-week period, with the health educators who developed the curricula alternating implementation with classroom health teachers. Thus, for each classroom of students, health educators and classroom teachers each delivered one half of the lessons. All of the project health educators were assigned to teach in equal numbers of social and affective curriculum schools.

All schools were randomly assigned to a condition prior to the 1982 implementation; that is, Project SMART used an experimental-like design. Because very few units were assigned to a condition in each year, however, the meaningfulness of random assignment was in question. In addition, some of the schools that were controls in the first year became treatment schools (for new seventh-grade cohorts) in the following year. The same procedure was used from Year 2 to Year 3 (Graham et al., 1990). For the 1982 cohort, two schools were affective (Schools 1-2), two schools were social (Schools 3-4), and four schools were controls (Schools 5-8). For the 1983 cohort, two schools were affective-social combined (Schools 5-6; changes in Year 2 program contents are discussed in the next section), two schools were social (Schools 7-8), and four schools were control (Schools 9-12). Finally, for the 1984 cohort, two schools were affective-social combined (Schools 9-10), two schools were social (Schools 11-12), and four schools were controls (Schools 13-16). Thus, the status of all but eight schools varied from one year to the next.

One-year posttest results from the first seventh-grade cohort showed that the social program was effective in delaying the self-reported onset of tobacco, alcohol, and marijuana use, but the affective program appeared to have a negative effect. Compared to controls, students who received the affective program reported significant increases in the onset of tobacco, alcohol, and marijuana use (Hansen et al., 1988). The investigators suggested that the outcomes of the affective program might be attributable to the fact that the control group's onset of drug use did not show the common pattern of increases (i.e., an artifact), the character of the program itself (i.e., it may have inadvertently encouraged experimentation), or the perceived difficulty of implementing the affective program relative to the social program (i.e., possibly poor or incomplete implementation).

Compared to the pilot test, which was limited to three tests of each curriculum lesson in both the affective and social programs, for each program with a different group of students, the first year of the experimental trial provided the health educators with much more extensive experience in delivering both programs. With time, the health educators found that there were elements of the social program—notably, role-plays and other highly interactive methods—that resulted in greater participation and involvement by students and that could not be replicated in the affective program. To the health educators, it seemed contrived to implement a curriculum (the affective program) that purposely did not address social factors related to drug use. Although teachers who were asked to deliver one half of the lessons did not complete written ratings of the curriculum lessons, their anecdotal reports to the health educators supported the finding that the affective program seemed contrived and difficult to implement and was less well received by students than was the social program. Teachers and health educators found the social program easier to implement because it purposely focused on social factors, which were more salient to the target age group, while de-emphasizing personal factors. In regard to the skills development components, program implementers found that peer pressure resistance skills training in the social program was more enjoyable and meaningful to the students than were the deep-breathing exercises, muscle tension relaxation training, and goal setting in the affective program.

Unfortunately, data on hypothesized program mediators were not available to determine whether the affective program had an impact on the specific beliefs and skills it was designed to change. Because the affective program showed no promise of being effective at prevention and, indeed, may have been harmful to students, at the end of the first year of program implementation, the research team decided to change the research design. The team chose to eliminate the affective program and instead compared the social-resistance training program to a combined program that included social-resistance training and particular affective components. In this sense, the first-year trial served as a large-scale pilot for a second phase of work.

▶ SECOND PHASE OF PILOT TESTING AND PROGRAM IMPLEMENTATION

The purpose of the second phase of pilot testing was to determine the workability of a combined version of the program that included selected lessons from the social and affective curricula. Approximately half of the activities from both the affective and social curricula were selected for the combined version (see Table 17.2). Project staff needed to make a decision about which lessons would go into the combined curriculum and which ones would be eliminated. The criteria used to determine which lessons would remain in the combined curriculum included (a) health educators' perceptions of the interest of the students in the lesson, (b) extent to which the lesson seemed to develop health-related skills (e.g., deep breathing did not seem very helpful or relevant to the kids at the time), (c) pacing of the lesson (i.e., lessons that seemed choppy or seemed to drag were dropped), and (d) balance of social and affective concepts. Similar to the first phase of pilot testing, the combined curriculum was tested in its entirety, and health educators recorded their impressions of the sequencing of activities, how well the lessons worked overall, and how students responded to them. At the end of the process,

TABLE 17.2   Summary of Lessons for Two Substance Abuse Prevention Curricula, Second Through Fourth Years of Implementation

Session	Social-Influences Curriculum	Social/Personal Skills Curriculum

1	Introduction
	    Program format
	    Sources of social influences
		Introduction
		    Program format
		    Sources of social influences
		    Introduction to stress and problem solving

2	Consequences
	    Consequences of using and not using drugs
	    Using consequences to resist peer pressure
		Consequences
		    Consequences of using and not using drugs
		    Using consequences to resist peer pressure

3	Peer pressure resistance skills
	    Techniques to say no
	    Scripting resistance to offers to use drugs
		Peer pressure resistance skills
		    Techniques to say no
		    Scripting resistance to offers to use drugs

4	Role-playing peer pressure resistance
	    Social situations that encourage drug use
	    Role-playing techniques
	    Role-playing resisting peer pressure to use drugs
	    Assertiveness
		Role-playing peer pressure resistance
		    Social situations that encourage drug use
		    Role-playing techniques
		    Role-playing resisting peer pressure to use drugs
		    Assertiveness

5	Normative expectations
	    Clarifying misperceptions regarding the prevalence of peer drug use
	    The nature of friends' influences
		Stress
		    Positive and negative stressors
		    Physical and emotional reactions to stress
		    Monitoring personal stressors

6	Adult influences
	    Role-playing resisting peer pressure to use drugs
	    The nature of modeling
	    Positive and negative parental influences
	    Talking to adults about drugs
		Coping with stress
		    Review of personal stressors
		    Strategies for coping with stress
		    Coping with stress without using drugs

7	Positive friendships
	    Qualities of good friends
	    Techniques to develop and keep good friends
	    Saying no (practice)
		Habit awareness
		    Identifying personal habits
		    Monitoring habits
		    Changing health-compromising habits

8	Entertainment influences
	    Influences to use and not use drugs in entertainment venues
	    Social activism on behalf of nondrug use in entertainment
		Decision making
		    The decision-making process (steps)
		    Deciding about drug use

9	Media influences
	    Media awareness
	    Advertising techniques
	    Evaluating advertising influences
	    Resisting media influences
		Decision-making skills
		    Role-playing decision making in drug-related situations

(continued)

TABLE 17.2 Continued

Session	Social-Influences Curriculum	Social/Personal Skills Curriculum

10	Antidrug commercials
	    Developing and demonstrating antidrug commercials
		Problem solving
		    Weighing the pros and cons of different solutions
		    How to get support in solving problems

11	Personal reasons for not using drugs
	    Identifying and role-playing personal reasons for not using drugs
		Personal reasons for not using drugs
		    Identifying and role-playing personal reasons for not using drugs

12	Public commitment
	    Videotaping of students' commitment to say no to pressure to use drugs
		Public commitment
		    Videotaping of students' commitment to say no to pressure to use drugs

the research team was confident that they had developed a curriculum that would be as acceptable to students and as easy to implement as was the social curriculum.

During the second through fourth years of the Project SMART intervention trial (1983-1984, 1984-1985), the relative efficacy of the social-resistance training versus combined social-resistance training and affective curriculum was tested. A different mechanism for program delivery was used in this phase of program implementation. Instead of having staff health educators and classroom teachers alternate teaching lessons for each classroom, health educators taught all lessons to one half of the classes in each school, and classroom teachers taught all lessons to the other half. One-year outcome results showed that both curricula produced significant reductions in cigarette and alcohol use and marginal reductions in marijuana use (Flay, Graham, et al., 1988). The curricula were equally effective in changing hypothesized program mediators such as behavioral intentions, beliefs about the prevalence of peer use, and resistance self-efficacy (Rohrbach et al., 1985).

▶ LESSONS LEARNED

When it was initiated, the Project SMART intervention trial was innovative in that it applied the social-influences approach to the prevention of multiple-substance abuse, tested the relative effectiveness of two distinct prevention approaches, and tested these approaches in schools that served ethnically diverse populations. Developing two theoretically distinct Project SMART curricula that would be equally well balanced in regard to the use of effective teaching methods, equally well received by students, and equally effective in meeting their respective educational objectives was a challenging task. Pilot testing of the curricula, though limited in scope, generated information that helped to refine the content of each curriculum.

HEALTH EDUCATOR TEAM APPROACH

One of the strengths of Project SMART's program development and pilot-testing approach was the use of a team of health educators whose professional preparation was in health behavior change theory and strategies. Often, researchers rely on one individual to write and test curriculum lessons. Use of a writing team is advantageous in that a broad range of activity ideas is generated, and health educators' diverse experiences may be applied. The brainstorming of ideas and extensive discussions after pilot testing not only results in more effective curricula but also makes the development process more enjoyable for the staff.

During Project SMART pilot testing, having each health educator teach some of the sessions and observe others provided more extensive information about the workability of specific lessons. Ultimately, the use of a team of health educators resulted in more creative and fresh curricula than might have been developed by a single educator. Another strategy may be to use external consultants, both researchers and educators, to generate curriculum ideas and check the accuracy of the content and the application of theory (e.g., Flay, Brannon, et al., 1988). However, external consultants may not be as well informed about the philosophy and goals of the program as internal staff who have been trained by the project investigators.

LENGTH OF PROGRAM DEVELOPMENT AND TESTING PROCESS

Sussman (1991) has suggested that school-based curricula be pilot tested through an empirical, building-block process in which parts of a curriculum are tested and refined prior to testing the full-draft curriculum. As is often the case in 4- and 5-year research projects, in Project SMART, there was limited time allocated to the development and pilot testing of curricula. The time frame allowed for testing of full-draft curricula only. Although a longer development phase would have provided the opportunity for more extensive piloting, it would have precluded collecting 2-year follow-up data during the same grant period. In retrospect, given that after 1 year of implementation we found that our two experimental curricula were not equivalent in regard to ease of implementation and receptivity by the students, it might have been better to extend the program development phase and reduce the number of posttest follow-ups. It is essential that investigators build in adequate time for program development and testing, particularly when an intervention trial is examining the relative efficacy of several program approaches, each of which needs to be developed.

COLLECTION OF PILOT-TEST DATA

Even within the limitations of pilot testing the curriculum activities only once, the process would have been improved by the collection of student self-report measures. One of the most important questions a pilot test can answer is whether the curriculum has an impact on the hypothesized mediators of behavioral effects, such as beliefs about the prevalence and acceptability of drug use, refusal self-efficacy, outcome expectancies, and so on (Sussman, 1991). There is evidence that mediators such as these predict drug abuse prevention program outcomes 1 or 2 years later (e.g., MacKinnon et al., 1991).

In the Project SMART pilot test, we might have used a single-group or between-groups pretest-posttest quasi-experimental design to assess program mediators as well as student receptivity to the lessons. Such data would have allowed us to determine whether the two curriculum approaches were comparable with regard to producing changes in hypothesized program mediators. As it was, we relied on health educators' judgments that both curricula were achieving their educational objectives effectively and that they were equally acceptable to students. Unfortunately, after the experience of delivering both programs during the first year of the intervention trial, it was the health educators' intuition that the affective program was not as effective or well received by students as was the social program. Overall, it was more difficult to implement. One-year follow-up student surveys supported these intuitions. At a minimum, we could have conducted informal discussions with the students after the pilot lessons to determine their impressions of both curricula.

The pilot-testing process also would have been enhanced if the health educator-observers and classroom teachers had completed quantitative measures of curriculum delivery. For example, multiple observers' ratings on scales assessing variables such as activity flow and student receptivity could have been compared to determine which activities needed refinement. Videotaping of pilot testing may have been useful because it would have allowed health educators and investigators to conduct post hoc ratings of curriculum delivery. In addition, it would have been helpful to involve classroom teachers in the ratings because they often have unique ideas about how to make new curriculum activities more workable.

PILOT-TESTING PROGRAM DELIVERY METHODS

Finally, we learned that the strategy for program delivery should be pilot tested in addition to the program itself. External classroom-based educational programs need to take into account the daily routines of classroom teachers. Our program implementation plan called for alternating lesson delivery between staff health educators and classroom teachers. We learned during the first year of program implementation that such a schedule did not work for at least some of the teachers. They were more accustomed to teaching programs as a unit, with one lesson every day, or once a week, rather than every other week. Furthermore, classroom teachers commonly devote time in the beginning of classroom sessions to taking attendance, reviewing homework assignments, and assigning new work. We designed each Project SMART session to take the entire classroom period, without allowing for these types of activities on the part of teachers. Another problem was that it was not uncommon for the health educator to arrive to teach a lesson only to find out that the previous lesson had not been taught by the regular classroom teacher. This resulted in one of two options: The health educator would either teach the previous lesson and return another day to teach the scheduled lesson, or the health educator would reschedule the visit for a later date (and wait for the regular teacher to deliver the lesson). One other problem was the lack of experience of the regular classroom teacher in teaching drug abuse prevention programs in general and, specifically, in using the variety of instructional strategies contained in Project SMART (e.g., teaching role-playing).

Flay, Graham, et al. (1988) found no significant effects for type of instructor on cigarette use, alcohol use, and marijuana use at 1- and 2-year follow-ups. However, we found that in terms of the completeness and efficiency of program implementation, health educator-led program delivery was more successful than teacher-led delivery. Ultimately, for the last 2 years of the project, it was decided that all lessons would be taught by a trained health education specialist. Had we pilot tested our program delivery methods, we would have found out that the proposed schedule would not work for some teachers. This might have eliminated some of the implementation difficulties we encountered in the first year of the experimental trial.

OTHER DESIGN CONSIDERATIONS

If the opportunity existed to begin Project SMART again today, a number of changes would be instituted immediately in the entire process of development and testing. In 1981, research in prevention was very limited. The early 1980s generally can be characterized as a period during which research ideas were just emerging. There were few traditions in program development or research design that researchers could rely on as guides to moving forward. The few examples of previous research that were available, many produced by members of the Project SMART research team, had been completed amid the discovery of many experimental design challenges. The full scope of issues that interventions needed to address and control for were not understood or fully appreciated. Indeed, at the time Project SMART was funded, the feeling among the research team was that the project was at the cutting edge of prevention research. In retrospect, the project served as a platform for moving the field forward, but the field eventually has moved well beyond what we were capable of at the time. The following is a partial listing of how the project might be reconsidered if completed today.

Program design has been markedly assisted with the development of word processing. Programs still go through a process that begins with the identification of ideas and drafting of interventions that eventually are used with a group of live participants. The initial period of writing in Project SMART was a struggle to complete on the part of participants. Processes were such that any change often required completely retyping the entire text of a session or activity. The luxury of word processing is often taken for granted in today's program design environment. Allowing multiple individuals to not only read but also edit a program would allow for significantly greater input and pretrial improvement.

In an environment in which word processing is operative, once a phase of pilot testing is initiated, program design changes are immediate. It is now even possible to write revised lesson plans on-site between sessions. Speed of revision contributes meaningfully to program design. Variations can be preprogrammed during pilot testing for resolution in the field. Such innovations would have significantly increased the flexibility of program design. If the two sets of variables (social and affective) were still of interest to the field, this flexibility would result in programming that would more easily allow versions of lessons to be refined and developed prior to a full-scale implementation, something that was not possible when Project SMART was initiated.

The process of program design would have been complemented with a variety of techniques such as the use of focus groups (Sussman, 1991) and multiple brief trials. Focus groups may be useful prior to program development, to determine the needs and interests of the target population, and after pilot testing to gather information regarding program acceptability. There also may have been an attempt to build in tailoring to the program based on demographic variables, pretest variables, or other sources of information. The goal of uniformity of implementation was intended to maximize program fidelity. This goal may have been replaced with one that emphasized maximized change in mediating variables (Hansen & McNeal, 1996). In other words, fidelity is likely to have been defined as the ability to create change in targeted mediators. Teachers would have been given an array of possible approaches in some lessons. This would have replaced an assessment of the ability of the teacher to stick to one approach when its applicability to a target audience may have been questionable. The program may have included rules for deciding about or prioritizing intervention alternatives.

The development of data analysis capabilities on personal computers significantly speeds the time of technical feedback about performance. With scanning and direct-input methods of encoding data, there is now the potential for a nearly immediate assessment of short-term program impact. A broad array of data, including process and performance data, would have been continuously collected. The concepts targeted by programming in Project SMART were understood conceptually, but measures for assessing changes in related variables and methods for completing appropriate analyses were not always available. We continue to learn about developmental changes in many of the variables targeted by intervention (Hansen & McNeal, 1999). Had the current potential for data-based feedback been available when Project SMART was under development, it would have significantly aided in the resolution of basic questions about program performance.

The field of prevention is now developed to the point where multiple sources of data can be used to answer many questions that emerge during program design. The concepts selected for targeting in Project SMART—affective or person-centered concepts and social or peer group-centered concepts—have now been articulated by a much wider array of etiologic studies. Furthermore, there are now meta-analytic studies (Gorman & Derzon, 1998) that would have been used to gain an understanding of statistical relationships that form the basis of concept selection. There would now be a requirement for some data-based evidence for association before concepts that made up *person centered* and *peer group centered* would be defined. It is likely that the research team would have given greater emphasis to understanding mediating variable data from the very beginning of the project. If specific meta-analytic data were not available, cross-sectional data would have been used to determine which variables appeared to go together and contribute to an understanding of drug use.

In short, the field has progressed in remarkable ways since the inception of Project SMART. Project SMART would have been designed differently in light of these advancements. However, it should be remembered that the need for many of these advancements was recognized only because projects such as Project SMART were willing to venture into prevention undertakings. Project SMART continued the long process of field development that had been started in the 1970s and that continues today. As noted by Sir Francis Bacon, "Truth emerges more readily from error than from confusion." Projects that continue to attempt the implausible will guarantee the advancement of the field into the future.

► CONCLUSIONS

The extent of program development and pilot testing in the Project SMART intervention trial, as well as the way in which it was conducted, was consistent with the standards for the prevention field in the early 1980s. At the time, there were few traditions in program development that researchers could rely on. Project SMART pilot testing emphasized observational methods and subjective judgments and was conducted without the benefit of current technologies such as word processing and personal computers. The project was considered to be the state-of-the-science in prevention research.

The prevention field has moved forward considerably since that time. There is now a recognition that program development is an iterative process that incorporates theory, review of extant program methods, assessment studies (both qualitative and quantitative), and feasibility testing (Sussman, 1991). With the advent of personal computers, program components can be written, pilot tested, and revised on the same day. Survey data can be processed quickly to answer questions regarding how well program components worked and whether they produced changes in the variables hypothesized to mediate program outcomes.

With the use of today's methods and technology, pilot testing of SMART could have been more extensive and might have precluded the finding, at the end of the first year of the intervention trial, that the two program approaches being tested were not equivalent in terms of ease of delivery, acceptance by students, and effectiveness. Nonetheless, the SMART trial made important contributions to the prevention field, and the program that was developed and tested served as a foundation for many effective prevention programs to follow (e.g., Flay, Brannon, et al., 1988; Flay, Graham, et al., 1988; Pentz et al., 1989; Sussman et al., 1993).

► REFERENCES

AJZEN, I., & FISHBEIN, M. (1980). *Understanding attitudes and predicting social behavior.* Englewood Cliffs, NJ: Prentice Hall.

ASCH, S. (1955). Opinions and social pressure. *Scientific American, 193,* 31-35.

BANDURA, A. (1977). *Social learning theory.* Englewood Cliffs, NJ: Prentice Hall.

BOTVIN, G. J., & ENG, A. (1982). The efficacy of a multi-component approach to the prevention of cigarette smoking. *Preventive Medicine, 11,* 199-211.

BOTVIN, G. J., ENG, A., & WILLIAMS, C. L. (1980). Preventing the onset of cigarette smoking through life skills training. *Preventive Medicine, 9,* 135-143.

BUREAU OF JUSTICE ASSISTANCE. (1988). *Implementing Project DARE: Drug Abuse Resistance Education.* Washington, DC: Bureau of Justice Assistance.

EVANS, R. I., ROZELLE, R. M., MITTELMARK, M. B., HANSEN, W. B., BANE, A. L., & HAVIS, J. (1978). Deterring the onset of smoking in children: Knowledge of immediate physiological effects and coping with peer pressure, media pressure, and parent modeling. *Journal of Applied Social Psychology, 8*, 126-135.

FESTINGER, L. (1954). A theory of social comparison processes. *Human Relations, 7*, 117-140.

FLAY, B. R., BRANNON, B. R., JOHNSON, C. A., HANSEN, W. B., ULENE, A. L., WHITNEY-SALTIEL, D. A., GLEASON, L. R., SUSSMAN, S., GAVIN, K. M., GLOWACZ, K. M., SOBOL, D. F., & SPIEGEL, D. C. (1988). The Television, School, and Family Smoking Prevention and Cessation Project: Theoretical basis and program development. *Preventive Medicine, 17*, 585-607.

FLAY, B. R., D'AVERNAS, J. R., BEST, J. A., KERSELL, M. W., & RYAN, K. B. (1983). Cigarette smoking: Why young people do it and ways of preventing it. In P. McGrath & P. Firestone (Eds.), *Pediatric and adolescent behavioral medicine* (pp. 132-183). New York: Springer-Verlag.

FLAY, B. R., GRAHAM, J. W., HOLT, L., HANSEN, W. B., JOHNSON, C. A., & ROHRBACH, L. A. (1988). *Social resistance versus personal and social skills for drug abuse prevention: Results from the 1983 cohort of Project SMART*. Los Angeles: University of Southern California Institute for Prevention Research.

GOODSTADT, M. S. (1980). Drug education: A turn on or turn off? *Journal of Drug Education, 10*, 89-99.

GOODSTADT, M. S., & SHEPPARD, M. A. (1983). Three approaches to alcohol education. *Journal of Studies on Alcohol, 44*, 362-380.

GOODSTADT, M. S., SHEPPARD, M. A., & CHAN, G. C. (1982). An evaluation of two school-based alcohol education programs. *Journal of Studies on Alcohol, 43*, 352-369.

GORMAN, D., & DERZON, J. H. (1998). *The relationship of negative affect, emotionality, and conventionality in predicting marijuana use, misuse, and abuse: A synthesis of evidence*. Report to the National Center for the Advancement of Prevention, Center for Substance Abuse Prevention, Rockville, MD.

GRAHAM, J. W., JOHNSON, C. A., HANSEN, W. B., FLAY, B. R., & GEE, M. (1990). Drug use prevention programs, gender, and ethnicity: Evaluation of three seventh-grade Project SMART cohorts. *Preventive Medicine, 19*, 305-313.

HANSEN, W. B., JOHNSON, C. A., FLAY, B. R., GRAHAM, J. W., & SOBEL, J. (1988). Affective and social influence approaches to the prevention of multiple substance abuse among seventh grade students: Results from Project SMART. *Preventive Medicine, 17*, 135-154.

HANSEN, W. B., & McNEAL, R. B., Jr. (1996). The law of maximum expected potential effect: Constraints placed on program effectiveness by mediator relationships. *Health Education Research, 11*, 501-507.

HANSEN, W. B., & McNEAL, R. B., Jr. (1999). Drug education practice: Results of an observational study. *Health Education Research, 14*, 85-97.

JOHNSON, C. A. (1982). Untested and erroneous assumptions underlying anti-smoking programs. In T. Coates, A. Peterson, & C. Perry (Eds.), *Promotion of health in youth* (pp. 149-165). New York: Academic Press.

KANDEL, D. B. (1975). Stages of adolescent involvement in drug use. *Science, 190*, 912-914.

LEUPKER, R. V., JOHNSON, C. A., MURRAY, D. M., & PECHACEK, T. F. (1983). Prevention of cigarette smoking: Three-year follow-up of an education program for youth. *Journal of Behavioral Medicine, 6*, 53-62.

MACKINNON, D. P., JOHNSON, C. A., PENTZ, M. A., DWYER, J. H., HANSEN, W. B., FLAY, B. R., & WANG, E. Y. (1991). Mediating mechanisms in a school-based drug prevention program: First-year effects of the Midwestern Prevention Project. *Health Psychology, 10*, 164-172.

McALISTER, A. L., PERRY, C. L., KILLEN, J., SLINKARD, L. A., & MACCOBY, N. (1980). Pilot study of smoking, alcohol, and drug abuse prevention. *American Journal of Public Health, 70*, 719-721.

PENTZ, M. A., DWYER, J. H., MacKINNON, D. P., FLAY, B. R., HANSEN, W. B., WANG, E. Y. I., & JOHNSON, C. A. (1989). A multi-community trial for primary prevention of adolescent drug abuse: Effects on drug use prevalence. *Journal of American Medical Association, 261*, 3259-3266.

ROHRBACH, L. A., SOBEL, J., HOLT, L., HANSEN, W. B., FLAY, B. R., & JOHNSON, C. A. (1985, November). *Process evaluation of a school-based drug abuse prevention program*. Paper presented at the annual meeting of the American Public Health Association, Washington, DC.

SCHAPS, E., DIBARTOLO, R., MOSKOWITZ, J., PALLEY, C. S., & CHURGIN, S. (1981). A review of 127 drug abuse prevention program evaluations. *Journal of Drug Issues, 22,* 17-44.

SUSSMAN, S. (1991). Curriculum development in school-based prevention research. *Health Education Research: Theory and Practice, 6,* 339-351.

SUSSMAN, S., DENT, C. W., STACY, A., SUN, P., CRAIG, S., SIMON, T. R., BURTON, D., & FLAY, B. R. (1993). Project Towards No Tobacco Use: 1-year behavior outcomes. *American Journal of Public Health, 83,* 1245-1250.

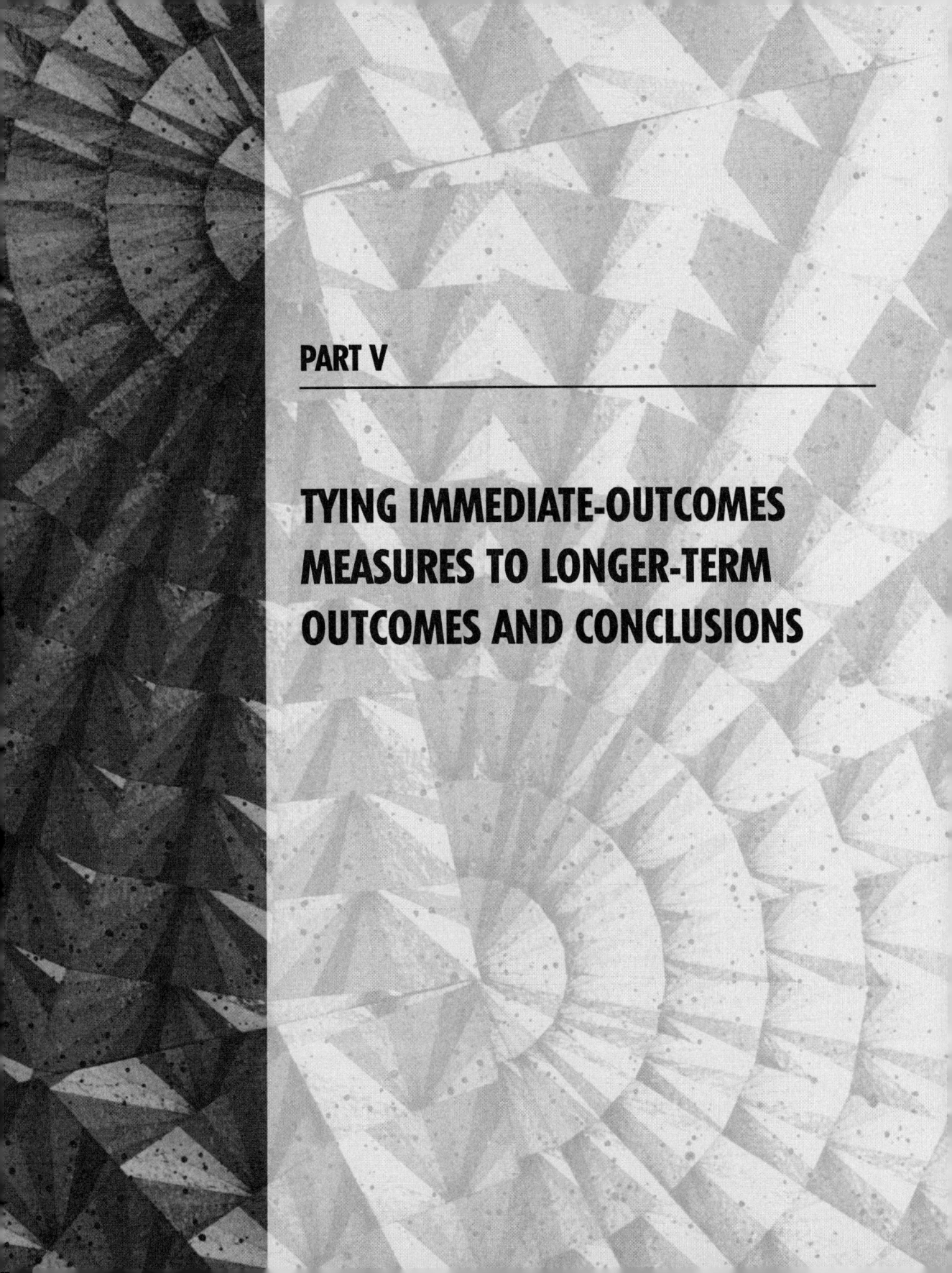

PART V

TYING IMMEDIATE-OUTCOMES MEASURES TO LONGER-TERM OUTCOMES AND CONCLUSIONS

CHAPTER 18

Using Meta-Analyses to Improve the Design of Interventions

Stewart I. Donaldson
Gordon P. Street
Steve Sussman
Nancy S. Tobler

Program development can be greatly enhanced by using systematically collected empirical data to guide design decisions. Empirical data may be used to complement hunches, observations, and anecdotal information gleaned from practice, and these data typically increase the program designer's confidence in the likelihood a program will succeed. This handbook describes in some detail how to use a theory-driven, empirically based approach to develop a program from its initial conception into full-scale program implementation and evaluation. The present chapter will discuss the potential benefits and pitfalls of using data that have been collected from previous research and practice to inform development of a health behavior program. Relevant empirical data from prior work can be used to make the initial conception of the program and selection of program activities as powerful as possible (also see Chapter 7, this volume, on pooling program information).

It may seem like a rather obvious suggestion to use the work of others in program development. That is, standing on the "shoulders of giants" or others who have been down the road one is about to travel forms the basis for most travel guides (this point is made in Chapters 4, 6, and 7, this volume). However, what is less obvious is how to accurately synthesize and apply this information to the design of a new intervention. A specific focus of this chapter will be placed on using meta-analysis, one of the newest techniques in the family of research synthesis strategies, to guide decisions being made during the program development phase of health behavior research and practice. In part, program development requires gathering and summarizing available data on the efficacy of variations in the contents and delivery modalities relevant to informed program planning. The purpose of meta-analysis is to provide a tight analytic structure to ensure that this process is conducted objectively and to produce results that are easy to interpret.

▶ META-ANALYSIS

Research synthesis attempts to illuminate consistencies and document variability in prior studies conducted within a defined program domain (Cooper & Hedges, 1994). Meta-analysis offers a range of statistical techniques that permit pooling findings from a variety of primary studies (i.e., single empirical works such as experiments, quasi-experiments, longitudinal measurement studies, and cross-sectional correlation studies). In contrast to traditional qualitative literature reviews, meta-analysis makes research synthesis an explicit scientific activity in its own right. That is, the meta-analyst goes through a similar set of stages required of any single scientific study: problem formulation, data collection, data evaluation, analysis and interpretation, and public presentation (Cook et al., 1992). Some of the primary characteristics of each of these stages are provided in Table 18.1.

STRENGTHS OF META-ANALYSIS

The advantages of using meta-analytic findings to inform program development may be best understood in comparison to the most common alternative sources of empirical information: the single health program study and the traditional qualitative literature review. The major advantage of using meta-analytic findings versus the single health program study is the potential for improved generalizability of findings or external validity (Hall, Rosenthal, Tickle-Degen, & Mosteller, 1994). Although single studies certainly vary on the degree to which findings are likely to generalize beyond their unique characteristics, findings from all primary studies are to some extent bound by the specific participant characteristics, situational factors, and research procedures used. By meta-analyzing findings over a number of primary studies, using different participants in different situations, and using different research procedures, one is able to get

TABLE 18.1 The Integrative Review as a Scientific Study

Stage of Research

Stage Characteristics	Problem Formulation	Data Collection	Data Evaluation	Analysis and Interpretation	Public Presentation
Research question asked	What evidence should be included in the review?	What procedures should be used to find relevant evidence?	What retrieved evidence should be included in the review?	What procedures should be used to make inferences about the literature as a whole?	What information should be included in the review report?
Primary function in review	Constructing definitions that distinguish relevant from irrelevant studies	Determining which sources of potentially relevant studies to examine	Applying criteria to separate "valid" from "invalid" studies	Synthesizing valid retrieved studies	Applying editorial criteria to separate important from unimportant information
Procedural differences that create variation in review conclusions	1. Differences in included operational definitions 2. Differences in operational detail	Differences in the research contained in sources of information	1. Differences in quality criteria 2. Differences in the influence of nonquality criteria	Differences in rules of inference	Differences in guidelines for editorial judgment
Sources of potential invalidity in review conclusions	1. Narrow concepts might make review conclusions less definitive and robust. 2. Superficial operational detail might obscure interacting variables.	1. Accessed studies might be qualitatively different from the target population of studies. 2. People sampled in accessible studies might be different from target population of people.	1. Nonquality factors might cause improper weighting of study information. 2. Omissions in study reports might make conclusions unreliable.	1. Rules for distinguishing patterns from noise might be inappropriate. 2. Review-based evidence might be used to infer causality.	1. Omissions of review procedures might make conclusions irreproducible. 2. Omission of review findings and study procedures might make conclusions obsolete.

SOURCE: Cooper (1982). Reprinted by permission.

a better estimate of the robustness or the external validity of a given finding or program effect. Thus, in most instances, meta-analytic findings should be a better source of information to use to shape one's understanding of program theory and to guide aspects of the design of a new intervention than findings from a single, primary study.

Meta-analysis also has important advantages over traditional literature reviews. Most traditional qualitative literature reviews use a "vote count" procedure to accumulate results across studies, which often does not account adequately for (a) statistical power issues (i.e., the ability to detect a true difference or program effect), (b) the methodological rigor of different primary studies, and (c) the possibility that other variables modify basic relationships between a program's inputs and its outcomes (Cook et al., 1992). For example, the traditional literature reviewer typically classifies how many studies show statistically significant results in the positive direction, negative direction, and how many are not statistically significant. The category with the most votes wins, and conclusions are drawn accordingly. In contrast, the meta-analyst estimates the magnitude of relationships between the intervention and outcomes regardless of whether statistical significance was found, differentially weights studies based on relevant factors such as quality of methodology and sample size, and controls for relevant variables that might influence the bivariate relationship between a program and outcome (e.g., dose, program fidelity). This results in an effect size estimate that can easily be used to determine the practical significance of the program. How to assess practical significance is discussed in more detail in a later section of this chapter on "Using Existing Meta-Analyses." In summary, meta-analytic reviews typically provide more precise estimates of the relationship between a program and its outcomes than traditional reviews because they overcome statistical conclusion validity problems that are likely to bias program effect estimates.

SOME LIMITATIONS OF META-ANALYSIS

Although meta-analysis has its virtues as a tool for synthesizing complex intervention research literatures, it is not without at least five potentially serious limitations. The main limitation of meta-analysis stems from the problem that it is usually impossible to access all relevant studies or to select a truly random sample of these studies in a particular program domain. For example, meta-analyses of the published literature may overestimate the magnitude of a program effect and possibly may even find a program effect when none exists. This would occur if positive evaluations in a particular area were more likely to be published and null or negative findings were more likely to remain in the investigators' file drawer, unavailable for research synthesis. In most program domains, it is believed that evaluations that fail to obtain effects often are not published and hence fail to be considered in research synthesis work, including meta-analysis (Matt & Cook, 1994). If one only synthesizes positive findings, assuming there are a substantial number of null or negative findings in an area, one could imagine finding a positive effect when none would exist if all studies were included. Therefore, it is critical to assess how well a particular meta-analysis has dealt with the "file drawer problem" (Rosenthal, 1995) and related sampling issues before using it to make key program design decisions (see Begg, 1994).

A related sampling problem is that only certain types of quantitative studies get included in meta-analyses. Even among published empirical works, many are excluded from a meta-analysis because the authors of these works fail to include basic statistics necessary for calculation of effect sizes (Sharpe, 1997). In other words, studies that use qualitative methods or that do not use quantitative techniques that easily convert to effect size estimates are systematically excluded from meta-analysis, thus limiting the generalizability of meta-analytic findings. Instead of simply excluding such studies from meta-analyses, corrective procedures and calculations have been used to produce an effect size estimator for a study. Ray and Shadish (1996) have demonstrated that some of these calculations produce overestimates of effect sizes, whereas others produce underestimates. Consequently, the methods of producing effect sizes for a meta-analysis also should be evaluated.

Another issue regarding different studies that are included in meta-analysis pertains to the study context dependence of effect size estimates. All else being equal (including the size of the true treatment effect), two studies that use different comparison groups will produce different effect size estimates. For example, some meta-analyses will combine studies that compare a treatment against no treatment (e.g., wait list control), but others will compare a treatment against an alternative treatment. The control group may show naturally occurring change or no change. However, the alternative treatment often will result in some change from baseline, which may result in a smaller effect size estimate. This is particularly important when evaluating meta-analyses that include single-group, pretreatment-posttreatment studies because they have no real comparison group at all. Instead, the pretreatment mean and standard deviation often are used as an estimate of a comparison group. Lipsey and Wilson (1993) found that effect sizes produced from single-group studies were 61% larger than those studies using control or comparison groups. Meta-analyses may or may not analyze and report separately these three types of comparisons to calculate an effect size (i.e., treatment vs. comparison, treatment vs. control, posttreatment vs. pretreatment).

Two other common threats to the validity of meta-analytic findings are problems due to mixing dissimilar studies and the inclusion of poor-quality studies (Sharpe, 1997). The first of these threats has been labeled mixing apples and oranges. Meta-analyses that combine statistical results from studies that manipulate and measure different variables among different participant populations may end up with a meaningless superordinate analysis. The key to overcoming this problem is to make sure the meta-analyst has selected a reasonable collection of studies to include in the pool—striking a balance between too broad and too narrow (Wartman, 1994). The second threat has been called "garbage in, garbage out" (Eysenck, 1978). In an effort to overcome study selection bias, some meta-analysts gather all available studies (e.g., Smith & Glass, 1977). Critics argue that including methodologically weak studies provides a distorted picture of the issue under investigation. It is important to consider how well a particular meta-analysis addresses the issue of variability in study quality. One other caveat: We cannot with any confidence ascribe causality to a relationship based on meta-analysis alone. The boundaries to how much we can learn about causation with meta-analysis are defined by the underlying primary studies (Wartman, 1994). Despite these potential limitations, meta-analyses that contain a thoughtful combination of qualitative and quantitative insights can dramatically improve the initial conception of a program, which can then be refined using an empirical program development approach (see Chapter 19, this volume; Sussman, Petosa, & Clark, 1996).

▶ META-ANALYSIS AND PROGRAM DEVELOPMENT

HOW TO INTERPRET THE RESULTS OF EXISTING META-ANALYSES

Calculations. This section describes the specifics of how to use meta-analysis for improving program development. In its best form, meta-analysis can provide program designers an accurate estimate of the relationships between a specific type of program and its desired outcomes across a range of implementation environments and participants. This estimate typically is expressed as an estimate of the effect size of the program on the outcome. The effect size is a population parameter that cannot be determined directly. Rather, it is an inference to a population based on sample distributions. It is estimated from the sample data collected as part of the primary studies. Statistical summaries of primary study data are used as single data points in a meta-analysis. Effect size is the ratio of the size of the difference between treatment (Mt) and control group (Mc) means over the common standard deviation (see Figure 18.1). Simply stated, the effect size estimate derived from a typical meta-analysis is the average effect size estimate across a range of primary studies.

It is important to evaluate the overall mean effect size of a treatment for variability and for appropriateness to the program that one hopes to develop. The standard deviation of the mean effect size and the range of the individual effect

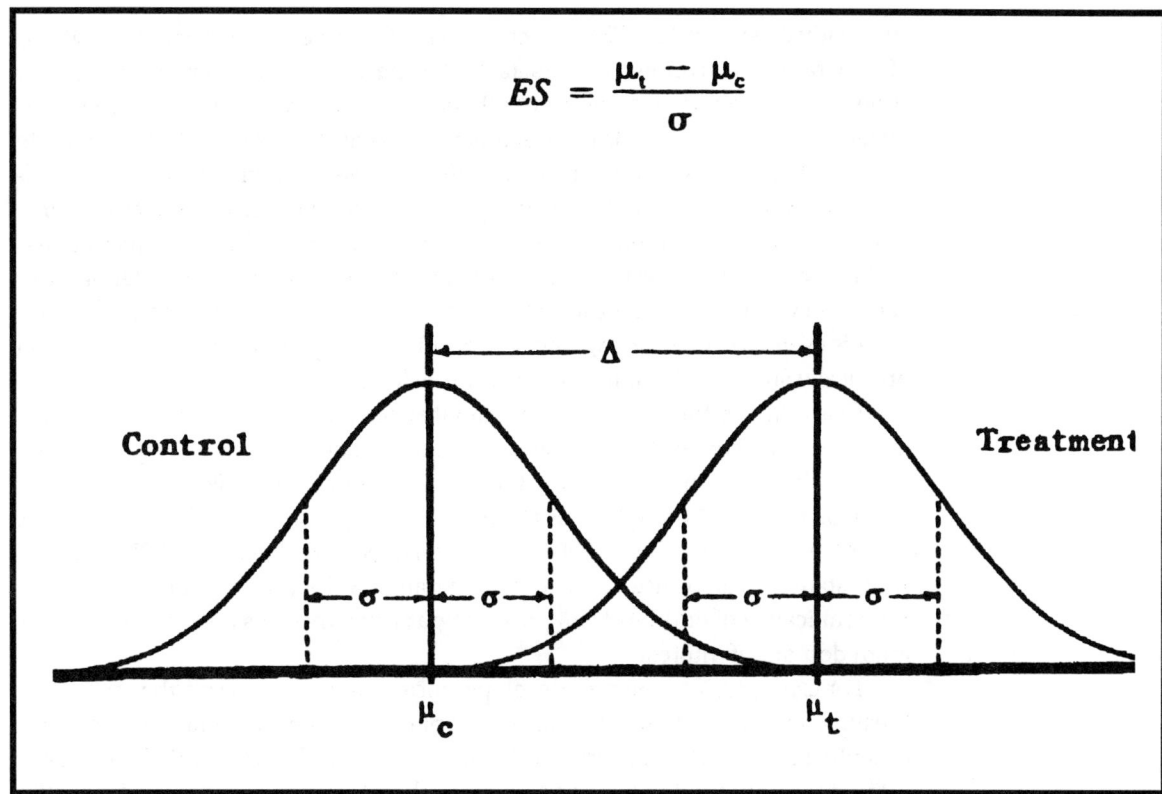

Figure 18.1. Effect Size (Lipsey, 1990)

sizes are typically presented in a meta-analysis. Also, the individual effect sizes and confidence intervals occasionally are presented for each study included in the meta-analysis. These data summaries can provide a rough indication of the range of outcomes that one might expect from a planned program. Sometimes, this variability may be considerable and raise concern that, despite a respectable overall effect size, a treatment may produce little to no benefit at all in certain contexts. One may want to examine the descriptions of the individual studies to determine which ones are more representative of the parameter that one's own program requires (studies that have similar populations, clinicians, etc.). Then one can examine the range and confidence intervals of these studies and calculate the mean effect size and standard deviation for this more focused subset of studies that are more relevant to one's program.

Once a program designer finds meta-analyses relevant to the new program being planned, she or he must be able to interpret the practical significance of these findings. Lipsey (1990) provides a framework for understanding the practical significance of effect size estimates of program effects. On the basis of the cumulative distribution of 102 selected mean effect sizes from 186 meta-analyses of program effectiveness studies (a meta-analysis of meta-analyses), Lipsey shows that an effect size between .00 and .32 should be considered small, between .33 and .55 should be considered medium, and between .56 to 1.20 should be considered a large effect in program effectiveness research. The wide, large effect category illustrates that some programs can have very strong effects. It is important to point out that this is a general framework for interpreting effect size estimates across a wide variety of program areas. The range for each category may vary somewhat based on the specific program domain. Nevertheless, this framework is useful to determine whether a specific type of program has demonstrated practically significant findings in previous evaluations.

One of the virtues of effect size estimates derived from meta-analyses is that they are easily converted into other common statistics, which is very useful for practical interpretation purposes. Table 18.2 provides effect size equivalents for common indices of strength of association (r^2 and r), Cohen's (1977) U3 measure, and Rosenthal and Rubin's (1982) "binomial effect size display" (BESD). Each of these statistics can be used to help the program developer understand the practical significance of findings from prior program effectiveness research in the program domain of interest.

For example, if a program developer locates a meta-analysis that estimates the effect size of a program similar to one planned to be .50 (a medium effect, as described earlier), she or he can use Table 18.2 to determine that this finding estimates that 6% of the variance ($r^2 = .06$) in the outcome is accounted for by the program. The planner can expect that his or her program will account for 6% of the variation in the health behavior. The next column shows that this statistic is equivalent to finding a correlation coefficient of $r = .24$ between the program and the outcome. Furthermore, Cohen's U3 measure (same row, third column in Table 18.2) estimates that 69% of the program or treatment group scored higher than the control group mean on the outcome measure of interest. (By comparison, if there was no effect [ES = .00], only 50% of the program group would have scored higher than the control group mean, and if ES = 1.2, 88% of the program group would have scored higher than the control group mean.)

A variation on Cohen's U3 percentage overlap index is the BESD (Rosenthal & Rubin, 1982). Rosenthal and Rubin suggest that for the purposes of illustrating ES, the success threshold can be presumed to be at the grand median for the combined treatment and control group distributions. This grand median standard presumes that when there is no effect (ES = .00), there will be a 50-50 success-failure split and a widening difference as the ES increases. In the example above, for an ES = .50, 62% of the program group would be considered successful, whereas only 38% of the control group would be successful (see column 4 in Table 18.2). Furthermore, this corresponds to a 24% differential between the two groups, as is shown in column 5. Consider a practical, concrete example for col-

TABLE 18.2 Effect Size Equivalents for ES, PV, r, and BESD (Lipsey, 1990)

ES	(1) PV (r²)	(2) r	(3) U3: % of T Above $\bar{X}_c$	(4) BESD C vs. T Success Rates		(5) BESD C vs. T Differential
0.1	.002	.05	54	.47	.52	.05
0.2	.01	.10	58	.45	.55	.10
0.3	.02	.15	62	.42	.57	.15
0.4	.04	.20	66	.40	.60	.20
0.5	.06	.24	69	.38	.62	.24
0.6	.08	.29	73	.35	.64	.29
0.7	.11	.33	76	.33	.66	.33
0.8	.14	.37	79	.31	.68	.37
0.9	.17	.41	82	.29	.70	.41
1.0	.20	.45	84	.27	.72	.45
1.1	.23	.48	86	.26	.74	.48
1.2	.26	.51	88	.24	.75	.51
1.3	.30	.54	90	.23	.77	.54
1.4	.33	.57	92	.21	.78	.57
1.5	.36	.60	93	.20	.80	.60
1.6	.39	.62	95	.19	.81	.62
1.7	.42	.65	96	.17	.82	.65
1.8	.45	.67	96	.16	.83	.67
1.9	.47	.69	97	.15	.84	.69
2.0	.50	.71	98	.14	.85	.71
2.1	.52	.72	98	.14	.86	.72
2.2	.55	.74	99	.13	.87	.74
2.3	.57	.75	99	.12	.87	.75
2.4	.59	.77	99	.11	.88	.77
2.5	.61	.78	99	.11	.89	.78
2.6	.63	.79	99	.10	.89	.79
2.7	.65	.80	99	.10	.90	.80
2.8	.66	.81	99	.09	.90	.81
2.9	.68	.82	99	.09	.91	.82
3.0	.69	.83	99	.08	.91	.83

umns 4 and 5. If one were talking about a smoking cessation program ($N = 200$ smokers in the program compared to $N = 200$ smokers in the control or comparison group), this would mean that 124 smokers who participated in the program of interest stopped smoking, in contrast to only 76 in the comparison program. In this context, a medium effect size of .50 appears "pragmatically" significant. It shows that 48 more people stopped smoking in the program group compared to the control group (i.e., the success differential shown in column 5 in Table 18.2).

Of course, presentation of these different estimates of effect sizes in the absence of other information can be misleading. A small effect may have enormous implications for health if it can save many lives. Because meta-analyses may overestimate effects of programming (null effects being less likely to appear in the literature), this problem is less likely to result from meta-analytic interpretation. However, if one simply looks at effect size as a rule for selection, other important information can get lost. For example, disseminability of a program is important to consider in addition to effect size. Certainly, effect size measures will continue to be a focus of discussion among statisticians and program developers. The measures provided herein are quite useful if one keeps in mind these other issues.

Using These Calculations to Plan New Programs. Having shown how to interpret the practical significance of effect size estimates, we will now consider the kinds of relationships a program designer might examine during program development. These relations provide a means to select feasible program components for new contexts. Four potential relations are identified here: strength of program effects over a range of program-constituent information, program-mediator links, mediator-outcome links, and moderator effects. The most common information available is the relationship between a specific type of program and its desired outcomes. The two most common aspects of a program that may be examined or varied are program content (e.g., consequences oriented vs. acquisition oriented) and type of delivery (e.g., didactic vs. interactive). Meta-analyses can be very useful for showing that over a range of implementation type and fidelity, specific content packages produce significantly stronger program effects. Of course, when these kinds of patterns emerge, they can be used to select or eliminate potential content areas and delivery approaches for the new program being planned (see Tobler & Stratton, 1997).

Many programs are conceptualized to consist of a number of components, often intended to lead to immediate or proximal changes (mediators) in participants that are presumed to later cause more distal intended outcomes (see Figure 18.2). Hansen and McNeal (1996) suggested that health behavior programs attempt to change these immediate factors, which, in turn, elicit desired outcomes. The outcomes typically studied are indirectly influenced by the program and are the result of whether the mediating factors are changed by the program and are

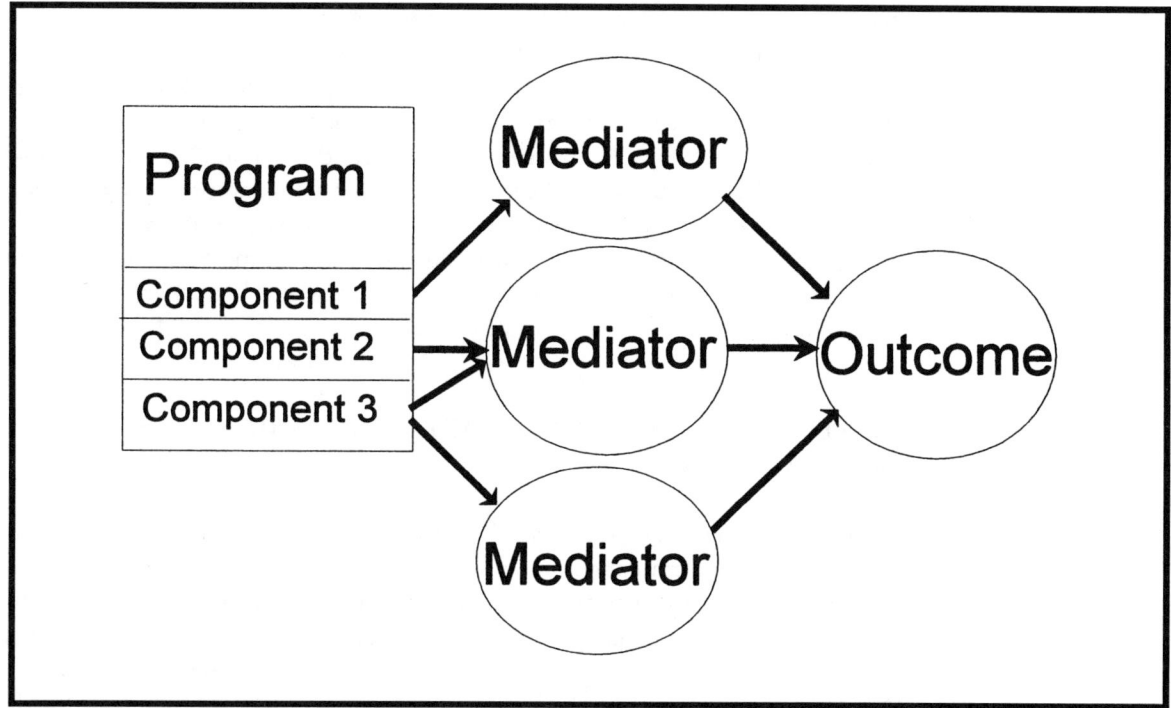

Figure 18.2. Three-Component Program

linked to the desired outcome. They call this the *law of indirect effect* in health behavior programming (see Chapter 19, this volume). Of course, some program, mediator, and outcome links occur quite proximally in time (e.g., smoking cessation), whereas other such links show long delays between changes in the mediator and observable changes on behavior (e.g., smoking prevention). Meta-analyses also can be useful for estimating the effect size between a program and its proximal outcomes (mediators) presumed to lead to desired health behavior change. Program-mediator "strength-of-link" information is very important to the program developer who is searching for program components that might alter hypothesized mediators of change in a certain context.

Meta-analyses also may help determine whether the link between the mediators (as shown in Figure 18.2) and the outcomes is likely to occur in a new program application. These links are critical because they ultimately determine how likely it is that a successful program, through changing mediator variables, is likely to produce health behavior change. Hansen and McNeal (1996) described this as the *law of maximum expected potential effect,* which suggests that the magnitude of change in a behavioral outcome that a program can produce is directly limited by the strength of relationships that exist between mediators and targeted behaviors (see Chapter 19, this volume). Meta-analyses of correlations or other measures of association between presumed mediators and outcomes, as opposed to the standardized difference effect sizes discussed in detail earlier, can be useful for estimating the maximum potential of a program to affect desired outcomes. Furthermore, Donaldson (Chapter 19, this volume) illustrates how moderator variables also are critical to an overall understanding of program development. Meta-analyses also may be used to estimate potential moderator effects in the new program. In particular, this information can be used to consider whether a program is likely to affect different genders or other subgroups within a population.

CONDUCTING ONE'S OWN META-ANALYSIS OF PREVIOUS RESEARCH

In some cases, previously published meta-analyses may have done much of the work if they overlap or contain a subset of studies that address one's area of interest. However, if one cannot find any meta-analytic reviews that adequately address the intervention program elements that one is attempting to assess, one may benefit from conducting a meta-analysis of one's own, if only a cursory one. Depending on the program development goals, this task may not be as difficult or time-consuming as it might sound, particularly if the focus is narrow. The procedures are fairly simple, and summaries of varying length and complexity have been published that can provide guidance (e.g., Durlak & Lipsey, 1991; Glass, McGaw, & Smith, 1981; Rosenthal, 1995).

Conducting a meta-analysis is much like conducting an individual study or evaluation of a program, except that the data are the effect sizes, and each subject is a study or evaluation rather than groups or individuals. Durlak and Lipsey (1991) conceptualize meta-analysis as composed of six major steps: (a) formulating the question, (b) searching for studies, (c) coding variables, (d) calculating effect sizes, (e) analyzing the data, and (f) drawing conclusions and interpretations. Tracking down all of the relevant studies for a meta-analysis for publication can take considerable time. In program development, one's time may be relatively limited, so one's sample of studies may be more skewed by ease of availability. Therefore, one should start as soon as possible to gather every study one can find relevant to the question, including unpublished studies. Excluding studies that failed to get published because they did not find significant results can result in a meta-analysis that overestimates the effectiveness of an intervention (Smith, 1980; as discussed previously herein). One should not rely only on computer database searches because researchers have found them unreliable, tending to miss as many as two out of three relevant studies (Durlak & Lipsey, 1991). One should supplement computer database searches by reviewing reference lists of relevant studies that one has already found and by contacting experts in the field for their published and unpublished studies and recommendations of additional studies to review.

Perhaps the most difficult and time-consuming step is coding the variables that will serve as the predictors and covariates in the meta-analysis. The more variables one determines are necessary to code, the longer this process can take, often averaging hours for each study in a published meta-analysis, so one should choose carefully. Variables that can be coded include demographic characteristics of participants (e.g., age, sex, ethnicity, education level, cognitive ability), intervention characteristics (e.g., duration, setting, mode of administration), and methodological considerations (e.g., research design, type of control group).

Because most intervention research compares data between groups, intervention study meta-analyses typically use a standardized group difference effect size statistic. Calculating this statistic actually can be quite easy if the studies provide three basic statistics for each group in the study: means, standard deviations, and sample sizes. The statistic is basically the difference between the means of two groups (e.g., a control or comparison group and a treatment group) divided by their pooled standard deviations. There are different ways to calculate the pooled standard deviations, depending on theoretical issues, but the most commonly used calculation is to multiply the standard deviation of each group by one less than its sample size, add the result, and then divide that by two less than the sum of both samples.

However, some studies do not report the necessary statistics. Alternative methods of calculating or estimating effect size must be used with recognition that the resulting effect sizes may not actually be equivalent to those produced using the basic formula (Ray & Shadish, 1996). If one is drawing studies from previously published meta-analyses that used standardized group mean effect sizes, one can borrow their effect size statistics rather than recalculating them with the recognition that the same cautions apply. Also, many studies may not use the same type of comparison group or sometimes any comparison group at all. In these cases, it will be important to include type of comparison group in the coding of variables so that differences between them can be analyzed and evaluated (i.e., separate analysis).

One analyzes effect sizes just like the dependent variables in individual studies. First, basic statistics (e.g., means, standard deviations, standard errors) should be calculated for the effect sizes across all studies and within important subsets of the studies. Rosenthal (1995) suggests calculating confidence intervals around each of the resulting average effect sizes to provide a sense of how big or small the overall effect of a treatment might really be across the studies or across subsets. Using a simple statistical calculator, one can enter the effect sizes of each study for the overall sample or subsets of the sample, and the mean and standard error can be produced. The 95% confidence interval is equal to the mean plus or minus two times the standard error. These confidence intervals allow quick evaluations regarding whether an effect size will be found significantly different from either another effect size or zero in further analyses.

Then, statistical analyses of the differences between those subsets can be conducted. For example, if differences in effectiveness between genders are a concern, an ANOVA could be conducted to determine if the effect sizes differed between studies that examined only women, those that examined only men, and those that included both men and women. *T* tests or contrasts could be used to assess differences between pairs or combinations of those subsets. Similarly, the same statistics could be run within studies that use different control groups (e.g., wait list control, pretest-posttest design) or other potentially influential methodological differences. Again, using the procedures described earlier can be very helpful when one cannot find any meta-analytic reviews that adequately address one's specific information needs.

USE OF META-ANALYSIS AS A MEANS OF EVALUATING COMPONENT OR PILOT STUDIES

Meta-analysis also presents program developers with new approaches for evaluating the success of a series of program components or pilot tests (these types of studies were discussed in Chapters 13 and 16, this volume). Such studies often are tested in the absence of a control group. A very simple approach would be to compare outcomes of program components or a pilot test directly to the BESD treatment group success rate estimates (see Table 18.2) that would be expected based on mean effect size for a treatment obtained from meta-analysis. As noted earlier, a treatment that is shown in meta-analysis to have ES = .50 would be expected to produce successful outcomes for 62% of those who received the treatment; a similar impact could be expected from a program component or pilot test. More realistically, variability due to random variation could be accounted for by determining ranges of expected outcomes. For a program component or pilot test that achieves an ES of .50 on a mediator variable and an ES standard deviation of .10, a successful outcome from 60% to 64% of program component or pilot test recipients might be expected to occur two thirds of the time. If the impact of the program component or pilot test has been determined, an estimated effect size can be determined for it from Table 18.2 and evaluated to determine if the obtained effect is falling within the expected effect size range. These comparisons would be quite rough, of course.

Another approach would be to conduct rudimentary meta-analysis on the component or series of components or the pilot test itself, using individual implementations (i.e., sequential trials) or components of the implementation (e.g., different sites, individual clinicians) to represent separate component or pilot studies. Pretreatment to posttreatment immediate-impact effects could be evaluated within each of these implementations, and effect sizes and confidence intervals could be calculated based on the differences between them. The purpose of evaluation is to determine how big or small the effects are for each component or pilot study implementation, how much variability there is between them, and how much consistency there is between them. If the implementations consistently produce positive effect sizes (subjects are changing in the desired direction on mediator variables) and the confidence intervals overlap above zero, the evidence of this meta-analysis suggests that the program component or pilot test version of a complete program is having some beneficial effect. If there are substantial differences between the effect sizes, the program developer can determine what is different between these implementations, determine which features promote better outcomes for clients, and modify existing or future implementations.

▶ SOME EXAMPLES OF META-ANALYSIS IN HEALTH BEHAVIOR RESEARCH AND PRACTICE

Over the past two decades, conventional qualitative analyses of the literature have not yielded convincing evidence for the efficacy of psychological, educational, and behavioral programs, collectively known as social programs. In fact, Rossi and Wright (1984) described the field of evaluation research as a "parade of close-to-zero effects." Rossi (1985) sardonically coined a series of laws that reflect the difficulties of producing social change through programs. The metallic laws of evaluation include the following:

1. *The iron law:* The expected value of any net impact assessment of any social program is zero.

2. *The stainless steel law:* The better designed the impact assessment of a social program, the more likely is the net impact to be zero.

3. *The copper law:* The more social programs are designed to change individuals, the more likely the net impact will be zero.

However, Lipsey and Wilson (1993) analyzed essentially the same evaluation literature using meta-analytic techniques and came to a very different conclusion about the field of program development. Meta-analytic reviews show a strong, dramatic pattern of positive overall effects that cannot readily be explained as artifacts of meta-analytic technique or generalized placebo effects.

More specifically, the most rigorous assessment of 156 meta-analyses, encompassing approximately 9,400 individual program effectiveness studies and more than 1 million individual participants, shows the average program effect size to be .47. Included in this work are a large number of health behavior meta-analyses, including, for example, the following:

1. patient education about treatment regimens, preventive behavior, self-care, and related topics—mean ES = .74 for all outcomes (Posavac, 1980);
2. physician-delivered smoking cessation/reduction programs—mean ES = .34 for quit rates (Dotson, 1990);
3. worksite smoking cessation/reduction programs—mean ES = .34 for quit rates (Fisher, 1990);
4. nonmedical psychologically based treatment of chronic pain—mean ES = 1.10 (Malone, Strube, & Scogin, 1989);
5. multidisciplinary treatments for chronic back pain—mean ES = 1.25 all outcomes (Flor, Fydrich, & Turk, 1992);
6. exercise interventions for depression—mean ES = .54 on depression (North, 1989);
7. educational interventions for diabetic adults—mean ES = .43 on knowledge, metabolic control, self-care, and psychological outcomes (Brown, 1990).

This research by Lipsey and Wilson (1993) is one of the most powerful examples of the value of meta-analysis for informing program development.

Other useful examples of the value of meta-analysis in health behavior programming can be found in the school-based drug abuse prevention area (see Tobler & Stratton, 1997). Meta-analysis in this arena has demonstrated knowledge and attitude changes for alcohol, tobacco, marijuana, and other illicit drug use. More important, although the magnitude for drug use behaviors is less, certain types of interventions are differentially effective in preventing, delaying, or decreasing the use of drugs. Combining short- and long-term effects across smoking and alcohol programs, Rundall and Bruvold (1988) showed a mean effect size for smoking behaviors of .25 ($n = 41$) and .14 ($n = 19$) for alcohol behaviors. Bangert-Drowns (1988) found a mean effect of .12 for 14 programs that included drug use measures. Tobler et al. (in press) meta-analyzed 207 programs and found that interactive programs that emphasize interactions and exchange with peers were statistically superior to noninteractive programs such as Drug Abuse Resistance Education (DARE) for all adolescents, including minority populations. In a subset of 93 high-quality, well-implemented programs, the interactive programs' mean effect size was .16 compared to .03 for the noninteractive programs. Using Rosenthal and Rubin's (1982) binomial effect size display, these modest effect sizes equal success rates of 8% and 1%, respectively. These meta-analytic findings suggest the value of designing future adolescent drug prevention programs to contain an interactive format.

CONCLUSION

Most would agree that developing effective health behavior programs is a challenging endeavor. It has been argued in this chapter that program development can be greatly enhanced by using meta-analyses of prior empirical studies to help guide program design decisions. Findings from systematic research syntheses should be used to complement, rather than replace, more qualitative descriptions and understanding of the new program content, context, participants, program delivery staff, and the like. This chapter has attempted to provide a balanced account of the strengths and weaknesses of using meta-analysis in program development. Furthermore, how to use existing meta-analyses and conduct one's own meta-analysis for program development purposes was described in some detail. Examples of meta-analyses from the health behavior literature were provided to illustrate many of the key points. It is hoped that the issues discussed in this chapter will be helpful toward the effort to develop more effective programs based on behavior science knowledge and principles, for the purpose of preventing and ameliorating some of our most pressing health and social concerns.

REFERENCES

BANGERT-DROWNS, R. L. (1988). The effects of school-based substance abuse education: A meta-analysis. *Journal of Drug Education, 18,* 243-264.
BEGG, C. B. (1994). Publication bias. In H. Cooper & L. V. Hedges (Eds.), *The handbook of research synthesis* (pp. 399-409). New York: Russell Sage.
BROWN, S. A. (1990). Studies of educational interventions and outcomes in diabetic adults: A meta-nalysis revisited. *Patient Education and Counseling, 16,* 189-215.
COHEN, J. (1977). *Statistical power analysis for the behavioral sciences.* New York: Academic Press.
COOK, T. D., COOPER, H., CORDRAY, D., HARTMAN, H., HEDGES, L. V., LIGHT, R. J., LOUIS, T. A., & MOSTELLER, F. (1992). *Meta-analysis for explanation: A casebook.* New York: Russell Sage.
COOPER, H. M. (1982). Scientific guidelines for conducting integrative research reviews. *Review of Educational Research, 52,* 291-302.
COOPER, H., & HEDGES, L. V. (1994). Research synthesis as scientific enterprise. In H. Cooper & L. V. Hedges (Eds.), *The handbook of research synthesis* (pp. 3-14). New York: Russell Sage.

DOTSON, J. H. (1990). Physician-delivered smoking cessation interventions: An information synthesis of the literature (Doctoral dissertation, University of Maryland, 1989). *Dissertation Abstracts International, 50,* 1953A.

DURLAK, J. A., & LIPSEY, M. W. (1991). A practitioner's guide to meta-analysis. *American Journal of Community Psychology, 19,* 291-332.

EYSENCK, H. A. (1978). An exercise in mega-silliness. *American Psychologist, 33,* 517.

FISHER, K. J. (1990). Worksite smoking cessation: A meta-analysis of controlled studies (Doctoral dissertation, University of Oregon, 1989). *Dissertation Abstracts International, 50,* 5007B.

FLOR, H., FYDRICH, T., & TURK, D. C. (1992). Efficacy of multidisciplinary pain treatment centers: A meta-analytic review. *Pain, 49,* 221-230.

GLASS, G. V., McGAW, B., & SMITH, M. L. (1981). *Meta-analysis in social research.* Beverly Hills, CA: Sage.

HALL, J. A., ROSENTHAL, R., TICKLE-DEGEN, L., & MOSTELLER, F. (1994). Hypotheses and problems in research synthesis. In H. Cooper & L. V. Hedges (Eds.), *The handbook of research synthesis* (pp. 17-28). New York: Russell Sage.

HANSEN, W. B., & McNEAL, R. B., JR. (1996). The law of maximum expected potential effect: Constraints placed on program effectiveness by mediator relationships. *Health Education Research, 11,* 501-507.

LIPSEY, M. W. (1990). *Design sensitivity.* Newbury Park, CA: Sage.

LIPSEY, M. W., & WILSON, D. B. (1993). The efficacy of psychological, educational, and behavioral treatment: Confirmation from meta-analysis. *American Psychologist, 48,* 1181-1209.

MALONE, M. D., STRUBE, M. J., & SCOGIN, F. R. (1989). Meta-analysis of non-medical treatments for chronic pain: Corrigendum. *Pain, 37,* 128.

MATT, G. E., & COOK, T. D. (1994). Threats to the validity of research synthesis. In H. Cooper & L. V. Hedges (Eds.), *The handbook of research synthesis* (pp. 399-409). New York: Russell Sage.

NORTH, T. C. (1989). The effect of exercise on depression: A meta-analysis (Doctoral dissertation, University of Colorado, 1985). *Dissertation Abstracts International, 49,* 5027B.

POSAVAC, E. J. (1980). Evaluations of patient education programs: A meta-analysis. *Evaluation and the Health Professions, 3,* 47-62.

RAY, J. W., & SHADISH, W. R. (1996). How interchangeable are different estimators of effect size? *Journal of Consulting and Clinical Psychology, 64,* 1316-1325.

ROSENTHAL, R. (1995). Writing meta-analytic reviews. *Psychological Bulletin, 118,* 183-192.

ROSENTHAL, R., & RUBIN, D. B. (1982). A simple, general purpose display of magnitude of experimental effect. *Journal of Educational Psychology, 74,* 166-169.

ROSSI, P. (1985, April). *The iron law of evaluation and other metallic rules.* Paper presented at State University of New York, Albany, Rockefeller College.

ROSSI, P. H., & WRIGHT, J. D. (1984). Evaluation research: An assessment. *Annual Review of Sociology, 10,* 331-352.

RUNDALL, T. G., & BRUVOLD, W. H. (1988). A meta-analysis of school-based smoking and alcohol-use prevention programs. *Health Education Quarterly, 15,* 317-334.

SHARPE, D. (1997). Of apples and oranges, file drawers and garbage: Why validity issues in meta-analysis will not go away. *Clinical Psychology Review, 17,* 881-901.

SMITH, M. L. (1980). Publication bias and meta-analysis. *Evaluation in Education, 4,* 22-24.

SMITH, M. L., & GLASS, G. V. (1977). Meta-analysis of psychotherapy outcome studies. *American Psychologist, 32,* 752-760.

SUSSMAN, S., PETOSA, R., & CLARK, P. (1996). The use of empirical curriculum development to improve prevention research. *American Behavioral Scientist, 39,* 838-852.

TOBLER, N. S., ROONA, M. R., OCHSHORN, P., MARSHALL, D. G., STREKE, A. V., & PARK, A. (in press). School-based adolescent drug prevention programs: 1998 meta-analysis. *Journal of Primary Prevention.*

TOBLER, N. S., & STRATTON, H. (1997). Effectiveness of school-based drug prevention programs: A meta-analysis of the research. *Journal of Primary Prevention, 18,* 71-128.

WARTMAN, P. (1994). Judging research quality. In H. Cooper & L. V. Hedges (Eds.), *The handbook of research synthesis* (pp. 97-110). New York: Russell Sage.

CHAPTER 18

Commentary

David Duncan

It has long been my belief that the most common reason for the failure of health behavior change programs has been poor choices of intervention strategies. Furthermore, I believe that these poor choices could have been avoided had the program planners done their homework in reading the available literature in the field. All too often, we seem not merely to persist in reinventing the wheel but to persevere in adopting the square model for our wheel in ignorance of others' past failures with square wheels. The general failure of planners and policymakers to use the available research has been discussed by many authors (Galster, 1999; *Getting Smart,* 1995; Hanson, 1997).

In teaching program planning, I have emphasized that a thorough literature review was an essential early step. I have found, however, that it is not enough simply to read the literature. It is necessary for planners to make a judgment based on that literature about what type of intervention is most likely to achieve the goals of their program with the population and setting they hope to serve.

Unfortunately, many planners seem to have little idea of how to make that judgment (*Getting Smart,* 1995). Some approach it as if they were choosing lunch in a cafeteria. One intervention looks particularly appetizing to them so they choose it. They do not examine the evidence for its effectiveness or seek any comparison between it and other alternatives. The literature, for them, is merely an array of choices from which they choose based on personal attraction.

Others behave like the carpenter whose only tool is a chisel. Just as the carpenter struggles to pound nails and cut lumber with his chisel, these persons try to achieve every goal with the same programmatic strategy. One may approach every problem armed with public service announcements, billboards, posters, and other mass media. Another tries to resolve every health problem with group training in stress management and self-esteem promotion. They search the literature only to find examples of the use of their favorite approach, not to compare the effectiveness of that approach to others.

Donaldson, Street, Sussman, and Tobler present meta-analysis as a systematic guide to making those critical choices among intervention strategies. I fully agree that meta-analysis can greatly enhance this process. There are, however, several additional points I think the reader should be aware of regarding the use of meta-analysis in selecting interventions. First, I want to revisit the issue of practical significance of meta-analysis findings. Most readers should be aware that a finding of statistical significance is quite a different thing from finding that the result is important. Significance only reflects our degree of confidence that there truly is a difference between two or more groups on some measure; it does not mean that the difference is great enough to be of any practical importance. In a large sample, one group of men may be found to be significantly taller than another group of men, but the mean difference in their heights could be as little as one inch.

Donaldson et al. describe effect sizes between .00 and .32 as small, between .33 and .55 as medium, and between .56 and 1.20 as large. An effect size greater than .55 certainly is likely to be statistically significant and very often also will have practical significance but not in all cases. In situations in which the preintervention variance was small, a change of one standard deviation may not be of much practical effect. Donaldson et al., for instance, note that an effect size of .50 represents only an explanation of 6% of the variance in outcomes. Although this may be perfectly adequate in some cases, 6% may be far too little bang for the bucks in other cases.

This is particularly true when the measure in use suffers from a plateau effect in the population or when the measure used has only a narrow range of possible scores. Take, for instance, an outcome measure of belief in the dangerousness of cocaine, which used a 6-point scale with points identified as very safe, safe, somewhat safe, somewhat dangerous, dangerous, and very dangerous. The preintervention mean might be 5.65 with a standard deviation of 0.40. An increase in the mean danger rating of 0.23 would be a large effect size and probably would be significant, but it would be only a change from an average rating of very dangerous to an average rating still of very dangerous (just a slightly more dangerous perception of cocaine).

Second, a rather more important problem is the likelihood that effect sizes found by meta-analysis will prove to be overestimates of the effect of the intervention in a real program. In the health care field, for instance, although Chalmers et al. (1987) report that meta-analytic conclusions about the effectiveness of treatments have been consistently supported by evidence from larger clinical trials, the impact of these treatments on the health of the population has been far less than predicted. The General Accounting Office (Silberman, Droitcour, & Scullin, 1992) has documented the consistent failure of new medical treatments to reduce death rates in the population to the extent predicted from the research data.

There are several possible explanations for these discrepancies between meta-analytic results and real-world experience. Subjects included in clinical trials and other studies often will have been carefully screened for suitability, resulting in the intervention being administered only to persons most likely to benefit from it. Being aware of the danger of Type III error (Basch, Sliepcevich, Gold, Duncan, & Kolbe, 1985; Steckler, 1989), the researchers may have taken careful precautions to guarantee that the intervention was fully implemented and that it was implemented by highly qualified personnel—conditions that may not be matched in the real world. It is also possible that the intensity of the intervention may have been greater in research settings than it will be in later community applications. Furthermore, studies in which the intervention failed to produce the expected results are less likely to have been published—the so-called file cabinet effect.

Finally, it is important for the planner to look at more than just the intervention and the outcomes studied in a meta-analysis. It also is important to examine the target populations and the settings in which the research studies were conducted and the impacts, if any, that these had on the effect sizes. It is important, for instance, that one should not select an intervention that has been found to be highly effective only for in-school populations of good readers if one's program will be community based and focused on academically unsuccessful adolescents.

Study design characteristics also should be considered in any meta-evaluation. These include all of the systematic aspects of the research design and procedure, except those that are part of the study context. Do not put your faith in an intervention that produced large effect sizes in only the weakest research designs but only small effect sizes in well-controlled experiments. Meta-analysis is a valuable tool for synthesizing the results of many studies in a way that can help us to make program-planning decisions. We need to be aware of the limitations of this approach to make intelligent use of it. With due regard for those limits, it will help us plan better interventions.

REFERENCES

BASCH, C. E., SLIEPCEVICH, E. M., GOLD, R. S., DUNCAN, D. F., & KOLBE, L. J. (1985). Avoiding Type III errors in health education program evaluations: A case study. *Health Education Quarterly, 12,* 315-331.

CHALMERS, T. C., LEVIN, H., SACKS, H. S., REITMAN, D., BERRIER, J., & NAGALINGAM, R. (1987). Meta-analysis of clinical trials as a scientific discipline: I. Control of bias and comparison with large co-operative trials. *Statistics in Medicine, 6,* 315-328.

GALSTER, G. (1999). The challenges for policy research in a changing environment. *Journal of Economic Perspectives, 9* [Online]. Available: http://www.urban.org/PERIODOCL/pubsect/pub_07.htm.

Getting smart, getting real: Using research and evaluation to improve programs and policies. (1995). Report of the Annie E. Casey Foundation's September, 1995 Research and Evaluation Congress [Online]. Available: http://www.aecf.org/aecpub/getsmart/aecget.htm.

HANSON, A. (1997). *Mental health parity: From research to policy* [Online]. Available: http://www.fmhi.usf.edu/parity/researchtopolicy.html.

SILBERMAN, G., DROITCOUR, J. A., & SCULLIN, E. W. (1992). *Cross design synthesis: A new strategy for medical effectiveness research* (Report No. GAO/PEMD-92-18). Washington, DC: General Accounting Office.

STECKLER, A. (1989). The use of qualitative evaluation methods to test internal validity. *Evaluation and the Health Professions, 12,* 115-133.

CHAPTER 19

Mediator and Moderator Analysis in Program Development

Stewart I. Donaldson

This chapter explores how mediator and moderator analysis can be used to help develop efficacious health behavior programs. Mediation analysis is most fruitfully employed in the analysis of previous main trial data and at the pilot-testing phase of program development, when multiple program components have been placed together into the same program and immediate-outcome mediator measures of these sets of components can be refined and tested with a relatively large sample. Thus, this chapter is placed toward the end of the text. Certainly, however, several of the lessons provided herein (in particular, a visual conceptual framework of main effects, mediator, and moderator models) are relevant to earlier stages of program development, including the advancement of theory development (Chapter 4, this volume), pooling programming (Chapter 7), and development of immediate-outcomes measures in perceived efficacy and component studies (Chapters 9, 11, and 13). Program conceptual frameworks hypothesizing mediator and moderator relationships among variables, in combination with empirical feedback, are used to guide program development. This approach promises to identify (a) which program components are most effective, (b) the mediating causal processes through which they work, and (c) the characteristics of the participants, service providers, settings, and the like that moderate the relationships between a program and its outcomes. Examples from the health behavior literature are used to illustrate the value of conceptualizing and analyzing mediator and moderator relationships in health behavior program development and evaluation.

Social programming in general—and, more specifically, health behavior intervention research—has a history filled with illustrations of "black-box," "input/output," or outcome-focused investigations. For example, Lipsey and Wilson (1993) meta-analyzed 111 meta-analyses of intervention studies across a wide range of program domains (representing evaluations of more than 10,000 programs) and reported that most of this literature is based on only crude outcome research with little attention to potential mediating and moderating factors. They suggested that the proper agenda for the next generation of program evaluation should focus on which program components are most effective, the mediating causal processes through which they work, and the characteristics of the participants, service providers, settings, and the like that moderate the relationships between a program and its outcomes.

It is argued in this chapter that this agenda should be broadened to aid in the development of better programs as well as their eventual evaluation. A basic premise is that health behavior interventions are much more likely to be successful if they are developed using a theory-driven, empirically based program development approach (see Chen, 1990; Donaldson, 1995a, 1995b; Sussman, 1991; Sussman, Dent, Burton, Stacy, & Flay, 1995; Sussman, Petosa, & Clarke, 1996). This approach rests on using empirical feedback to guide program development. Succinctly stated, first the *process* through which program components are presumed to affect outcomes and the *conditions* under which these processes are believed to operate are conceptualized. For example, a *mediator* is a variable that is affected by the program, which in turns affects the outcome of interest. In contrast, a *moderator* variable affects the direction or strength of the relationships between the program and a mediator or a mediator and an outcome. Next, hypothesized mediator and moderator relationships are examined by piloting the program or components of the program and conducting rather small-scale data collection efforts (see Chapters 13 and 16, this volume). Data about the program are used to refine the conceptual framework, and the data collection process is repeated until the program developer decides the program is worthy of full-scale implementation and evaluation (see Figure 19.1). The definitions and use of mediator and moderator variables in program development are described in more detail in this chapter.

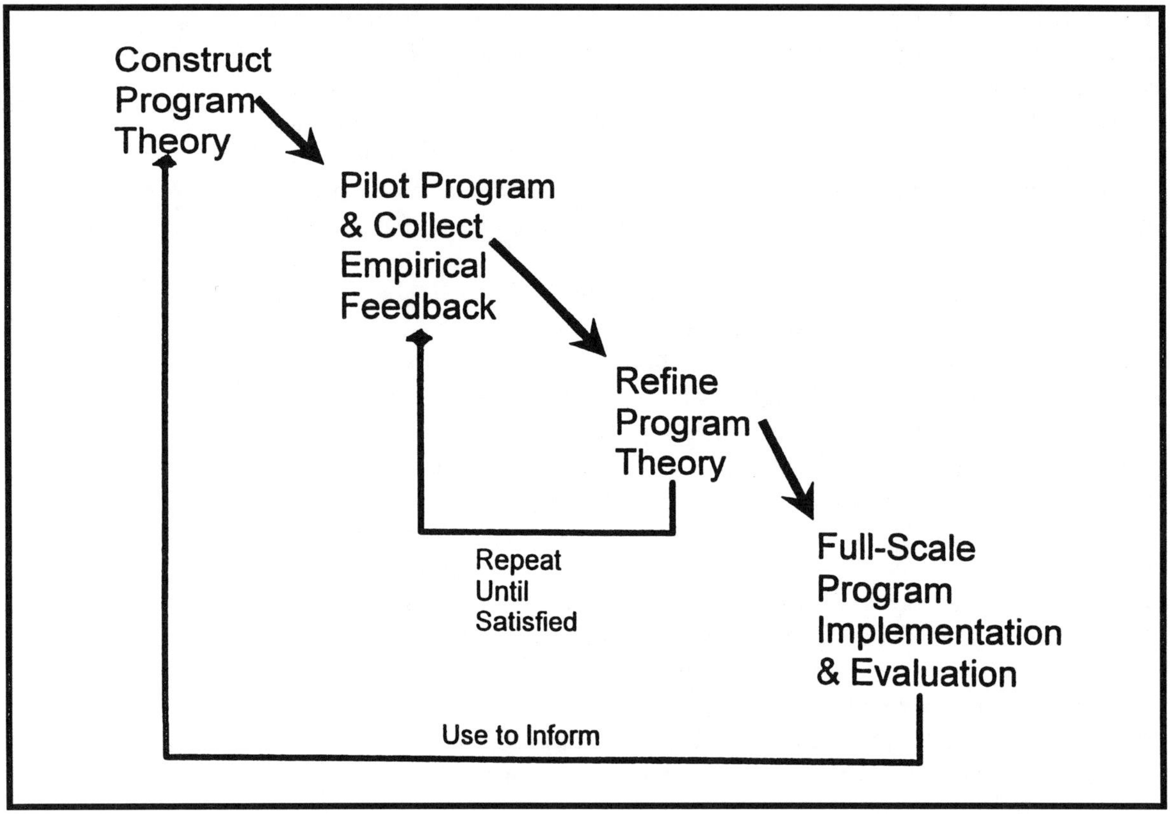

Figure 19.1. Program Theory Development

▶ DEVELOPING CONCEPTUAL FRAMEWORKS

Many health behavior programs represent practitioners' best guesses or opinions about how to improve desired outcomes. Although practitioners' perspectives are certainly important, they often can be made much more potent when they are used as a starting point in a systematic program development process (see Chapter 1, this volume). Using a theory-based evaluation framework (Chen, 1990), the first task of systematic program development is to develop a conceptual framework of how the program intends to achieve its objectives. In some cases, this may be purely the program designers' view of the program. Often, this view is implicit, and the task is to make this view or program theory explicit and testable. However, it is often possible and highly desirable to base this conceptual framework on multiple sources of information such as (a) prior theory and research in the program domain (see Chapters 4-6), (b) implicit theories held by those closest to the operation of the program (program personnel such as health educators or other human service providers), (c) observations of the program in action, and, in some cases, (d) exploratory research to test critical assumptions about the nature of the program (see Donaldson, 1995a, 1995b; Lipsey & Pollard, 1989; Weiss, 1997).

Programs can be conceptualized to take on many theory forms (Lipsey & Pollard, 1989). However, in the health behavior domain, variable-oriented models are the standard. Variable-oriented theory forms depict a causal process presumed to work in terms of variables and the covariation among those variables. For example, a health education program might be postulated to improve dietary knowledge, which is presumed to improve dietary behavior. This simple model asserts that the program is related to both dietary knowledge and dietary behavior and that they are related to each other. Of course, it is easy to conceptualize some programs to include a large number of variables and various types of relationships among variables. Part of the task of developing a conceptual framework during the program development phase is to find a parsimonious model that is likely to account for a large percentage of the variance in the desired outcome variables. That is, a model is needed that explains why participants who receive the program would do better on the desired outcomes than those who receive a control or comparison program.

Although some program conceptual frameworks can be complex and contain a large number of variables within the framework, relationships among variables are typically described as one of three basic types: (a) direct or main effects, (b) indirect or mediator relationships, or (c) moderator relationships. That is, program conceptualization in health behavior programming usually breaks down into direct, mediator, and moderator relationships between variables. Below, I describe how each type of relationship is used to represent health behavior programs.

DIRECT EFFECT

In the past, the standard and most common conceptualization of a health behavior program was known as a direct effect. That is, a program was typically conceived to affect an outcome or outcomes (see Figure 19.2). Health behavior programs were focused on outcomes such as increased physical activity, improving eating habits, weight loss, smoking cessation, and the like. The focus of most program developers was to include as many activities as possible in the program in an effort to make sure outcomes were in fact improved. The task of the evaluation researcher was to demonstrate whether a program did improve desired outcomes. Reviews of the program evaluation literature over the past two decades have found that, in most studies, programs are conceptualized as undifferenti-

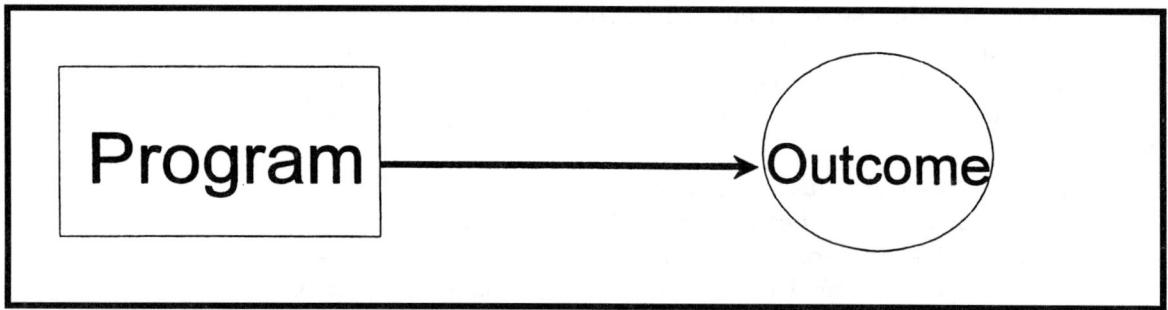

Figure 19.2. Direct-Effect Program Conceptualization

ated "black-box" treatment packages and only report information about direct effects (Lipsey, 1988; Lipsey, Crosse, Dunkel, Pollard, & Stobart, 1985; Lipsey & Wilson, 1993).

One main limitation of the direct-effect conceptualization and evaluation is that little is learned when there is no overall program effect. For example, the researcher is not able to disentangle the success or failure of program implementation from the validity of the conceptual model on which the program is based (Chen, 1990; Donaldson, 1995a, 1995b). Similarly, there is no way to sort out which components of a program are efficacious and which are ineffective or actually harmful. Another serious problem with the direct-effect conceptualization is that, arguably, behavioral interventions have only indirect effects. Hansen and McNeal (1996) call this the *law of indirect effect*:

> This law dictates that direct effects of a program on behavior are not possible. The expression or suppression of a behavior is controlled by neural and situational processes over which the interventionist has no direct control. To achieve their effects, programs must alter processes that have the potential to indirectly influence the behavior of interest. Simply stated, programs do not attempt to change behavior directly. Instead they attempt to change the way people think about the behavior, the way they perceive the social environment that influences the behavior, the skills they bring to bear on situations that augment risk for the occurrence of the behavior, or the structure of the environment in which the behavior will eventually emerge or be suppressed. The essence of health education is changing predisposing and enabling factors that lead to behavior, not the behavior itself. (p. 503)

Another way to restate this law is to say that a program affects immediate-outcome variables directly (which may include changes in attitudes or results of behavioral skills training) and long-term outcome variables indirectly (the targeted health behavior). Therefore, the direct-effect conceptualization alone adds

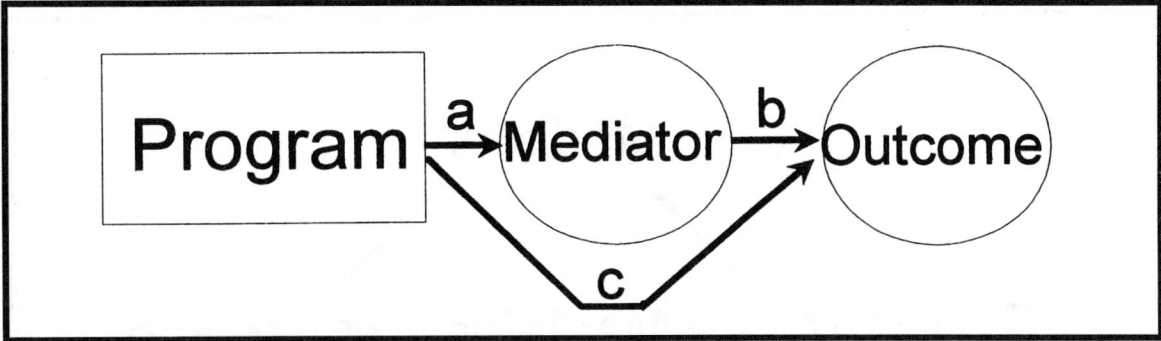

Figure 19.3. Indirect-Effect Program Conceptualization

little value to the process of theory-driven, empirically based program development.

MEDIATION MODELS

In contrast, using an indirect-effect conceptualization of a program can dramatically improve understanding about a program's functioning. I will illustrate this point first by modestly adding only one additional variable to the direct-effect conceptualization shown in Figure 19.2. Figure 19.3 illustrates a basic two-step mediation model. This model shows that the program affects the mediator (Path a), which in turn affects the behavioral outcome (Path b). Path c represents the residual direct effect. Theoretically, if Path c is zero, the mediator variable is the lone cause of the outcome. If Path c is nonzero, there are believed to be additional mediators (as yet unexplained) that explain the link between the program and the outcome. It is important to note that with just this additional variable, a researcher is now in a position to determine (a) whether the program was effective enough to alter its target (i.e., success or failure of program implementation) and (b) whether the program is aimed at the right target (the validity of the conceptual model; i.e., does the mediator variable in fact improve the outcome variable?).

Most health behavior programs are considered to be multiple-component interventions, which are more accurately conceptualized to contain multiple-mediator variables (e.g., see Figure 19.4). In the practice of program development, it is probably most often the case that program components reflect the program developer's view of how to optimize the chances of obtaining desired outcomes, rather than a combination of components shown to be effective (cf. Hansen, 1993). West and Aiken (1997) described fundamental tensions between

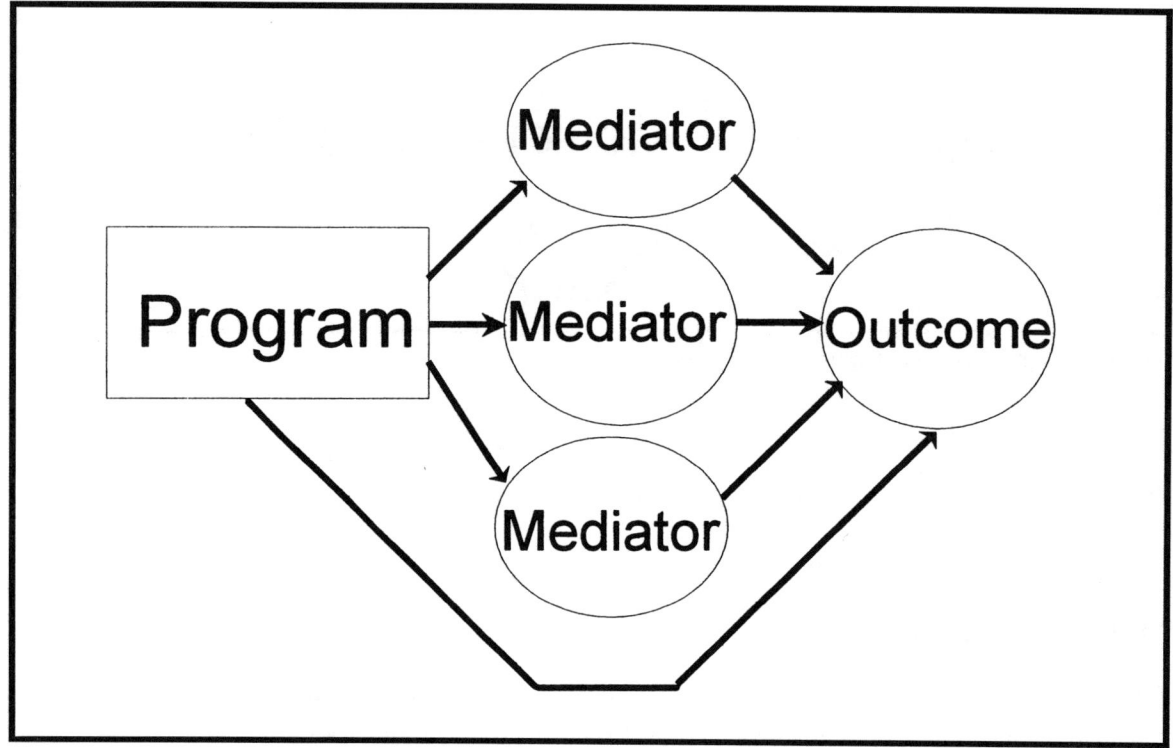

Figure 19.4. Multiple-Mediator Model

program developers and evaluation researchers associated with the development of multicomponent programs. Put simply, although program developers are primarily concerned with maximizing the efficacy of the entire program, evaluation researchers have become increasingly concerned with how each component affects targeted mediators or risk factors and which, in turn, produce their effects on the desired outcomes.

I submit that more complex multiple-mediator model conceptualizations of health behavior programs are usually necessary to accurately reflect the multicomponent nature of programs. These conceptualizations can enhance the program development process by more precisely identifying the program characteristics that are presumed to influence each target mediator. Pilot empirical work can then be conducted to estimate whether it is likely that each individual program component will have a large enough effect on the targeted mediators to have an effect on desired outcomes when the program is actually implemented. Carefully selecting mediators to explain and maximize the effects of the program should be the common goal of program developers and evaluators.

Another important benefit of conceptualizing a program in this way is that it exposes often implicit theoretical program mechanisms. That is, the paths going from the mediators to the outcomes represent the conceptual foundation of the program. In some cases, the link between the assumed risk factor (mediator) and outcome has been well established in prior research. In other cases, there is considerable ambiguity about the links. It is not uncommon for program developers who use this approach to modify the program dramatically because the original conceptual links appear very unrealistic once they are exposed. It is important to keep in mind that the magnitude of change in a behavioral outcome that a program can produce is directly limited by the strength of the relationships that exist between mediators and outcomes, according to Hansen and McNeal (1996). Hansen and McNeal describe this as the *law of maximum expected potential effect*:

> The magnitude of change in a behavioral outcome that a program can produce is directly limited by the strength of relationships that exist between mediators and targeted behaviors. The existence of this law is based on the mathematical formulae used in estimating the strength of mediating variable relationships, not from empirical observation, although we believe that empirical observations will generally corroborate its existence. An understanding of this law should allow intervention researchers a mathematical grounding in the selection of mediating processes for intervention. An added benefit may ultimately be the ability to predict with some accuracy the *a priori* maximum potential of programs to have an effect on targeted behavioral outcomes, although this may be beyond the current state-of-the-science to achieve. (p. 502)

This does not mean that a program might not achieve strong effects without knowledge of all its mediators of effects. However, better control over programming would be achieved by such knowledge. Furthermore, this does not mean that composite, diffuse mediators such as perceived program quality are not adequate for some program development purposes. Certainly, perceived program quality is affected by the impact of the program, and it predicts later behavior change. However, knowledge of specific mechanisms of change provides better prediction of ultimate, behavioral program effects. Therefore, it is critical to make sure that the program is aiming at the right targets (mediators) if it is going to have any chance of achieving outcomes.

PATH MODERATORS

In general, a moderator is a qualitative (e.g., gender, ethnicity, socioeconomic status, intelligence) or quantitative (e.g., program attendance, integrity of the program) variable that affects the direction or strength of the relationships

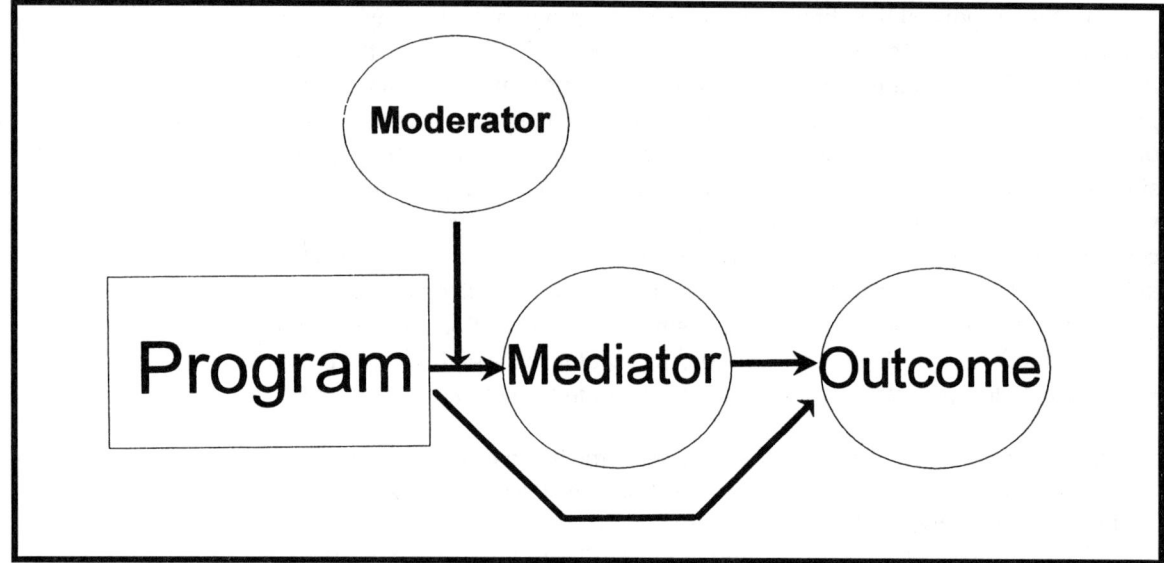

Figure 19.5. Moderator of Program-Mediator Relationship

between the program and mediator or mediator and the outcome (see Baron & Kenny, 1986). Figure 19.5 illustrates that Moderator 1 conditions or influences the path between the program and the mediator. This means that the strength or the direction of the relationship between the program and the mediator is significantly affected by the moderator variable. This type of moderator relationship is of primary importance in program development. Program developers can benefit greatly from considering if potential moderator variables such as participant characteristics, provider characteristics, characteristics of the setting of program implementation, strength of the programs, and program fidelity significantly influence the program's ability to affect target mediators.

Figure 19.6 illustrates that Moderator 2 conditions the path between the mediator and outcome. This type of relationship addresses the generalizability of the presumed program mechanism. For example, is the relationship between the mediator and the outcome the same for (a) females versus males, (b) inner-city children versus children living in the suburbs, or (c) Latinos, African Americans, Asian Americans, and European Americans? Although it is most often the case that the relationships between the mediators and program are presumed to generalize across all participants, in some cases it is possible that participant characteristics condition the relationships between the mediators and outcomes. Assessing this type of moderator relationship is usually not feasible during the program development phase. Nevertheless, it is important to identify significant moderators of all paths when conceptualizing how a program is presumed to

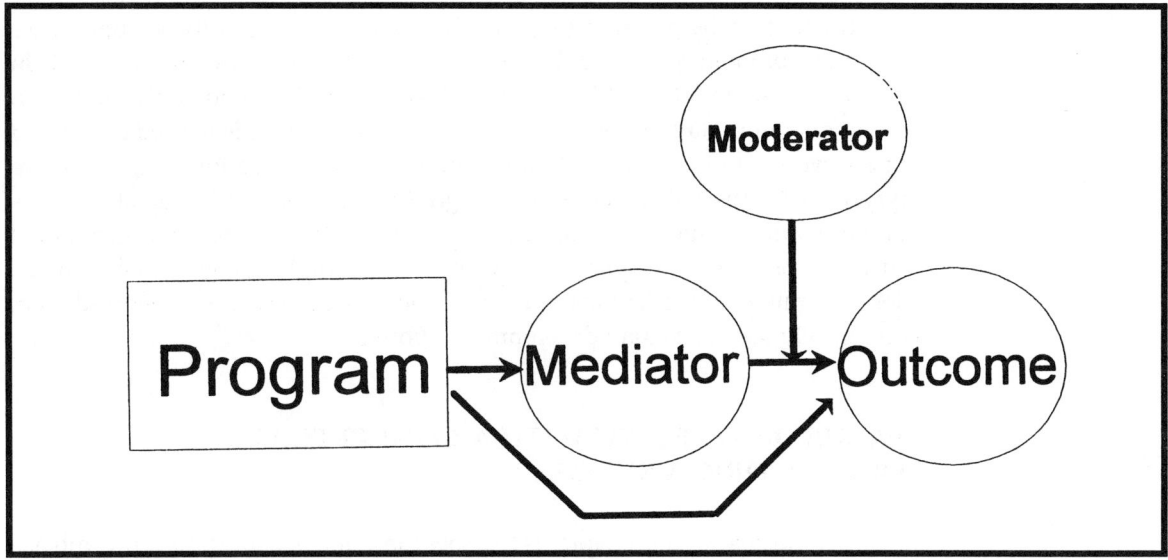

Figure 19.6. Moderator of Mediator-Outcome Relationship

work. These relationships may be critical to understand the program effects, or the lack thereof, later on when the program is being evaluated.

ALTERNATIVE CONCEPTUALIZATIONS

This chapter is focused on analyzing mediator and moderator relationships during program development. However, it is worth mentioning that there are alternative ways programs may be conceptualized. First, Lipsey and Pollard (1989) pointed out that although variable-oriented thinking is ubiquitous in the social sciences, much of what is of interest in program development and evaluation is not the status of variables but the status of persons (e.g., are they healthier?). They illustrate person-oriented conceptual frameworks by describing stage state models, including a concrete example provided by Runyan (1980). Furthermore, Collins, Graham, Rousculp, et al. (1994) have introduced a relatively new methodology, latent transition analysis, which allows for the examination of stage-sequential development of persons. Examples of stage-sequential program models are presented in Collins, Graham, Rousculp, and Hansen (1997) and Collins, Graham, Long, and Hansen (1994). Although person-oriented models represent a promising alternative for conceptualizing programs, this approach is still relatively new, and its value in program development is yet to be demonstrated.

Others have discussed how to develop more complex logic models to graphically represent management objectives, actual project operations, and the logical structure of the program (e.g., see Smith, 1989). Most of these approaches share the ultimate goal of developing a conceptualization of the program in which measurements could be taken to test assumptions and verify mediation and moderator relationships. Finally, the discussion above is limited to cases of one wave (set) of mediators. More complex conceptualizations might involve two or more waves of mediators. Although these models may be valuable in certain program evaluation situations, it is important to note that testing a model such as this typically requires a very large and complex longitudinal data set. Testing multiwave mediation models is beyond the scope of most theory-driven, empirically based program development efforts.

VALUE OF STARTING WITH A CONCEPTUAL FRAMEWORK: A SUMMARY

The purpose of this chapter is to show the value of conceptualizing and assessing mediator and moderator relationships during program development. I argue that there is great value in thinking through the logic or rationale for the various program activities prior to implementation and evaluation. This conceptual framework or program theory, often a refined set of mediator and moderator relationships, ultimately can be used

1. to disentangle the success or failure of program implementation (*action theory*) from the validity of program theory (*conceptual theory*);
2. as a basis for informed choices about evaluation methods;
3. to identify pertinent variables and how, when (e.g., dose-response and intervention-decay functions), and on whom they should be measured;
4. to carefully define and operationalize the independent (program) variables;
5. to identify and control for extraneous sources of variance;
6. to alert the program developer and evaluator to potentially important or intrusive interactions (e.g., differential participant response to the intervention);
7. to dictate the proper analytical or statistical model for data analysis and the tenability of the assumptions required in that model; and
8. to make a thoughtful and probing analysis of the validity of program evaluation in a specific context and provide feedback that can be used to improve the program under investigation while developing a cumulative wisdom about how programs work and when they work (cf. Baranowski,

Lin, Wetter, Resnicow, & Hearn, 1997; Bickman, 1987; Chen, 1990; Donaldson, 1995a, 1995b; Lipsey, 1993; Lipsey & Pollard, 1989).

EMPIRICAL CONFIRMATION ◄

So far, I have described only the first step of conceptualizing the program under investigation, which is shown as constructing program theory in Figure 19.1. Once we have done our best initial thinking about the program, it is time to test some of the assumptions of the framework. That is, the next challenge is to obtain empirical data to assess if initial mediator or moderator relationships match the reality of the participant experiences. As illustrated in Figure 19.1, empirical feedback (data) is used to refine program theory in an iterative fashion. That is, small-scale studies are conducted during program development in an effort to confirm or refine program theory and to strengthen the program.

Others have discussed in some depth systematic strategies (West & Aiken, 1997) and models (Sussman, 1991; Sussman et al., 1995, 1996) for empirically testing hypothesized program mediators and moderators during program development. For example, Sussman (1991) proposed a four-step empirical curriculum development model that consists of (a) adopting and extending a theoretical knowledge base on prior research in the program domain; (b) pooling curriculum activities from similar programs shown to be effective, as well as developing new activities to target potential mediators (risk factors) not previously addressed; (c) testing individual activities using focus groups, theme studies, and experimental and quasi-experimental component studies; and (d) combining activities and lessons to produce a full curriculum to be tested using feasibility and pilot studies. Results from a model such as Sussman's can provide valuable information for refining program theory and for strengthening a program before it is fully implemented. (An updated "chain model" is presented in Chapter 1, this volume.)

PROGRAM-MEDIATOR RELATIONSHIPS

When using empirical data to refine or confirm the program conceptualization during program development, one must focus on the program-mediator relationships. That is, the emphasis is on assessing whether the program is able to change target mediators. For example, Figure 19.7 illustrates a multicomponent (three-component) program designed to affect three mediators. Note that although program Components 1 and 2 are presumed to affect one specific mediator, Component 3 is theorized to affect both Mediators 2 and 3. This is meant to illustrate that program activities may be designed to affect more than one mediator, and one mediator may be targeted by more than one program component. As described by Sussman (1991) and West and Aiken (1997), quantitative or qualitative methods can be employed to give some indication of how well the program appears to be affecting the mediators by using a small sample of participants receiving a component, some combination of program components, or the entire program curriculum. However, it is important to note that one of the greatest challenges of empirical confirmation or disconfirmation during program development is to obtain trustworthy empirical information. The risks and concerns about data quality are discussed below.

MODERATORS

Investigating the extent to which program-mediator relationships are affected by key moderator variables also can yield important information during program development. For example, participant characteristics such as gender, ethnicity, socioeconomic status, relevant experience, and the like may affect how well the program is received and consequently the program's ability to change target mediators in some subgroups. In Figure 19.7, it can be seen that program Component 1 may significantly affect Mediator 1 among female participants but not among male participants. This would suggest that adjustments in program content are necessary if the goal is to change the behavior (outcome) of both female and male participants.

Service provider characteristics, characteristics of the setting of program implementation, strength of the program, and program fidelity are other common moderators that can be examined during program development. Identifying the optimal strength of a program or dose-response function can be a critical issue to examine in program development (Lipsey, 1990). The dose-response function describes the relationship between the dose of the program delivered to participants (e.g., weak dose, moderate dose, strong dose) and the targeted mediators. It is not uncommon for a relatively strong dose of a program (e.g., 8-week curriculum) to affect mediators significantly more than a relatively weak version of the program (e.g., 1-day workshop). This would indicate that the strength of the program is a significant moderator variable. However, in other cases, a relatively weak dose may have the same effect on mediator variables as stronger doses, indicating that the additional time and resources needed to provide the higher dose of the program are not needed or cost-effective. Obviously, finding the optimal dosage of a program during program development can dramatically increase the chances that the program eventually will be shown to be effective.

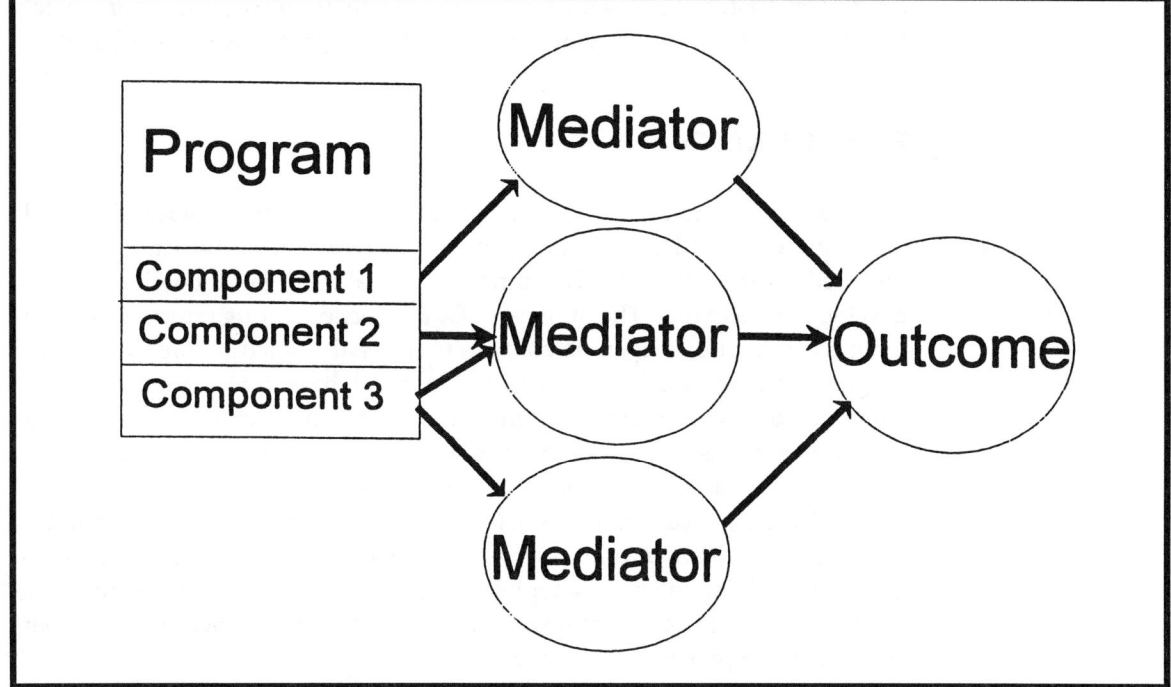

Figure 19.7. Three-Component Program

MEDIATOR-OUTCOME RELATIONSHIPS

It is typically much more difficult to test mediator-outcome relationships using empirical evidence collected during program development than it is to examine program-mediator relationships. In many situations, mediators are measured immediately following the program, whereas outcomes are measured at later points. That is, once a program has changed its targeted mediating variables, it usually takes some time before the mediators produce changes in health behavior. Although there certainly are exceptions, it is usually more fruitful to review prior research establishing the strength of the relationships between a program's target mediators and target outcomes (see also Chapter 7, this volume). If previous studies on the whole suggest weak or nonexistent relationships, it is important to think carefully about how likely previous findings generalize to the program under development. If it seems highly likely that negative findings could generalize, it might be worth abandoning those target mediators that are unlikely to affect outcomes. In addition, evidence showing strong moderator relationships between target mediators and outcomes may suggest the conditions under which the program should be implemented. Again, due to time and resource constraints, it is usually not feasible to gather quality data to adequately test mediator-outcome relationships while the program is being developed.

DATA QUALITY

I have been careful not to advocate a specific method or methods of data collection that should be used during program development. Rather, I have emphasized the development of a strong conceptual framework to guide program development activities. The purpose of data collection during program development is to examine, as rigorously as possible given the practical constraints of the program development context, the likelihood that the components of the framework will hold up when the program is fully implemented and evaluated. The inherent dilemma is that program developers most often must rely on data that could have serious limitations by common evaluation research standards. Nevertheless, by using focus groups, theme studies, interviews, surveys, experimental and quasi-experimental component studies, and the like to gather some data to examine mediator and moderator relationships, one can shed light on the feasibility of program assumptions and ultimately help program developers strengthen the program (see Sussman, 1991).

In my experience, data collection efforts during program development are particularly useful for uncovering serious program flaws. For example, if a program is implemented to a sample of people with similar characteristics to the target population, and pilot data suggest that program activities are not affecting specific mediators, this alerts the program developer to areas where program activities may need to be strengthened or changed. However, it is also possible that null findings are simply due to research design sensitivity problems (Lipsey, 1990). Similarly, positive findings that appear to confirm the model can be in error due to threats to internal, construct, or external validity (see Cook & Campbell, 1979; Donaldson, 1995a, 1995b). The challenge of empirical program development is to probe and consider these issues in an effort to make empirically informed decisions about improving the program. Again, the underlying premise is that it is more likely to develop a strong program with limited data than with no data at all.

ANALYTIC TECHNIQUES

There has been significant advancement in statistical techniques for testing mediation in intervention research over the past two decades (Folmer, 1981; MacKinnon & Dwyer, 1993; Sobel, 1982). Common structural equation modeling statistical packages such as EQS (Bentler, 1995) and LISREL (Jöreskog &

Sörbom, 1993) can now be used to test complex mediation models when rather large and complex databases are available. Moreover, mediation also can be established using a series of simple regression equations (Baron & Kenny, 1986; MacKinnon, 1994; West & Aiken, 1997). Although it is often unrealistic to imagine conducting full-scale mediation analyses during program development, the logic behind these statistical tests is worth reviewing in anticipation of what a program must eventually achieve to be considered effective.

There are five steps or tests commonly used to assess mediation (Baron & Kenny, 1986; Judd & Kenny, 1981a, 1981b; MacKinnon, 1994). To establish mediation, the following relationships (tests) typically are examined:

1. The program causes the outcome (regressing the outcome variable on the program variable).
2. The program causes the mediator (regressing the mediator variable on the program variable).
3. The mediator causes the outcome variable (regressing the outcome variable on the mediator variable) (Baron & Kenny, 1986).
4. The mediator causes the outcome variable controlling for exposure to the program (regressing the outcome variable on both the program and mediator variable).
5. The mediated effect is significant (see MacKinnon, 1994).

It is important to point out that subtle nuances must be considered when testing for mediation. For example, it is possible that mediation still exists even if Test 1 is not positive (program causes mediator) because a suppressor effect could be present (e.g., one mediator variable is effective, and another is counterproductive, leaving the appearance of no effect of the program on the outcome). Furthermore, Test 5 is particularly important when there are multiple mediators of program effects (MacKinnon, 1994; West & Aiken, 1997). Fortunately, there have been some very good full-length treatments in recent years of how to use statistical approaches to test for mediation in intervention research (see MacKinnon, 1994; MacKinnon & Dwyer, 1993; West & Aiken, 1997).

Statistical approaches for testing moderators in intervention research are also well established (Aiken & West, 1991; Baron & Kenny, 1986). Again, a moderator variable is a third variable that affects the strength and direction of the statistical relationship (e.g., zero-order correlation) between two other variables (e.g., program and mediator variable). Figure 19.8 illustrates how to test whether dosage level moderates the relationship between the program and its target mediator. Path a represents the effect of the program on the mediator. Path b represents the relationship between dosage level (moderator) and the target mediator. Path c represents the products of Paths a and b (known as the interaction). In this

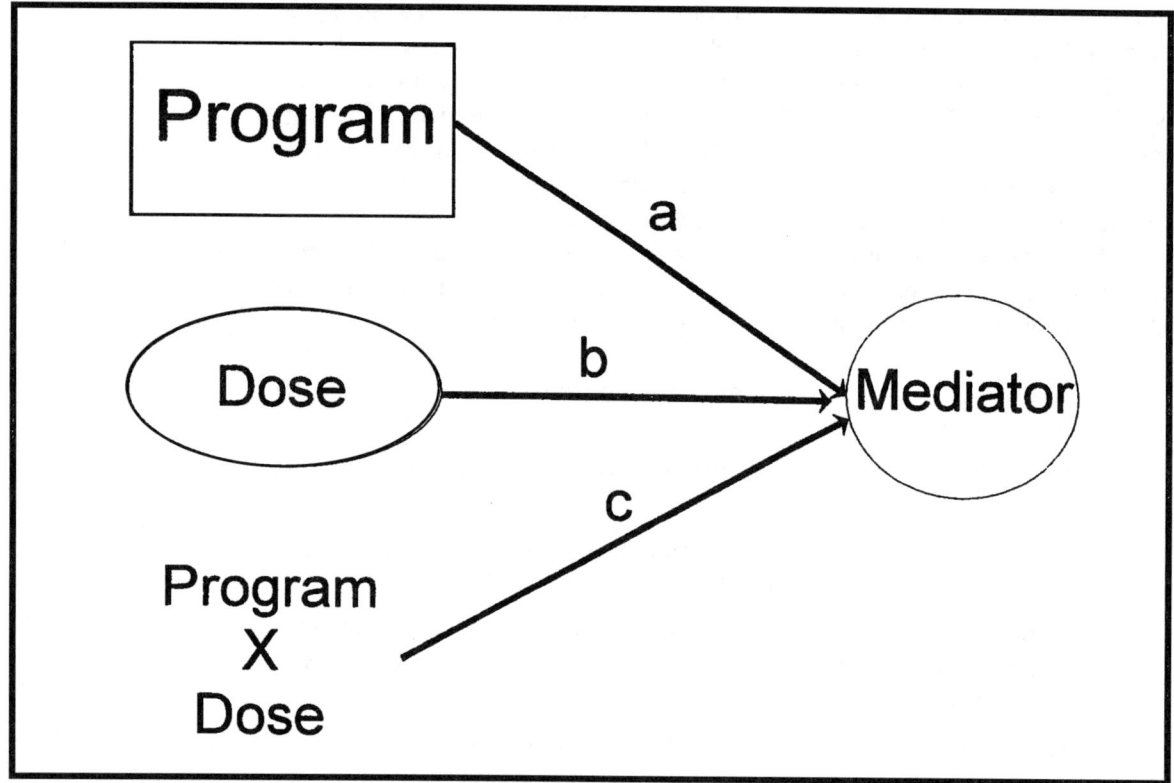

Figure 19.8. Testing a Moderator Relationship

example, dosage level moderates the relationship between the program and the mediator if the interaction term is statistically significant (Path c). Paths a and b are superfluous to the test of moderation. However, it is easier to interpret the interaction term when the moderator is not related to the program or mediator variables (Baron & Kenny, 1986). For in-depth discussions on using statistical approaches for testing moderator models and statistical interactions, see Aiken and West (1991) and Baron and Kenny (1986).

In all but the rare situation, program developers are forced to analyze mediator and moderator relationships with limited empirical data. For example, if we assume a medium effect size (ES = .40) and set alpha at .05 and power at .80, we would need to implement our program to at least 200 participants (e.g., 100 randomly assigned to treatment and 100 randomly assigned to a comparison group) to have confidence in statistical tests such as the ones described earlier (see Lipsey, 1990). It is unlikely that this level of time and resources is available for data collection during program development. Of course, when it is, the statistical approaches described earlier can be used to confirm or modify the program's conceptual framework (see Chapter 16, this volume).

However, it is more likely that trends in a more limited set of data collected from fewer participants will have to be used to estimate the likelihood that program components will have their desired effects when the program is fully implemented. Under these conditions, quantitative or qualitative data from participants who experience all or some aspect of the program can be used to assess trends between (a) the program and the target mediators and (b) the potential moderators of those trends (e.g., did the program appear to work better for certain subgroups?). Again, these analyses can be used to modify aspects of the program in an effort to strengthen its impact on target mediators, which should ultimately lead to more robust program effects.

LIMITATIONS

An accurate conceptual framework can go a long way toward improving the chances of program success. Most program frameworks can be reduced down to a series of mediator and moderator relationships. Empirical confirmation or disconfirmation of these relationships and the framework as a whole are often essential for building effective program theory and, consequently, effective health behavior programs. Unfortunately, the process of good program theory development is often rather long term and ongoing. Although assessing mediators and moderators during program development can be useful, it also carries the risk of misleading program developers. I have argued that this risk is due largely to the dangers associated with making decisions about the program based on limited data. But acknowledging and understanding these limitations can improve decisions about program modification in response to the limited data collected. In the best-case scenario, one can assess mediators and moderators in program development by using some version of an empirical curriculum or program development model, which promises to dramatically improve the overall quality of program development in health behavior research and practice (Sussman, 1991; Sussman et al., 1996).

SOME HEALTH BEHAVIOR EXAMPLES

In the final section of this chapter, I will provide several examples of mediator and moderator relationships presented in previous health behavior research. This section is meant to be an illustrative rather than an exhaustive review of the literature. It is probably safe to say that the prototypical program theory in health behavior research is Knowledge ➥ Attitude ➥ Health Behavior (cf. Weiss, 1997).

That is, a health behavior program increases knowledge (e.g., of the benefits of regular physical activity, nutrition, safe sex, or cancer screening), more knowledge leads to changes in attitudes (e.g., about exercise, diet, condom use, or preventive health services), and changes in attitudes lead to changed health behavior. However, the literature is now replete with examples that deviate from this popular basic framework.

MacKinnon (1994) provides a table illustrating a wide variety of mediators of health behavior outcomes found across a diversity of prevention studies. For example, educational achievement and parent-child communication are listed as mediators of unintentional pregnancy and unprotected intercourse in teenage pregnancy prevention (Dryfoos, 1990), safer-sex practices mediate the prevalence of sexually transmitted diseases in AIDS/HIV prevention programming (Coyle, Boruch, & Turner, 1991), the quality of parent-child relationships and active coping skills mediate outcomes of conduct and mental health problems in divorce prevention research (Sandler, Wolchik, & Braver, 1988), awareness of hotline services and referrals to general psychiatric care mediate outcomes of reduced suicide ideation and deaths due to suicide in suicide prevention research (Shaffer, Philips, Garland, & Bacon, 1989), and social norms mediate anabolic steroid use in adolescent steroid use prevention (Goldberg, Bents, Bosworth, Trevisan, & Elliot, 1991). Furthermore, an application of mediation analysis with a multicomponent health behavior program targeting multiple mediators recently has been described in some detail by West and Aiken (1997). Using data from a breast cancer screening trial based on the health belief model (Aiken, West, Woodward, Reno, & Reynolds, 1994), the benefits of screening mammography, the severity of breast cancer, a woman's perceptions of her susceptibility to breast cancer, and the barriers to screening mammography are hypothesized to influence a woman's intention to get a screening mammography. West and Aiken (1997) concluded that perceptions of susceptibility and knowledge about benefits were the key mediators of intentions to get screening, and they show the reader in detail how they arrived at that conclusion through mediation analysis. Below, I will further illustrate mediator and moderator relationships in health behavior research by highlighting examples from the exercise, occupational mental health promotion, and adolescent drug abuse prevention literatures.

PHYSICAL ACTIVITY

The direct benefits of regular physical activity and fitness are well documented. Regular physical activity can increase life expectancy and prevent obesity, coronary heart disease, hypertension, diabetes, osteoporosis, colon cancer, stroke, and depression (U.S. Department of Health and Human Services, 1991). What is probably less well known is that physical activity appears to also buffer or

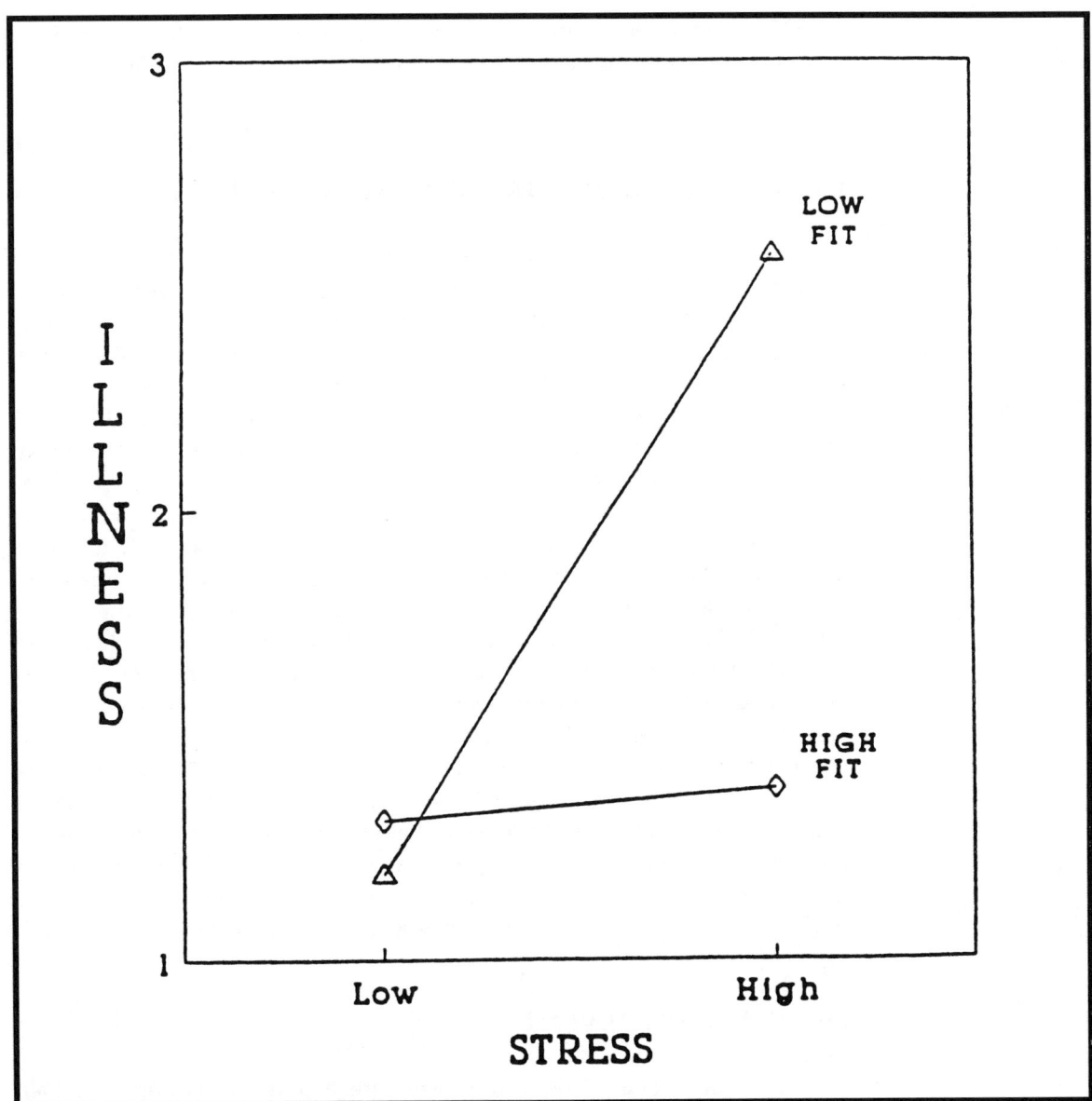

Figure 19.9. Fitness as a Moderator of the Stress-Illness Relationship (Brown, 1991)

moderate the relationship between stress and illness. Research conducted by Brown (1991) illustrates this moderator relationship clearly. In summary, under periods of high stress, people who are not physically fit report significantly more health center visits (illness) than those who are physically fit (see Figure 19.9). However, fitness itself was not significantly related to health center visits, illustrating the importance of conceptualizing and testing for interactions or moderators in health behavior program development and research (see Brown, 1991; Brown & Siegel, 1988).

OCCUPATIONAL MENTAL HEALTH PROMOTION

The nature of one's work (e.g., the presence or absence of work, conditions of work) is often a substantial determinant of health status, well-being, and overall quality of life (Donaldson, Gooler, & Weiss, 1998). A decade of reengineering, downsizing, or "right-sizing" has caused many loyal workers to lose stable, well-paying jobs (Donaldson & Weiss, 1998). Many displaced workers remain unemployed for long periods, suffering a variety of psychosocial and physical health consequences. Preventive interventions for the recently unemployed have been shown to enable unemployed workers to avoid depression, anxiety, and adverse health behaviors while seeking reemployment (Price, van Ryn, & Vinokur, 1992; Vinokur, Price, Caplan, van Ryn, & Curran, 1995; Vinokur, van Ryn, Gramlich, & Price, 1991). Another illustrative example of mediators and moderators of health behavior programs comes from the occupational health promotion literature and is shown in Figure 19.10. Figure 19.10 illustrates that the JOBS program affects the target mediators of job search self-efficacy, self-mastery, and inoculation against setbacks and that these mediators lead to better reemployment and mental health outcomes. However, it also was discovered that mental health status at pretest moderated the relationships between the mediators and outcomes. That is, the program worked much better for people who were not depressed or showing signs of other mental illnesses before receiving the program. This is a good example of mediators and a moderator operating together in one prevention program, and the findings suggest that different types of programs are needed for those already depressed or experiencing mental illness symptoms.

DRUG ABUSE PREVENTION

One health behavior domain in which mediation analyses have received much attention in recent years is adolescent drug abuse prevention programming (Donaldson et al., 1996). Hawkins, Catalano, and Miller (1992) conducted a thorough review of this literature and presented 17 risk factors (potential mediators of prevention program effects) with corresponding prevention findings. These risk factors included laws and norms, availability, extreme economic deprivation, neighborhood disorganization, physiological factors, family drug behavior, family management practices, family conflict, low bonding to family, early and persistent problem behaviors, academic failure, low commitment to school,

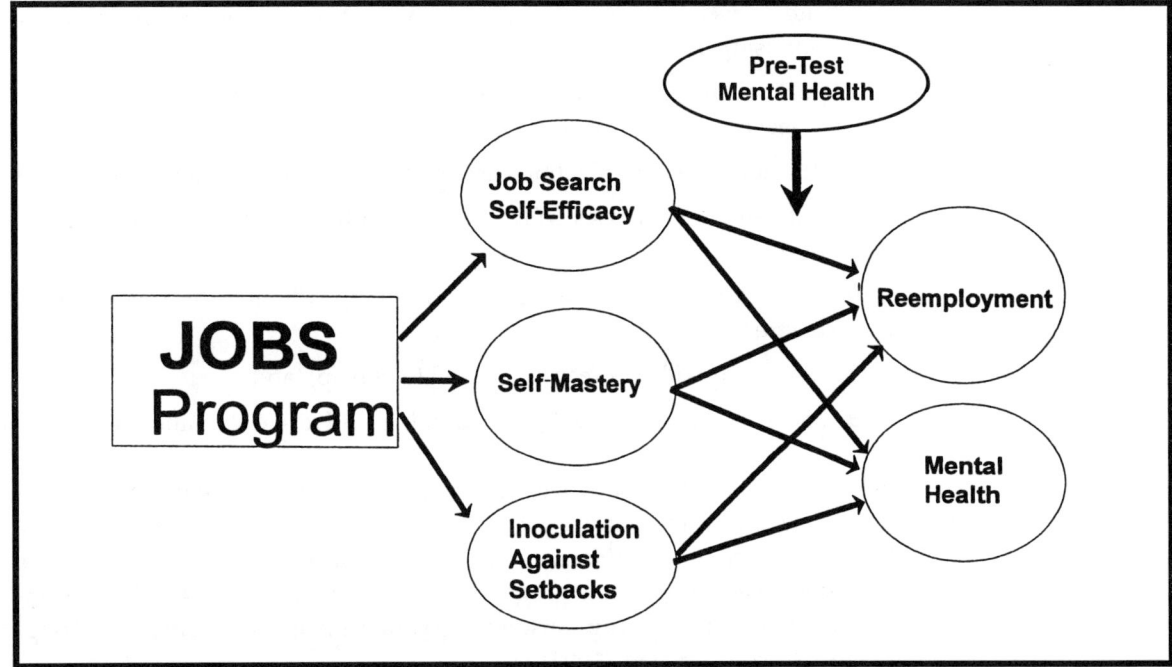

Figure 19.10. Mediators and Moderator of the JOBS Program

peer rejection in elementary grades, association with drug-using peers, alienation and rebelliousness, attitudes favorable toward drug use, and early onset of drug use. Interventions designed to prevent these risk factors are presumed to lower rates of adolescent drug abuse (see also Chapter 6, this volume).

Hansen (1993) summarized the 12 most popular drug abuse prevention strategies (and their presumed theoretical program or mediating mechanisms):

1. normative education (decreases perceptions about prevalence and acceptability beliefs, establishes conservative norms),
2. refusal assertion training (increases the perception that one can deal effectively with pressure to use drugs if they are offered, increases self-efficacy),
3. information about consequences of use (increases perceptions of personal vulnerability to common consequences of drug use),
4. personal commitment pledges (increases personal commitment and intentions not to use drugs),
5. values (increases perception that drug use is incongruent with lifestyle),

6. alternatives (increases awareness of ways to engage in enjoyment without using drugs),
7. goal-setting skills (increases ability to set and achieve goals, increases achievement orientation),
8. decision-making skills (increases ability to make reasoned decisions),
9. self-esteem (increases feeling of self-worth and valued personal identity),
10. stress skills (increases perceptions of coping skills, reduces reported level of stress),
11. assistance skills (increases availability of help), and
12. life skills (increases ability to maintain positive social relations).

Although most drug abuse prevention programs still reflect the program developers' view of how to optimize prevention effects rather than a combination of strategies proven to work (Hansen, 1993), mediation analyses suggest that social influences-based prevention programming is one of the most effective approaches for preventing drug abuse among young adolescents from general populations (Donaldson et al., 1996).

For example, MacKinnon et al. (1991) found that social norms, especially among friends, and beliefs about the positive consequences of drug use appeared to be important mediators of program effects in project STAR (Students Taught Awareness and Resistance). The program did not appear to have effects through resistance skills (refusal training). The notion that social norms are a potent aspect of prevention programming was subsequently tested in a randomized prevention trial known as the Adolescent Alcohol Prevention Trial (AAPT) (Donaldson, Graham, & Hansen, 1994; Donaldson, Graham, Piccinin, & Hansen, 1995; Hansen & Graham, 1991). Figure 19.11 represents a summary of the findings from project AAPT and shows the following:

(a) Normative education lowered beliefs about drug use acceptability and prevalence estimates (in seventh grade), which predicted cigarette, marijuana, and cigarette use (in eighth grade). This pattern of results was virtually the same across potential moderators of gender, ethnicity, context (public vs. private school), drugs, and levels of risk and was durable across time (Donaldson et al., 1994). MacKinnon, Weber, and Pentz (1988) also failed to find strong moderator relationships across drug abuse prevention programs using gender, ethnicity, grade, socioeconomic status, and urbanization.

(b) Resistance skills training did improve refusal skills, but refusal skills did not predict subsequent drug use (Donaldson et al., 1994).

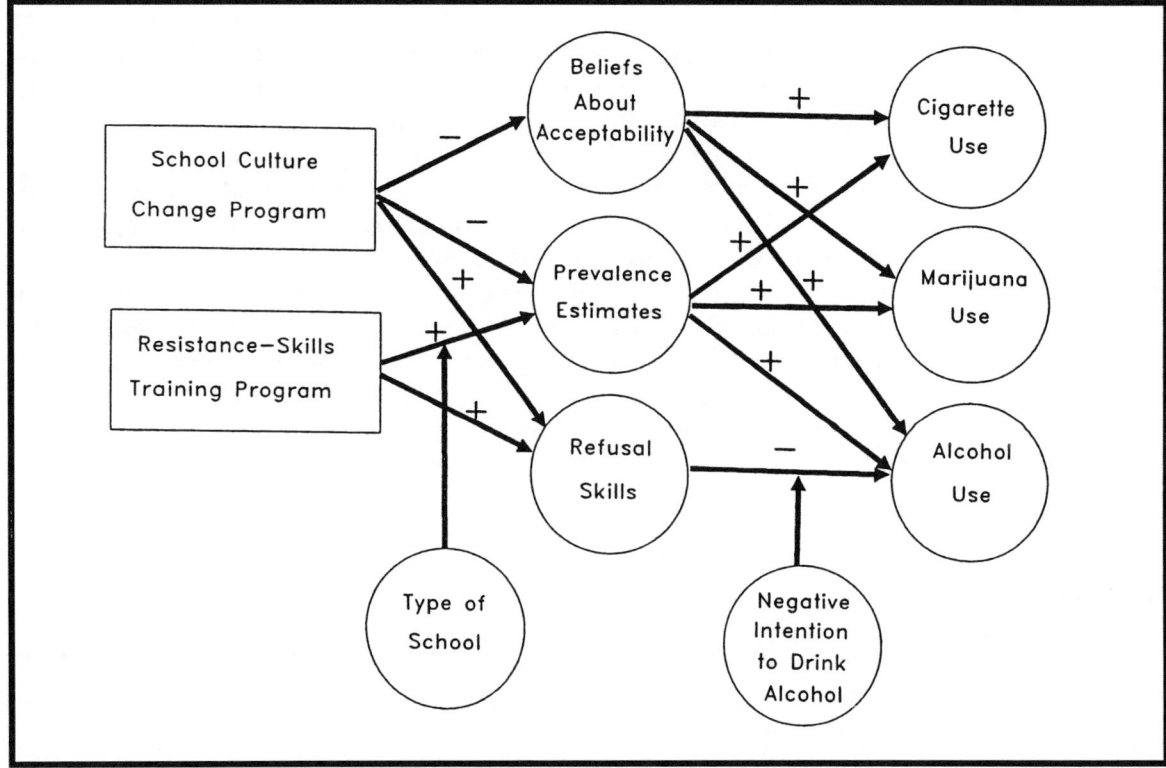

Figure 19.11. Summary of Findings From the Adolescent Alcohol Prevention Trial

(c) Those who received only resistance skills in public schools actually had higher prevalence estimates (a harmful effect; type of school is shown as the moderator) (Donaldson et al., 1995).

(d) Refusal skills did predict lower alcohol use for those students who had negative intentions to drink alcohol (negative intention to drink is the moderator) (Donaldson et al., 1995).

This example is meant to illustrate that some health behavior programs are quite complex, and mediator and moderator analyses conducted over a series of studies are sometimes needed to aid understanding of program effects.

CONCLUSION

Many health behavior interventions involve rather complex relationships among program, mediator, moderator, and outcome variables. Throughout this chapter,

I have provided a range of examples of mediator and moderator relationships found in the health behavior intervention research literature. It now should be clear that traditional black-box program conceptualizations and evaluations fail to capture the complexity of most health behavior programs.

It has been argued in this chapter that using conceptual frameworks consisting of hypothesized mediator and moderator relationships during program development, in combination with empirical feedback, promises to improve our ability to develop efficacious programs. Although limited data collection efforts conducted during program development are particularly useful for uncovering serious program flaws, design sensitivity and threats to validity problems must be carefully considered when using an empirical program development approach. Nevertheless, analyzing mediator and moderator relationships using limited data, in contrast to no data at all, is much more likely to result in the development of programs that do indeed improve health behavior and ultimately the human condition.

▶ REFERENCES

AIKEN, L. S., & WEST, S. G. (1991). *Multiple regression: Testing and interpreting interactions.* Newbury Park, CA: Sage.

AIKEN, L. S., WEST, S. G., WOODWARD, C. K., RENO, R. R., & REYNOLDS, K. D. (1994). Increasing screening mammography in asymptomatic women: Evaluation of a second generation, theory-based program. *Health Psychology, 13,* 526-538.

BARANOWSKI, T., LIN, L. S., WETTER, D. W., RESNICOW, K., & HEARN, M. D. (1997). Theory as mediating variables: Why aren't community interventions working as desired? *Annals of Epidemiology, 7,* 89-95.

BARON, R. M., & KENNY, D. A. (1986). The moderator-mediator variable distinction in social psychological research: Conceptual, strategic, and statistical considerations. *Journal of Personality and Social Psychology, 51,* 1173-1182.

BENTLER, P. M. (1995). *EQS structural equations model program manual.* Encino, CA: Multivariate Software.

BICKMAN, L. (1987). The functions of program evaluation theory. *New Directions for Program Evaluation, 33,* 5-18.

BROWN, J. D. (1991). Staying fit and staying well: Physical fitness as a moderator of life stress. *Journal of Personality and Social Psychology, 60,* 555-561.

BROWN, J. D., & SEIGAL, J. M. (1988). Exercise as a buffer of life stress: A prospective study of adolescent health. *Health Psychology, 7,* 341-353.

CHEN, H.-T. (1990). *Theory-driven evaluation.* Newbury Park, CA: Sage.

COLLINS, L. M., GRAHAM, J. W., LONG, J., & HANSEN, W. B. (1994). Crossvalidation of latent class models of early substance use onset. *Multivariate Behavioral Research, 29,* 165-183.

COLLINS, L. M., GRAHAM, J. W., ROUSCULP, S. S., FIDLER, P. L., PAN, J., & HANSEN, W. B. (1994). Latent transition analysis and how it can address prevention research questions. In L. M. Collins & L. Seitz (Eds.), *Advances in data analysis for prevention intervention research* (NIDA Research Monograph No. 142). Washington, DC: Government Printing Office.

COLLINS, L. M., GRAHAM, J. W., ROUSCULP, S. S., & HANSEN, W. B. (1997). Heavy caffeine use and the beginning of the substance use onset process: An illustration of latent transition analysis.

In K. J. Bryant, M. Windle, & S. G. West (Eds.), *The science of prevention: Methodological advances from alcohol and substance abuse research* (pp. *000-000*). Washington, DC: American Psychological Association.

COOK, T. D., & CAMPBELL, D. T. (1979). *Quasi-experimentation design and analysis issues for field settings.* Skokie, IL: Rand McNally.

COYLE, S. L., BORUCH, R. F., & TURNER, C. F. (1991). *Evaluating AIDS prevention programs.* Washington, DC: National Academy Press.

DONALDSON, S. I. (1995a). Peer influence on adolescent drug use: A perspective from the trenches of experimental evaluation research. *American Psychologist, 50,* 801-802.

DONALDSON, S. I. (1995b). Worksite health promotion: A theory-driven, empirically based perspective. In L. R. Murphy, J. J. Hurrel, S. L. Sauter, & G. P. Keita (Eds.). *Job stress interventions* (pp. 73-90). Washington, DC: American Psychological Association.

DONALDSON, S. I., GOOLER, L. E., & WEISS, R. (1998). Promoting health and well-being through work: Science and practice. In X. B. Arriaga & S. Oskamp (Eds.), *Addressing community problems: Psychological research and intervention* (pp. 160-194). Thousand Oaks, CA: Sage.

DONALDSON, S. I., GRAHAM, J. W., & HANSEN, W. B. (1994). Testing the generalizability of intervening mechanism theories: Understanding the effects of school-based substance use prevention interventions. *Journal of Behavioral Medicine, 17,* 195-216.

DONALDSON, S. I., GRAHAM, J. W., PICCININ, A. M., & HANSEN, W. B. (1995). Resistance-skills training and onset of alcohol use: Evidence for beneficial and potentially harmful effects in public schools and in private Catholic schools. *Health Psychology, 14,* 291-300.

DONALDSON, S. I., SUSSMAN, S., MacKINNON, D. P., SEVERSON, H. H., GLYNN, T., MURRAY, D. M., & STONE, E. J. (1996). Drug abuse prevention programming: Do we know what content works? *American Behavioral Scientist, 39,* 868-883.

DONALDSON, S. I., & WEISS, R. (1998). Health, well-being, and organizational effectiveness in the virtual workplace. In M. Igbaria & M. Tan (Eds.), *The virtual workplace* (pp. 22-44). Harrisburg, PA: Idea Group.

DRYFOOS, J. G. (1990). *Adolescents at risk: Prevalence and prevention.* New York: Oxford University Press.

FOLMER, H. (1981). Measurement of the effects of regional policy instruments by means of linear structural models and panel data. *Environmental Planning Annual, 13,* 1435-1448.

GOLDBERG, L., BENTS, R., BOSWORTH, E., TREVISAN, L., & ELLIOT, D. L. (1991). Anabolic steroid education and adolescents: Do scare tactics work? *Pediatrics, 87,* 283-286.

HANSEN, W. B. (1993). School-based alcohol prevention programs. *Alcohol Health & Research World, 17,* 54-60.

HANSEN, W. B., & GRAHAM, J. W. (1991). Preventing adolescent alcohol, marijuana, and cigarette use among adolescents: Peer pressure resistance training versus establishing conservative norms. *Preventive Medicine, 20,* 414-430.

HANSEN, W. B., & McNEAL, R. B., JR. (1996). The law of maximum expected potential effect: Constraints placed on program effectiveness by mediator relationships. *Health Education Research, 11,* 501-507.

HAWKINS, J. D., CATALANO, R. F., & MILLER, J. M. (1992). Risk and protective factors for alcohol and other drug problems in adolescence and early adulthood: Implications for substance abuse prevention. *Psychological Bulletin, 112,* 64-105.

JÖRESKOG, K. G., & SÖRBOM, D. (1993). *LISREL 8: User's reference guide.* Chicago: Scientific Software.

JUDD, C. M., & KENNY, D. A. (1981a). *Estimating the effects of social interventions.* New York: Cambridge University Press.

JUDD, C. M., & KENNY, D. A. (1981b). Process analysis: Estimating mediation in treatment evaluations. *Evaluation Review, 5,* 602-619.

LIPSEY, M. W. (1988). Practice and malpractice in evaluation research. *Evaluation Practice, 9,* 5-24.

LIPSEY, M. W. (1990). *Design sensitivity.* Newbury Park, CA: Sage.

LIPSEY, M. W. (1993). Theory as method: Small theories of treatments. *New Directions for Program Evaluation, 57,* 5-38.

LIPSEY, M. W., CROSSE, S., DUNKEL, J., POLLARD, J. A., & STOBART, G. (1985). Evaluation: The state of the art and the sorry state of the science. *New Directions for Program Evaluation, 27,* 7-28.

LIPSEY, M. W., & POLLARD, J. A. (1989). Driving toward theory in program evaluation: More models to choose from. *Evaluation and Program Planning, 12,* 317-328.

LIPSEY, M. W., & WILSON, D. B. (1993). The efficacy of psychological, educational, and behavioral treatment: Confirmation from meta-analysis. *American Psychologist, 48,* 1181-1209.

MACKINNON, D. P. (1994). Analysis of mediating variables in prevention and intervention research. In A. Cazares & L. A. Beatty (Eds.), *Scientific methods for prevention intervention research* (NIDA Research Monograph No. 139, pp. 127-154). Rockville, MD: National Institutes of Health.

MACKINNON, D. P., & DWYER, J. H. (1993). Estimating mediated effects in prevention studies. *Evaluation Review, 17,* 144-158.

MACKINNON, D. P., JOHNSON, C. A., PENTZ, M. A., DWYER, J. H., HANSEN, W. B., FLAY, B. R., & WANG, E. Y. (1991). Mediating mechanisms in a school-based drug prevention program: First-year effects of the Midwestern prevention project. *Health Psychology, 10,* 164-172.

MACKINNON, D. P., WEBER, M. D., & PENTZ, M. A. (1988). How do school-based drug prevention program work and for whom? *Drugs and Society, 3,* 125-143.

PRICE, R. H., VAN RYN, M., & VINOKUR, A. D. (1992). Impact of a preventive job search intervention on the likelihood of depression among the unemployed. *Journal of Health and Social Behavior, 33,* 158-167.

RUNYAN, W. K. (1980). A stage-state analysis of the life course. *Journal of Personality and Social Psychology, 6,* 951-962.

SANDLER, I. N., WOLCHIK, S., & BRAVER, S. L. (1988). The stressors of children's post-divorce environment. In S. Wolchik & P. Karoly (Eds.), *Children of divorce: Empirical perspectives in adjustment.* New York: Garden.

SHAFFER, D., PHILIPS, I., GARLAND, A., & BACON, K. (1989). Prevention issues in youth suicide. In D. Shaffer, I. Philips, & N. B. Enzer (Eds.), *Prevention of mental disorders, alcohol and other drug use in children and adolescents* (DHHS Pub. No. (ADM)90-1646, pp. 225-271). Washington, DC: Government Printing Office.

SMITH, M. F. (1989). *Evaluability assessment: A practical approach.* Boston: Kluwer.

SOBEL, M. E. (1982). Asymptotic confidence intervals for indirect effects in structural equation models. In S. Leinhart (Ed.), *Sociological methodology 1982* (pp. 290-312). San Francisco: Jossey-Bass.

SUSSMAN, S. (1991). Curriculum development in school-based prevention research. *Health Education Research: Theory and Practice, 6,* 339-351.

SUSSMAN, S., DENT, C. W., BURTON, D., STACY, A. W., & FLAY, B. R. (1995). *Developing school-based tobacco use prevention and cessation programs.* Thousand Oaks, CA: Sage.

SUSSMAN, S., PETOSA, R., & CLARKE, P. (1996). The use of empirical curriculum development to improve prevention research. *American Behavioral Scientist, 39,* 838-852.

U.S. DEPARTMENT OF HEALTH AND HUMAN SERVICES. (1991). *Healthy People 2000: National health promotion and disease prevention objectives* (DHHS Pub. No. PHS 91-50212). Washington, DC: Government Printing Office.

VINOKUR, A. D., PRICE, R. H., CAPLAN, R. D., VAN RYN, M., & CURRAN, J. (1995). The JOBS I preventive intervention for unemployed individuals: Short- and long-term effects on reemployment and mental health. In L. R. Murphy, J. J. Hurrel, S. L. Sauter, & G. P. Keita (Eds.), *Job stress interventions* (pp. 125-138). Washington, DC: American Psychological Association.

VINOKUR, A. D., VAN RYN, M., GRAMLICH, E. M., & PRICE, R. H. (1991). Long-term follow-up and benefit-cost analysis of the Jobs Program: A preventive intervention for the unemployed. *Journal of Applied Psychology, 76,* 213-219.

WEISS, C. H. (1997). How can theory-based evaluation make greater headway? *Evaluation Review, 21,* 501-524.

WEST, S. G., & AIKEN, L. S. (1997). Toward understanding individual effects in multicomponent prevention programs: Design and analysis strategies. In K. J. Bryant, M. Windle, & S. G. West (Eds.), *The science of prevention: Methodological advances from alcohol and substance abuse research* (pp. 167-209). Washington, DC: American Psychological Association.

CHAPTER 19

Commentary

David P. MacKinnon

Donaldson does a fine job outlining the importance of mediator and moderator analysis and its uses in program development. He provides an important practical and theoretical perspective by including discussion of these issues from a variety of disciplines, including psychology, program evaluation, and sociology. There are many of us who agree with Donaldson. Mediation and moderator analysis has the potential to increase scientific understanding of behavior as well as to improve the effectiveness of programs. Also, program development is a critical phase for the application of moderator and mediator methodology. Given the many reasons for use of these approaches to program development, it is surprising that they are not used more often. At least part of the reason for this failure is a lack of understanding of the usefulness of these approaches. Donaldson's chapter should help remedy this situation.

The purpose of this commentary is to expand on several points in the chapter and raise a few new ones. I start with several comments on the variables suitable for moderator and mediation analysis, and then I discuss some topics specific to mediation analysis. As mentioned in the chapter, it is not yet clear whether programs have differential effects across subgroups of subjects. Because most programs are delivered to persons who differ in gender, age, and ethnicity, these are likely candidates for moderator effects in most studies. The socialization and cultural effects of ethnicity and gender are important to consider in program development (Pinderhughes, 1989). Age is another critically important moderator variable because of the different maturational processes involved at different ages, particularly among children. Programs designed for elementary schoolchildren, for example, are obviously different from programs for high school students. The mediators targeted also may have different meaning across levels of the moderator variable (e.g., age).

Often, however, it is difficult to determine whether a variable is a moderator or a mediator. For example, gender, age, and ethnicity are clearly potential moderator variables because they are immutable, at least for most reasonable programs. Other variables, especially personality variables, could potentially be changed by a health behavior program and, as a result, may be thought of as mediator variables. However, for most health behavior programs, the program intensity required to change these variables is often unrealistic. In this quandary, variables such as risk-taking tendency and antisocial personality, for example, may be best thought of as moderator variables. That is, the determination of whether a variable is a mediator or moderator depends, in part, on the mutability of the variable.

One important moderator of program effects is the level of the outcome variable before the program is delivered. Probably the best example is the moderator variable of drug use with subgroups such as never users, experimenters, and regular drug users. Prochaska, DiClemente, and Norcross (1992) suggest that there are different stages of drug addiction, and programs that target each stage must focus on different mediating variables to be effective. A program designed to prevent the onset of drug abuse may affect only the subgroup of never users and may not affect experimental or regular users. Any major outcome of a study can be conceptualized in this manner (e.g., educational achievement, fitness, and body image). In prevention research, these different levels of the outcome variable have been called primary, secondary, and tertiary prevention (or, similarly, universal, selective, and indicated prevention), corresponding to preventing a behavior that has not yet occurred, prevention of a behavior before it becomes more serious, and prevention of further symptoms among persons who are at the riskiest level on the outcome, respectively (Last & Wallace, 1992). Effective programs are presumably those that address the specific mechanisms of these three different types of prevention.

However, to make matters more confusing, it is possible that a variable could serve as both a moderator and a mediator. A program may change a mediating variable, which then changes the outcome variable. At the same time, the effect of the program may depend on the level of the mediator. Statistical methods to examine these types of variables are only now beginning to appear (Merrill, 1996). The relevance for program development is that some individual differences variables are most reasonably conceptualized as moderator variables but also may act as mediators.

A critical decision in the consideration of moderators in program development is how to incorporate significant moderator effects into a new prevention program. For the case of gender, ethnicity, and age, it is often not difficult. At least for gender and age, it is reasonable to separate the subgroups prior to the delivery of special programs. Most prevention programs are appropriately delivered to different age groups, and there are situations when programs are delivered to one gender (e.g., high school football players) (Goldberg et al., 1996). Separation of persons by ethnic groups seems a bit more problematic but may be reasonable in some situations.

Tailoring a program to most other moderator variables, however, is very difficult. For example, it may be impractical for a prevention study to separate persons merely depending on their level of drug use. This strategy actually may be counterproductive if the subgroup of regular users, for example, reactively develops its own even more extreme prodrug use norms. Labeling of students by other students in the school also would be counterproductive. Separation of persons, depending on their risk taking or other personality characteristics, has a similar risk of negative labeling and may not be practical for ethical and other reasons. Larger unit-level measures of these variables (e.g., school, clinic, hospital) may be more useful in the delivery of specialized prevention programs to high-risk youth, for example, as the labeling of these youth has occurred naturally.

There is a lack of receptivity to the moderator approach to program development, perhaps due in part to the above-stated ethical issues. Typically, the criterion for a successful theory is that it applies across many settings and across subgroups, including subgroups defined by moderators. Theories that are inaccurate when applied to subgroups usually are discarded. Very few studies have included a theoretical analysis of subgroup characteristics that is detailed enough to predict different program effects across subgroups. Such an analysis might lead to more effective programming, however. Program development is the ideal stage to develop these types of hypotheses based on theory.

In my opinion, mediation analysis is a more fruitful area for program development than moderator analysis primarily because of the difficulty of including moderators in program development and the limitations just discussed. From the mediation perspective, program design is based on the commonsense notion that a program that changes a variable causally related to the outcome variable will lead to a change in the outcome variable.

There are two important steps in program development based on the mediation hypothesis. First, the theoretical and empirical evidence for how the proposed mediators are related to the outcome must be described. Theoretical and empirical research should be used to identify mediators. It is useful to create a conceptual theory table consisting of the mediators across the top of a table and the outcome variables listed along the side of the table. The entries in this table correspond to the mediator and its relationship to the outcome variable. Ideally, some measure of effect size, such as the partial correlation squared (Cohen, 1988, pp. 412-421), for the mediator-outcome relationship is included in the table. It is important to list all mediating variables, including ones that are unreasonable to change in a short program, such as personality or risk-taking behavior. The purpose of this conceptual theory table is to clearly list the theory and other backgrounds from which the mediators were selected, thereby providing a perspective on the program.

A second important task of program development is to create an action theory table consisting of the mediators targeted by the program and the program components designed to change the mediators. Here, the mediators are listed across the top of the table, and the program components or sessions are listed on the side of the table. The entries in the table are the indicators of which components target which mediator. Often, the table demonstrates that a program actually targets only one mediator, and the program can be improved by targeting additional mediators. Another important addition to this table is to provide some estimate of the amount of change in a mediator (e.g., the partial correlation squared effect size) that can be expected from a particular program component. Reliable measures of this type of information are likely to be achieved far in the future, but attempts to identify these values serve a useful purpose of gauging approximately just how much of an effect can be expected from the program. It is critical to consider whether the program can reasonably change the mediator using the planned program components.

Both the conceptual theory and action theory tables provide critical insight into the extent to which a program component can change a mediator and the extent to which the mediator is related to the outcome variable. By carefully completing these tables, the theoretical and empirical rationale of the program is clearly laid out. Besides clarifying the program mechanisms for the program developers, the basis of the program is clarified for others; furthermore, the mediating processes identified in these tables can help guide the data analysis plan.

As described in the chapter, use of mediator and moderator analysis is important whether or not a significant overall program effect is obtained (Chen, 1990). Mediation analysis can provide insight as to why the program did not work. If there are no program effects on the mediators targeted by the prevention program, then it is not surprising that program effects were not observed on the dependent variable. This is an action theory failure described by Chen, corresponding to the action theory table described earlier. If there are significant program effects on the mediator but not on the dependent variable, then there is evidence that the theoretical and empirical basis for the prevention program is faulty because the mediators targeted by the program were changed, yet the dependent variable was not changed. This is a conceptual theory failure described by Chen, corresponding to the conceptual theory table described earlier. In the case of no overall program effects, moderator analysis can help identify subgroups in which the program had differential effects.

There are at least three limitations to the mediation approach to program development aside from the focus on variable- versus person-oriented models mentioned in the chapter. First, if the delivery of the intervention is randomized, then the relationship between exposure to the randomized manipulation and the mediator is a reasonable estimate of the causal effect of the program on the mediator. This is not true for the relationship between the mediator and the dependent variable, which is based on a correlational relationship. It is possible that the dependent variable causes the mediator, rather than the mediator causing the dependent variable, the latter relation being hypothesized in the mediation model. Careful consideration of these issues is important for accurate interpretation of results.

Another problem is that the relationship between the mediator and the outcome may be changed by the intervention. In this case, methods to examine this differential correlation across groups are necessary. Finally, several researchers have conducted a detailed causal analysis of the mediation model (Holland, 1988), showing that it is often difficult to demonstrate causal relations among the independent variable, the mediator, and the outcome variable. The action theory and conceptual theory tables described earlier and replication studies can further clarify the roles of these variables and address these limitations.

The statistical methods to estimate mediation effects and their standard errors are widely available in major computer software packages such as EQS (Bentler, 1997) and LISREL (Jöreskog & Sörbom, 1993).

Calculation of the mediated effect and its standard error is relatively easy to compute by hand from ordinary regression analysis (MacKinnon, 1994), and these models are easily extended to multiple-mediator models and longitudinal models. As described in the article, the number of studies applying these analyses has increased. Future studies should greatly increase our understanding of program mechanisms that will further inform program development.

In summary, mediation and moderator analysis holds great promise for the development of program evaluation as a science. Explicit detail regarding the mediators targeted and how the program will change the mediators improves theory and enhances the practical effects of programs. It is hoped that mediators and moderators found in one study will apply across studies and that theory used to explain program effects for one outcome variable also will explain program effects for other variables. Although it is too early to tell, mediation and moderator analysis has the potential to significantly increase our understanding of health behavior, as well as improve health behavior programs. The success of these methods depends on continued theoretical work in program development.

▷ REFERENCES

BENTLER, P. M. (1997). *EQS for Windows (version 5.6)* (Computer program). Encino, CA: Multivariate Software.

CHEN, H. -T. (1990). *Theory-driven evaluation.* Newbury Park, CA: Sage.

COHEN, J. (1988). *Statistical power for the social sciences.* Hillsdale, NJ: Lawrence Erlbaum.

GOLDBERG, L., CLARKE, G., ELLIOT, D., MaCKINNON, D. P., MOE, E., ZOREF, L., GREEN, C., WOLF, S. L., GREFFRATH, E., MILLER, D. J., & LAPIN, A. (1996). Effects of a multidimensional anabolic steroid prevention intervention: The Adolescents Training and Learning to Avoid Steroids (ATLAS) program. *Journal of the American Medical Association, 276,* 1555-1562.

HOLLAND, P. W. (1988). Causal inference, path analysis, and recursive structural equation models. *Sociological Methodology, 18,* 449-484.

JÖRESKOG, K. G., & SÖRBOM, D. (1993). *LISREL (version 8.12)* [Computer program]. Chicago: Scientific Software International, Inc.

LAST, J. M., & WALLACE, R. B. (1992). *Public health & preventive medicine.* Norwalk, CT: Appleton & Lange.

MACKINNON, D. P. (1994). Analysis of mediating variables in prevention and intervention studies. *National Institute on Drug Abuse Research Monograph Series, 139,* 127-153.

MERRILL, R. (1996). *Statistical tests for variables that serve as moderators and mediators.* Doctoral dissertation, Arizona State University.

PINDERHUGHES, E. (1989). *Understanding race, ethnicity, and power: The key to efficacy in clinical practice.* New York: Free Press.

PROCHASKA, J. O., DICLEMENTE, C. C., & NORCROSS, J. C. (1992). In search of how people change: Applications to addictive behaviors. *American Psychologist, 47,* 1102-1114.

CHAPTER 20

Needs for the Future of Program Development

Steve Sussman
Rick Petosa
Howard Leventhal

One needs to learn to walk before one can run. Also, one can be *taught* to walk and then to run, which has been the ultimate purpose of this book. We wrote it to try to impart several lessons to program developers. It presented the importance of using empirical methods in program development, introduced examples of how it is done, and reviewed principles and specific strategies that enable the reader to "run with it." We hope that we have presented these lessons comprehensively and persuasively. We designed this book for a variety of audiences, with some of the material being more complex than other parts. For the practitioner, we hope you were able to see the forest even though some of the trees might be a bit thick. Partner with local researchers or have program-planning staff receive training in the behavioral sciences, if needed. Perhaps this volume helped you identify sufficiently what your agency needs to know to engage in effective program development. Your target audience deserves effective programming, and your staff will surely enjoy developing and implementing effective programs.

The following section of this chapter includes a consideration of the pitfalls of using as empiricist program development process, a review of the chain model, and a consideration of the need for future research on methods classification, prediction of larger-term outcomes, and technological advances.

▶ OBSTACLES TO MAINTAINING AN EMPIRICAL PROGRAM DEVELOPMENT PROCESS

There are at least four potential pitfalls pertaining to the maintenance of an empirical program development regimen. First, once an empirically based program is developed, people may not want it changed. One might assume that through the use of an empirical program development process, the program so developed will be eternal in effectiveness. Also, policymakers may not want to endorse additional expenditures after a decision to select a data-driven program is made. Furthermore, program-setting supervisors may not want a new program because a change in programming may necessitate at least a temporary increase in workload for in-house staff. However, we all know that the social climate changes. A period of ongoing empirical program adaptation will be needed once every several years. Even though the same health behavior contents or messages may remain relevant over long spans of time, the community will change. In particular, as language evolves, technology advances, and cultural symbols change, examples used in training materials will need to change. Use of slang, clothing styles, music, celebrity names, and current events depicted in programs need to be reasonably current. Of course, it is also possible that with evolving community needs, core elements of programming also may have to change to remain effective. Empirical program development instituted on a regular cycle will enable continuous program evolution to adapt to changing community needs.

Second, if empirical program development methodology continues to gain respect, one should beware of programs that provide only lip service to empirical program development to achieve approval of decision makers. Program decision makers will need to be informed consumers of programs, focusing on the nature and intensity of the development procedures used to produce a program. A means of assessing quality control of program development methods is needed. All we can say right now, however, is that use of one method is better than use of intuition, and use of multiple methods is likely to be better than use of only one method. Also, we would argue that the use of both perceived and immediate-impact studies is needed. However, we are only beginning to think about means of achieving quality control.

One particular type of data might be of concern to the program developer who is trying to use the contents of this text. Beware of testimonials. When a person says a program worked for him or her, he or she is pledging allegiance to the program. Retrospective biases, interpretation biases, conformity pressures, and editing of information may cloud assessments of the effectiveness of these types of data. Do not let someone pass such information off as high quality; they are selling you their program. Such data can be used as one type of program development support. For example, individuals can provide evidence of program acceptability or feasibility. But one should be wary of testimonials that make claims regarding program effectiveness. A health program should gather assessments using different target sample sources and methods of data collection to provide a complete and converging picture of the truth.

Third, pragmatic, political decision making sometimes may influence the goals or content of programs on which we use empirical program development methods. Some practitioners, researchers, or community members may believe that some health issues should not be addressed by institutions; they feel, rather, that such issues should be the sole realm of the family. The limitations of receptivity due to moral concerns can and should be assessed through the use of program development studies—and some modalities of programming may not become used for a specific purpose due to a wall of moral resistance. We all have our own opinions on the need for social change. If we can develop programs systematically that work within the norms of community moral standards (e.g., "tips for parents to educate their children on sex"), at least effective messages are getting used. Flexible use of program development methods can show favorable health behavior returns.

Finally, there is an issue of different frameworks for evaluating cost-effectiveness of programming. Policymakers may question whether placing money up front for program development is worth the trade-off in terms of money spent later for program delivery. Unfortunately, cost-benefit, in at least some public policy terms, may include consideration of meeting public demand with highly acceptable, noncontroversial programming that involves powerful implementation forces that can assist with the maintenance of delivery. The program "solves" the pressures placed on the policymakers, addresses the image needs of third parties, and addresses the general demands of the public. Of course, the program may not work. But who cares? It "works" for the public. The cost-benefit in terms of public policy may favor not engaging in program development, whereas the cost-benefit to the targets of programming probably would favor its use (Bukoski & Evans, 1998). To protect against superfluous programming, policymakers need to be educated in a long view of health promotion. An eye on saving lives in the future should go hand in hand with an eye on getting votes now (see Chapter 3, this volume, for a detailed discussion of related issues). Also, it is likely that relatively favorable program judgments provided by a target audience are relatively likely to be accurate and could be used to sway public officials to use programs that work rather than ones that do not.

Also, three pitfalls of an "illusion of failure" can lead people to close their eyes and shut their ears to concepts of program development. One is a question of language, the second is a question of methods, and the third is a question of application. First, we need to remember that jargon in the scientific and practice realms needs two-way translation for better mutual application of program development principles. For example, many practitioners refer to *research* as meaning "to think about" or "look up information in a book," whereas most researchers refer to research as a systematic information-building process. An *intervention* may be thought to mean family confrontation of a drug abuser to a practitioner in a mental health context, whereas it may mean a health behavior trial to a researcher. Clarification of terms is needed, or else this Tower of Babel issue will lead to thoughts that program development is not feasible.

Second, program development work involves oftentimes relatively simple research methods. Researchers should remember to show a little tolerance regarding use of scientific designs if they are to develop programs using multiple steps with limited funds. Although experimental work may be ideal, documentation of one's own and others' work and replication work can assist in making even simple designs, such as single-group pretest-posttest designs, useful to decision makers (e.g., Sussman, Dent, Burton, Stacy, & Flay, 1995).

Finally, some researchers and practitioners may question the scope of application of program development models, such as the chain model. They may wonder if we are only conveying ideas that are useful for the health education of individuals. Indeed, a lot of demand reduction-type material was offered in this text. Can these same program development steps be used in what might be called supply reduction, policy-oriented, environmental modification, or health protection-type programming? For example, how does one develop programming that might include price measures, legal blood alcohol concentration (BAC) levels, control of sales, or control of advertising as a means of decreasing the prevalence of alcohol abuse? It might be pondered whether these same six steps apply. Sure they do! Theory and assessment work can apply—"Where in the environment are the key problem units?" would be the question (e.g., Pentz, Bonnie, & Shopland, 1996). Perceived efficacy studies would be very important and would involve policymakers, gatekeepers of regulatory mechanisms, and the consumer. Component or pilot studies could involve contrasts of single environmental strategies on a small scale. Such contrasts may be easier in the arena of supply control (e.g., bartender behavior) as opposed to price control. However, such work could and has been completed in this arena. Certainly, the results of previous studies could be used to inform future work. The key here is to select the proper theory (molar level), the proper target subjects (regulators, suppliers, consumers), and a realistic methodology (perhaps perceived efficacy studies need to be relied on more than component studies). We believe that these three additional pitfalls are just illusions of failure. Program development is a robust, hard-nosed, multiapplication methodology to help people build the best health behavior programs possible.

A REVIEW OF THE CHAIN MODEL

The groundwork for a science of program development has been laid in this book. In brief, we believe that health behavior programs should be evaluated as they are being constructed to make sure the programs are theoretically sound and will achieve stated goals. The early phase of program development should focus on the theoretical processes that determine why a program is needed and how to modify behavior. Middle phases should examine individual program component contents and modalities of implementation. Later phases should combine program components and pilot test a complete program, using as criteria of efficacy immediate mediator and outcome measures that are likely to predict longer-term outcomes (Sussman, Petosa, & Clarke, 1996).

We proposed a six-step program development chain model. First, one would develop a theory of target group needs and link these to program activities. In other words, concurrent with the assessment of a target population need, a theory of program mediation would be developed to address this need (Chapters 1-6, this volume). When one delineates a target population, a health problem within this group, and the parameters of the health problem, one begins to develop a theory for solving the health problem. Program activities that plausibly address health needs are then generated. These activities indicate the beginnings of a theory of how to solve the health problem.

We suggest that needs assessments are never separated from theory. For example, study of a remote population in need of achieving healthier lifestyles, as determined by level of heart disease risk, cannot be examined separately from theoretical notions of health lifestyles, quality of life, and cultural traditions. Likewise, program activities to reduce the problem cannot be separated from notions such as cultural sensitivity. One may think of a program as affecting variables (e.g., farming techniques, culture) that mediate the relationship between antecedent variables (e.g., food availability and types of foods) and consequence variables (e.g., unhealthy diet).

Second, there is a need to systematically pool and warehouse promising activities for new uses (see Chapters 7 and 8, this volume). The theory of program mediation developed in the prior step leads one to search for promising activities or activity ideas to test (e.g., instruction in farming that is consistent with cultural norms). One should be able to go through a library of activities or activity ideas and pull out useful information. However, proprietary interests need to be addressed and potential conflicts overcome. In many cases, creative, innovative ideas are needed. Thus, it is likely that program staff may need to generate plausible novel activity ideas as well.

Third, there is a need to systematize a set of perceived efficacy studies that can screen among promising activity ideas gathered in the last step for additional program development work (see Chapters 9-12, this volume). Numerous ideas gathered during the previous step should be able to be contrasted using methods that are relatively time-saving and cost-effective. This could be viewed as a program activity screening step. Activities may be verbal or written in administration or completion; myriad tools are available, as was documented in previous chapters.

Fourth, there is a need to systematize a set of immediate-impact studies that can provide a means of determining workability of individual program components (see Chapters 13 and 14, this volume). Possibly, the top half of the most favorably rated activities from the previous perceived efficacy study step would be retained for this one. Fifth, there is a need to systematize program construction and pilot testing of a complete program (see Chapters 15-17). Perhaps 50% of activities from the previous step are retained for the complete program. Sequencing of activities and sessions is considered. Finally, there is a need to refine a set of immediate posttreatment measures that predict longer-term outcomes (see Chapters 18 and 19). Meta-analytic and other statistical modeling work are promising directions to take to identify important mediators and moderators.

We think this program development chain model is promising. But there are many challenges to this and other program development models. This text has met many of these challenges, but much work remains. In the following section, we would like to present some of these challenges for future program development research and practice.

▶ FUTURE RESEARCH NEEDS

Several research needs have been pointed out earlier in this text. We wish to highlight two of them. First, there is too little systematization of methods. We present a brief systematization scheme based on previously presented chapter material. Perhaps this scheme only cuts the surface of what is needed in elaborating and refining future program development methods. Second, there is some uncertainty about what mediators or moderators should target. We present a 12-variable scheme as a heuristic start on this search.

LITTLE SYSTEMATIZATION OF METHODS

In previous program development work, there has been too little systemization of methods. In the present text, we began this work of systematization. We wish to quickly summarize chapter material to provide the skeleton of a systematization of methods.

Theory to Activity Ideas. There are three main approaches to theory-activity linking. First, *acquisition-oriented theorizing* focuses on counteracting etiologic variables. Self-report questionnaires or use of methods such as focus groups can help identify what these etiologic variables are (e.g., poverty) and help identify program needs (e.g., increase access to health care, teach literacy), which may mediate positive subsequent changes in behavior (health care seeking, environmental advocacy). Second, *behavior-targeted theorizing* focuses on manipulating changes in health behavior and is derived from learning theories; changes in behavior data often are collected through a functional analysis of behavior. A functional analysis of behavior can involve interview or observational data. Stimuli (i.e., immediately proximal antecedent information), concurrent events, and consequences of behavior are the data collected. Finally, *consequences-oriented theorizing* focuses on minimizing consequences of one's behavior through means of health protection. For example, in addition to teaching parents to place medication out of reach of their children, they may make use of safety caps. The practitioner or researcher might consider all three types of theoretical approaches when generating program activities. In the future, perhaps an integration of these theories will be recognized or realized (see Chapter 4 for a detailed presentation).

Pooling and Warehousing. Several methods of pooling program outcomes information were mentioned, including (a) literature synthesis, (b) expert panel consensus ratings, (c) consensus meetings, (d) grant agency reports on grantees, and (e) creation of ongoing consortiums. One may argue that pooling should consist of unpublished and published literature synthesis by research experts, followed up by expert panel ratings produced as the result of a consensus meeting. However, an incomplete literature synthesis could result in a biased selection. Warehousing materials can be accomplished through private-company catalogues, as Web site collections, or through technical reports or materials made available through research collaborators. This area needs much work because copyright and proprietary consideration may make access to works or potential target clients limited. Certainly, careful selection of activities (or development of new activity ideas) is necessary for subsequent tests that fit well one's theory of behavior change and are likely to be acceptable to the current target population (see Chapter 7 for a detailed presentation).

Perceived Efficacy Studies. There are numerous means to establish the overall perceived quality, as well as perceived effect on a specific hypothesized mediator, of a program activity. The methods to be used depend on the target population (e.g., level of literacy, access to the population). Verbal methods include (a) unstructured and semistructured interviews of key informants or at key locations (intercept), (b) community forums, (c) use of consensus methods such as the Delphi technique, (d) role-playing as a behavioral means of expressing approval for an activity, (e) focus groups, or (f) use of a Thematic Apperception Test (TAT)-like protocol (describe a picture or cartoon of the activity). Verbal methods are appropriate for illiterate populations or those who prefer not to write down their responses (see Chapter 9 for a detailed presentation). Written methods include (a) draw a situation (draw the activity), (b) sorting tasks, (c) use of open-ended and closed-ended questionnaires, (d) use of theme studies, (e) sentence completion tasks, and (f) use of word association-like tasks. Written methods are appropriate for mute populations or in relatively traditional educational settings. Some methods can be presented in either a verbal or a written modality (e.g., use of the TAT-like story protocol, word association; see Chapter 11 for a detailed presentation). By using any of the above methods, perceived quality of numerous activities may be screened. Perceived program quality generally is measured as a quantitative index of ratings of perceived interest, potential learning, and perceived helpfulness of activity ideas. Effects on hypothesized mediators of change (e.g., specific beliefs or skills) also can be measured. After establishing and ranking activities on perceived program quality or perceived effects on desired mediators, around half of the activities can be retained for further testing.

Component Studies. These studies involve actually implementing activities with subjects or groups of subjects. There are four main types of component relations: (a) Multiple components may impart the same content using a different process (traditional component relation), (b) components may build on each other (building-block components), (c) components with different contents may strengthen each other (complementary components), and (d) components may be tailored to different community populations (constellation components). When developing a program, certain components may be tested for the best repetition of similar information. If so, the traditional component study, perhaps using an iterative single-group design, may be used. Multiple-activity processes (games, role-plays, lectures, debates) may be contrasted, and the best two or three activities may be retained. For example, a lecture on physical consequences of unsafe sex and a "stages of unsafe sex" role-playing activity may be retained for use in a pregnancy prevention curriculum.

However, when beginning a program, teaching a behavioral skill, and ending a program, a building-block design is used in general. Sets of components over a 2-day sequence generally are compared to best impart relationship development between health educators and target persons, learning and practice of skills, and decision making and making a commitment. When developing cognitive and behavioral-type components, one must ensure that these components reinforce each other in general—they tend to be complementary. For example, learning what are popular prohealth norms and then practicing skills that support those norms are complementary tasks. Finally, when tailoring a component for different audiences, often a comparison evaluation study is used. The component is compared across different groups to assess their reactions to the component. In addition, as a variation on this constellation approach, the component may be tailored specifically and differentially to the perspective of the different target participants. For example, a city leader as a target participant may be taught how to motivate others to use refusal assertion training (a type of training of trainers), whereas a youth may be taught refusal assertion training. Rules of thumb for evaluating program activity quality ("three quarters" up the scale) and retention ("keep half") also might be offered (see Chapter 13 for a detailed presentation).

Sequencing. Several factors need to be considered when sequencing program components into a complete package. Before providing detailed information, aside from the general purposes of the project, a positive relationship needs to be established between the program facilitator (health educator) and the audience (target population). Trust and willingness to listen are key attitudes to instill in the audience. Next, general information about the health behavior should be provided to orient the audience to the issues in the topic area. Then the mediators should be counteracted. Learning of skills should precede practice of those skills. Direct instruction, rehearsal, role-play, and feedback are used in a sequence to instill behavioral changes. Cognitive activities should be interspersed with behavioral activities to maintain interest and to provide a complementary effect. Inconsistencies between individual perceptions, social consensus, and objectively established facts can be made explicit to help produce cognitive changes. These changes should facilitate bonding with a social and physical environment conducive to the desired change. Generally, toward the end of the program, decision making and making a commitment should help facilitate the desired lifestyle change.

The instruction of the program components should be interactive. In other words, the audience should engage in a fair amount of discussion with the facilitator and with each other. In this way, the audience becomes an active participant in its own change. The program should flow smoothly, producing experiences that indicate motivation to change, insight regarding the desirability and possibility of achieving healthier behaviors, and practice of behaviors that lead to better health. Multiple sensory modalities should be used to facilitate learning. Material should be summarized at the beginning and end of session reviews. Finally, the audience should be followed through with birthday cards, notes, phone calls, session summaries, or other means to indicate that the supportive group relationship remains in spirit.

Another look at sequencing is based on the assumption that health behavior research programs can be constructed for persons at different ages and contexts and that developmental levels and readiness for change can induce a sequence of whole-program packages. Much work is needed to identify sequencing of programming at this molar level (see Chapter 15 for a detailed presentation).

Piloting. Pilot studies provide a means to test the whole program after its parts have been assembled—to work out timing of activities, revise draft measures, and the like—before actually carrying out the trial. Pilot studies are among the most popular of program development steps. Although previous steps are imperative, the pilot study is the practice run before the main race. If a careful regimen of training is not completed beforehand, at least the runner will know the course.

Several designs can be used to test a whole program. Single-group designs provide a means of examining changes in responses of subjects before and after receiving a program. Subjects serve as their own controls. However, numerous confounds exist that compromise the interpretation of changes achieved. Repeating single-group studies, with subtle variations in program contents or process and with replications across groups (iterative single-group studies), can provide some means of control for confounds, such as the effects of time, testing, maturation, regression to the mean (internal validity confounds), or time-by-program interactions (external validity confounds). Quasi-experimental designs provide comparison groups and control for the when and where of measurement, but self-selection effects could still bias the interpretation of program effects. Experimental designs provide the clearest results but sometimes cannot be arranged administratively and sometimes are limited in terms of external validity (generalizability).

Small sample sizes in pilot studies could limit statistical power. Thus, some careful thought is needed to decide how many subjects are needed for this type of study. Effects on immediate-impact measures with large effect sizes and directional hypotheses permit reasonable empirical tests for pilot studies.

As with other studies, measures in pilot studies are of implementation, process, and immediate outcomes. Implementation includes the degree to which a program was delivered as designed (adherence), which aspects of the program were not delivered (omissions), and changes made while delivering the program (reinvention). Process evaluations are of program receptivity and perceived program quality—that is, of interest, perceived learning, believability, and perceived helpfulness (see Chapter 16 for a detailed presentation).

PREDICTING LONGER-TERM OUTCOMES

We argued that a rigorous program development process might permit the identification of mediators and moderators of program effects. Mediators are measures that, when effected, affect later behavior through substantive or content-related pathways and procedural or process-related pathways. Moderators are measures that affect the relations of the program with its mediators (e.g., leaving out key aspects of a program when instructing it, institutional support) or affect the relations of the mediators with program outcomes (e.g., trying to elicit attitude changes on persons who already hold the desired attitude; see Chapter 19 for a detailed presentation about program mediation).

Unfortunately, we know only a little about program moderation and mediation. With respect to moderators, there is evidence that pretest or immediate-outcome variables such as specific differences in social environmental support (e.g., institutional efficacy or support for the target persons) modulate the effects of the mediators on later behavior across a wide variety of health behavior contexts (e.g., Sussman et al., 1995). However, we view many moderator variables as invariant—they can be studied statistically but generally are not subject to manipulation. (As another example, gender and ethnicity are typical moderators and are invariant to immediate change.)

We should get an idea on key mediators that might be important across health behavior contexts. Without measurements of mediators, it is difficult to tell why a program worked or did not work. With a reasonably consistent set of mediators, we may be able to discern why programs work across many contexts. That being said, we have learned enough to suggest that there are several reasonably consistent known mediators of health behavior change. Perceived program quality may mediate program effects in several domains. Arguably, this is a higher-order combination of other mediators, which is good for predicting whether a program is likely to work but is bad in terms of identifying specifics regarding why it worked. Also, degree of group interaction in processing program material may mediate change; this variable identifies specific processes of material but not its contents. On the other hand, an increase in negative attitudes toward unhealthy target behaviors is a content-related mediator of the relations of programming to behavioral outcomes in several health domains, such as drug abuse prevention (Hansen, 1992; Tobler & Stratton, 1997).

We posit that there are six main specific "content" mediators of program effects in health behavior programs. These mediators are likely to be relevant to health programs one may design. If they are on target with one's program goals and objectives, they should be measured with an immediate posttest or as differences between pretest and posttest:

1. *Social skill:* ability to act on one's social environment. These skills include assertiveness, clarity of communication, ability to listen, and ability to ask questions. These skills often are instructed in comprehensive social influences programming and can be measured through self-reports or role-play assessments.

2. *Social support:* strength and number of relationships that can support one in difficult times. Several attempts to manipulate social support have led to equivocal results. However, joining social support groups, trying to achieve social support through phone calling, and trying to arrange contracts of support with significant others are methods of achieving social support that might be tried. Social support can be measured through gross measures of one's social network (e.g., marital status) or through perceived satisfaction with one's social support, as examples.

3. *Social norms:* large social norms or perceptions of such norms that steer one toward healthy behavior. Very successful strategies to counteract unhealthy behavior norms include behavior prevalence overestimates reduction and normative restructuring. Health behavior prevalence estimates and perceived acceptability estimates among one's peers are reasonable measures to use.

4. *Learning skill:* ability to learn quickly and accurately material needed to help one adapt to changing circumstances or to surmount difficult environments. In particular, one needs to learn how, where, and for whom to obtain resources; how to keep or invest resources; and how to protect oneself from the influence of inaccurate information. Mastery of procedures for enacting health behaviors may reflect, in part, learning skill. Often, functional assessments are completed to tap such skill.

5. *Self-control:* the ability to regulate one's own thoughts and actions. This involves the ability to set goals and plan methods to prompt desirable behavior or the ability to edit out undesirable or self-defeating verbal and nonverbal behavior. Often, this type of mediator is counteracted through instruction in decision making, self-talk, and relaxation skills and can be measured through self-reports of one's tendency to act on impulse or through behavioral observation.

6. *Outcome expectancies:* what an individual believes will be the results of engaging in a certain behavior. Creation of explicit outcome expectancies often involves estimating the perceived costs and benefits of engaging in a healthy versus an unhealthy behavior. Consideration is needed of the temporal scope of outcomes, consideration of all relevant benefits and costs simultaneously in working memory, and ability to actively seek out new potential costs and benefits infor-

mation. Motivation interventions, which clarify discrepancies between where one is in goal achievement and where one wants to be, also may be perceived as a means to make explicit and perhaps change one's outcome expectancies regarding engaging in a health behavior. Often, outcome expectancies are established through use of open-ended responses to questionnaires or through use of interviewing techniques.

Please note that the first three mediators involve social skills or perceptions. One's ability to favorably process one's social world and obtain support when needed indicates the capacity to cushion stresses and change behavior with support from others. Awareness of social norms may influence and shape individuals' perceptions about health and health behavior. The second three mediators involve intrapersonal skills or perceptions. One's motivation and ability to regulate one's behavior and learn material that assists in adaptation to life circumstances indicate the capacity to change from within.

In addition, we posit that four main program process mediators should be measured, particularly at immediate posttest, and will predict longer-term outcomes. These are the following:

1. *Motivation of the target population to participate in the whole program:* Motivation of target population may be measured through high attendance, high homework returns, low rate of tardiness, or self-report indicators that the target group was motivated to participate in the program. One can manipulate cooperation by maximizing the quality of program materials, encouraging participant involvement, engaging in relationship-building activities among participants and program facilitator, and appropriate pacing of homework and other participant demands.

2. *Smooth delivery of program:* Delivery of a program should flow from topic to topic with little disruption from extraneous sources. One can assess smooth delivery through gross measures of disruption (e.g., changes in scheduling of sessions, starting sessions at different times, interference through nonprogram events such as fire alarms). Smooth program delivery can lead participants to trust the information source, enhances program credibility, and maximizes one's ability to integrate program information together. One can maximize smooth delivery through the cooperation of key persons in the delivery environment and by engaging in program delivery at a convenient location.

3. *High level of planned participant interaction during program (e.g., Socratic style, group discussions):* High interaction between health educator and target group, as well as members of the target group with each other, permits rich transmission of information and norms relevant to the establishment of change. Direct participant involvement tends to build perceived program relevance, enhance retention of learning, and improve participant ratings of the program. Use

of this interaction style requires facilitator training but is incorporated into many effective programs. This variable can be measured (a) by recording what percentage of questions asked by the facilitator are answered by the facilitator or the target group or (b) by recording the percentage of people in the program who speak during each session.

4. *Providing memorable programming:* This can be measured by letters of support written by program participants or by recall of program name or activities. Indications of commitment to program or memory for program contents indicate a long-term effect of the program on target sample receptivity. Memora- bility can be manipulated by using novel strategies (e.g., videotaping public commitment), although memory of correct messages may require use of booster sessions and elaboration of learned information to a trained facilitator. It should be recognized that mediators of behavior change might not be the same variables as mediators of the *maintenance* of behavior change. Possibly this last mediator is most relevant to maintenance of change.

Please note that each process mediator is relatively important at different phases of program implementation. Relationship building and motivation are important at the beginning of the program, smooth delivery and participant interaction are important from the first session on, and making the program memorable is particularly important toward the end of the program or in follow-up sessions.

We also do not wish to underestimate the importance of high perceived quality ratings to discern how well the program development model is doing overall. We assume that effects on both content and process mediators are reflected in adjectives of perceived program quality—beliefs that a program is interesting, leads to learning, is credible, and is relevant and helpful to achieve desired health outcomes. We recommend use of this higher-order mediator construct—to use along with other mediator measures. Possibly, this measure will tap the important mediators and will reflect how well all the content and process mediators are working together to elicit health behavior effects (integration). In summary, we presented six content mediators (three interpersonal and three intrapersonal), four process mediators, and one higher-order mediator. We hope these mediators provide a good start for program developers who are wondering what are likely to be important mediators to target in their programs.

TECHNOLOGICAL ADVANCES

Who can anticipate the future of the means of program delivery? How will rapidly changing information technologies shape and influence consumer preferences and health program delivery systems? Right now, computer technology permits interactive health programming over the World Wide Web, through electronic mail, or through use of compact-disc technologies. Visual interaction features continue to develop and promise to involve greater person-to-person contact. Programming can be delivered from and to any part of the world. Program development approaches will need to involve these modalities to an increasing extent in the future. Electronic mail permits immediate delivery of manuscripts and communications, which can facilitate coordination among different agencies involved in programming. Thus, technology permits better community-wide program development efforts.

There is no question that information technologies will increase our collective capacity to store and disseminate information. The challenge is to learn how to integrate these technologies into future health programs and increase the effectiveness of these programs. For example, Prochaska, DiClemente, Velicer, and Rossi (1993) report that computer-based health counseling may be more appealing and effective for some individuals than human counselors. This is particularly true if the computer-based intervention is carefully matched to individual stage of change. Although information technologies hold promise as tools for health programs, in most cases, the potential has yet to be tested. Empirical program development methods would be an ideal approach to the careful integration and testing of these technologies.

The first leap in behavioral health focused on means to elicit changes in behavior to achieve better health status (Matarazzo, 1984). The recent desire to integrate behavioral approaches with biomedical (e.g., pharmacological treatments) and biogenetic engineering approaches suggests that program development will need to consider how to piece together questionnaire, behavioral observation, and related approaches to assessment with blood metabolytes analysis. Such work has been conducted in the field of behavioral pharmacology for years, but this technology has not been applied much to health programming. This biopsychosocial approach is likely to gain increasing importance over the next 100 years.

CONCLUSIONS ◄

It is an exciting time for program planners. As part of multidisciplinary teams, they can now use empirical methods and work together toward the improvement of health behavior programs. Inherent in these methods is the means to carefully assess the degree of effectiveness of both program elements and complete coordinated programs. The empirical process would yield a cumulative, self-correcting body of knowledge directly linked to solving the health problems communities seek to address. Consistent use of empirical program development methods would allow us to directly and specifically answer the question, "What works?" Furthermore, we would possess a knowledge base that would allow elaboration on "what works with whom, under what conditions, and for what price." Answers to these questions will empower professionals, policymakers, and consumers to make informed decisions regarding the appropriate role for health promotion in each community for each health concern.

Some skeptics may claim that health program development processes have little to no relevance to long-term impacts because generally only perceived impact or immediate impact is assessed. Still, a systematic process of program development is better than relying on the subjective judgments of a few people. At minimum, a program that is well received has a better chance of achieving compliance by recipients. At maximum, and quite likely, a program that changes a variety of proposed mediators and moderators in desired directions will achieve effects on long-term behavior. Clearly, this approach paves the way for documenting program effects. Program planners will be able to test assumptions regarding the relationships between short-term health program effects, changes in health behavior, and, ultimately, changes in health status. We hope this handbook empowers decision makers with information necessary for the efficient allocation of resources and the establishment of sound health policy.

▶ REFERENCES

BUKOSKI, W. J., & EVANS, R. I. (Eds.). (1998). *Cost-benefit/cost-effectiveness research on drug abuse prevention: Implications for programming and policy* (NIH Pub. No. 98-4021). Washington, DC: U.S. Department of Health and Human Services, National Institutes of Health, Superintendent of Documents, Government Printing Office.

HANSEN, W. B. (1992). School-based substance abuse prevention: A review of the state of the art in curriculum, 1980-1990. *Health Education Research: Theory and Practice, 7,* 403-430.

MATARAZZO, J. D. (1984). Behavioral health: A 1990 challenge for the health professions. In J. D. Matarazzo, S. M. Weiss, J. A. Herd, N. E. Miller, & S. M. Weiss (Eds.), *Behavioral health: A handbook of health enhancement and disease prevention* (pp. 3-40). New York: John Wiley.

PENTZ, M. A., BONNIE, R. J., & SHOPLAND, D. R. (1996). Integrating supply and demand reduction strategies for drug abuse prevention. *American Behavioral Scientist, 39,* 897-910.

PROCHASKA, J., DICLEMENTE, C. C., VELICER, W. F., & ROSSI, J. S. (1993). Standardized, individualized interactive and personalized self-help programs for smoking cessation. *Health Psychology, 12,* 399-405.

SUSSMAN, S., DENT, C. W., BURTON, D., STACY, A. W., & FLAY, B. R. (1995). *Developing school-based tobacco use prevention and cessation programs.* Thousand Oaks, CA: Sage.

SUSSMAN, S., PETOSA, R., & CLARKE, R. (1996). The use of empirical curriculum development to improve prevention research. *American Behavioral Scientist, 39,* 838-852.

TOBLER, N. S., & STRATTON, H. H. (1997). Effectiveness of school-based drug prevention programs: A meta-analysis of the research. *Journal of Primary Prevention, 18,* 77-128.

CHAPTER 20

Commentary 1
Richard I. Evans

The authors of this chapter understandably have a difficult task to cull from the vast amount of literature, relating to a great variety of health promotion programs, a scientific perspective for future researchers and program developers on how to launch *truly* effective theory-based programming. Such a *general* scientific perspective, as described in this chapter, does provide a functional model for investigators in many diverse and often disparate arrays of *specific* health promotion-targeted behaviors. However, the chapter's general prescription for future program development might need to cross many hurdles to be fulfilled in specific instances of health behavior-oriented programming. The difficulties encountered in developing HIV prevention programs for adolescents, in which the present author currently is involved, might be briefly examined to further explore the contingencies related to health behavior programs that might present particular challenges to applying the chain model as reviewed in this final chapter.

Although health behavior programs, by their very nature, may be related to serious health threats to individuals, they generally do not involve many of the social sanctions related to the initiation or continuance of active sexual behavior that presents the major threat of HIV exposure for adolescents. Prevention of at-risk sexual behavior obviously involves a more complex decision-making process for adolescents than is involved in most health behaviors and one that is affected by biological, psychological, and social/economic mediators or moderators. The behavior that places typical adolescents at risk for AIDS is sexual intercourse (heterosexual or homosexual) that involves an exchange of body fluids, obviously quite different from circumstances that place adolescents at risk for substance abuse, which does not, in the final analysis, require contact between two individuals. (This would apply, of course, to most other health behavior programs, as generally discussed by the authors of this chapter.)

Safer-sex options available to adolescents include (a) abstinence from sexual intercourse, (b) engaging in sexual intercourse but exercising care in the selection of sexual partners, and (c) the correct use of latex condoms during each sexual encounter that involves a possible exchange of body fluids. Training adolescents to follow such prescriptions, considering the normal developmental state of physiological sexual arousal and the spontaneity of sexual behavior for typical adolescents, presents a difficult challenge to behavioral scientists attempting to develop AIDS risk prevention programs. Furthermore, safer-sex decision making among adolescents is too often influenced by the concurrent use of alcohol and other drugs that may impair judgment (Dryfoos, 1990). The relationship between use of drugs and sexual behavior is a particularly good example of why AIDS prevention programs are far more difficult to develop than those directed at most other health behaviors. For adolescents, the problems of responding to physiological sexual arousal and social pressures to engage in sexual behavior may be further complicated by problems related to prior or concurrent use of alcohol or other substances or, for that matter, other health-related behaviors. This constellation of behaviors, each component of which places adolescents at risk in its own right, has important consequences for the transmission of HIV. Although all possible causal or even correlational connections between substance use and HIV risk sexual behavior have not been documented empirically, it can be argued that both direct and indirect causal relations, as discussed in this chapter, might exist at each of three levels: biological, psychological, and social/economic.

At the biological level, there is the direct transmission of HIV via needle sharing among IV drug users. A possible indirect, interactive effect connecting drug use to HIV transmission might involve alcohol or other drug use that leads to impaired immune response, resulting in easier acquisition of HIV when exposure occurs during unsafe sexual behavior.

At the psychological level, one might suggest a direct effect in the form of antecedent trait predispositions (e.g., risk taking) that have a causal impact on both drug use and unsafe sexual behavior. A potential indirect linear effect might involve use of alcohol or other drugs to the extent that decision making related to perceived vulnerability to HIV is impaired, resulting in unsafe sexual behavior.

At the social/economic level, adolescent drug users may engage in prostitution in exchange for drugs or to obtain money to purchase drugs. This places them in one of the most disturbing "at risk for AIDS" sexual relationship networks. Furthermore, adolescents who are consistently exposed for any reason (e.g., runaways, low socioeconomic status, school or family dysfunction) to an environment in which drug-related sexual activity is common may conform to such an environment even in the absence of direct economic pressure. Although the above discussion does not attempt to state, exhaustively, all conditions that must be addressed in programs designed to prevent HIV transmission, it does illustrate many of the problems faced in preventing AIDS in adolescents that would rarely be involved in other health-related behaviors.

Probably, most closely paralleling interventions designed to prevent teenagers' use of tobacco, alcohol, illegal drugs, or other health-threatening behaviors would be the promotion of abstinence (i.e., zero tolerance), which is advocated by many individuals and institutions in our culture. However, the use of such an approach to prevent the spread of AIDS among adolescents is, unfortunately, in contradiction to a well-established finding. Approximately 50% of young men and 21% of young women have engaged in sexual intercourse by the time they are 16 years old (Miller, Turner, & Moses, 1990). Although well-planned interventions might be expected to increase the number of adolescents who choose abstinence as a prevention strategy, pragmatically, such an approach would not affect the behavior of a significant number of adolescents at high risk for HIV exposure because they are already sexually active and would continue to be so.

Successfully "inoculating" adolescents with the wisdom and perspicacity to be selective in choice of sexual partners is also difficult. Mays and Cochran (1993) explored this behavior in an investigation involving 394 young adults. Results indicated that partner questioning about AIDS risk histories was not reliable. Risk minimization in partners by respondents was especially prevalent among African American and Hispanic young adults. Males were relatively likely to minimize the AIDS risk histories they reported to partners. In addition, a substantial proportion of the young adults surveyed apparently use partner questioning to reduce their HIV risk, at least in their minds (perhaps as a sort of rationalization), resulting in less frequent condom use when compared to others who did not question partners. Thus, it would appear to be unlikely to expect adolescents to seek information or to receive truly valid responses concerning sexual history or HIV status of potential partners.

Of all of the alternatives presented, persuading adolescents to use latex condoms correctly, particularly if used together with a spermicidal foam, may represent the most plausible prevention strategy presently available to sexually active adolescents. Well-planned intervention programs must address most of the perceived negative factors associated with condom use. Adolescents may resist the use of condoms because of the supposedly decreased sensitivity to the sexual experience and interference with the spontaneity involved in the sexual act. The dangers inherent in unprotected sexual intercourse must be addressed to offset such concerns. Negative community reaction to encouraging condom use also must be addressed. Specific community education programs must be integrated within such prevention programs.

It is evident, then, that the adolescent decision-making process as it relates to sexual activity must, of necessity, consider a number of circumstances that would not be operative in a decision related to tobacco, alcohol, illegal drug use, or, for that matter, most other health-related behaviors. Even if one is able to effectively inoculate adolescents with strategies to resist social influences to engage in risky sexual activity, conflicts within individuals exposed to an AIDS prevention program may be difficult to resolve. To illustrate internal conflicts within the individual involved in decision making related to engaging in sex, we might consider a hypothetical best-case scenario. For illustrative purposes, we might use the case of a White 16-year-old male who has been exposed to an HIV risk behavior prevention program in a high school health class. He has learned about the AIDS virus and its mechanisms of transmission. He has come to perceive himself as more vulnerable to acquiring the virus than he had previously believed. Furthermore, his parents and older brother have encouraged him to take seriously what he has learned in his health class and to read the surgeon general's mail-out on AIDS his family received. He respects the values and opinions of his parents and older brother. Even within the network of discussion among his peers and the social norms to which he might be expected to conform, the importance of engaging in safe sexual practices is reinforced.

This young man has now made several resolutions (i.e., has engaged in a decision-making process leading to some specific intentions concerning his sexual practices and drug use). First, he will not use IV drugs or any other illegal drugs; this was not a difficult decision because he and his friends have never tried them, and drug use is not approved within the adolescent subculture of his community. Second, although he enjoys drinking alcohol with his friends and engages in sexual intercourse (recently initiated with his new girlfriend), he will have learned the importance of avoiding the use of alcohol during a sexual encounter. Third, when engaging in sexual intercourse, he will have learned the importance of using condoms. Last, assuming this young man possesses considerable self-efficacy, it would seem that this individual is not predisposed to engage in HIV risk behavior.

However, let us examine his impression management style. He presents himself as an independent, vigorous, virile, experientially oriented person. He is predisposed toward risk taking as a manifestation of his impression management style (consistent with a "macho" image). The youth's father and older brother have durable symbols of male identity such as athletic trophies, financial accomplishments, and occupations conveying imagery associated in American culture with the hard-driving, risk-taking male gender role (Gollwitzer & Wicklund, 1985; Wicklund & Gollwitzer, 1982). In contrast, at his stage of development as an adolescent, unlike an adult, our subject has only more transitory behaviors at his disposal with which to symbolize the "macho" identity he chooses to convey. Thus, despite his specific rational intention to engage in safe sex, on a particular occasion the youth might well spend the evening drinking with his girlfriend and engaging in unprotected sexual intercourse as he acts out this "macho" role. A predisposition toward such "macho" risk taking can moderate an intention to engage in safe sex, even with such a relatively high level of perceived individual self-efficacy and safe-sex knowledge.

The case just presented suggests that even under ideal circumstances, an intervention program that appears to have an effective impact on the intention to engage in safe-sex behaviors must still address the problem of intrapersonal predispositions within the individual. Such intrapersonal predispositions and even the contingencies that lead to the intention to engage in safe-sex behaviors may be quite different in the case of females, members of minority groups who suffer various social and economic deficits, and homosexual or bisexual individuals, as examples. Therefore, any HIV prevention program obviously must be extremely sensitive to the subcultural characteristics of the targeted adolescent population. In our current investigation involving a large tri-ethnic study population, we have determined that even with adolescents most receptive to AIDS prevention programs, an array of contingencies must be addressed that block the conversion from knowledge to intention to safe-sex behavior. Contingencies differ from group to group and from individual to individual. In health programming, each psychosocial moderator must be specifically considered and specifically related to the realistic context of the sexual act. To be successful, prevention and other health behavior programs must address each component of the biological, psychological, and social/economic moderators that are indigenous to the population target group of adolescents.

In the development phase of health behavior programs, such as outlined in the chapter, the overall impact of the program might be increased if attention is given to the fact that any general model often may be very difficult to apply under various field contingencies in unique health behavior problems such as those involving AIDS prevention, as I have encountered. The bottom line: Moderator variables need careful consideration in program development.

▷ REFERENCES

DRYFOOS, J. G. (1990). *Adolescents at risk*. New York: Oxford University Press.

GOLLWITZER, P. M., & WICKLUND, R. A. (1985). The pursuit of self-defining goals. In J. Kuhl & J. Beckmann (Eds.), *Action control: From cognition to behavior* (pp. 61-85). New York: Springer-Verlag.

MAYS, V. M., & COCHRAN, S. D. (1993). Ethnic and gender differences in beliefs about sex partner questioning to reduce HIV risk. *Journal of Adolescent Research, 1*(1), 77-88.

MILLER, H. G., TURNER, C. F., & MOSES, L. E. (Eds.). (1990). *AIDS: The second decade*. Washington, DC: National Academy Press.

WICKLUND, R. A., & GOLLWITZER, P. M. (1982). *Symbolic self-completion*. Hillsdale, NJ: Lawrence Erlbaum.

CHAPTER 20

Commentary 2
Stan Maes

Although the chapter on "Needs for the Future of Program Development," based on the chain model, contains a lot of valuable ideas concerning program development, some underlying assumptions are open to discussion. The chapter seems to concentrate on specific health behavior change at an individual level, induced by experts. Although this is a defensible perspective, additional considerations are in need of comment. First, I am not certain that concentrating on specific isolated health behaviors such as quitting smoking or reducing alcohol or food intake is the most effective way to promote healthy lifestyles or to discourage unhealthy lifestyles. Second, because behavior is the result of an interaction between the individual and the environment, the analysis of environmental factors is an important issue in the development of a health behavior change program. Third, it is not clear what *need assessment* really means in the proposed model. The need to change seems to be defined externally or normatively in terms of recommended health behaviors; humans, however, are self-regulatory, which implies that they must experience a need to change. As a consequence, an important step in the development of a program might be to explore positive and negative relationships that exist within the target population between the target health behaviors and personal goals. I will elaborate on these three remarks in the following paragraphs.

The idea that health behavior change might concentrate on isolated targets such as smoking, consumption of sugar or fat, physical exercise, seat belt use, alcohol consumption, condom use, driving safely, or relaxation suggests that these behaviors are basically unrelated and that it is a defensible strategy to tackle them separately. As Leventhal, Prohaska, and Hirschman (1985) have pointed out, these behaviors are surface phenomena, which are highly influenced by underlying processes involving emotional or stress control, cognitive control, symptom control, and social control processes. In other words, different unhealthy behaviors share the same underlying mechanisms. Smoking, drinking too much alcohol, eating salty or sweet snacks, or risk-taking behavior all may have a similar function in stress reduction, may be supported within certain social reference groups, may be used to control similar symptoms, and may be rooted in common underlying beliefs or expectancies. Thus, one could argue that health promotion and disease prevention programs should concentrate more on the regulation of psychological processes, rather than on changing surface behaviors. Although this point of view does not invalidate many of the suggestions for program development made in the chapter, the steps suggested in the chain model may become a lot more complex if the program is targeted at influencing these underlying mechanisms. One might then conclude that we need more comprehensive programs directed at broader lifestyle changes or that specific health behavior change programs should at least share basic common characteristics. In other words, although there is most probably no magic bullet for change, programs should target these common psychological mechanisms that underlie the onset and maintenance of health behaviors. It is possible that the model could get focused more on surface elements (e.g., need for a behavioral change; detailed analysis of the problem behavior) than on comprehensive lifestyle changes and their underlying determinants. In contrast, some writers would argue that a few of the most important successes in the history of health promotion have come from comprehensive programs within community, work, school, health care, family, or leisure settings, which address these underlying mechanisms (Tilford & Tones, 1994).

The chapter seems to concentrate on behavioral change at an individual level and neglects, to some extent, the fact that behavior is a function of an interaction between the individual and the environment. By environment, I mean not only the social environment, to which the chapter gives credit by stressing the importance of social support. Behavior is also influenced by environmental measures of a different nature, such as introducing healthy food in canteens at school and at work, restricting smoking in public areas, creating facilities for physical exercise in the immediate environment of the individual, providing condoms, or designing roads. Some authors have even argued that environmental factors play the most important role in health behavior change (Altman, 1990). In other words, besides behavioral analysis and examination of the role of behavioral mediational processes, a screening of supportive or discouraging characteristics of the environment should be an important phase in the development of a program.

This screening of environmental risks (or protective factors) also should include characteristics of the larger environment, which may seem unrelated to these health behaviors at first sight. There is, for example, a lot of evidence that characteristics of the work environment (e.g., high demands in combination with a lack of control and low social support from boss and colleagues) can have adverse health effects, including cardiovascular disease, negative pregnancy outcomes, and psychosomatic complaints (Van der Doef & Maes, 1998). Such an ecological perspective is equally valid in other contexts such as school settings (Trickett & Birman, 1989). Unhealthy behaviors probably mediate the positive and negative effects of environmental factors because they can be seen as a means to cope with environmental demands or challenges. For this reason, interventions directed at changes in these environmental characteristics should parallel interventions that focused on direct health behavior change (Maes, Kittel, Scholten, & Verhoeven, 1996; Maes, Verhoeven, Kittel, & Scholten, 1998). It is, in my view, overly optimistic to believe that people can change on their own. Although this may be partly true for early adopters, as, for example, the masses who spontaneously stopped smoking decades ago, current smokers are "die-hards" who are resistant to behavioral change strategies and therefore require interventions that are supported by environmental changes. Moreover, interventions that concentrate only on individual behavioral change may elicit resistance in the target group because most people do not like to be treated as "blamed victims."

An important threat to program efficacy is the fact that most health behavior change programs tend to define the target of change in an external way: Quitting smoking, reducing alcohol intake, or starting physical exercise may be externally imposed goals, which makes internalization of these goals by the target population a very important issue. Adoption of an external goal can be defined as the integration of this goal into the existing goal hierarchy of the individual. The hierarchical organization of goals implies that movement toward a goal is more likely if this goal is in line with (and less likely if it is in conflict with) higher-order goals. Approximation toward many health behaviors, however, can create important conflicts at a level of higher-order goals. Losing weight, reducing alcohol consumption, quitting smoking, starting a vigorous exercise program, and avoiding snacks between meals are examples of health goals that undoubtedly serve higher-order health goals but are frequently in conflict with higher-order well-being goals. Within a specific behavioral episode, there also may be important interactions between goals at the same level. At the behavioral level, conflicts also can occur because of energy or time scarcity. In other words, there are different things that one might want to do at a certain moment, but one cannot do them all at once. Therefore, the occurrence of one behavior may limit the occurrence of a whole sequence of other behaviors because of limited capacity or energy. For these reasons, quitting smoking may interfere with studying for an exam, and engaging in physical exercise three times a week may conflict with spending time with a new romantic partner. In a study of 528 employees responsible for providing residential spending time with a new romantic partner. In a study of 528 employees responsible for providing residential care at seven nursing homes, we showed that competing personal goals are particularly important predictors for the initiation and maintenance of regular exercise (Maes & Gebhardt, in press). As a consequence, the efficacy of a program as perceived by the target group will depend on negative and positive relationships between the target health behavior(s) and existing personal (higher-order and behavioral) goals. It may, therefore, be wise to include an assessment of possible supportive, conflicting, and competing goals in the development of a program.

The authors of the chapter are aware of these issues, which have been alluded to in earlier chapters. Nevertheless, they should give more credit to these issues. On the other hand, there is also a danger of accepting these remarks too easily: Their adoption will undoubtedly complicate the development of a health behavior program, and, in some cases (as in the analysis of environmental factors or relevant personal goals), they raise a lot of methodological problems. Last but not least, this commentary would have been much longer if it had concentrated on all the merits of the proposed model and the many invaluable ideas on program development that it contains.

REFERENCES

ALTMAN, D. G. (1990). The social context and health behavior: The case of tobacco. In S. A. Shumaker, E. B. Schron, & J. K. Ockene (Eds.), *The handbook of health behavior change* (pp. 241-269). New York: Springer.

LEVENTHAL, H., PROHASKA, T. R., & HIRSCHMAN, R. S. (1985). Preventive health behavior across the life span. In J. Rosen & L. Soloman (Eds.), *Prevention in health psychology* (pp. 191-235). New York: University Press of New England.

MAES, S., & GEBHARDT, W. (in press). Self-regulation and health behavior: The health behavior goal model. In M. Boekaerts, P. R. Pintrich, & M. Zeidner (Eds.), *Handbook of self-regulation*. San Diego, CA: Academic Press.

MAES, S., KITTEL, F., SCHOLTEN, H., & VERHOEVEN, C. (1996). Health promotion at the worksite, a European perspective. *Japanese Health Psychology, 4,* 73-83.

MAES, S., VERHOEVEN, C., KITTEL, F., & SCHOLTEN, H. (1998). Effects of a Dutch work-site wellness-health program: The Brabantia Project. *American Journal of Public Health, 88,* 1037-1041.

TONES, K., & TILFORD, S. (1994). *Health education, effectiveness, efficiency and equity.* San Diego, CA: Singular Publishing Group, Inc.

TRICKETT, E. J., & BIRMAN, D. (1989). Taking ecology seriously: A community development approach to individually based preventive interventions in schools. In L. A. Bond & B. E. Compad (Eds.), *Primary prevention and promotion in schools* (pp. 361-390). Newbury Park, CA: Sage.

VAN DER DOEF, M., & MAES, S. (1998). The job demand-control (-support) model and physical health outcomes: A review of the strain and buffer hypotheses. *Psychology and Health, 13,* 909-936.

Author Index

Aaker, D. A., 289
Abbott, G. K., 8
Abelson, A. G., 239
Adams, G. L., 73
Agar, M., 140
Ager, C. R., 143
Agosti, V., 143
Aiken, L. S., 125, 135, 475, 481, 482, 485, 486, 488
Ajzen, I., 411, 427
Alcoholics Anonymous, 8
Almeida, P. M., 268, 269
Alterman, T., 179
Altman, D. G., 239, 242, 253, 522
Ames, G. M., 139
Ames, S. L., 110, 112, 120, 291, 295
Amodeo, M., 143
Anderson, J. R., 109, 113, 124
Anderson, P., 73
Andrews, J. A., 73-74
Annis, H. M., 114
Annon, K., 388
Antaki, C., 104
Aono, J. Y., 305
Aral, S. O., 210
Arguello, M., 101, 102
Argyris, C., 173
Asch, S., 427
Aspen Reference Group, 328, 329
Astin, J. A., 134
Aubrey, L. L., 269
Axelli, T., 392
Azzoni, A., 139
Bachman, J. G., 268, 349

Backer, T. E., 71, 200
Bacon, K., 488
Baer, J. S., 388
Bagehot, W., 61
Baker, E., 373, 377
Baker, T. B., 127
Balanda, K. P., 400
Balch, G., 265
Balka, E. B., 137
Banaji, M. R., 108, 109
Bandura, A., 35, 37, 427
Bangert-Downs, R. L., 143, 464
Baranowski, T., 7, 480-481
Barckley, M. F., 73-74
Barnhardt, T. M., 112
Baron, R. M., 134, 478, 485, 486
Barr, D., 173
Barth, R. P., 73
Bartholomew, L. K., 158
Basch, C. E., 18, 247, 257, 258, 259, 270, 271, 397, 468
Bates, G. W., 297
Baxter, T., 415
Beatty, P. A., 114
Begg, C. B., 453
Bein, T. H., 388
Bell, R. M., 412
Belloc, N. B., 10, 50
Bem, D. J., 294
Bennetti, R., 392
Benson, G., 16
Benson, H., 308, 309
Bentler, P. M., 134, 137, 484, 499
Bents, R., 488

Berg, B. L., 243, 249, 257, 259
Berk, R. A., 413
Berkowitz, G., 140
Bernard, H. R., 247, 252, 260
Bernard, L. C., 87
Berry, J. W., 265
Bertrand, J. T., 261
Besselman, L., 256
Best, J. A., 427
Bhattacharyya, K., 16, 93
Bice, T. L., 297
Bickman, L., 143, 481
Biederman, J., 139
Biglan, A., 74, 98, 99, 170, 176
Birman, D., 522
Black, N., 207
Blair, G., 392
Blanchard, E. B., 10
Blankenship, A. B., 289
Bloom, J. R., 163
Bolles, R. C., 121
Bonewasser, M., 100
Boney-McCoy, S., 15
Bonnie, R. J., 87, 179, 504
Borenstein, M., 333
Boroughs, J. M., 388
Boruch, R. F., 488
Bosworth, E., 488
Bosworth, K., 338
Botvin, E. M., 373, 377
Botvin, G. J., 373, 377, 425
Bouchet, C., 417
Bowers, J., 115
Bradburn, M., 293
Brannon, B. R., 439, 444
Bransford, J. D., 115, 121
Braver, S. L., 488
Braverman, M. T., 6
Breen, G. E., 289
Breslow, L., 10, 50
Breslow, N., 10
Briancon, S., 417
Bridger, J. C., 87
Brieger, W. R., 239
Brindis, C., 140
Brink, S. G., 372
Brody, G. H., 15
Brook, J. S., 137
Brook, L., 293
Brotman, R., 339
Broussard, B., 397, 399
Brown, B., 87
Brown, J., 116-117, 118
Brown, J. D., 489, 490
Brown, J. M., 388

Brown, L. F., 261
Brown, R., 240
Brown, S. A., 109, 114, 137, 464
Brown-Collins, A., 104
Brownell, K. D., 7
Brudenell, I., 139
Brune, C. M., 115
Brunswick, A. F., 137
Bruvold, W. H., 464
Bry, B. H., 133
Bryant, A., 269
Bryant, K. J., 73, 132, 134
Bryk, A. S., 134
Bukowski, W. J., 503
Bureau of Justice Assistance, 426
Burgess, P. M., 297
Burke, R., 285
Burnette, K. D., 388
Burton, D., 6, 7, 15, 16, 24, 82, 85, 87, 158, 170, 180, 257, 258, 268, 269, 271, 273, 276, 284, 289, 290, 293, 326, 328, 331, 333, 335, 346, 349, 350, 354, 368, 377, 403, 408, 417, 471, 481, 504, 511
Bush, P. J., 409
Bushman, B. J., 143
Bussiere, M. T., 143
Butcher, J. N., 300
Byrne, C., 87

Cadet, J. L., 265
Caetano, R., 137
California Department of Education, 184
Campbell, D. T., 6, 336, 337, 398, 399, 408, 484
Campbell, I. M., 297
Campbell, J., 140
Campbell, T. F., 71
Candelaria, J., 139
Caplan, R. D., 490
Card, J. J., 210, 215, 222-223, 226
Carey, M. P., 388
Carnine, D., 74
Carr, P. A., 158, 190
Carr, T. H., 112, 116
Carroll, A., 140
Carter, L. J., 366
Castro, F., 254
Catalano, F. R., 110, 133, 362, 490
Catania, J., 322
Catford, J., 208
Cattarello, A. M., 412
Centers for Disease Control and Prevention (CDC), 158, 180, 190, 334
Cetingok, M., 87
Chaiken, S., 411
Chalmers, T. C., 468

Chambless, D. L., 74
Chan, G. C., 427
Chassin, L. A., 84-85, 87, 88, 89, 137
Chatham, L. R., 388
Chavez, L. R., 247
Cheadle, A., 406
Chen, H.-T., 471, 472, 474, 481, 499
Chen, K., 366
Chesney, M. A., 10
Chevillard, I., 143
Christiansen, B. A., 109
Churgin, S., 426, 427
Cicchetti, D., 133, 134, 140
Claffey, A., 142
Clark, N., 7
Clarke, P., 285, 307, 454, 471, 481, 487
Clarke, R., 6, 12, 19, 505
Clayson, Z., 140
Clayton, R. R., 412
Cleary, S. D., 15, 16
Cluss, P. A., 9
Coates, T. J., 322
Cochran, S. D., 101, 173, 518
Coffman, S. G., 297
Cohen, A., 139
Cohen, E., 139, 140
Cohen, J., 333, 405, 456, 498
Cohen, R., 100
Coie, J. D., 132, 133
Colby, S. M., 388
Collins, H. M., 104
Collins, J. L., 252
Collins, L. M., 366, 369, 479
Collins, M., 293
Conte, H. R., 253
Cook, C. W., 255
Cook, T. D., 336, 337, 347, 399, 408, 450, 452, 453, 484
Cook, T. J., 409
Cooper, H., 143, 450
Cooper, H. M., 143
Cooper, K. H., 9
Costa, F. M., 7
Cowen, E. L., 85
Coyle, K., 167
Coyle, S. L., 488
Craig, S., 6, 7, 271, 272, 273, 278, 289, 322, 335
Creer, T. J., 392, 397, 410, 413
Crippens, D. L., 265
Crosse, S., 474
Curran, J., 490
Cutter, G., 7

Dagenbach, D., 112, 116
D'Angelo, L. J., 214

Daniel, M., 11, 16
Dannenberg, A. L., 336
Dansereau, D. F., 388
D'Avernas, J. R., 427
Davidson, K. C., 134
Davies, M., 137
Davison, G. C., 296, 297
Day, G. S., 289
De Leon, G., 389
Dean, A. G., 333
DeCicco, I. M., 18, 257, 258, 259, 271
Dees, S. M., 388
DeJong, W., 35, 38
Delsky, A. S., 179
Dembo, R., 137
DeMoor, C., 271, 354
Denham, J. W., 8
Dent, C. W., 6, 7, 15, 16, 18, 24, 82, 85, 87, 110, 112, 113, 119, 120, 158, 170, 174, 180, 257, 258, 268, 269, 271, 272, 273, 276, 278, 284, 287, 288, 289, 290, 291, 293, 295, 296, 307, 309, 322, 326, 328, 329, 331, 333, 335, 346, 349, 350, 354, 368, 377, 403, 407, 408, 417, 444, 471, 481, 504, 511
DeQuattro, V. L., 297
Derzon, J. H., 443
Detsky, A. S., 414
Dey, I., 18, 272
DHEW. See U.S. Department of Health, Education, and Welfare
DHHS. See U.S. Department of Health and Human Services
Diaz, T., 373, 377
DiBartolo, R., 426, 427
DiClemente, C. C., 329, 364, 497, 515
DiClemente, R. J., 214
Diehr, P., 406
Dignan, M. B., 158, 190, 392
Dinh, K. T., 411
DiTecco, D., 35
Diwan, V. K., 406
Dobson, D., 409
Doebler, M. K., 87
Doherty, K. T., 110
Dolan-Mullen, P., 179
Donaldson, S. I., 23, 331, 471, 473, 474, 481, 484, 490, 492, 493
Donnelly, G., 168
Donner, A., 406
D'Onofrio, C. N., 173, 200
Donohew, L., 378
Donovan, J. E., 7, 110
Dorfman, L., 74
Dotson, J. H., 464
Downs, S. H., 207
Droitcour, J. A., 468
Drop, M. J., 139
Drug Strategies, 18

Dryfoos, J. G., 180, 322, 488, 517
DuBois, D. L., 73
Duffy, A., 139
Duncan, D. F., 468
Duncan, S. C., 134
Duncan, T. E., 134
Dunkel, J., 474
Dunlap, E., 139
Dupuy, T. N., 371
Durlak, J. A., 143, 144, 147, 460
Dusenbury, L., 373, 377
Duval, S., 309
Dwyer, D. P., 6, 24
Dwyer, J. H., 267, 363, 484, 485

Eagly, A. H., 411
Eakle, K., 380
Earleywine, M., 15, 110
Edelman, M., 105
Edwards, R. W., 372
Elder, J. P., 85, 241, 242, 254, 365
Elixhauser, A., 414
Elkin, I., 424
Ellickson, P. L., 412
Elliot, D. L., 488
Eng, A., 425
Englemann, S., 73
Ennett, S. T., 412
Epstein, L. H., 9
Eriksson, B., 406
Ernster, V. L., 183
Eron, L. D., 73
Evans, R. I., 15, 425, 503
Eysenck, H. A., 454

Fagan, J., 137
Fairbanks, J., 139
Fairchild, H. H., 139
Family Life Council of Greater Greensboro, Inc., 189
Farmer, J., 392
Farquhar, J. W., 10
Farrell, W. S., 215
Farrington, D. P., 132
Fazio, R. H., 112
Feldman, J. M., 109
Feldman, R. H. L., 10
Fendrich, M., 139
Ferrell, B. A., 392, 397, 400
Ferrell, B. R., 392, 397, 400
Festinger, L., 427
Fetro, J. V., 73
Feyerabend, P., 104
Fielding, J., 179

Filer, M., 16
Fillmore, K. M., 143
Fishbein, M., 16, 93, 208, 411, 427
Fisher, J. D., 210, 214
Fisher, K. J., 464
Fisher, R. P., 120
Fisher, W. A., 210, 214
Fishkin, S. A., 267
Fitzpatrick, B., 337
Flay, B. R., 6, 7, 15, 16, 17, 24, 35, 38, 82, 85, 87, 110, 133, 158, 170, 180, 257, 258, 267, 268, 269, 271, 273, 276, 284, 288, 289, 290, 293, 326, 328, 331, 333, 335, 345, 346, 347, 349, 350, 354, 368, 377, 392, 397, 403, 408, 417, 425, 427, 434, 435, 438, 439, 441, 444, 471, 481, 504, 511
Fletcher, J. M., 134
Fletcher, R. H., 416
Fletcher, S. W., 416
Flor, D. L., 15
Flor, H., 464
Flora, J. A., 11, 87
Flynn, B. S., 35, 37, 414
Foege, W., 50
Folmer, H., 484
Ford, D. H., 134, 140
Forrest, J. D., 210
Fowler, R. D., 252
Fox-Cardomone, L., 240
Francis, D. J., 134
Freeman, H. E., 7
Freimuth, V. S., 87, 240, 257, 258
Friedman, M. J., 424
Frost, J., 210
Fry, A. F., 115
Fuchs, R., 267
Funder, D. C., 294
Fydrich, T., 464

Gabriel, R. M., 323
Gal, C., 143
Galaif, E. R., 16, 18, 265, 287, 288, 291, 293, 296, 307, 335
Galster, G., 467
Gardner, H., 381
Garland, A., 488
Gebhardt, W., 523
Gee, M., 425, 435
Geiselman, R. E., 120
Geller, E. S., 241, 242, 254
Gentry, J. H., 73
Georgoudi, M., 99
Gergen, K., 100
Gergen, M., 100
Gerrard, M., 15
Ghez, M., 140
Gibbons, F. X., 15

Gill, M. M., 288, 291, 295, 296
Gingiss, P. L., 372
Glantz, M., 133
Glanz, K., 173
Glasgow, R. E., 73, 88, 98, 99
Glass, G. V., 454, 460
Gleason, G. R., 16
Gleghorn, A., 137
Glynn, S., 89
Glynn, T., 178, 188
Golaszewski, T., 173
Gold, R. S., 468
Goldberg, L., 488, 498
Goldberg, M., 208
Goldman, M. S., 109
Gollwitzer, P. M., 519
Goodman, B., 64
Goodman, R., 62, 66
Goodstadt, M. S., 427
Gooler, L. E., 490
Gordon, J. R., 112, 113, 114
Gordon, J. S., 73-74
Gorman, D., 443
Goshen-Gottstein, Y., 116
Gottfredson, G. F., 208
Gottlieb, N. H., 372
Grady, M. L., 71
Grady, R., 388
Graf, P., 115, 116, 121
Graham, J. W., 6, 15, 23, 331, 366, 369, 372, 409, 425, 434, 435, 438, 441, 444, 479, 492, 493
Gramlich, E. H., 490
Gratz, R. R., 142
Gray, J. A., 112
Green, L. W., 11, 16, 50, 52, 57, 58, 64, 158
Greenblat, C. S., 100
Greenwald, A. G., 108, 109
Grills, C., 388
Groff, J. Y., 179
Grosch, J. W., 179
Gross, N. C., 369
Groves, R. M., 413
Grube, J. W., 139
Gruenewald, P., 110
Guarneccia, P. J., 87
Guillemin, F., 417
Gupta, J. N. D., 256
Gurgevich, E. A., 87
Gursen, M. D., 137
Guthrie, B. J., 392, 397

Haaga, D. A. F., 297
Hache, G., 256

Haggerty, R. J., 132, 133
Hahlweg, K., 73
Hahn, G. L., 366
Hakanson, M., 392
Haley, N., 74
Hall, J. A., 450
Hammar, S. L., 305
Hansen, W. B., 6, 15, 21, 23, 24, 89, 331, 362, 363, 366, 369, 372, 375, 378, 380, 409, 425, 434, 435, 442, 443, 458, 459, 474, 475, 477, 479, 491, 492, 493, 511
Hanson, A., 467
Hanson, M., 270
Hanson, R. K., 143
Harlow, L. L., 388
Harr, J., 190
Harre, R., 100
Harris, M., 102
Harsh, L., 401
Hartman, R. J., 257
Harvey, D. R., 392
Haseleu, J. A., 240
Haskins, M., 323
Hauck, W. W., 322
Hawkins, J. D., 110, 133, 362, 490
Hayes, L. J., 98, 99
Hayes, S. C., 85, 87, 92, 98, 99
Hays, W. L., 377
Heaney, C. A., 14, 80, 87, 88, 91, 92
Hearn, M. D., 480-481
Heather, N., 389
Heckhausen, J., 134
Hedges, L. V., 143, 450
Heimann-Ratain, G., 270
Heise, D. R., 80
Heisey, J. G., 116, 122
Henkin, I., 139
Henningfield, J. E., 265
Herd, J. A., 33
Herity, B., 392
Higgins, D. L., 17, 18, 247, 248
Higgins, P., 181, 188
Hill, A. B., 110
Hinkle, S., 240
Hintzman, D. L., 113
Hirayama, H., 87
Hirayama, K. K., 87
Hirschman, R. S., 521
Hochbaum, G. M., 173
Holder, H., 345
Holland, H. L., 120
Holland, P. W., 499
Holland, R. R., 414
Hollett-Wright, N., 15
Hollon, S. D., 74

Holtgrave, D. R., 210, 414
Hopfield, J. J., 109, 112, 113
Hops, H., 288
Hopson, T., 323
Hornsby, J. S., 256
Horowitz, L. M., 121
Horst, S., 116
Houghton, S., 140
Hovell, M. F., 241, 242, 254
Howard, D. V., 115, 116, 122
Howard, J., 178, 188
Hubbell, F. A., 247
Hugdahl, K., 110
Hughes, A. S., 410
Huizinga, D., 137
Hunsaker, P. L., 255
Hussong, A. M., 137

Independent Evaluation Consortium, 330
Inn, A., 110
Institute of Medicine, 134, 210, 268
Irwin, L. M., 240
Isaac, S., 7

Jaccard, J., 110
Jackson, P., 269
Jacobs, D. R., Jr., 110
Jacoby, L. L., 109, 116-117, 118
Jaffe, J. H., 110
James, L. E., 176
Jansen, M. A., 178, 188
Jarvis, M., 269
Jasechko, J., 116-117, 118
Jeffery, G., 256
Jenkins, C. N. H., 176
Jernigan, D., 74
Jessor, R., 7
Joe, G. W., 388
Joe, K. A., 140
Joffe, J., 176
Johnson, B. D., 139
Johnson, C. A., 6, 24, 179, 346, 425, 428, 434, 435
Johnson, M., 296
Johnson, P. B., 139
Johnson, V., 134
Johnston, J., 305
Johnston, L. D., 268, 349
Johnstone, B. M., 143, 412
Jöreskog, K. G., 134, 484-485, 499
Judd, C. M., 485

Jumper-Thurman, P., 372
Jung, C. G., 295

Kabat-Zinn, J., 168
Kalton, G., 293
Kandel, D. B., 137, 366, 426
Kann, I., 252
Kannel, W., 133
Kaplan, C. D., 140
Kaplan, H. B., 137
Kaplan, R. M., 81
Kaskutas, L. A., 137
Kastel, S., 380
Kaufmann, C. L., 392
Kayser, E., 100
Kazdin, A. E., 137, 148
Keita, G. P., 142
Kelleher, C., 208
Kelley, C. M., 109, 116-117, 118
Kelley, M., 222-223, 226
Kelly, J. A., 211
Kenny, D. A., 134, 402, 478, 485, 486
Kersell, M. W., 427
Kessler, R. C., 413
Kettner, P. M., 7
Khurshid, A., 406
Kihlstrom, J. F., 109
Killen, J., 285, 426
King, A. C., 239, 242, 253
Kirby, D., 73, 210
Kittel, F., 522
Klar, N., 406
Klein, E., 140
Klepp, K., 110
Klinger, D. A., 139
Klitzer, M. D., 110
Klonoff, E. A., 104
Knibbe, R. A., 139
Knorr, K. D., 104
Knowles, J., 50
Koegel, P., 139
Koepsell, T., 406
Kohlberg, L., 365, 367
Kohler, C. L., 257, 258
Kok, G., 158, 392, 397, 412
Kolbe, L. J., 252, 468
Kornhaber, M. L., 381
Kotke, T. E., 73
Krank, M. D., 117
Kreuter, M. W., 11, 50, 52, 57, 158
Krohn, R., 104

Krueger, R. A., 140, 257, 259
Krupat, E., 87
Kushi, L. H., 257
Kyle, J., 180

Labaw, P., 293
L'Abbe, K. A., 179
Labouvie, E. W., 137
LaChance, P., 176
Lacy, L., 265
Landers, C., 74
Landis, S. E., 402
Landrine, H., 104
Lapin, A., 337
Lashley, K. S., 9
Lasswell, M., 100
Lasswell, T., 100
Last, J. M., 498
Latour, B., 104, 105
Lawendowski, L. A., 388
Ledda, M. A., 247, 397
Lee, M., 163
Lefebvre, R. C., 11, 87
Lehman, R. M., 305
Lehr, R., 256
Leigh, B. C., 110, 111
Leino, E. V., 143
Leland, N., 73
Lenneweber, V., 100
Lettieri, D. J., 133
Leupker, R. V., 425, 428
Leventhal, H., 15, 521
Levine, I. S., 140
Lewin, K., 33
Lewis, F. M., 173
Lichtenstein, E., 73-74
Lichtman, K., 268, 271, 272, 288, 349
Lin, L. S., 480-481
Lippert, P., 267
Lipsey, M. W., 143, 144, 147, 453, 455, 456, 460, 463, 464, 471, 473, 474, 479, 481, 482, 484, 486
Little, G. L., 388
Little, R. J., 413
Littlefield, J., 121
Liu, X., 137
Lloyd, L., 328
Loeber, R., 132, 133, 137
Loh, L., 328
Lombard, D. N., 392, 410
Long, J. D., 369, 479
Longshore, D., 112, 388

Lonner, W. J., 265
Lopes, C., 265
Lorch, E., 378
Lorig, K., 173
Lorion, R., 180
Loschper, G., 100
Loue, S., 328
Lovato, C., 58
Lowe, J. B., 400
Lubich, L., 139
Luce, B. R., 414
Luck, D. J., 293
Lynch, J. G., 109
Lytle, L. A., 409

Maccoby, N., 10, 285, 426
MacDonald, J., 140
MacFadden, B., 8
Mackesy-Amiti, M. E., 139
MacKinnon, D. P., 6, 24, 82, 120, 179, 346, 363, 411, 440, 484, 485, 488, 492, 500
Maes, S., 522, 523
Magana, J. R., 247
Mahler, H. I. M., 337
Mahler, K. A., 214
Malfetti, J. L., 18, 257, 258, 259, 271
Mallari, A., 215
Malone, M. D., 464
Manfredi, C., 265
Mant, D., 208
Marconi, K. M., 87
Marcus, S. H., 9
Marín, B. V., 252, 255, 261
Marín, G., 252, 255, 261, 403
Markman, H. J., 73
Marks, G., 15
Marlatt, G. A., 112, 113, 114
Martin, D. C., 406
Martin, L. L., 7
Maslow, A., 373
Masson, M., 112
Masson, M. E. J., 109, 112, 115, 116, 121
Matarazzo, J. D., 5, 9, 10, 33, 515
Matt, G. E., 453
Mayer, J. A., 241, 242, 254
Mays, V. M., 101, 518
McAlister, A. L., 426
McCarthy, P. R., 257
McCaul, K. D., 88
McClelland, J. L., 112
McCoy, J. K., 15

McCuller, W. J., 271, 288
McFarland, B. H., 392
McGaw, B., 460
McGinnis, J., 50, 179
McGlynn, S. M., 115, 116
McGrath, E., 142
McGuigan, K., 412
McKenna, H. P., 255, 256
McKeon, P., 133
McLain, A., 173
McLeroy, K. R., 7, 87
McNeal, R. B., Jr., 362, 363, 378, 442, 443, 458, 459, 474, 477
McNeill, A. D., 269
Meertens, R., 392, 397, 412
Merrill, R., 498
Messeri, P., 137
Mesters, I., 392, 397, 412
Mettger, W., 87, 240, 257, 258
Meyer, D., 109
Micco, A., 115, 116, 121
Michael, W. B., 7
Middlestadt, S. E., 16, 93
Miller, B. C., 210
Miller, D. C., 7
Miller, H. G., 518
Miller, J. G., 104, 134
Miller, J. Y., 110, 133, 362, 490
Miller, N. E., 33
Miller, T. Q., 15, 87, 110, 133, 346
Miller, W. R., 269, 351, 375, 387, 388, 389
Miln, R., 139
Mischel, W., 294
Mishra, S. I., 247, 309
Mitchell, C. M., 139
Moffitt, T. E., 133
Montgomery, S. B., 200
Moore, C. M., 255
Moore, K., 210
Moore, R. S., 139
Morawski, J. G., 103
Moroney, R. M., 7
Morris, E. K., 98, 99
Morrison, K., 339
Morse, E., 127
Mosbach, P., 15
Moses, L. E., 518
Mosher, D. L., 296
Moskowitz, J., 407, 426, 427
Mosteller, F., 450
Mott, L. A., 142
Mrazek, P. J., 74, 132, 133
Mueller, D., 181, 188
Mummendey, A., 100

Munoz, R. F., 132
Murphy, L. R., 179
Murray, D. M., 407, 425, 428

Namerow, P., 210
National Education Association, 185
National Institute of Justice, 388
National Institute on Drug Abuse, 134, 139, 142
National Institutes of Health (NIH), 99, 100, 104
Nevo, D., 18, 24
Newcomb, M. D., 15, 110, 112, 137
Nezami, E., 269, 297, 308, 309, 351
Nguyen, T., 189
Niego, S., 215, 222-223, 226
NIH. *See* National Institutes of Health
Nisbett, R. E., 108
Nissinen, A., 31
Norcross, J. C., 329, 364, 387, 497
North, T. C., 464
Nutbeam, D., 208

Ockene, I. S., 168
Ockene, J. K., 168
Odgers, P., 140
Oetting, E. R., 372
O'Leary, K. D., 10
Olson, J. M., 411
O'Malley, P. M., 137, 268, 349
O'Nell, T. D., 139
Onstad, L. E., 411
Orlandi, M. A., 74
Orleans, C. T., 339
O'Rourke, K., 179
Ostwald, S. K., 392, 399, 413
Otero-Sabogal, R., 176
Oxendine, J., 189

Paikoff, R., 210
Palley, C. S., 426, 427
Pallonen, U. E., 268, 269, 272, 285, 349, 388
Palmgreen, P., 378
Pandina, R. J., 132, 133, 134, 137, 140
Parcel, G. S., 73, 74, 158, 392, 397, 412
Parerny, D. M., 305
Park, J., 222-223, 226
Park, R. J., 257
Parker, H., 139
Parker, P., 337
Parker, V. C., 292
Pasick, R. J., 176

Paskett, E. D., 366, 392
Paynter, S., 110
Pearson, H. W., 133
Pechacek, T. F., 425, 428
Peck, R. C., 144
Pederson, L. L., 208
Pentz, M. A., 6, 24, 87, 179, 269, 308, 324, 346, 351, 407, 408, 426, 444, 492, 504
Pepper, S. C., 98
Peregoy, S. M., 270
Pérez-Stable, E. J., 176
Perry, C. L., 73, 74, 110, 285, 426
Persampieri, M., 121
Petersen, M. R., 179
Peterson, A. V., 411
Peterson, J. L., 210, 222-223, 226, 322
Petosa, R., 6, 12, 19, 57, 64, 285, 307, 454, 471, 481, 487, 505
Petraitis, J., 15, 87, 110, 133, 346
Philips, I., 488
Philliber, S., 210
Phillips, K. A., 414
Piaget, J., 365, 367
Piccinin, A. M., 492, 493
Pickens, R. W., 133, 265
Pierce, J. P., 15
Pike, K., 102, 105
Pinch, T. J., 104
Pinderhughes, E., 497
Piserchia, P., 179
Plested, B., 372
Poggie, J., 249
Polanyi, M., 105
Pollack, K., 104
Pollard, J. A., 473, 474, 479, 481
Popay, J., 207
Posavac, E. J., 464
Powell, K. E., 323
Presson, C. C., 84-85, 87, 88, 89
Price, R. H., 132, 180, 490
Prochaska, J. O., 268, 269, 329, 364, 365, 387, 388, 497, 515
Prohaska, T. R., 521
Prokhorov, A. V., 388
Pruitt, B. T., 256
Pryor, J. B., 401
Prytulak, L. S., 121
Puska, P., 31
Putnam, R., 173

Rabinow, P., 104
Raja, M., 139
Ramírez, G., 179
Ramos-McKay, J., 180

Rapaport, D., 288, 291, 295, 296
Rather, B. C., 109
Raudenbush, S. W., 134
Ray, J. W., 453, 461
Reblando, J., 414
Redding, C. A., 388
Reeder, G. D., 401
Reinecke, M. A., 73
Reingold, E. M., 116
Reiss, D., 132
Reno, R. R., 488
Resnicow, K., 480-481
Reynolds, K. D., 488
Rhiner, M., 392, 397, 400
Richardson, J. L., 15
Richmond, R. L., 73
Rieger-Ndakorerwa, G. E., 267
Rimer, B. K., 173
Risser, J., 305
Ritt, A., 268, 272, 349
Rittel, H. W., 166
Robins, C., 296
Robinson, K. D., 388
Robison, J. I., 179
Rodriguez, O., 87
Roediger, H. L., 109, 113, 115, 124
Rog, D. J., 143
Rogers, E. M., 62, 71, 73, 74, 349, 369
Rohrbach, L. A., 200, 372, 409, 438
Rollnick, S., 269, 351, 375, 387
Romer, D., 305
Rosario, M., 214
Rose, L. A., 369
Rosenbaum, J., 16, 93
Rosenthal, R., 252, 256, 450, 453, 456, 460, 461, 465
Rosnow, R. L., 99, 252, 256
Rossi, J. S., 268, 269, 388, 515
Rossi, P. H., 7, 463
Rothenberger, J., 392, 399, 413
Rotheram-Borus, M. J., 214
Rousculp, S. S., 366, 479
Rubin, D. B., 456, 465
Rubin, R. S., 293
Rudner, R. S., 80, 91
Rudzinski, K. A., 87
Rumelhart, D. E., 112
Rundall, T. G., 464
Runyan, W. K., 479
Russo, N. F., 142
Ryan, B., 369
Ryan, K. B., 427
Ryan, N. E., 73

Sabini, J., 104
Sabogal, F., 176
Sahai, H., 406
Salomaa, V., 31
Sanchez, M. V., 87
Sandler, I. N., 488
Sarason, I. G., 411
Sayers, M., 133
Scarbrough, M. L., 402
Schacter, D. L., 109, 115, 116, 121
Schafer, R., 288, 291, 295, 296
Schaps, E., 426, 427
Schatzkin, A., 133
Schlegel, P., 73
Schlegel, R. P., 35
Schnurr, P. P., 424
Schofield, R., 87
Scholten, H., 522
Schooler, N. R., 424
Schorr, L., 180
Schramski, T. G., 392
Schreibman, D., 16
Schuckit, M. A., 137
Schulenberg, J. E., 137
Schulz, R., 134
Schuster, E., 257
Schvaneveldt, R., 109
Schwartz, C. E., 134
Schwarz, N., 103, 104, 264
Scogin, F. R., 464
Scrimshaw, N. S., 16
Scullin, E. W., 468
Sechrist, L., 71
Secker-Walker, R. H., 414
Segal, S. D., 139
Segall, M. H., 265
Seigal, J. M., 490
Selye, H., 104
Semmer, N. K., 267
Severson, H. H., 73-74, 170, 268, 269, 276
Shadish, W. R., 453, 461
Shaffer, D., 488
Shamdasani, P. M., 270
Shapiro, D. H., 134
Sharpe, D., 453
Shaughnessy, J. J., 252
Shaw, R. J., 116, 122
Shepherd, M., 16, 93
Sheppard, M. A., 427
Sherman, J. E., 127
Sherman, S. J., 84-85, 87, 88, 89
Shiffman, S., 264
Shinar, O., 16

Shipley, T. E., 139, 140
Shopland, D. R., 87, 179, 504
Sifaneck, S. J., 140
Sikkema, K. J., 392, 410
Silberman, G., 468
Silver, M., 104
Silvestri, B., 17
Simon, T. R., 89, 288, 322, 326, 329, 335
Simpson, D. D., 388
Simpson, J. M., 406
Singer, G., 98, 99
Singleton, E. G., 265
Slavin, R. E., 143
Sliepcevich, E. M., 468
Slinkard, L. A., 426
Smith, B. N., 256
Smith, C., 208
Smith, D., 173
Smith, G. T., 109
Smith, M. F., 480
Smith, M. L., 454, 460
Smith, N. F., 268, 269, 388
Smith, T. W., 305
Smitham, D. M., 372
Snow, D. L., 402
Snyder, S. E., 392, 397, 410, 413
Sobel, J., 425, 434, 435
Sobel, M. E., 484
Soler, E., 140
Solomon, D. S., 10
Sörbom, D., 134, 484-485, 499
Sorensen, G., 168
Sorenson, J. R., 173
Spencer, T. J., 139
SPSS, Inc., 333
Squire, L. R., 109
Stacy, A. W., 6, 7, 15, 16, 18, 24, 82, 85, 87, 89, 110, 111, 112, 113, 120, 127, 137, 158, 170, 180, 257, 258, 268, 269, 271, 272, 273, 278, 284, 287, 288, 289, 290, 291, 293, 295, 296, 307, 322, 326, 328, 331, 333, 335, 346, 349, 350, 354, 368, 377, 403, 408, 417, 471, 481, 504, 511
Stahler, G. J., 139, 140
Stanley, J. C., 398, 399
Steckler, A., 62, 66, 468
Stein, B. S., 115, 121
Stein, J., 112
Stephenson, W., 294
Sterky, G., 406
Stern, R. A., 85, 365
Stetson, B. A., 114
Stevens, M. M., 142
Stewart, B., 257, 258
Stewart, D. W., 270

Stewart, S. L., 163
Stobart, G., 474
Stoolmiller, M., 134
Stormark, K. M., 110
Stouthamer-Loeber, M., 133
Stratton, H., 458, 464
Stratton, H. H., 6, 18, 21, 24, 330, 362, 405, 410, 411, 511
Strickland, B. R., 142
Strube, M. J., 464
Stuebing, K. K., 134
Sudman, S., 293
Suffet, F., 339
Sullivan, W. M., 104
Sussman, S., 6, 7, 12, 15, 16, 18, 19, 20, 24, 82, 85, 87, 89, 92, 119, 120, 139, 158, 170, 174, 180, 257, 258, 265, 268, 269, 271, 272, 273, 276, 278, 284, 285, 287, 288, 289, 290, 291, 292, 293, 295, 296, 307, 308, 309, 322, 326, 328, 329, 331, 333, 335, 346, 349, 350, 351, 354, 368, 377, 392, 271, 288, 397, 403, 408, 410, 417, 428, 439, 440, 442, 444, 454, 471, 481, 482, 484, 487, 504, 505, 511
Swift, R., 117
Swinger, T., 100
Szalay, L. B., 110

Taggart, V. S., 409
Tank, D. W., 109, 112, 113
Tatum, C., 392
Taylor, C., 103, 104
Taylor, C. A., 389
Taylor, R. B., 8
Taylor, W. C., 73, 74
Taylor, W. R., 414
Tebes, T. K., 402
Tedeschi, T., 100
Telch, M. J., 285
Theiss, P. K., 409
Themba, M., 74
Thompson, N. M., 134
Thoresen, C. E., 6, 11
Thornberry, T. P., 137
Tickle-Degen, L., 450
Tiffany, S. T., 109, 112
Tilford, S., 522
Timmreck, T. C., 328
Tjerandsen, C., 188
Tobler, N. S., 6, 18, 21, 24, 143, 330, 362, 405, 410, 411, 458, 464, 511
Tolman, E. C., 121
Tomson, G., 406
Tones, K., 522
Torgerson, W. S., 298
Torrestad, A., 392

Toth, S. L., 133, 134, 140
Tourangeau, R., 305
Trebow, E., 407, 408
Trevisan, L., 488
Trickett, E. J., 522
Tuchfeld, B. S., 9
Tulving, E., 109, 124
Tuomilehto, J., 31
Turk, D. C., 464
Turkheimer, E., 134
Turner, C. F., 488, 518
Turner, G. E., 405, 408
Turrisi, R., 110
Tyas, S. L., 208

Unfried, P., 73
U.S. Department of Health and Human Services (DHHS), 9, 10, 50, 167, 168, 181, 182, 268, 488
U.S. Department of Health, Education, and Welfare (DHEW), 50, 181
Ureda, J. R., 8

Vaccaro, D., 16
Valdez, R. B., 247
Van de Goor, L. A., 139
Van der Doef, M., 522
van Ryn, M., 14, 80, 87, 88, 91, 92, 490
Vartiainen, E., 31
Vegega, M. E., 110
Velez, R., 392
Velicer, W. F., 365, 388, 515
VERDICT Brief Biannual Newsletter, 71
Verhoeven, C., 522
Vicary, J. R., 87
Vinokur, A. D., 490
Vogel, R. S., 297
Voorberg, N., 87

Wadden, T. A., 7
Wadsworth, K. N., 137
Wagner, E. H., 416
Wake, W. K., 381
Waldrop, M. M., 361
Waligora-Serafin, B., 256
Walker, E. A., 247, 397
Wallace, R. B., 498
Wallach, L., 74
Wallerstein, N., 87
Walter, H. J., 397
Walton, C., 305

Ward, V. M., 261
Ward-Colasante, C., 392
Warnecke, R., 265
Wartman, P., 454
Watson, J. B., 9
Webber, M. M., 166
Weber, M. D., 492
Weeks, K., 400
Weinberger, M., 260
Weiner, M. D., 271, 288
Weingardt, K. R., 110, 111
Weiss, C. H., 473, 487
Weiss, R., 490
Weiss, S., 33
Weiss, S. M., 33
Wells-Parker, E., 143
West, R. J., 269
West, S. G., 73, 125, 132, 134, 135, 475, 481, 482, 485, 486, 488
Weston, R., 74
Wetter, D. W., 480-481
White, H. R., 137
Whitley, R., 104
Wicklund, R. A., 309, 519
Widaman, K. F., 113
Widiger, T. A., 142
Wilens, T. E., 139
Williams, C. J., 112
Williams, C. L., 425
Williams, G., 207
Williams, L., 137
Williams, M. E., 297
Wills, T. A., 15, 16
Wilson, A., 392
Wilson, D. B., 453, 463, 464, 471, 474

Wilson, G. T., 10
Wilson, R., 58
Wilson, T. D., 108
Winder, J. A., 392, 397, 410, 413
Windle, M. T., 73, 132, 134
Windsor, R. A., 7, 400
Winett, R. A., 239, 242, 253, 392, 410
Winston, J. A., 35, 38
Wise, R. A., 110
Wislar, J. S., 139
Witte, K., 339
Wolchik, S., 488
Wolkenstein, B. H., 366, 409
Woloshyn, V., 117
Woodby, L., 400
Woodward, C. K., 488
Woolgar, S., 104, 105
Worden, J. K., 11, 18, 35, 37, 38, 87, 271, 288, 414
World Health Organization, 31
Wright, J. D., 463
Wynder, E. L., 397

Yamaguchi, K., 366
Youells, F., 142

Zanna, M. P., 411
Zapka, J. G., 178, 190
Zechmeister, E. B., 252
Zighelboim, V., 297
Zimmerman, J. D., 140
Zoref, L., 176
Zuckerman, A. E., 409

Subject Index

AAPT. *See* Adolescent Alcohol Prevention Trial
Acceptability of components, 328, 329-330, 332, 339-341, 409-410, 503
Accessibility of components, 329-330, 332, 339-341
Action theory tables, 499
Activities:
  role-playing to test, 256-257
  screening. *See* Perceived efficacy studies
  selecting, 175-176
  sequencing. *See* Sequencing
  See also Components
Activity acceptance. *See* Perceived efficacy studies
Activity pooling and warehousing, 17-18
  benefits, 159-162, 207, 208-209
  case study, 41-42
  conducting searches, 193-197, 205
  contacting program developers, 193
  evaluation issues, 208
  for pilot studies, 428
  for theme studies, 309
  future research needs, 507
  information sources, 17, 177-193
  justifying concepts, 164-169
  literature searches, 22, 214-215
  making program information available, 200-201
  planning searches, 162-164
  reviewing information, 197-199, 204-205
  tracking sheets, 194-196
  use in planning interventions, 169-177
  See also Program Archive on Sexuality, Health, and Adolescence (PASHA)
Add Health Survey, 223, 226
Administrators, 290, 304, 332

Adolescent Alcohol Prevention Trial (AAPT), 492-493
Adolescents:
  alcohol prevention programs, 388, 492-493
  effective behavioral change programs, 210-211
  health behavior approaches, 7
  health surveys, 223, 226
  high-risk behavior, 378, 517, 518
  HIV prevention programs, 101, 210-211
  interviewing, 252
  misperceptions of prevalence of substance use, 433
  parental consent procedures, 170
  pregnancy prevention programs, 210, 216-217, 488
  sexual activity, 517, 518
  smokers, 267-268, 271-272, 365, 368
  targeting mass media campaigns to, 37-38
  See also Drug use prevention programs; Participants; Pregnancy prevention programs; Smoking prevention programs
Affective education approach:
  components, 427-428
  pilot study, 425-426, 429-434
  results, 435-436
  theoretical basis, 427
African Americans, 265, 276
  See also Ethnic groups
Agency for Health Care Policy and Research, 183
AIDS. *See* HIV prevention programs
Alcohol use:
  as gateway drug, 426
  clearinghouses, 186
  focus groups on, 260-261
  motivations, 109
  prevention programs, 230, 388, 492-493

program types, 504
recovery programs, 388
response bias, 264-265
See also Drug use; Project SMART
Alcoholics Anonymous, 8
All Stars program, 375, 376, 380-381
American Association of Health Plans, 183
American Medical Association, 183
American Psychological Association Task Force, 74, 180
American Public Health Association (APHA), 8, 192
Amherst Wilder Foundation, 181
APHA. *See* American Public Health Association
Archives. *See* Program archives
Articulated thoughts in simulated situations (ATSS), 296-298
Asian American adolescents, 276
See also Ethnic groups
Assessment studies:
 data collection methods, 138
 design types, 136, 137-138
 domains, 131
 ethnographic, 139-140
 in prevention science, 131-132
 level of observation, 136, 140-141
 literature reviews, 144-148
 literature searches, 22, 144-146
 measurement probes, 147-148
 pooling multiple information sources, 142-144
 purposes, 135
 questions of inquiry, 135-136
 structure of observations, 136, 138-140
 subject characteristics, 136-137, 141, 146-147
 unit of analysis, 136, 140-141
Assessments, needs, 14-15, 36-37, 142-143, 505, 521
Association strength measures:
 binomial effect size display (BESD), 456-458
 U3, 456
Asthma, 410-411, 412, 413-414
ATSS. *See* Articulated thoughts in simulated situations
Attitudes, 411-412
Attitudinal theories, 15

Bacon, Francis, 443
Behavior:
 antecedents, 85
 association with outcomes or cues, 111-112, 124
 consequences, 86, 507
 contexts, 99-100
 functional analysis, 15
 mechanistic conception, 98-99, 101
 proximal and distal determinants, 346, 458-460
 stages of change models, 364-366, 387-388
 theories of, 85-86
 See also Health behavior
Behavioral health movement, 9-11

Beliefs, 411
BESD (binomial effect size display), 456-458
Biopsychosocial theory, 134, 155
Booster programming, 119-124, 377-378, 379, 389, 412
Breast cancer screening programs, 163-164, 488
Brochures, 189

California, continuation high schools, 271-272, 308, 349, 350, 354
California Department of Education, 184
California Department of Health Services, 187
Cambridge Scientific Abstracts, 191
Cancer:
 testicular self-examination, 399, 413-414
 See also Breast cancer
Card sorting assessments, 294-295
Case studies, 138-139
CATCH. *See* Child and Adolescent Trial for Cardiovascular Health
Causal histories. *See* Theories
Causal models. *See* Theories
Causes, 81-82, 87-88
Centers for Disease Control and Prevention (CDC), 9, 183, 200, 264
Chain Model, 12-13, 505-506
 activity pooling and warehousing (step 2), 17-18, 41-42
 benefits, 49, 52
 case study, 34-36
 challenges in applying, 517-520
 component studies (step 4), 19-20, 43-44
 perceived efficacy studies (step 3), 18-19, 42-43
 precede-proceed planning, 11-12
 predicting longer-term outcomes (step 6), 21-22, 45-46
 program construction and pilot testing (step 5), 20-21, 44-45
 research-to-practice cycle, 212, 232-234
 scope of application, 504
 steps, 13-14
 use of theory (step 1), 14-17, 36-41
Change:
 diffusion of innovations, 61-62, 369
 financial incentives, 71
 institutional readiness for, 372
 models of, 364-366
 strategies, 169
Child and Adolescent Trial for Cardiovascular Health (CATCH), 409
Children:
 attitudes toward smoking, 411-412
 parental consent procedures, 170
 safety programs, 174
Cholera, 8
Chronic diseases, 31-33, 180
Cigarettes. *See* Smoking

Clearinghouses, 185-187
Clinical guidelines, 183
Clinical psychology, 74
Cognitive development, 365-366, 367, 373
Cognitive theories, 15, 35, 108-109
  See also Memory
Commercial health behavior programs, 190-191
Communities:
  access to university research, 266
  changing needs, 502
  concerns, 24
  controversial topics, 58, 332, 503
  definition, 57, 253
  factors in health program development, 57-58, 69
  moral standards, 503
  participation in program development, 24, 261-262, 265, 332
  political issues, 503
  readiness for change, 372
Community forums, 253-255
Community programs, 189-190
Community surveillance studies, 142
Complex logic models, 479-480
Component studies, 19-20, 321-322, 348-349
  benefits, 327, 346-347, 358
  case study, 43-44
  community involvement, 332
  delivering components, 333-334
  designs, 335-337
  differences from outcomes evaluations, 322-323
  documentation, 342
  evaluation criteria, 328-331, 339-341
  evaluation forms, 355
  future research, 508-509
  group comparison evaluations, 326
  interpretation of results, 338-341, 356-358
  limitations, 358-360
  measurement strategies, 337-338
  mediators assessed, 330-331, 341
  meta-analysis of, 462-463
  order based, 325-326, 333
  process, 328, 350-351, 354-356
  Project EX, 350, 351, 354-360
  questions asked, 326-327
  research phase, 345-346
  sample sizes, 332-333
  statistical power issues, 332-333
  substantive contrasts, 325
  supplemental groups, 332
  target groups, 331-333
  types, 325-326
  uses, 504
Components:
  acceptability, 328, 329-330, 332, 339-341, 409-410, 503
  accessibility, 329-330, 332, 339-341
  building blocks, 324, 325-326, 334, 341
  complementary, 324
  constellation, 324-325
  definition, 321
  effectiveness, 327
  feasibility, 358
  goals, 323, 330, 331, 346
  integration in pilot studies, 423
  interactive methods, 509, 513
  linking to mediators addressed (action theory table), 499
  multiple, 322
  relations among, 323-325, 359, 508
  selecting, 175-176
  transitions between, 341
  See also Sequencing
Computers:
  data analysis, 443, 484-485, 499-500
  future capabilities, 514-515
  interviews using, 252-253, 262
  nonverbal methods of perceived efficacy studies, 298-300, 305
  use for Delphi technique, 255-256
  word processing, 442
  See also Internet
Concept evaluation. See Perceived efficacy studies
Concepts, 80
Conceptual frameworks:
  alternatives, 479-480
  developing, 472-473
  direct effects, 473-475
  importance, 480
  mediators, 475-477
  moderators, 477-479
Conferences, 182, 189
Conflict resolution techniques, 323
Contextualism, 99-100, 101
Continuation high schools, 271-272, 308, 349, 350, 354
Coronary heart disease. See Heart disease
Correlations, 456
Critical thinking errors, 89
Curriculum development:
  four-step model, 12
  See also Health behavior program development

DAPT. See Draw-a-picture test
DARE. See Drug Abuse Resistance Education
Data analysis:
  methods, 134, 484-487, 499-500
  multidimensional scaling, 298
  software, 443, 484-485, 499-500
Data collection:
  amount of data, 486-487
  methods, 138
  pilot studies, 440
  quality, 484

unobtrusive methods, 65-66
  See also Validity
Databases:
  bibliographic, 182
  online, 22, 192, 194, 214, 392, 460
Debates, 381
Delphi technique, 255-256, 508
Depression, 464
Designs:
  longitudinal, 137, 147, 155, 226, 413
  quasi-experimental, 335-336, 337, 401-402
  selecting, 504
  single-group pretest-posttest, 335, 336, 397-398, 399-400, 405
  true experimental, 138, 336, 337, 397, 398, 400-401, 405
  types, 136, 137-138
DHHS. *See* U.S. Department of Health and Human Services
Diabetes, 180, 464
Diffusion of innovations. *See* Innovations
Direction motivation, 269-270, 308, 351
Disease prevention. *See* Prevention programs
Diseases. *See* Chronic diseases; Infectious diseases
Divorce prevention, 488
Dose-response function, 482, 485-486
Drama, 380, 382
Draw-a-picture test (DAPT), 120
Driving under influence (DUI), 108, 113
Drug Abuse Resistance Education (DARE), 204, 378, 412, 426, 464
Drug use:
  clearinghouses, 186
  driving under influence (DUI), 108, 113
  gateway drugs, 369, 426
  recovery programs, 388
  research, 109-110
  response bias, 264-265
  sequence of behaviors, 366, 369
  stages, 121
  See also Alcohol use
Drug use prevention programs:
  affective education approach, 425-426, 427
  approaches, 491-493
  archive, 230
  boosters, 119-124, 377-378, 412
  cognitive theories used, 110-112, 113-119
  in continuation high schools, 354
  mediators, 490-493
  meta-analyses, 464-465
  moderators, 497-498
  normative education, 324
  refusal assertion skills training, 23
  research, 108, 109-110
  sequencing, 375, 377-378, 380-381

social-influences model, 16-17, 425, 426, 427, 492
steroids, 488
theme studies, 293-294
  See also Project SMART
DUI. *See* Driving under influence

Ecology of health behavior programs, 54-55, 67, 73
Educational Resources Information Center (ERIC), 186, 194
Educators. *See* Practitioners
Effects:
  direct, 473-475
  indirect, 458-460, 474-475
  sizes, 454-458, 461-462, 468
  See also Outcomes
Elaborative processing, 115-116, 118, 119, 120-122
Elicitation questionnaires, 15-16
Emic approach, 102
  See also Contextualism
Empirical curriculum development model, four-step, 12
Empirical data. *See* Data
Empirical program development. *See* Chain Model
Energy motivation, 269, 270, 308-309, 351
Environmental context, 367, 370-374
EQS, 484, 499
ERIC (Educational Resources Information Center), 186, 194
Ethnic groups:
  acceptability of components, 329-330, 403
  adapting interventions to, 98, 99, 100, 105
  cross-population research, 265-266
  cultural norms, 329
  health problems, 180, 399
  participant characteristics as moderator, 478, 497
  See also specific groups
Ethnographic studies, 139-140
Etic approach, 102
Etiologic research, 15-16, 93
  importance, 132-135, 155
  in prevention, 156-157
  methods, 17, 134
  pooling multiple information sources, 142-144
  uses in program development, 156-157
  See also Assessment studies; Research
Europe, 8
Evaluation:
  acceptability, 328, 329-330, 332, 339-341, 409-410, 503
  accessibility, 329-330, 332, 339-341
  additional steps, 63-64
  communicating results, 64-65
  component studies, 328-331, 339-341
  cost-effectiveness, 32, 74, 414-415, 503
  criteria, 213-214, 215
  difficulties, 208

"file drawer problem," 453
formative and developmental, 64, 70
goals, 323
lack of, 50
methods, 53-54
of instructors, 423
of longer-term outcomes, 21-22, 458-460
PASHA programs, 225-228
pilot studies, 407-415, 423
planning, 162
program effects on mediators, 481-482
researchers' focus on, 61, 234
texts, 7
training in procedures, 65
validity, 148, 398, 402, 484
See also Outcomes; Perceived efficacy studies
Exercise, 9, 488-490, 523
Experimental study designs, 138, 336, 337, 397, 398, 400-401, 405
Explicit cognition, 108, 110

Family interaction theory, 15
Family members, 290, 304, 332
Federal Security Agency, 9
Femininity, 103
  See also Gender
Fixed aggregation problem, 208
Flow, 380-381, 382
Flyers and brochures, 189
Focus groups, 19, 140, 257-261
  advantages, 258, 271, 284
  analysis of results, 260
  examples, 260-261, 265
  facilitators, 259-260
  interview guides, 259
  method, 272-276
  participants, 257, 258, 272, 273-276
  planning mass media campaigns, 39
  questions, 259, 272, 273, 274-275, 284, 285
  results, 276-284
  setting up, 258
  uses, 257-258, 270-271, 442
Forsyth County (North Carolina), 368
Freedom of Information Act, 188
Funding agencies, 56, 188

Gender:
  adapting programs, 99
  as moderator, 478, 497
  behaviors related to, 103
General Accounting Office, 468

Government agencies, 181, 183-184, 185, 188
Government Information Locator Service, 186
Grant-making agencies, 188
Guidelines and recommendations, 183-184
Guttman models, 366, 379

Hawthorne effect, 416-417
Health behavior:
  antecedents, 85
  attitudes, beliefs, and intentions, 411-412
  changing multiple, 346, 521-522
  complex causation, 87-88
  consequences, 86, 507
  environmental context, 522
  influencing, 33
  motivations, 109-110
  multiple problems caused by same behavior, 167, 346
  risk factors for chronic diseases, 31-33
  target behaviors, 81, 98
  texts, 8, 10
  underlying factors, 521-522
Health behavior program development:
  assumptions, 167-168
  community factors, 57-58, 69
  construction, 20
  costs, 24
  detailed planning, 160-162, 169-177
  formal methods, 51-52
  history, 8-11
  importance of improved methods, 5-7
  justification of concepts, 164-169
  organizational factors, 55-56, 69
  practitioner factors, 58-60, 69-70
  quality control, 502
  research needs, 506-515
  researcher factors, 60-61, 70
  resources needed, 56
  reviewing existing programs, 158, 159-162
  shortcomings, 208
  systemization of methods, 506-510
  time and resource requirements, 161-162
  training, 230
Health behavior program development models, 11-12
  benefits, 49, 52
  empirical curriculum development, 12
  implementation challenges, 23-25, 54-61, 69-70, 73-75
  need for, 50
  overcoming obstacles, 61-66, 70-71
  precede-proceed planning, 11-12
  social marketing/formative evaluation, 11
  See also Chain Model; Theory-based program development
Health behavior programs:

adaptations over time, 502
adapting to specific groups, 98, 99, 100, 105
adopting existing programs, 205-206
behavioral objectives, 172
budgets, 177
change strategies, 169
commercial, 190-191, 221
content, 173-174
cost-effectiveness, 32, 74, 414-415, 503
definition, 4
distributing information about, 200-201
ecology of, 54-55, 67, 73
effectiveness measurements, 53, 74, 215, 502-503
failures, 467, 499, 522-523
feasibility and effectiveness, 53-54
implementation issues, 73-75, 161
instruction methods, 59, 174-175, 179, 509
lack of evaluation, 50
length and duration, 171
materials, 176
modalities, 173, 176
names, 167
participants. *See* Participants
personnel, 176-177
rationale, 50, 160, 166
schedules, 177
selecting existing interventions, 149-150
sequencing. *See* Sequencing
settings, 55-56, 170-171, 304, 482
shortcomings, 48-49
support for, 162
target populations. *See* Target populations
theoretical bases, 84-86, 172-173, 204, 220
See also Components; Prevention programs
Health departments:
  community surveillance studies, 142
  mass media campaigns, 35-36, 37-46
  resources, 35
Health educators. *See* Practitioners
Health Information Network, National Education Association, 184
Health protection model, 86
Heart disease, 5, 31, 409, 415
High schools, continuation, 271-272, 308, 349, 350, 354
Hispanic adolescents, 101
  See also Ethnic groups
HIV prevention programs, 388
  for adolescents, 210-211, 218-219, 517-520
  for young Latinas, 101
  implicit cognition theory, 110
  mediators, 488
  pilot studies, 400-401
  See also Program Archive on Sexuality, Health, and Adolescence (PASHA)

ICT. *See* Implicit cognition theory
Idealism, 378
Immediate-outcome studies, 19-20, 327
  See also Component studies; Outcomes, immediate
Immunizations, 9, 10, 402
Imoyase, 388
Implementation:
  adaptations, 502
  costs, 415
  evaluation in pilot studies, 407-409, 441
  issues, 23-25, 161, 208-209
  of empirical development methods, 54-61, 69-70, 73-75
  of existing programs, 205-206
  results different from pilot tests, 416-417
Implicit cognition theory (ICT), 108-109, 110-114, 126
  See also Memory
In-depth interviews, 250-251
Infectious diseases, 8, 9, 10, 31
Inflection points, 373
Information technology. *See* Computers
Informed consent, 170
Innovations:
  adoption rates, 62-66
  compatibility, 63-64
  complexity, 64-65
  diffusion of, 61-62, 73-75, 369
  observability of results, 66
  trialability, 65-66
Institute for Program Development and Evaluation, 230
Instruction methods, 59, 174-175, 179, 509
Instructors. *See* Practitioners
Insurance, 9
Intellectual development. *See* Cognitive development
Intentions, 411
Intercept interviews, 251
Internet:
  community action Web sites, 190
  database searches, 22, 192, 194, 214, 392, 460
  disseminating information through, 71
  evaluating information on, 192
  government agency Web sites, 181, 182, 183, 186
  research uses, 305
  searching, 191-192
  use for Delphi technique, 256
Interventions:
  meanings of term, 504
  See also Health behavior programs
Interviews:
  computerized, 252-253, 262
  conducting, 243
  in-depth, 250-251
  intercept, 251
  key informant, 248-250
  locations, 251-252
  modes, 252-253

of adolescents, 252
prerecorded questions, 252, 264-265
probes, 247
selecting interviewers, 249
semistructured, 243, 247-248
stimuli, 243
structured, 243, 246
telephone, 249, 252
unstructured, 243, 246-247

JOBS program, 490
Join Together, 190
Journal articles, 178-179, 180, 192

Key informant interviews, 248-250
Kids Act!, 184-185
Knowledge:
　acquisition, 59
　as mediator, 410-411

Language issues, 265, 504
Latent transition analysis, 479
Latinas, 101
　See also Ethnic groups
Law of indirect effect, 459, 474-475
Law of maximum expected potential effect, 459-460, 477
Learning methods, 381-382
Learning theory, 88
　See also Social learning theories
Leventhal, Howard, 9
Lind, James, 8
LISREL, 484-485, 499
Literature searches:
　assessment studies, 22, 144-146
　conceptual issues, 144-146
　for programs, 22, 178-179, 180, 192, 214-215, 467
　limitations, 452
　methods, 146-148, 460-461
　perceived efficacy studies, 23
　pilot studies, 23, 392, 393-396
　program development methods, 22-23
　selection criteria, 144-146
　See also Meta-analyses
Lombardi, Vince, 48
Longitudinal studies, 137, 147, 155, 223, 226, 413

Mammography, 488
Marijuana, 271, 426
　See also Drug use
Masculinity, 103
　See also Gender

Mass media campaigns, 35-36, 37-46, 414-415
Materials:
　developing, 16-17
　in PASHA, 211, 220-222, 224-225, 232
　reviewing existing, 176
　revising, 220-221
　testing, 242
　vendors, 57-58, 190-191
　See also Perceived efficacy studies
Measurement probes, 147-148
Mediating variable analysis, 363
Mediators:
　actions, 81-82
　addressing multiple, 374, 475-476, 488
　content, 511-513
　definition, 471
　distinguishing from moderators, 497, 498
　empirical confirmation, 16, 481-482, 483-484, 485
　examples in health behavior research, 488-493
　failure analysis, 499
　future research, 511-514
　hypothesizing, 14, 15, 470-471, 498-499
　importance in prevention, 107-108
　knowledge, 410-411
　lack of attention in research, 471
　measuring changes, 440, 511-514
　memory, 110, 126
　models, 475-477
　multiple waves, 480
　of substance use, 428, 440
　program process, 513-514
　relationship to longer-term outcomes, 458-460, 477, 510-511
　use in program development, 498-499
　See also Component studies
MedINFO, 22, 392
MEDLINE, 192, 214
Memory:
　activating concepts, 110-111, 113-114, 115
　as mediator, 110, 126
　elaborative processing, 115-116, 118, 119, 120-122, 124-125
　implicit, 109
　recall studies, 295
　repetitive testing, 116, 122
　research on, 108-109
　unintended effects, 116-118
Men:
　testicular self-examination, 399, 413-414
　See also Gender
Mental health:
　meta-analyses, 464
　occupational promotion, 490
　pilot studies, 424
Meta-analyses:
　advantages, 450-452

as information sources, 179
component or pilot studies, 462-463
examples, 463-465, 471
goals, 450
interpreting, 454-460, 467-468
issues in, 208
limitations, 452-454, 467-468
process, 143-144, 450, 460-462
risk of effect overestimation, 452-453, 468
techniques, 450
Metacognition, 108
Metropolitan Life Insurance Company, 9
Midwestern Prevention Project, 324-325
Minority groups. *See* Ethnic groups
Models. *See* Conceptual frameworks; Theoretical models
Moderators:
  accessibility of component, 330
  actions, 82
  between mediators and outcomes, 478
  between programs and mediators, 478
  definition, 471, 477-478
  distinguishing from mediators, 497, 498
  empirical confirmation, 481, 482-484, 485-486
  examples, 488-493
  future research, 511
  hypothesizing, 470-471
  lack of attention in research, 471
  level of outcome variable before program delivery, 497-498
  measuring, 46
  models, 477-479
  participant characteristics as, 478, 482, 497
Moral reasoning, development of, 365-366
Moral reconation therapy, 388
Motivation:
  direction/goal, 269-270, 308, 351
  effort/energy, 269, 270, 308-309, 351
  for alcohol and drug use, 109
  for smoking cessation, 269-270, 277-278, 279-283, 308-309
  health behavior, 109-110
  of participants, 58
Musashi, Miyamoto, 361
Music, 380, 382

National Cancer Institute, 345, 349
National Clearinghouse for Alcohol and Drug Information, 186
National Diabetes Prevention Center, 180
National Education Association, 184
National Guidelines Clearinghouse, 183
National Health Lunch and Blood Institute, 345
National Institute of Diabetes and Digestive and Kidney Disease, 180
National Institute on Drug Abuse, 17
National Institutes of Health (NIH), 8

National League of Cities, 180
National Longitudinal Survey of Adolescent Health (Add Health), 223, 226
National Technical Information Service, 182
National Women's Health Information Center, 186, 192
Native Americans, 180, 189, 329, 399
  See also Ethnic groups
Nebraska Council to Prevent Alcohol and Drug Abuse, 375
Needs, hierarchy of, 373
Needs assessments, 14-15, 36-37, 142-143, 505, 521
Newsletters, 189
NIH. *See* National Institutes of Health
Node link mapping, 388-389
Nonverbal methods of perceived efficacy studies, 19, 287, 508
  card sorting, 294-295
  computerized, 298-300, 305
  data analysis, 298
  directive, semidirective, and nondirective, 291
  memory recall, 295
  projective techniques, 295-298
  self-report questionnaires, 292-293
  strengths and weaknesses, 300, 301
  target groups, 289-291, 300, 304
  See also Theme studies
Nutrition, 9

Obesity prevention programs, 399
Observational studies, 139
Older Americans Act, 9
Operator variables. *See* Mediators
Organizational factors in health behavior program development, 55-56, 69
Outcomes:
  measuring, 483-484
  target, 81
Outcomes, immediate:
  as predictors of longer-term outcomes, 24, 458-460
  attitudes, beliefs, and intentions, 411-412
  behavioral, 412
  direct effects of programs, 474
  evaluation, 410-412
  knowledge, 410-411
  literature searches, 23
  measuring, 21-22, 172
  objectives, 172
  studies, 19-20, 327
  See also Component studies; Effects
Outcomes, long-term:
  indirect effects, 458-460, 474-475
  literature searches, 23
  measuring, 46, 413-414
  predicting, 21-22, 24, 510-514

PAHO. *See* Pan American Health Organization
Pain, chronic, 464
Pan American Health Organization (PAHO), 8, 9
Paper-and-pencil methods. *See* Nonverbal methods of perceived efficacy studies
Paradigms. *See* Theories
Parental consent procedures, 170
Participants:
   characteristics, 136-137, 141, 146-147, 169-170, 519-520
   characteristics as moderators, 478, 482, 497
   in focus groups, 257, 258, 272, 273-276
   informed consent, 170
   interactive instruction, 509, 513
   interpretations of own behavior, 104
   minors, 58, 170
   recruiting, 170
   relationships with instructors, 60, 375-376, 378-379, 388, 509, 513
   See also Adolescents; Target populations
PASHA. *See* Program Archive on Sexuality, Health, and Adolescence
Perceived efficacy, definition, 240
Perceived efficacy studies, 18-19
   applications, 303-304, 504
   case study, 42-43
   comparing settings, 304
   future research, 305, 507-508
   goals, 18
   importance, 261, 288-289, 303
   limitations, 242
   literature searches, 22
   nonverbal methods. *See* Nonverbal methods
   planning, 241-242
   process, 240, 288-289
   purpose, 242
   verbal methods. *See* Verbal methods
Perceived program quality, 410, 511, 514
Person-oriented conceptual frameworks, 479
Physical activity. *See* Exercise
Pilot studies, 21
   benefits, 391, 416, 422
   comparing program formats, 400-401
   control and comparison groups, 403-404
   cost-effectiveness analysis, 414-415
   data analysis, 406, 440, 443
   definition, 391
   differences from large-scale trials, 391-392, 416-417
   evaluation measures, 407-415, 423, 442-443
   future research, 510
   goals, 397
   implementation, 407-409, 441
   literature searches, 23, 392, 393-396
   mass media campaigns, 44-45
   meta-analysis of, 462-463
   methods, 397-402, 405
   of program delivery methods, 441
   outcome variables, 405, 410-412
   process evaluation, 409-410, 423
   sample sizes, 392, 404-405, 407, 423-424
   subjects, 403-407
   timeframes, 422-423, 439-440
   unit of analysis, 405-407
   uses, 504
   weaknesses, 392
   See also Project SMART
PMEDS. *See* Prevention Minimum Evaluation Data Set
Polio vaccine, 9
Pooling. *See* Activity pooling and warehousing
Poverty cycle of health education, 50
Practitioner/researcher relationships:
   building, 64
   collaboration, 70, 212, 229, 232-234, 342
   communication issues, 69, 70-71, 206
   dialogue during pilot studies, 423
   different backgrounds, 59
   different time perspectives, 61, 70, 71
   partnerships, 501
   terminology issues, 504
Practitioners:
   attitudes toward theory, 86-88
   backgrounds, 52, 58
   characteristics as moderators, 482
   competence, 423
   delivery of health behavior programs, 58-60, 69-70, 176-177
   lack of experience with empirical methods, 59-60
   relationships with participants, 60, 375-376, 378-379, 388, 509, 513
   training in program development methods, 63, 64, 230
Precede-proceed planning model, 11-12
Pregnancy prevention programs, 210, 216-217, 488
   See also Program Archive on Sexuality, Health, and Adolescence (PASHA)
Prevention Minimum Evaluation Data Set (PMEDS), 221
Prevention programs:
   assessment studies, 131-132, 148-149, 155-156
   booster programming, 119-124, 377-378, 379, 389, 412
   cognitive theories used, 110-119
   cost-effectiveness, 414-415, 503
   diabetes, 180
   HIV, 101, 210-211, 218-219, 388, 400-401, 488, 517-520
   infectious diseases, 8, 9, 10, 31
   mediators, 107-108
   processing confounds, 118-119
   sexually transmitted diseases, 210-211, 218-219
   theoretical models, 135
   See also Drug use prevention programs; Health behavior programs; Smoking prevention programs
Prevention science, 131-132, 441-442
Privacy issues, 240-241, 252-253, 264-265

Professional meetings, 182, 189
Program Archive on Sexuality, Health, and Adolescence (PASHA), 187-188, 211
 effectiveness evaluation, 225-228
 expanding on, 228-231
 field tests, 222-228, 229-230, 232
 goals, 211-212
 identification of promising programs, 213-220
 implementation issues, 223, 231-232
 lessons learned, 231-232
 Practitioner Advisory Panel, 222, 229, 230
 program packages, 211, 220-222, 224-225, 232
 Scientist Expert Panel, 213, 233
 technical support, 224
Program archives, 187-188, 230
Program champions, 66
Program development. See Health behavior program development
Program for Appropriate Technology in Health, 189
Programs. See Health behavior programs; Prevention programs
Project EX, 349, 350
 component study, 350, 351, 354-360
 components, 351, 352-353, 354
Project SMART (Self-Management and Resistance Training):
 activity pool, 428
 combined version, 436-438
 curriculum development, 426-429
 data collection, 440
 goals, 425-426
 health educator team, 426-427, 439
 implementation, 434-436
 lessons learned, 438-443
 pilot test (phase 1), 429-434, 439-440
 pilot test (phase 2), 436-438
 results, 435-436, 438
Project STAR (Students Taught Awareness and Resistance), 426, 492
Project Towards No Drug Abuse (TND), 354
Project Towards No Tobacco Use (Project TNT), 293, 349-350, 359
Projective techniques, 295-298
Protective factors, 81, 133
Psychological time-sharing, 379-380
Psychology, 74
Psychosocial development levels, 367-368, 387-389
Psychosocial variables, 269
PsycINFO, 22, 192, 214, 392
Public health:
 behavior change programs, 50
 community surveillance studies, 142
 cost-effectiveness, 32, 503
 history, 5, 8, 31
 in developing world, 31
 U.S. national objectives, 181

Qualitative methods, 207, 337-338
 See also Verbal methods of perceived efficacy studies
Quantitative methods, 207, 338
 assessment of mediators and moderators, 485-486
 in meta-analyses, 462
 software packages, 443, 484-485, 499-500
Quasi-experimental study designs, 336, 337, 401-402
Questionnaires, 292-293

Recursiveness, 377-378, 379, 382, 389
Refusal assertion skills training, 16-18, 23, 491
Regression equations, 485
Reinforcement. See Booster programming
Reinforcement control approaches, 86
Relative advantage, 62-63
Reliability, 148
Research:
 community access to, 266
 etic and emic approaches, 102
 future needs, 506-515
 levels of interpretation, 104-105
 meanings of term, 504
 phases, 345-346
 qualitative methods, 207, 337-338
 quantitative methods, 207, 338, 484-486, 499-500
 whole-system approach, 207-208
 See also Assessment studies; Designs; Etiologic research
Research synthesis. See Meta-analyses
Researchers:
 information useful to practitioners, 206
 interpretations of behavior, 104
 issues in health behavior program development, 60-61, 70
 See also Practitioner/researcher relationships
Research-to-practice cycle, 212, 232-234
Resource books, 184-185
Resource centers, 185-187
Response bias, 264-265
Response control approaches, 86
Risk factors, 31-33, 81, 133, 155
Robert Wood Johnson Foundation, 184, 188
Role-playing:
 activities, 432-433
 in perceived efficacy studies, 256-257, 262

Salk polio vaccine, 9
Schools:
 as settings for health behavior programs, 55-56, 285, 371, 404-405
 continuation high schools, 271-272, 308, 349, 350, 354
 institutional issues, 370-374
Self-Enhancement, Inc., 323
Self-Management and Resistance Training. See Project SMART

Self-report questionnaires, 292-293
Semistructured interviews, 243, 247-248
Senses, used in learning, 381-382
Sentence completion, 296
Sequencing, 361-362
  by intuition, 364
  conceptual approaches, 363-366
  definition, 362
  development level of target group, 367-370, 373, 387
  diffusion of innovations, 369
  environmental context, 367, 370-374
  flow, 380-381, 382
  future research, 509-510
  gaining trust of participants, 375-376, 388
  in existing programs, 176
  institutional issues, 370-374
  lack of research, 362-363
  logical ordering, 377, 378
  multiple interventions, 374-379
  processes, 377
  recursiveness, 377-378, 379, 382, 389
  research needs, 383
  within single topics, 379-382
Sexual activity:
  of adolescents, 517, 518
  sequence of behaviors, 366
Sexually transmitted diseases (STDs):
  prevention programs, 210-211, 218-219
  See also HIV prevention programs; Program Archive on Sexuality, Health, and Adolescence (PASHA)
Single-group pretest-posttest study designs, 335, 336, 397-398, 399-400, 405
SMART (Self-Management and Resistance Training). See Project SMART
Smoking:
  as gateway drug, 426
  behavior patterns, 368, 388
  by adolescents, 267-268, 271-272, 365, 368
  by African Americans, 265
  children's attitudes toward, 411-412
  clearinghouses, 187
  dependence, 269
  response bias, 264-265
  surgeon general's report, 9
Smoking cessation programs:
  chemical dependency issues, 350
  clinics in high schools, 349-350
  component studies, 335, 349
  focus groups, 271, 272-284
  for adolescents, 268, 285, 349-350
  history, 9
  meta-analysis, 464
  motivations, 269-270, 277-278, 279-283, 308-309, 351
  Project EX, 349, 350, 351-360
  Project TNT, 293, 349-350, 359

  psychosocial issues, 350
  reasons for failure to quit, 268-269
  stages of change, 388
  theme studies, 308, 309-317
  theoretical frameworks, 269
  withdrawal symptoms, 269
Smoking prevention programs:
  advocacy of, 74-75
  archive of programs, 230
  component studies, 335
  for adolescents, 35-36, 388
  mass media campaigns, 35-36, 37-46, 414-415
  mediators, 16-17
  refusal assertion skills training, 17-18
  theoretical basis, 35
  See also Project SMART
Social cognitive theory, 35, 37, 38
Social construction of reality, 103-105
Social learning theories, 15, 88, 427
Social marketing/formative evaluation approach, 11
Social-influences model:
  components, 427-428
  pilot study, 425, 426, 429-434
  results, 435-436, 492
  theoretical basis, 427
  use in smoking prevention, 16-17
Sociofile, 214
Sociometrics Corporation, 17, 187, 229, 230
Software. See Computers
Special interest groups, 57
Spencer Foundation, 17
Stages of change models, 364-366
Stage-sequential program models, 479
STAR (Students Taught Awareness and Resistance), 426, 492
Statistical power:
  in component studies, 332-333
  in pilot studies, 404-405
Statistical significance, 338-339, 467-468
Statistics:
  descriptive, 338
  inferential, 338
  software packages, 443, 484-485, 499-500
  See also Meta-analyses; Quantitative methods
STDs. See Sexually transmitted diseases
Stepped-care approach, 7
Steroid use prevention, 488
Stimulus control approaches, 86
Stress, 104, 489
Structured interviews, 243, 246
Students Taught Awareness and Resistance (STAR), 426, 492
Study designs. See Designs
Substance use prevention programs, 322, 371, 404-405, 490-493
  See also Drug use prevention; Project SMART
Suicide prevention, 334, 488

Surveys, 39
Surviving in Recovery program, 388
Synergistic group effect, 258

Tanglewood Research, 371-375, 376, 378
Tape recorders, 252, 264-265
Target populations:
   acceptability of components, 6, 329-330, 403
   component studies, 331-333
   development level, 367-370, 373, 387-389
   for nonverbal methods of perceived efficacy studies, 289-291, 300, 304
   mass media campaigns, 38-39
   motivations, 58
   selecting, 168-169
   time commitment, 58
   See also Participants
Task forces, 142
TAT. *See* Thematic Apperception Test
TCU. *See* Texas Christian University
Teachers. *See* Practitioners
Technical reports, 181-182
Technology:
   future capabilities, 514-515
   See also Computers; Internet
Teenagers. *See* Adolescents
Telephone interviews, 249, 252
Television, School, and Family Project, 335
Testicular self-examination, 399, 413-414
Texas Christian University (TCU), 388-389
Thailand, 208
Thematic Apperception Test (TAT), 296
Theme studies, 19, 293-294, 307-308
   analysis, 314
   benefits, 307
   for smoking cessation programs, 308, 309-317
   procedure, 313-314
   results, 315-317
Theoretical models:
   confirming, 93
   developing, 472-473
   direct effects, 473-475
   elements, 80-83
   for prevention programs, 135
   selecting, 91
   variables, 473
Theories:
   ABCs approach, 85-86, 507
   applications, 88, 92-94, 172-173
   attitudes of practitioners, 86-88
   attitudinal, 15
   building, 93-94, 95-96
   cognitive, 15, 35, 108-109
   cultural sensitivity, 98, 105

   definition, 80
   elicitation questionnaires, 15-16
   etiologic research, 15-16
   explicit, 85
   family interaction, 15
   heuristic value, 91
   implicit, 84-85
   levels, 83-84, 94-95
   linking to materials development, 16-17
   literature searches, 22
   measurement, 83-84
   selection criteria, 90-92, 105
   social construction of reality, 103-105
   social learning, 15, 88, 427
   testability, 85, 91
Theory-based program development, 79-80, 94, 472-473
   approaches, 507
   conceptual frameworks, 472-481
   empirical confirmation, 481
   examples, 487-488
   importance, 88-90, 480
   in Chain Model, 14-17, 36-41
   limitations, 94-95
   pitfalls, 502-504
Time-sharing, psychological, 379-380
TND. *See* Project Towards No Drug Abuse
TNT. *See* Project Towards No Tobacco Use
Tobacco. *See* Smoking
Tobacco Education Clearinghouse, 187
Transtheoretical model (TTM), 364-365, 387-388, 389
TRAP (stages of drug use involvement), 121
True experimental study designs, 138, 336, 337, 397, 398, 400-401, 405
TTM. *See* Transtheoretical model

U3 measure, 456
Unemployment, 490
U.S. Congress, 8
U.S. Department of Education, 186
U.S. Department of Health and Human Services (DHHS), 10, 182, 186
U.S. Department of Health, Education, and Welfare (DHEW), 9
U.S. Department of Justice, 182
U.S. Department of Veterans Affairs, 71
U.S. Marine Corps, 260-261
U.S. Public Health Service, 8, 9, 181
University of California, Los Angeles Drug Abuse Research Center, 388
Unstructured interviews, 243, 246-247

Vaccines, 9
Validity, 148

construct, 484
internal and external, 398, 402, 484
Variables, 80-81, 473
antecedent, 81
measuring, 95
See also Mediators; Moderators
Verbal methods of perceived efficacy studies, 19, 239, 240, 507-508
advantages and disadvantages, 240-241, 245-246
community forums, 253-255
Delphi technique, 255-256
interviews, 243, 246-253, 262
language issues, 265
privacy issues, 240-241, 252-253, 264-265
reducing response bias, 264-265
role-playing, 256-257, 262
types, 244
See also Focus groups
Violence:
conferences on, 182
prevention programs, 323

Warehousing. See Activity pooling and warehousing
Web. See Internet
WHO. See World Health Organization
Women:
health information center, 186, 192
See also Breast cancer; Gender
Word association, 295-296
Word processing, 442
Work environment, 490, 522
World Health Organization (WHO), 9, 10
Written methods of perceived efficacy studies. See Nonverbal methods
Written responses to pictures, 296

Youth Risk Behavior Survey, 252

Youths. See Adolescents

About the Contributors

David G. Altman, Ph.D., is Professor of Public Health Sciences at the Wake Forest University School of Medicine. Before arriving at Wake Forest University in 1994, he spent 10 years at the Stanford Center for Research in Disease Prevention, Stanford University School of Medicine. He has conducted a variety of studies in the general area of community health promotion. He is a past president of Stop Teenage Addiction to Tobacco (STAT) and serves as National Program Director of the Robert Wood Johnson Foundation Substance Abuse Policy Research Program. In 1997, he was selected as a Fellow of the W. K. Kellogg Foundation National Leadership Program. He is a Fellow of the American Psychological Association and the Society of Behavioral Medicine (SBM) and a member of the American Public Health Association, Council on Epidemiology and Prevention of the American Heart Association, and the Society of Public Health Education. He received his doctorate in social ecology from the University of California, Irvine, in 1984.

Susan L. Ames, M.A., is a research assistant and predoctoral student at the Institute for Health Promotion and Disease Prevention Research, Department of Preventive Medicine, University of Southern California. Her research interests include implicit cognition and substance use in high-risk populations, impact of memory on addictive behaviors, developing prediction models of substance use, prevention and harm reduction of addictive behaviors, and psychosocial correlates of drug use and other risk behaviors. She received an M.A. in Psychology from California State University, Los Angeles, in 1994.

M. Douglas Anglin, Ph.D., is involved in more than 50 federal-, state-, and county-funded research projects dealing with multiple aspects of drug abuse, including prevalence estimation, needs assessment, and resource allocation; the evaluation of community treatment and other interventions for drug abusers; HIV/AIDS epidemiology and high-risk behavior in drug users; and social policy analysis. He has served as an adviser for a number of organizations, including the Los Angeles County

Alcohol and Drug Programs Administration, the California State Department of Alcohol and Drug Programs, the California Department of Corrections, the Federal Bureau of Prisons, the Office of National Drug Control Policy, the National Institute on Drug Abuse, the Center for Substance Abuse Treatment, and the National Association of State Alcohol and Drug Abuse Directors. Among his current activities, Dr. Anglin is Director of the UCLA Drug Abuse Research Center (Neuropsychiatric Institute). He received his doctorate in social psychology from the University of California, Los Angeles, in 1980.

Guadalupe X. Ayala, M.A., is an evaluation and data manager on several NIH-funded research projects with a focus on Latino health. She received her master's degree in psychology from California State University, San Marcos in 1995 and is pursuing a doctoral degree in clinical psychology/behavioral medicine at SDSU-UCSD. She has more than 7 years of experience in the health research field, including 5 years working with Spanish-dominant populations. Her research experiences have been in the area of health promotion with Latinas, treatment compliance among cardiovascular patients, instrument development, acculturation and intergenerational issues, theory development, and nutrition assessment.

Kris Bosworth, Ph.D., is a faculty member in the College of Education at the University of Arizona, where she holds the Smith Endowed Chair in Substance Abuse Education. She has been involved in prevention research for more than 20 years, with a focus on development, implementation, and evaluation of theory-based interventions for middle schools. A hallmark of her research is the appropriate use of technology as a tool for delivery of prevention interventions. Previously, she has held positions as Associate Research Scientist at the University of Wisconsin–Madison Center for Health Systems Research and Analysis, Associate Professor and Director at the Center for Adolescent Studies at Indiana University, and Visiting Scientist at the Centers for Disease Control and Prevention's Youth Violence Prevention Team. She received her doctorate of education in the Department of Continuing Adult and Vocational Education, School of Education, at the University of Wisconsin–Madison in 1988.

Brian Colwell, Ph.D., CHES, is Associate Professor in the Department of Social and Behavioral Health at the Texas A&M School of Rural Public Health. Prior to that, he was Associate Professor of Health Education at Texas A&M University. He is actively involved in research and service related to improving school health education and reducing adolescent risk behaviors. He is the codeveloper, with Dr. Dennis Smith, of the Adolescent Tobacco Use Awareness and Cessation Program that is used by the state of Texas. He is a member of the Board of Directors of the Texas Division of the American Cancer Society. He earned his doctorate in health behavior at Indiana University in 1992.

Gerald C. Davison, Ph.D., has been on the University of Southern California faculty since 1979 as Professor of Psychology. From 1979 to 1984, he was Director of Clinical Training and, from 1984 to 1990, department chair. From 1994 to 1996, he served as interim dean of the Annenberg School for Communication. His research interests are in cognitive assessment and cognitive behavior therapy, with particular focus on the application of his articulated thoughts in a simulated situations paradigm to a variety of emotional/behavior phenomena, including anxiety, depression, Type A behavior, borderline hypertension, safer sexual behavior, and dating violence. He received his doctorate in psychology from Stanford University in 1965.

Clyde W. Dent, Ph.D., is Associate Professor of Research in the Department of Preventive Medicine and the Institute for Health Promotion and Disease Prevention Research at the University of Southern California. His interests include evaluation of drug abuse prevention programs, especially as pertaining to Hispanic populations. He received his doctorate in psychology from the University of North Carolina in 1984.

Stewart I. Donaldson, Ph.D., is Associate Professor of Psychology and Organizational Behavior at the School of Organizational and Behavioral Sciences, Claremont Graduate University. He currently serves as co-chair of the Theory-Driven Evaluation and Program Theory Topical Interest Group of the American Evaluation Association. He is principal investigator on several program development and evaluation research grants, including the evaluation of the California Wellness Foundation's $20 million Work & Health Initiative. His interests include theory-driven program design and evaluation, substance abuse prevention, and worksite health promotion, including employee assistance programming. He received his doctorate in psychology from the Claremont Graduate University in 1991.

Carol N. D'Onofrio, Dr.P.H., is Professor Emerita at the School of Public Health, University of California, Berkeley; Adjunct Research Scientist at the Northern California Cancer Center; and freelance consultant. Her work concentrates on the development and evaluation of public health programs for vulnerable populations, including youth, ethnic minority groups, people with disabilities, the poor, and the sick. Her research focuses on tobacco use prevention, breast and cervical cancer screening, and, more recently, the needs of cancer patients and the delivery of health services in managed care environments. She also has conducted research on survey methodology. She is past president of the Society for Public Health Education and has served on the Governing Council and the Program Development Board of the American Public Health Association. She received her doctorate in public health from the University of California, Berkeley, in 1973.

Ronald S. Drabman, Ph.D., is Professor of Psychiatry and Human Behavior and Director of the clinical psychology training programs at UMC. His interests include all aspects of child behavior. He has published in the areas of child behavior modification and the effects of television violence and behavioral pediatrics. His research has been supported by several grants from NIMH. He is a fellow of the APA (Divisions 12 and 25). He served as finance chairperson and on the publications board of *Behavior Therapy*. Currently, he is an associate editor of *Behavior Therapy* and secretary-treasurer of AABT. He has been executive secretary of the Mississippi State Board of Psychological Examiners and associate editor of the *Journal of Applied Behavior Analysis*. The program he directs received the first annual outstanding training program award from

AABT. He received his doctorate from the State University of New York at Stony Brook in 1972.

David Duncan, Dr.P.H., is Senior Study Director in the Substance Abuse Research Group, at Westat, an employee-owned research corporation that performs contract research primarily for the federal government. He has extensive experience as a researcher, administrator, and academic in the areas of substance abuse, public health, and health education. His interdisciplinary doctorate in behavioral science, epidemiology, biostatistics, and program evaluation was awarded in 1976 by the University of Texas at Houston.

John P. Elder, Ph.D., is Professor and Head of the Division of Health Promotion at San Diego State University in the Graduate School of Public Health. His research has included smoking prevention and tobacco control, heart health nutrition in the Latino community, and international child survival programs. He has published 190 articles and chapters as well as three books. He received an M.P.H. degree from Boston University and a Ph.D. in Psychology from West Virginia University.

Jill English, Ph.D., is Assistant Professor of Health Science at California State University, Fullerton. She has been working in the area of health education curriculum development, implementation, and evaluation for the past 15 years. In addition, she had conducted research in drug prevention programs, provided technical assistance throughout the nation in the field of drug prevention, and taught health education in schools. Her interests are in the areas of curriculum development and school health. She graduated from the University of Southern California in 1988 with a doctorate in education.

Richard I. Evans, Ph.D., is Distinguished Professor in the Department of Psychology at the University of Houston and Director of the Social Psychology Program and the Social Psychology/Behavioral Medicine Research Group. He was the principal author of the "U.S. Surgeon General's Report on Smoking in Children and Adolescents"; he pioneered the social influence conceptualizations on prevention of smoking and other health risk behaviors, which generated the social inoculation model that encompasses resistance skills training and other prevention strategies; and he contributed the technique for increasing the validity of self-reports of risky health behaviors. He directs the NSF–supported Oral/Visual History Project, which includes videotaped dialogues and books reflecting those dialogues with the world's notable psychologists. His interests include social influence processes, measurement of smoking behavior, and social inoculation models for tobacco, alcohol, and HIV prevention. He graduated from Michigan State University in 1950 with a doctorate in social psychology.

Brian R. Flay, D.Phil., is Professor of Public Health at the University of Illinois–Chicago, and Director of the Health Research and Policy Centers, a cluster of university-wide centers focusing on health behavior, health promotion and disease prevention, health in the elderly, health services, and public policy. He continues his research on smoking and drug abuse etiology and prevention, as well as AIDS and violence prevention. He received his doctorate in social psychology from Waikato University in New Zealand in 1976. After receiving postdoctoral training in evaluation research and social psychology at Northwestern University (Evanston, Illinois) under a Fulbright/Hays Fellowship, he started research on smoking prevention at the University of Waterloo (Ontario, Canada). In 1987, he moved to the University of Illinois at Chicago to start the Prevention Research Center in the School of Public Health. In 1993, he was recognized by the Research Council of the American School Health Association for outstanding research.

Shirley M. Glynn, Ph.D., is Clinical Research Psychologist at the West Los Angeles VA Medical Center and Associate Research Psychologist in the Department of Psychiatry and Behavioral Sciences at UCLA. She received her Ph.D. in clinical/social psychology in 1985 from the University of Illinois in Chicago. After completing her clinical internship at Camarillo, California, State Hospital, she accepted a position as the psychologist on the Clinical Research Unit at the UCLA NPI&H Clinical Research Center for the Study of Schizophrenia at Camarillo State Hospital. In 1987, she joined the Research Service at the West Los Angeles VA Medical Center to conduct clinical trials of psychosocial interventions for serious psychiatric disorders. She has published extensively in the areas of schizophrenia, posttraumatic stress disorder, behavioral interventions, and family treatment. She is a licensed psychologist in California and, in addition to her research interests, has a small private practice.

Lawrence W. Green, Dr.P.H., is Distinguished Fellow/Visiting Scientist in the Office on Smoking and Health at the Centers for Disease Control and Prevention (CDC). From 1991 to 1999, he was Director of the Institute of Health Promotion Research and Professor of Health Care and Epidemiology at the University of British Columbia. He served as the first director of the U.S. Office of Disease Prevention and Health Promotion. That office coordinated the first "Surgeon General's Report on Health Promoion and Disease Prevention" and the "1990 Objectives for the Nation." His honors include the Award of Excellence and the Distinguished Career Award, American Public Health Association; the Jacques Perisot Medal of the International Union for Health Promotion and Education; the Distinguished Fellow Award of the Society for Public Health Education; the Presidential Citation, Scholar Award, and Distinguished Service Award of the Association for the Advancement of Health Education; and Honorary Fellow of the American School Health Association. He received his degree in public health at the University of California at Berkeley in 1968.

Stephen L. Hamann, M.P.H., Ed.D., is Assistant Dean for Medical Education in the Faculty of Medicine at Rangsit University, and he is founder of the Tobacco Control Policy Research Network in Thailand (http:\\www.ash.or.th). Subareas of particular focus include program implementation and evaluation research and practice, evidence-based medicine, and tobacco cessation and control among the populace in Thailand. He received his doctorate in education from the University of Hawaii at Honolulu in 1992. He previously received his M.P.H. from the University of Illinois at Chicago in 1976.

William B. Hansen, Ph.D., is President of Tanglewood Research. He has written numerous curricula for school-based prevention, including Project SMART, Project STAR, and All Stars. He has authored more than 80 articles in scientific journals. He has served on the faculty at the University of California at Los Angeles (1978-1984), the University of Southern California (1980-1989), and Bowman Gray School of Medicine (1989-1996). Groups that have relied on him for advice about prevention include the U.S. Congress' Office of Technology Assessment, the U.S. Department of Education, the National Institute on Drug Abuse, the Center for Substance Abuse Prevention, the United Nations, and the U.S. Information Agency. He received his doctorate in psychology from the University of Houston in 1978.

Jack E. Henningfield, Ph.D., is Vice President, Research and Health Policy, Pinney Associates, Bethesda, Maryland, and Associate Professor of Behavioral Biology, Department of Psychiatry and Behavioral Sciences, Johns Hopkins University School of Medicine, Baltimore. He has conducted research on the effects of a wide range of psychoactive drugs on animals and humans, with a continuous emphasis on the validity and generality of the methods and measures used. His interests in obesity research have led to approximately 300 publications in the archival literature. He received his doctorate in Experimental Psychology with a psychopharmacology emphasis from the University of Minnesota in 1977.

Beth Rachael Hoffman, B.A., has been a teaching assistant and predoctoral student at the Institute for Health Promotion and Disease Prevention Research, Department of Preventive Medicine, University of Southern California, since 1998. Her research interests include the effects of culture, ethnicity, and socioeconomic status on high-risk behaviors, particularly drug use and sexual practices, in adolescents. She received her degree in Psychology from the University of Maryland, Baltimore County in 1998.

C. Anderson Johnson, Ph.D., is the Sidney Garfield Professor in the Department of Preventive Medicine and Director of the Institute for Health Promotion and Disease Prevention Research at the University of Southern California. He has more than 30 years of experience in health behavior research, including school-based and community-based prevention trials. He currently is overseeing components of the Independent Evaluation of the California Tobacco Control Program. Recently, he became Director of one of the NIC-sponsored TTURC centers, which involves collaboration with the Department of Public Health in Wuhan, China, to develop and deliver smoking prevention programs to Chinese adolescents. His interests include the etiology of health-related lifestyles and approaches to the prevention of behavioral risks for disease, including drug abuse, nutritional practices, physical exercise, and communication strategies. He received his doctorate in Psychology from Duke University in 1974.

Valerie Johnson, Ph.D., is Associate Professor of Sociology with the Center of Alcohol Studies at Rutgers University. Currently, she is a coinvestigator on a longitudinal study, funded by the National Institute on Drug Abuse, on vulnerability to drug abuse as well as a principal investigator on a study funded by the National Institute on Alcoholism and Alcohol Abuse on familial transmission of alcohol and related problems.

Her research focuses primarily on the etiology, familial transmission, and consequences of alcohol and drug use, especially among adolescents and young adults, as well as evaluation research. She received her doctorate in Sociology from Rutgers University in 1985.

Jeffrey L. Kibler, Ph.D., is a postdoctoral fellow specializing in clinical psychology and behavioral medicine at the University of Mississippi Medical Center. He is currently examining the role of cognitive, emotional, and physiological factors in posttraumatic stress disorder and depression. He received his doctorate in 1999 from the University of Miami, specializing in clinical health psychology. His doctoral dissertation focused on pain perception in Type 1 diabetes mellitus. His research interests include behavioral, psychological, and physiological markers for cardiovascular disease and psychophysiological bases for pain, psychopathology, and sleep disorders.

Elizabeth A. Klonoff, Ph.D., is Professor of Psychology and Co-Director of Clinical Training in the University of California-San Diego/San Diego State University Joint Doctoral Program in Clinical Psychology, and Executive Director of the Behavioral Health Institute at San Diego State University. From 1988-2000, she was Professor of Psychology and executive director of the Behavioral Health Institute at California State University–San Bernardino. Her research focuses on smoking among and the health behavior of ethnic minorities, women, and children. She is a Fellow in the American Psychological Association Divisions 35 (Women) and 45 (Ethnic Minorities). She received her doctorate in clinical psychology from the University of Oregon in 1977.

Hope Landrine, Ph.D., is Research Professor at California State University–San Diego State University Joint Docoral Program in Clinical Psychology, and R & D Director of the Behavioral Health Institute at San Diego State University. She was Associate Professor of Psychology at California State University–San Bernardino from 1986 to 1992, and Senior Research Scientist at Los Angeles County Public Health Foundation from 1993 to 2000. Her research focuses on smoking among and the health behavior of ethnic minorities and the health behavior of ethnic minorities, women, and children. She received her doctorate in clinical psychology from the University of Rhode Island in 1983, postdoctoral training in social psychology at Stanford University, and postdoctoral training in cancer control as a National Cancer Institute Fellow at the University of Southern California Medical School. She is a Fellow in the American Psychological Association, Divisions 9 (Social Issues), 35 (Women), and 45 (Ethnic Minorities).

Howard Leventhal, Ph.D., is the Board of Governor's Professor of Health Psychology at Rutgers University. He was former chair of the Department of Psychology at the University of Wisconsin–Madison. He was president of the Division of Health Psychology (38) of the American Psychological Association (1996-1997). He has served as chair of the Behavioral Medicine Study Section of NIH. Among other activities, he currently is a member of the advisory board of the Research Institute for Psychology and Health (at Lieden, Utrecht, and Tilburg). His theoretical and empirical contributions, in more than 200 articles and book chapters, span the fields of the emotions, illness behavior, and illness attribution, including patient compliance with treatment regimens, interventions to minimize pain, strategies for smoking intervention and prevention, and strategies to control hypertension. He has been recently inducted into the National Academy of Science Institute of Medicine. He received his doctorate in Psychology from the University of North Carolina in 1956.

Kara Lichtman, B.A., is Project Manager for Project EX, a motivation-enhanced adolescent tobacco cessation study funded by the Tobacco-Related Disease Research Program of California. Over the past 2 years, she has obtained broad experience in the field of curriculum development research. As program specialist, her responsibilities have included curriculum development and implementation as well as data collection, management, and analysis. Project EX has become the most effective experimental teen tobacco use cessation trial to date.

Douglas Longshore, Ph.D., is Associate Research Sociologist and Associate Director at the UCLA Drug Abuse Research Center and also is Associate Behavioral Scientist at RAND, Santa Monica, California. He has been a research associate and project manager in the Studies and Evaluation Department of System Development Corporation, Santa Monica, California. He also has worked as a social science analyst and project manager in the Program Evaluation and Methodology Division of the U.S. General Accounting Office, Washington, D.C. He received his doctorate in Sociology from University of California, Los Angeles, in 1981.

Michael Lynskey, Ph.D., 1997, is a lecturer in the National Drug and Alcohol Research Centre at the University of New South Wales in Sydney, Australia, and is working in a number of areas, including the etiology of illicit drug use and drug-related harm, the comorbidity of substance use and mental health problems, and the prevention of substance-related harm. He received his doctorate in Psychology from Otago University in 1996. Between 1991 and 1997, he worked at the Christchurch Health and Development Study, a longitudinal study of 1,265 children born in Christchurch (New Zealand) who have been studied from birth to the age 18.

David P. MacKinnon, Ph.D., is Professor in the Psychology Department at Arizona State University, Tempe. His interests include statistical methods in prevention research and health psychology, such as investigation of mediation effects and information processing of warning labels. He received his doctorate in psychology from the University of California, Los Angeles, in 1986.

Stan Maes, Ph.D., is Professor of Health Psychology at Leiden University, the Netherlands. He received his doctorate in psychology and educational sciences from Gent State University (Belgium) in 1976. He served on the Faculty of Psychology and Educational Sciences at Gent State University from 1971 to 1973, at Antwerp University on the Medical Faculty from 1973 to 1981, and at Tilburg University (the Netherlands) from 1981 to 1990, where he became the first chair in this discipline outside of the United States. He was cofounder and the first president of the European Health Psychology Society (1986-1992), president of the Health Psychology Division of the International Association of Applied Psychology (1990-1994), and, since 1998, president of the International Society on Health Psychology Research. He is a member of the editorial board of eight journals in the field of health psychology. He has published more than 150 scientific publications, including 5 books, in various languages, concerning health promotion in school and work settings, doctor-patient communication, and psychological aspects of and interventions with chronic disease patients.

Suzanne M. McMurphy, Ph.D., is Assistant Professor at the University of New Hampshire in the Department of Social Work. From 1988 to 1990, she was a Fulbright Scholar in Sweden, after which she remained working with the Swedish National Council for Crime Prevention and the Swedish Ministry of Justice through 1993. After returning to the United States, she has continued to collaborate internationally on substance abuse and criminal justice issues. Most recently, she has worked with the BIOMED project in the Netherlands, developing instruments on evaluating substance abuse treatment programs within Europe. She is currently the principal investigator of a number of evaluation projects, including an NIJ-sponsored evaluation of substance abuse treatment programs in the New Hampshire Department of Corrections. She received her doctorate in social policy from Bryn Mawr College in 1993.

Kim T. Mueser, Ph.D., is a licensed clinical psychologist and Professor in the Departments of Psychiatry and Community and Family Medicine at the Dartmouth Medical School in Hanover, New Hampshire. He completed his psychology internship, training at Camarillo State Hospital, California, in 1985. He was on the faculty of the Psychiatry Department at the Medical College of Pennsylvania in Philadelphia from 1985 until 1994. His clinical and research interests include research on the treatment of persons with severe mental illness and substance use disorders ("dually diagnosed" clients), family treatment and social skills training for severe mental illness, and other aspects of psychiatric rehabilitation. He has lectured widely on psychiatric rehabilitation and has published more than 100 articles in refereed journals and numerous books. He received his doctorate in clinical psychology from the University of Illinois at Chicago in 1984.

Elahe Nezami, Ph.D., is Research Assistant Professor and Director of the undergraduate program in the Department of Preventive Medicine. She completed a 3-year postdoctoral fellowship, funded by the National Cancer Institute. Her research interests include tobacco use prevention and cessation, cross-cultural interpretation of mental health measures, and international health. She received her doctorate in psychology from the University of Southern California in 1993.

Starr Niego, Ph.D., is a developmental psychologist who specializes in designing, implementing, and evaluating education and health promotion programs, particularly for at-risk youth. She is a Senior Research Associate at Sociometrics, where she is Project Director for the Program Archive on Sexuality, Health, and Adolescence (PASHA), a collection of effective teen pregnancy and STD/HIV/AIDS prevention programs. She received her doctorate in psychology from the Department of Human Development and Family Studies at Cornell University in 1995.

Robert J. Pandina, Ph.D., is a developmental neuropsychologist with specialty training in experimental and clinical psychopharmacology. His current research, which focuses on understanding the biopsychosocial origins and consequences of alcohol and drug use, abuse, and dependence, emphasizes a life span developmental perspective and employs longitudinal methodology. Other areas of expertise include mechanisms of drug action, development and assessment of prevention and treatment interventions, drug testing in the workplace, and forensic psychology. He is Director of the Rutgers University Center of Alcohol Studies, the principal investigator of the National Institute on Drug Abuse–funded Health and Human Development Laboratory, and Professor of Psychology in the Graduate School of Applied and Professional Psychology at Rutgers. He received his doctorate in psychology from the University of Vermont in 1973.

Mary Ann Pentz, Ph.D., is Professor of Preventive Medicine at the Institute for Health Promotion and Disease Prevention Research at the University of Southern California. She has chaired the NIDA Epidemiology and Prevention Studies section and has served on advisory boards for the Robert Wood Johnson Foundation and OSAP in the area of community substance abuse prevention. Her interests include community approaches to substance abuse prevention, policy effects on drug abuse, and stress prevention. She received her doctorate in psychology from Syracuse University in 1978.

Brian Perrochet, B.A., is an independent writer and editor specializing in social sciences and medical research. He has worked with researchers from the UCLA Drug Abuse Research Center since 1989. He was lead editor of a collection of comprehensive articles on drug abuse and its consequences among pregnant and parenting women in California (published as a special volume of the *Journal of Psychoactive Drugs*). He is the founding editor of *Futures in Drug Abuse Research,* the quarterly newsletter and Web site serving the 44 research training programs funded by the National Institute on Drug Abuse since 1995.

James Peterson, Ph.D., has been Vice President of Sociometrics Corporation since 1996. He has directed the Data Resources Program of the National Institute of Justice, the Outreach Demonstration Evaluation project for the Social Security Administration, and the evaluation of the Option for Pre-Teens program. Previously, he served as study director at Temple University's Institute for Survey Research. There, he directed more than 20 studies, focusing primarily on research on drug use, fertility, and child development. He currently is directing the Contextual Data Archive and the American Family Data Center projects, among others. He received his doctorate in sociology from the University of Chicago in 1972.

Rick Petosa, Ph.D., is Associate Professor in the Department of Health Behavior and Health Promotion in the School of Public Health at The Ohio State University. He is the author of 55 journal articles and 59 research presentations on the design, implementation, and evaluation of health behavior change programs. He has served as principal investigator on school-based interventions funded by the W. T. Grant Foundation and the American Heart Association. Currently, he is an evaluation consultant on a project designed to disseminate an empirically based curriculum for HIV prevention. Also, over the past 4 years, he has completed several investigations related to physical activity among youth, adults, and postretirement adults. He received his doctorate in health education and behavioral science from Southern Illinois University in 1980.

Pekka Puska, M.D., M.Pol.Sc., Ph.D., is Professor and Director of the Department of Epidemiology and Health Promotion at the National Public Health Institute of Finland. He also is Director of the Division of Health and Chronic Diseases for the National Public Health Institute of Finland and Deputy to the Director General of the National Public Health Institute of Finland. He has been a member of the World Health Organization (WHO) permanent panel of experts on cardiovascular diseases from 1978 to the present, and he was given the WHO Annual Health Education Award in 1990. He also was a member of the Finnish National Parliament from 1987 to 1991. He has more than 400 publications in the fields of public health, epidemiology, disease prevention, and health promotion. He received his M.Pol.Sc. and doctorate in medicine from the University of Turku in 1968 and 1971 and his doctorate in Public Health from the University of Kuopio in 1974.

Louise Ann Rohrbach, Ph.D., M.P.H., is Research Assistant Professor in the Department of Preventive Medicine at the University of Southern California. Her research interests include theory-based program evaluation, development and evaluation of school- and community-based tobacco control and substance abuse prevention programs, diffusion of effective prevention programs, and gender differences in adolescent substance abuse. She received her doctorate in Health Behavior Research from the Department of Preventive Medicine at the University of Southern California in 1989. She received her master's in public health from the University of California, Los Angeles in 1980.

Herbert H. Severson, Ph.D., is Associate Professor of Counseling Psychology at the University of Oregon–Eugene and is Senior Research Scientist at the Oregon Research Institute (formerly its director). He has been Professor of Psychology at the University of Northern Colorado and University of Oregon. He has been a contributing author to three surgeon general reports and coauthor of the Institute of Medicine report, "Growing Up Tobacco Free." His interests include the importance of substance abuse cessation programming for adolescents and treatment of aggressive behavior in adolescents. He has more than 80 publications. He received his doctorate in psychology from the University of Wisconsin–Madison in 1973.

Thomas R. Simon, Ph.D., is a behavioral scientist with the Division of Violence Prevention in the National center for Injury Prevention and Control of the Centers for Disease Control and Prevention (CDC). His current research is focused on understanding risk and protective factors for violence and suicide. He serves as a scientific advisor on several CDC-funded longitudinal evaluations of violence and suicide prevention programs. He also conducted program development and evaluation research in the areas of adolescent tobacco use and substance abuse. He received his Ph.D. in preventive medicine at the University of Southern California in 1996.

Edward G. Singleton, Ph.D., is Visiting Research Scholar-in-Residence at the Howard University Center for Drug Abuse Research in Washington, D.C. From 1991 to 1994, he was a Senior Fellow for the National Institute on Drug Abuse (NIDA) Intramural Research Program. He has been a Maryland-licensed psychologist since 1986, and a Diplomate Board-Certified Forensic Examiner since 1996. He was awarded status as a Diplomate by the American Board of Psychological Specialties in June 1997. Other honors include the NIDA Director's Award of Merit for Exemplary Achievements as part of the Historically Black Colleges and Universities (HBCU) Task Force (1994) and the 1998 Lonnie E. Mitchell Award for Outstanding Contributions to Research, Prevention, and Treatment of Alcohol and Drug Addiction. Research interests are psychometric applications to substance abuse research. He received a doctorate in Psychology from Howard University in 1985.

Dennis W. Smith, Ph.D., is Chair of the Department of Health and Human Performance, University of Houston, Texas. He received his doctorate in health education from The Ohio State University in 1985. From 1987 to 1990, he held a postdoctoral appointment at the Universities of North Carolina at Greensboro and Chapel Hill working on an NCI-funded project on tobacco curriculum diffusion in schools. He has won numerous awards, including Outstanding Leadership in Comprehensive School Health Education and Cancer Prevention, American Cancer Society, Texas Division, Inc., 1996-1997, and he was elected Fellow by the American School Health Association in 1994.

Alan W. Stacy, Ph.D., is Research Associate Professor at the University of Southern California, Department of Preventive Medicine, and Research Psychologist in the Department of Psychology at the University of California, Los Angeles. He has published numerous articles on cognitive processes in health behavior (including alcohol, tobacco, and other drug use), and HIV-related and diet behavior. He has been the principal or coprincipal investigator on a number of federally funded projects on the etiology of alcohol and other drug use, on prevention of tobacco and other drug use in adolescents, and on effects of alcohol advertising. His main theoretical focus is on understanding how associations in memory influence health behavior implicitly, without one's conscious deliberations of the pros and cons of alternative activities. He received his doctorate in psychology from the University of California at Riverside in 1986.

Gordon P. Street, Ph.D., is a research instructor specializing in biostatistics and clinical research at the Center for Treatment and Study of Anxiety at MCP/ Hahnemann University in Philadelphia. He graduated in June 1998 from the California School of Professional Psychology in San Diego, where his research explored the application of a scientific approach to the professional practice of psychology. In one study, he found that counselors-in-training were more likely to display confirmation bias within an interviewing task when encouraged to use an intuitive approach than when encouraged to use a scientific approach. He is currently involved in research into the course and treatment of posttraumatic stress disorder and social phobia.

Alan N. Sussman, Ph.D., is Adjunct Professor, Daley College and College of Lake County, Department of Social Sciences and Humanities and Department of Communication Skills. He has served on the faculty of Departments of Philosophy in the United States (including Indiana University, Northwest; State University of New York, College at Buffalo) and abroad (Universities of Calabar, Ghana, Sierra Leone, Zimbabwe) over the past 35 years. He has published several articles pertaining to philosophy of mind, logic, and philosophy of science in journals, including the *Journal of Philosophy.* Sub-areas of particular focus are in the areas of epistemology, metaphysics, the philosophy of language, and theory development. He received his doctorate in philosophy from the University of Chicago in 1974.

Steve Sussman, Ph.D., is Professor in the Department of Preventive Medicine and Institute for Health Promotion and Disease Prevention Research at the University of Southern California. He served on a clinical psychology residency at Jackson Veterans Administration and University of Mississippi Medical Centers. He has published more than 160 articles, chapters, or books in the area of drug abuse prevention and cessation. He was the principal investigator of the Project Towards No Tobacco Use (TNT), a tobacco use prevention project that is recognized by CDC, NIDA, CSAP, the California Department of Education, and Sociometrics, Inc. as a model program. Sub-areas of particular focus are prediction of tobacco and other drug use, school-based tobacco and other drug abuse prevention and cessation (e.g., Project TND, indicated drug abuse prevention; Project EX, teen tobacco use cessation), other research with high-risk populations, and an emphasis on the use of program development methods. He received his doctorate in psychology from the University of Illinois at Chicago in 1984.

Nancy S. Tobler, Ph.D., has held a joint associate professorship in the Schools of Social Welfare and Public Health, Department of Biometry and Statistics, from the State University of New York at Albany. Her research interests include the use of quantitative and qualitative methods in the systematic integration of research-based evaluations of adolescent substance abuse prevention programs. Her previous experiences included work as a science teacher and as a therapist in sexual abuse prevention. She was principal evaluator on a Center for Substance Abuse Prevention High Risk Youth grant. Her meta-analytic work, as well as other works, has been published in numerous peer-reviewed journals, and she has been a frequent invited speaker at national conferences. She received her doctorate in Social Welfare from the School of Social Welfare, State University of New York at Albany.

Jennifer B. Unger, Ph.D., is Research Assistant Professor in the Department of Preventive Medicine. She currently is overseeing a portion of the evaluation of the California Tobacco Control Program, a statewide education, community, and media effort. She also is a coprincipal investigator of the newly funded NCI TTURC grant. She has conducted research on the psychosocial predictors of health behaviors such as physical activity, substance use, unprotected sex, and needle sharing. She is especially interested in the role of social networks in determining health behaviors and health outcomes. She received her doctorate in health behavior research from the Department of Preventive Medicine at the University of Southern California in 1996.

Thomas Ashby Wills, Ph.D., is Associate Professor in the Health Psychology Training Program, conducted jointly by the Ferkauf Graduate School of Psychology and the Albert Einstein College of Medicine. He is a Fellow of the American Psychological Association Divisions 8 and 38 (social and health psychology). His research interests include social support and health, stress and coping processes, and adolescent substance abuse. Currently, he is conducting a cohort study on the role of temperament processes in adolescent substance use escalation. He received his doctorate in Psychology from the University of Oregon–Eugene in 1974. He received postdoctoral training in epidemiology at the Columbia University School of Public Health.

John K. Worden, Ph.D., has served in the Office of Health Promotion Research in the College of Medicine at the University of Vermont, reaching the rank of Research Professor in 1991. Since 1979, he has developed and evaluated community-based health promotion interventions. One of these interventions was a smoking prevention program funded by the National Cancer Institute, comprising an intensive mass media campaign designed for youth in Grades 5 through 10 along with a school program. For this project, Dr. Worden and colleagues received the C. Everett Koop National Health Award in 1996 and the Best Paper Award, *Health Education and Behavior,* from Sage Publications in 1997. Dr. Worden and colleagues also have developed and evaluated community-based and mass media interventions to promote breast cancer screening, help young adults quit smoking, and prevent alcohol use by adolescents. He received his doctorate in Mass Communication from Syracuse University in 1971.